Stahl's Essential Psyc

Prescriber's Guid and Adolescents

Child and adolescent psychopharmacology is a rapidly growing field with psychotropic medications used widely in the treatment of this patient group. However, psychopharmacological treatment guidelines used for adults cannot simply be applied for children or adolescents, thus presenting healthcare professionals with assessment and prescribing challenges. Based on the world's best-selling resource *Stahl's Prescriber's Guide*, this new book provides a user-friendly step-by-step manual on the range of psychotropic drugs prescribed for children and adolescents by healthcare professionals.

The medications are presented in the same design format in order to facilitate rapid access to information. Each drug is broken down into a number of sections, each designated by a unique color background thereby clearly distinguishing information presented on therapeutics, safety and tolerability, dosing and use, what to expect, talking to patients and caregivers, special populations, and the art of psychopharmacology, and followed by Suggested Readings.

This book is intended to be genuinely helpful for practitioners of psychopharmacology by providing them with the mixture of facts and opinions selected by the authors. Ultimately, prescribing choices are the reader's responsibility. Every effort has been made in preparing this book to provide accurate and up-to-date information in accord with accepted standards and practice at the time of publication. Nevertheless, the psychopharmacology field is evolving rapidly and the author and publisher make no warranties that the information contained herein is totally free from error, not least because clinical standards are constantly changing through research and regulation. Furthermore, the author and publisher disclaim any responsibility for the continued currency of this information and disclaim all liability for any and all damages, including direct or consequential damages, resulting from the use of information contained in this book. Clinicians recommending and patients using these drugs are strongly advised to pay careful attention to and consult information provided by the manufacturer.

Stephen M. Stahl is Clinical Professor of Psychiatry and Neuroscience at the University of California, Riverside School of Medicine; Adjunct Professor of Psychiatry at the University of California, San Diego; and Honorary Visiting Senior Fellow in Psychiatry at the University of Cambridge, UK. He has conducted various research projects awarded by the National Institute of Mental Health, Veterans Affairs, and the pharmaceutical industry. Author of more than 500 articles and chapters, Dr. Stahl is also the author of the bestseller *Stahl's Essential Psychopharmacology.*

Jeffrey R. Strawn is a tenured Professor in the Department of Psychiatry and Behavioral Neuroscience and has a secondary appointment in the Department of Pediatrics, Division of Clinical Pharmacology and the Division of Child & Adolescent Psychiatry. He is also a Clinical Psychiatrist at University of Cincinnati Medical Center, UC Health and at Cincinnati Children's Hospital Medical Center, Division of Child & Adolescent Psychiatry. In his clinical practice, he works with youth with anxiety and related disorders and their families and supervises residents and fellows. Dr. Strawn has authored more than 220 peer-reviewed publications. He is a distinguished fellow of the American Academy of Child & Adolescent Psychiatry and has received multiple awards for teaching, mentorship, and research.

Stahl's Essential Psychopharmacology

Prescriber's Guide – Children and Adolescents

Stephen M. Stahl

University of California at San Diego
San Diego, California

Jeffrey R. Strawn

University of Cincinnati College of Medicine
Cincinnati, OH

Editorial assistant

Meghan M. Grady

With illustrations by

Nancy Muntner

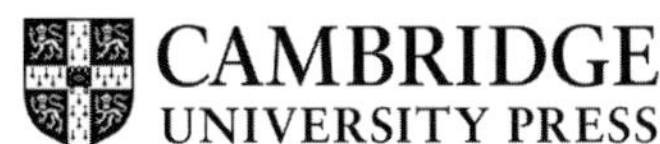

CAMBRIDGE
UNIVERSITY PRESS

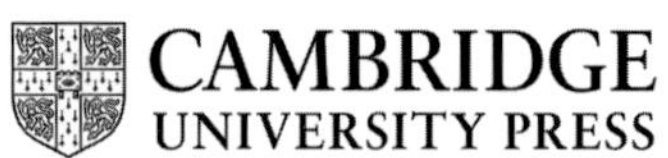

Shaftesbury Road, Cambridge CB2 8EA, United Kingdom

One Liberty Plaza, 20th Floor, New York, NY 10006, USA

477 Williamstown Road, Port Melbourne, VIC 3207, Australia

314–321, 3rd Floor, Plot 3, Splendor Forum, Jasola District Centre, New Delhi – 110025, India

103 Penang Road, #05–06/07, Visioncrest Commercial, Singapore 238467

Cambridge University Press is part of Cambridge University Press & Assessment, a department of the University of Cambridge.

We share the University's mission to contribute to society through the pursuit of education, learning and research at the highest international levels of excellence.

www.cambridge.org
Information on this title: www.cambridge.org/9781009267502

DOI: 10.1017/9781009267526

First published 2019
Second edition 2024

Printed in Mexico by Litográfica Ingramex, S.A. de C.V.

A catalogue record for this publication is available from the British Library

Library of Congress Cataloging-in-Publication Data
Names: Stahl, Stephen M., 1951– author.
Title: Stahl's essential psychopharmacology prescriber's : children and adolescents / Stephen M. Stahl, University of California at San Diego, San Diego, California, Jeffrey R. Strawn, University of Cincinnati College of Medicine, Cincinnati, OH ; ediitorial assistant, Meghan M. Grady with illustrations by Nancy Muntner.
Other titles: Essential psychopharmacology prescriber's
Description: Second edition. | Cambridge, United Kingdom ; New York, NY, USA : Cambridge University Press, [2024] | Includes bibliographical references and index.
Identifiers: LCCN 2023051817 | ISBN 9781009267502 (paperback) | ISBN 9781009267526 (ebook)
Subjects: LCSH: Psychotropic drugs. | Psychopharmacology. | MESH: Psychotropic Drugs – pharmacology – Handbooks.
Classification: LCC RM315 .S835 2024 | DDC 615.7/8–dc23/eng/20231215
LC record available at https://lccn.loc.gov/2023051817

ISBN 978-1-009-26750-2 Paperback

Contents

Introduction

Psychotropic medications have a vital role in the treatment of psychiatric disorders among children and adolescents (Strawn et al., 2022). However, using these medications effectively and appropriately demands a deep understanding of pediatric pharmacokinetics and pharmacodynamics alongside the nuanced findings from double-blind, placebo-controlled trials. Within the context of developmental psychopharmacology, this Introduction highlights general principles that apply to the medication monographs that follow. Beyond this, we introduce you to specific changes that we have made in the *Second Edition* to help you understand how metabolism, drug–drug interactions, and pharmacogenetics are relevant to specific medications.

Not Just Little Adults: Developmental Pharmacology

The landscape of pharmacokinetics and pharmacodynamics in children and adolescents diverges significantly from that of adults, thereby necessitating differences in dosing and producing differences in response patterns and tolerability. It is crucial to recognize the interplay between pharmacokinetic and pharmacodynamic factors, as these factors influence one another and differ from adults. Such differences include variations in side effects (e.g., akathisia and drug-induced parkinsonism, hyperprolactinemia, weight gain) (Correll et al., 2010; Maayan and Correll, 2011; Koch et al., 2023), dosing (e.g., lithium) (Findling et al., 2011), and efficacy (e.g., benzodiazepines) among children, adolescents, and adults (Dobson et al., 2019).

Pediatric Pharmacokinetics

At birth, metabolic capacity in children is lower than in adults, gradually reaching adult levels by around 2 years of age (Strawn and Ramsey, 2024). However, near puberty, metabolism may surpass the levels observed in adults. In addition to developmental differences in hepatic metabolism, changes in renal function and fat distribution during childhood and adolescence influence the pharmacokinetics of various medications in the pediatric population. Furthermore, children and adolescents possess a greater total body water content and relatively less adipose tissue compared to adults, impacting the distribution of many medications and the accumulation of lipophilic substances and their metabolites.

Absorption and Bioavailability: The Journey Within

The route of administration greatly influences the absorption of drugs, with oral medications being particularly influenced by gastric pH and the presence of food in the stomach (Strawn and Ramsey, 2024). Bioavailability, on the other hand, represents the fraction of a drug that enters systemic circulation, which can be influenced by concomitant medication use and first-pass metabolism. Young children may also absorb some drugs faster than adults do, leading to higher peak drug levels and peak-related side effects. For this reason, once-a-day drugs for adults may occasionally have to be given twice or three times a day in children.

Drug Distribution: Mapping the Pathways

As drugs travel through the blood, they distribute throughout the body, with the distribution to their site of action being influenced by protein binding and how they cross the blood–brain barrier (Strawn and Ramsey, 2024). The volume of distribution (V_D) serves as an indicator of the extent to which a drug is distributed within bodily tissues rather than remaining in the plasma. Higher V_D values signify greater tissue distribution, whereas lower V_D values indicate a more plasma-centric concentration. The V_D is influenced by factors such as high lipid solubility (e.g., certain benzodiazepines), low rates of ionization, and low plasma protein binding. Moreover, the V_D varies across development, and age-related changes in body composition can further influence drug distribution. Prepubertal children have more body water and less fat (where lipid-soluble drugs are stored) compared to adults. Prepubertal children also tend to have less protein binding of drugs compared to adults, leaving a greater proportion of the biologically active drug in the plasma.

Metabolism: Unraveling the Enzymatic Pathways

Hepatic enzyme activity develops early, and the rate of drug metabolism is related to liver size, which is proportionately larger in children than in adults. Because the liver parenchyma is also larger in children than in adults relative to body size, children may require a larger dose per kilogram of body weight of drugs that are primarily metabolized by the liver.

Various psychotropic medications undergo metabolism mediated by cytochrome P450 enzymes, namely CYP3A4, CYP2C19, or CYP2D6, within the liver (Hicks et al., 2015). While CYP2D6 activity remains relatively constant from the age of 1 through adulthood, CYP2C19 and CYP3A4 activities may be increased in children compared to adults (Strawn et al., 2018; Ramsey et al., 2019). Drug–drug interactions can occur through the inhibition or induction of these enzymes. Furthermore, younger children may exhibit increased hepatic clearance due to greater liver blood flow in relation to total body mass, resulting in a larger first-pass effect for certain drugs.

Excretion: Bid Farewell to the Medication

The renal and hepatic pathways serve as the primary routes for the excretion of drugs and their metabolites. Renal clearance is substantially higher in pediatric populations compared to adults and experiences a decline from ages 2 to 20 (Strawn and Ramsey, 2024) and this has implications for several medications, including lithium.

Pharmacogenetics in Children and Adolescents: Deciphering Genetic Variability

Variations within genes encoding metabolizing enzymes, such as *CYP2C19* and *CYP2D6*, influence the activity of these enzymes, including in children and adolescents (Ramsey et al., 2019). Consequently, patients can fall into different metabolizer groups, including poor metabolizers (with minimal to no enzyme activity), intermediate metabolizers, normal metabolizers, rapid metabolizers, or ultrarapid metabolizers (with increased enzyme activity). Dosing recommendations tailored to these metabolizer types are available from the Clinical Pharmacogenetics Implementation Consortium (CPIC) (Hicks et al., 2015), the Dutch Pharmacogenetics Working Group, and some are incorporated within US Food and Drug Administration (FDA) labels. The systemic concentration of a medication can be influenced by the activity of CYP2C19 and CYP2D6 enzymes, requiring dose adjustments. Poor metabolizers may require lower doses, while ultrarapid metabolizers may necessitate higher doses. It is imperative to focus on individual genes for medication dosing adjustments, avoiding the temptation of employing pharmacogenetic testing for medication selection.

While pharmacogenetic tests offer valuable insights, certain limitations must be acknowledged. First, these tests may overpromise by asserting the ability to predict medication effectiveness and optimal drug concentrations. Second, the strength of evidence for gene–drug associations may vary across different tests, with limited or absent data available for certain pharmacogenetic variants in the pediatric population. Hence, caution is advised when applying such tests to children and adolescents without empirical grounding (Ramsey et al., 2020). Moreover, numerous clinical factors must be taken into account when selecting appropriate medications for individual patients, considering developmental effects on pharmacokinetically related enzymes (Ramsey et al., 2020). While we discourage relying solely on pharmacogenetics for medication selection, dismissing clinical factors or the evidence base for medications is equally problematic (Ramsey et al., 2020).

No consensus has yet been reached regarding the utility of pharmacogenetic testing in child and adolescent psychiatry. Nevertheless, dosing recommendations based on pharmacokinetic genes are included in FDA labels and Clinical Pharmacogenetics Implementation Consortium (CPIC) consensus guidelines (Bousman et al., 2023), and these guidelines are employed in many institutions across adult and child and adolescent psychiatry. However, it is crucial to exercise caution when extrapolating pharmacokinetic models from adults to youth, considering the influence of developmental factors on medication metabolism. Prospective and retrospective pediatric studies have provided insights into the impact of variation in these pharmacokinetic genes on drug concentration, tolerability, and response for several classes of medication metabolized by these enzymes (Aldrich et al., 2019; Strawn et al., 2020). Dose adjustments based on CYP2C19 metabolizer status are supported by modeling studies in adolescents for citalopram, escitalopram, and sertraline (Strawn et al., 2019), as well as by CPIC recommendations. Similarly, dose adjustments for atomoxetine, fluvoxamine, and paroxetine based on CYP2D6 metabolizer status are also supported by evidence.

The FDA recommends dosing based on product insert information for CYP2C19 for citalopram and CYP2D6 for aripiprazole and atomoxetine. These dosing recommendations aim to balance exposure levels (area under the concentration–time curve) and hold the potential to mitigate side effects associated with high exposure or treatment failures associated with low exposure to these medications. However, establishing a clear relationship between medication blood levels and efficacy can be challenging, as it may be confounded by tolerability and other factors. In certain cases, increased metabolism observed in rapid and ultrarapid metabolizers may lead to patients appearing "treatment resistant" due to sub-therapeutic medication blood concentrations. This phenomenon was observed in the Treatment of SSRI-resistant Depression in Adolescents Study (TORDIA) concerning fluoxetine and sertraline (Sakolsky et al., 2011). Finally, it is worth noting that a boxed warning in carbamazepine's product insert advises screening patients with ancestry in genetically at-risk populations (Asians) for the presence of HLA-B*1502 prior to initiating treatment. Due to the high risk of severe dermatological reactions, including Stevens–Johnson syndrome, carriers should refrain from receiving carbamazepine unless the benefits clearly outweigh the risks.

These insights into pharmacogenetics should not overshadow the importance of thorough clinical evaluations and the consideration of various clinical factors when deciding on medication usage. The choice of medication should be based on available evidence, and when pharmacogenetic testing is conducted, it should inform dosing adjustments, monitoring levels, or the selection of medications within the evidence-based class for a specific condition.

Hold On to Your Seat: What Is Different About Treating Children and Adolescents Compared to Adults?

Diagnoses in children and adolescents can be less stable than in adults; thus, at each follow-up visit, clinicians should look for morphing from one diagnosis to another and for emerging comorbidities that have changed since the last visit. In reality, there are at least two patients when treating a child/adolescent: the child/adolescent and the caregiver, each involved in different ways in the diagnosis and treatment of the patient, and each with different needs for information and explanation. Family dynamics, school environment, and social interactions with peers can also affect symptoms and behaviors.

Even more so than in adults, there is a need for "triangulation" of information when treating children and adolescents, particularly to assess improving or deteriorating symptoms, that is, not only the child or adolescent's perspective and any of the clinician's perspective at the time of the visit, but also a third observer who can confirm what the clinician observes or what the child says (particularly the primary caregiver, but also a teacher or other family members). Clinicians should be even more prepared to change/adjust/discontinue dosage of medications in children as diagnosis and symptoms change, as side effects occur, and as development progresses.

Additionally, clinicians should be alert to how the disorders that are the focus of treatment as well as the treatments change over the course of development. For example:

Attention Deficit Hyperactivity Disorder (ADHD) Medications:

- More hyperactivity may be observed in younger patients
- In younger patients, ADHD may be seen as irritability, aggressive behaviors, and school refusal instead of inattention, potentially resulting in diagnosing/treating inattention
- Clinical presentation in children with inattention without hyperactivity may be dismissed as immaturity or "spaciness," especially in young girls
- Younger children tend to be more sensitive to the effects of stimulants
- Since young children may absorb drugs faster than adults, immediate-release formulations may need to be given several times (3–4) a day. And because intestinal transit times are faster in younger children and absorption differs, the "actual" duration of action of some medications may differ in younger children compared to older ones.

Antidepressant Medications:

- Clinical presentation of depression in children and adolescents may be different than in adults, that is, with irritability, and school refusal
- For selective serotonin reuptake inhibitors (SSRIs), children can have a two- to threefold higher incidence of vomiting than adolescents, who have a somewhat higher incidence than adults (Strawn et al., 2023)
- Treatment-emergent activation syndrome (TEAS) may be more common in children compared to adolescents and adults (Luft et al., 2018)

Practical Notes

Conduct a thorough diagnostic evaluation and consider utilizing evidence-based psychosocial and behavioral interventions prior to psychotropic medications, especially in milder cases and when available and practical. However, the majority of children who receive psychosocial treatments that are not evidence-based interventions do not demonstrate improvement and may deteriorate.

Whenever possible, treat with one medication at a time and have clear goals and expectations. Align expectations for improving grades with the child/adolescent's strengths, empowering them to improve. Be cognizant of excessive pressure from some parents to improve grades that can lead to low self-esteem. Consider use of objective rating scales with special attention to teacher comments. These rating scales can be employed to assist in screening and diagnosing certain psychiatric disorders. However, it is crucial to note that these scales should not replace a comprehensive clinical assessment conducted by trained professionals. Standardized measures typically offer normative data that enable clinicians to compare a patient's symptoms to those of children of similar age. Be cautious in refilling medications without seeing patients. Integrate information from the child, parent, and teachers. In most cases, don't have the child/adolescent take medication at school to prevent stigma and avoidance of medication and in the case of stimulants, diversion. Suicide is one of the leading causes of death in the child/adolescent age group, especially for those without treatment of an underlying mental health disorder, so be vigilant to the onset of depression in patients with comorbid psychiatric conditions. Surveys by the Centers for Disease Control and Prevention (CDC) show that 15–20% of high school students in the past year have had serious thoughts of suicide and that 8–10% made a suicide attempt.

Comorbid Psychiatric Disorders / Managing Comorbidity

When it comes to children, psychiatric comorbidity is the rule rather than the exception (Masi et al., 2004, 2006; Ghuman et al., 2007; Cardoso et al., 2017), and comorbidity may be more common in children and adolescents compared to adults. For these reasons, it is essential to collect a current symptom portfolio at each visit and re-diagnose or add diagnoses as necessary. It is important to treat each individual symptom, as well as the diagnosis as a whole. Summarized in the accompanying table are some common psychiatric comorbidities in children and adolescents.

Disorder	Common comorbidities
ADHD	Mood and anxiety disorders, substance use and nicotine dependence
Depressive / Mood Disorders	Anxiety disorders, substance abuse, eating disorders, autism spectrum disorders, and ADHD
Psychotic Disorders	Mood and anxiety disorders, substance abuse, and ADHD

Comorbid Intellectual / Developmental Disabilities / Brain Injury

Patients with intellectual and developmental disabilities are almost always excluded from clinical trials. The administration of medications in this population is based on expert consensus and clinical expertise rather than on controlled trials. Modern pediatric psychopharmacology requires adequate diagnosis and treatment of specific symptoms of that diagnosis. Psychotropic medications should be used with caution in this population and be vigilant about reduced tolerability compared to other children. As many psychotropic drugs reduce the seizure threshold, be aware of possible induction of seizures in at-risk patients and in those with known seizure disorders. In this population, common sense and experience suggest "start low; go slow."

Antipsychotic Medications in This Population:

- Meta-analysis suggests that short-term antipsychotic use can help reduce challenging behaviors in children with intellectual disabilities, but the quality of existing evidence is low and significant side effects have also been reported

- Second generation antipsychotics (particularly risperidone) show moderate to large effects in decreasing irritability, disruptive behaviors, and aggression in children with and without autism spectrum disorders and developmental disabilities for short-term treatment
- Use of antipsychotics in this population in the past was encouraged by approval of a related drug, haloperidol, for severe behavior problems in children of combative, explosive hyperexcitability, symptoms common in this population
- No new atypical antipsychotics are approved for "severe behavior problems in children of combative, explosive hyperexcitability"
- Use of antipsychotics for nonspecific tranquilization in this population is not consistent with best medical practices

"Highly Vulnerable" Population / Foster Children

According to the World Bank, a "highly vulnerable" child refers to a child who faces a significant risk of inadequate care and protection. It is estimated that approximately 20% of children in the United States fall into this category. Foster care data suggest that around half of these children have psychiatric diagnoses, while two-thirds of children in juvenile detention centers and foster care settings also have psychiatric diagnoses. Among children with developmental disabilities, about 40% have comorbid psychiatric diagnoses, particularly depression, ADHD, and anxiety disorders. Psychological trauma is prevalent among approximately 90% of children in residential treatment centers. To address the needs of highly vulnerable populations more effectively, interventions should focus on improving living and educational environments, reducing repetitive stress, poverty, abuse, and neglect, and minimizing exposure to community violence and extreme poverty. Implementing trauma-informed care can be especially beneficial for these children and adolescents.

To avoid irrational polypharmacy, it is important to simplify medication regimens whenever possible instead of adding more medications. Highly vulnerable children enrolled in Medicaid are prescribed psychotropic medications at a rate 2–5 times higher than other children. Furthermore, a significant proportion of low-income children and those in foster care or with disabilities are prescribed two or more psychotropic medications. For children with autism spectrum disorders covered by commercial insurance, one-third receive two or more psychotropic medications, and 15% receive three or more. Even infants under the age of 1 with autism are being prescribed psychotropic medications. Vulnerable children, who often have more psychiatric disorders, are seldom the focus of research, resulting in standards of care being established based on the practices of those currently treating such children without the benefit of sufficient studies or research on similar populations.

The diverse and severe symptoms experienced by maltreated youth may lead caregivers to employ treatment strategies that result in significant polypharmacy. In a recent retrospective evaluation of Medicaid-enrolled or foster care children, up to one-third receive "high-level psychotropic polypharmacy" (Keeshin and Monson, 2022), which involved taking at least four psychotropic medications for a duration of at least 30 days. The majority of children with high-level polypharmacy had "disruptive behavior disorders," along with other comorbid diagnoses. These disruptive behavior disorders often include ADHD, oppositional defiant disorder, and conduct disorder, which have been associated with or speculated to be misdiagnosed as traumatic stress (Keeshin and Monson, 2022). Such prescribing patterns are not isolated incidents, as elevated prescribing rates have been observed in groups exposed to childhood maltreatment or at high risk for traumatic stress.

We must understand the underlying pressures influencing these prescribing practices and develop strategies for safe and effective de-prescribing when possible. However, in addressing polypharmacy in these populations and de-prescribing, it is crucial to consider the needs of each individual and recognize that the goal is not necessarily to discontinue all medications but to prioritize thoughtfully and reduce or discontinue medications with limited efficacy or high risk. Contextual factors such as the current medication regimen, access barriers to alternative treatments, and the perspectives of the patient and other stakeholders should also be considered.

Polypharmacy may arise from pressure to deviate from guidelines due to unrealistic expectations or the need for quick solutions from stakeholders such as parents or schools. It can also result from inadequate access to evidence-based treatments or insufficient mental health resources. Recent attention has been directed toward de-prescribing in this population, as described by Keeshin and Monson (2022). They outline a process that involves:

- collecting a comprehensive medication history,
- prioritizing medications with high risks or unclear rationales,
- developing and implementing a specific plan for reduction or discontinuation, and
- using a stepwise approach with sufficient observation time for adverse effects or symptom reemergence.

Comorbid Medical Conditions and Substance Use

Many children and adolescents with chronic medical conditions may be depressed or anxious or have other comorbid psychiatric conditions and need to take psychotropic medications. For antidepressants such as SSRIs, no dose adjustment is needed for patients with mild to moderate renal impairment but should be used cautiously in patients with severe renal impairment. When patients have hepatic impairment, SSRIs should be given at a lower dose (perhaps by half dose). Preliminary research suggests that most SSRIs are safe in patients with cardiac impairment, although some have been associated with QT prolongation in pediatric populations. When prescribing SSRIs, exercise caution if the patient is taking drugs for medical conditions that are metabolized by CYP2D6, CYP2C9/CYP2C19, or CYP3A4, and these effects are now highlighted throughout the *Second Edition* (Figure 1).

For patients taking ADHD medications, dose adjustment is not generally necessary for renal impairment. For patients with moderate liver impairment, the dose of ADHD medications should be reduced to 50%; for those with severe liver impairment, the dose should be lowered to 25% of the normal dose. Some ADHD medications can increase heart rate and blood pressure, so use with caution in patients with cardiac impairment and do not use in patients with structural cardiac abnormalities.

When prescribing antipsychotics, use this class of medication with caution if patients have renal, hepatic, or cardiac impairment, particularly with QT prolongation with this class of medication. For all psychotropic medications, for guidelines during pregnancy and breast feeding consult the adult prescriber's guide (*Stahl's Essential Psychopharmacology: Prescriber's Guide*).

Substance use, and in particular cannabis use, is increasing in adolescents (Weinberger et al., 2020) and has important treatment implications. For example, cannabis, which inhibits CYP2C19 in addition to other cytochromes, has been shown to increase concentrations of some antidepressant medications in youth (Vaughn et al., 2021) (Figure 2) and across disorders has been associated with reduced treatment response, raising the possibility that substance use needs to be treated independently from the

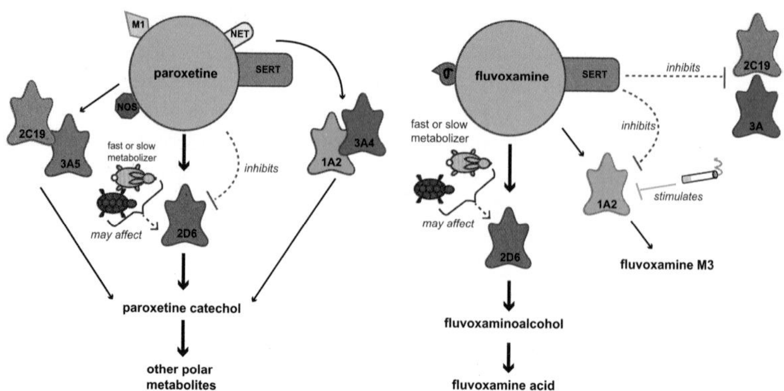

Figure 1 Examples of pharmacogenetic and environmental (e.g., smoking) factors influencing medication and the effects of medication on cytochromes that are highlighted in the Second Edition.

primary mood or anxiety disorder that is often the focus of our psychopharmacological interventions.

Potential Ethical Issues and Informed Assent

Children should have their condition explained to the extent that they can understand. Consent for medication in children and young adolescents can be made more difficult if the parents are in conflict, such as in custody disputes and divorce; it is recommended to obtain consent from both legal guardians, no matter the percentage breakdown of custody or who has "medical decision-making authority." Informed consent and assent are an ongoing, iterative process, a dynamic conduit. Regularly review the treatment plan, documenting the review process and accommodating any modifications that may prove necessary, ensuring the treatment remains aligned with the patient's evolving needs. Finally, try to get children and adolescents to agree to go along by respecting their input and, whenever possible, gaining their informed "assent," as legally, they cannot give informed consent under the age of 18. In doing this, ask questions such as "What would you want this medicine to help with?" or "What things make you worried about taking medicine?"

When engaging in the informed consent process with patients and their families, it is paramount to imbue the discussion with clarity, transparency, and comprehensive information. To facilitate this, we recommend incorporating the following components:

- **Target symptoms, prioritized:** Discuss specific symptoms that will serve as the focal point of the treatment, ensuring patients and families grasp the objectives of the proposed intervention.
- **Proposed medication plan:** Present a cogent outline encompassing the medication name, dosage, timing, and any intended adjustments that may arise during the course of treatment.
- **Specific rationale and risks:** Offer justification for the chosen medication plan, highlighting its anticipated benefits. Simultaneously, describe the potential risks and side effects, including any pertinent boxed warnings.
- **Alternatives to medication:** Engage in a thoughtful exploration of alternative treatment options, embracing the possibility of nonpharmacological approaches and engaging patients and families in the decision-making process.

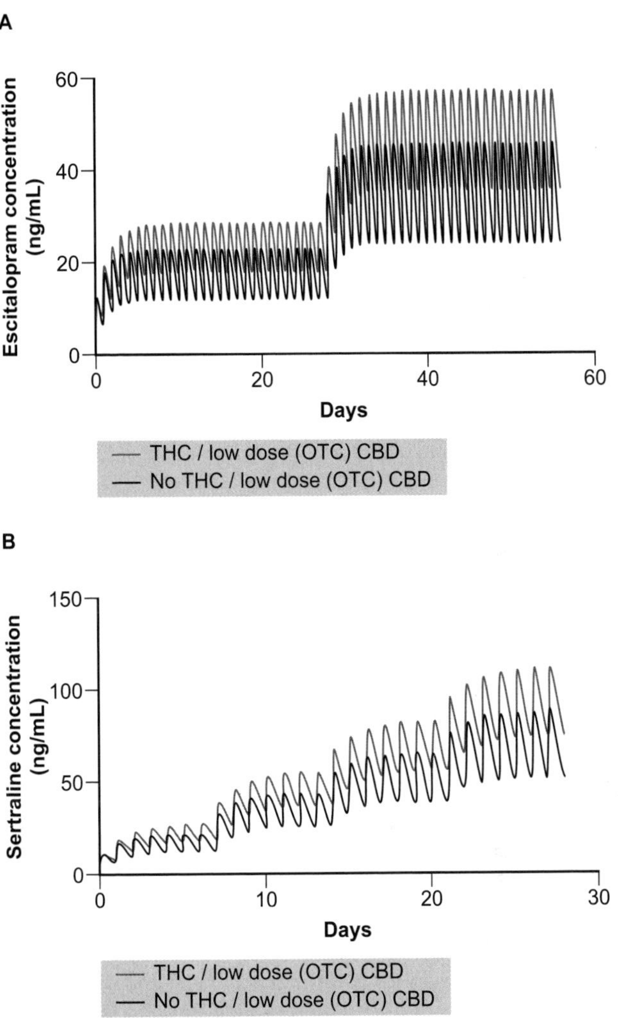

Figure 2 Simulated concentrations of escitalopram and sertraline in adolescents using and those not using cannabis (adapted from Vaughn et al., 2021).

- **FDA-approved use versus off-label use:** Distinguish between FDA-approved usage and off-label use. Articulate how medical professionals, while granted leeway in prescribing practices, may venture beyond the confines of FDA endorsement, often driven by empirical evidence and clinical rationale. Provide a glimpse into common off-label applications, bolstered by supportive research, and outline strategies to manage any potential challenges that may arise.
- **Cost of care:** Address the financial aspect of treatment, including the choice between brand names and generics, follow-up visits, and potential cost-saving measures.
- **Monitoring plan:** Establish a monitoring framework, delineating the necessary laboratory tests and the frequency of follow-up visits to ensure a vigilant and adaptive approach to treatment.

- **Concurrent treatment and intervention:** Emphasize the importance of a holistic treatment paradigm, integrating complementary therapies, school plans, and other interventions to maximize therapeutic outcomes.

Throughout these discussions, it is crucial to bear in mind the following considerations:

- Check state laws pertaining to the age of consent for mental health care, particularly in relation to medication treatment, ensuring legal compliance and ethical practice.
- Extend the conversation to include the child's perspective, fostering their assent and encouraging their participation as valued partners in the decision-making process, with due consideration to their age and cognitive development.
- Establish an ongoing communication channel, unequivocally conveying your availability and providing clear instructions on how patients or their families can reach you or designated coverage in the event of inquiries or concerns.

When children or adolescents refuse to take medications:

- Make sure the problem is not something manageable like side effects or problems swallowing or even the taste of the medication.
- Monitor what the patient actually does, not what they say or complain about; many children complain, yet they take their medication.
- Most families are not "democracies," so enlist the help of caregivers to explain and when it's necessary to exert some influence on getting the patient to take the medication.
- Giving medication in food without the patient's knowledge is unethical and should be discouraged.

Engaging Primary Care with Mental Health Professionals

More psychotropic drugs are prescribed for children and adolescents by primary care clinicians than by mental health clinicians, especially stimulants. Get written consent to mutually share information with the primary care clinician and make sure they are aware of the diagnosis and the medications. Make sure you know all the diagnoses and medications being managed in primary care or specialty care. Once the patient is stable, the primary care clinician can often take over from a mental health practitioner as the prescriber and refer back if problems emerge. If recommending the discontinuation of psychotropic drugs being prescribed by primary care and changing to something else, it is best to inform the clinician directly rather than through the parents to facilitate communication, reduce misunderstandings, and foster collaboration.

Summary

In sum, for psychiatric disorders and symptoms in children and adolescents, conducting thorough and developmentally sensitive assessments is critical before and throughout psychopharmacological treatment. Treatment plans should stem from comprehensive and accurate diagnostic evaluations, taking into account comorbidity, sub-syndromal symptoms, family factors, personality/temperament, and learning issues, including learning disorders and weaknesses. Addressing these factors may enhance the benefits of pharmacotherapy and decrease the incidence of "medication treatment resistance."

References

Aldrich SL, Poweleit EA, Prows CA et al. Influence of CYP2C19 metabolizer status on escitalopram/citalopram tolerability and response in youth with anxiety and depressive disorders. Front Pharmacol 2019;10(February):99; doi:10.3389/fphar.2019.00099.

Bousman CA, Stevenson JM, Ramsey LB, et al. Clinical Pharmacogenetics Implementation Consortium (CPIC) guideline for CYP2D6, CYP2C19, CYP2B6, SLC6A4, and HTR2A genotypes and serotonin reuptake inhibitor antidepressants. Clin Pharmacol Ther. 2023;114(1):51–68. doi:10.1002/cpt.2903.

Cardoso TDA, Jansen K, Zeni CP et al. Clinical outcomes in children and adolescents with bipolar disorder and substance use disorder comorbidity. J Clin Psychiatry 2017;78(3):e230–e233; doi:10.4088/JCP.15m10293.

Correll CU, Sheridan EM, DelBello MP. Antipsychotic and mood stabilizer efficacy and tolerability in pediatric and adult patients with bipolar I mania: a comparative analysis of acute, randomized, placebo-controlled trials. Bipolar Disord 2010;12(2):116–41; doi:10.1111/j.1399-5618.2010.00798.x.

Dobson ET, Bloch MH, Strawn JR. Efficacy and tolerability of pharmacotherapy for pediatric anxiety disorders: a network meta-analysis. J Clin Psychiatry 2019;80(1):17r12064; doi:10.4088/JCP.17r12064.

Findling RL, Kafantaris V, Pavuluri M et al. Dosing strategies for lithium monotherapy in children and adolescents with bipolar I disorder. J Child Adolesc Psychopharmacol 2011;21(3):195–205; doi:10.1089/cap.2010.0084.

Ghuman JK, Riddle MA, Vitiello B et al. Comorbidity moderates response to methylphenidate in the Preschoolers with Attention-Deficit/Hyperactivity Disorder Treatment Study (PATS). J Child Adolesc Psychopharmacol 2007;17(5):563–80; doi:10.1089/cap.2007.0071.

Keeshin BR, Monson E. Assessing and responding to the trauma of child management. Focus 2022;20(2):176–83; doi:10.1176/appl.focus.20210033.

Koch MT, Carlson HE, Kazimi MM et al. Antipsychotic-related prolactin levels and sexual dysfunction in mentally ill youth: a 3-month cohort-study. J Am Acad Child Adolesc Psychiatry 2023;62(9):1021–50; doi:10.106/j.jaac.2023.0.007.

Luft MJ, Lamy M, DelBello M et al. Antidepressant-induced activation in children and adolescents: risk, recognition and management. Curr Probl Pediatr Adolesc Health Care 2018;48(2):50–62; doi:10.1016/j.cppeds.2017.12.001.

Maayan L, Correll CU. Weight gain and metabolic risks associated with antipsychotic medications in children and adolescents. J Child Adolesc Psychopharmacol 2011;21(6):517–35; doi:10.1089/cap.2011.0015.

Masi G, Perugi G, Toni C et al. Obsessive-compulsive bipolar comorbidity: focus on children and adolescents. J Affect Disord 2004;78(3):175–83; doi: 10.1016/S0165-0327(03)00107-1.

Masi G, Perugi G, Toni C et al. Attention-deficit hyperactivity disorder – bipolar comorbidity in children and adolescents. Bipolar Disord 2006;8(4):373–81; doi:10.1111/j.1399-5618.2006.00342.x.

Ramsey LB, Bishop JR and Strawn JR. Pharmacogenetics of treating pediatric anxiety and depression. Pharmacogenomics 2019;20(12):867–70; doi:10.2217/pgs-2019-0088.

Ramsey LB, Namerow LB, Bishop JR et al. Thoughtful clinical use of pharmacogenetics in child and adolescent psychopharmacology. J Am Acad Child Adolesc Psychiatry 2020;60(6):660–4; doi:10.1016/j.jaac.2020.08.006.

Sakolsky DJ, Perel JM, Emslie GJ et al. Antidepressant exposure as a predictor of clinical outcomes in the Treatment of Resistant Depression in Adolescents (TORDIA) study. J Clin Psychopharmacol 2011;31(1):92–7; doi:10.1097/JCP.0b013e318204b117.

Strawn JR, Mills JA, Poweleit EA, Ramsey LB, Croarkin PE. Adverse effects of antidepressant medications and their management in children and adolescents. Pharmacotherapy 2023;43(7):675–90; doi:1002/phar.2767.

Strawn JR, Mills JA, Schroeder H et al. Escitalopram in adolescents with generalized anxiety disorder: a double-blind, randomized, placebo-controlled study. J Clin Psychiatry 2020;81(5):20m13396; doi:10.4088/JCP.20m13396.

Strawn JR, Poweleit EA, Ramsey LB. CYP2C19-guided escitalopram and sertraline dosing in pediatric patients: a pharmacokinetic modeling study. J Child Adolesc Psychopharmacol 2019;29(5):340–7; doi:10.1089/cap.2018.0160.

Strawn JR, Ramsey LB. Chapter 53.5. Pediatric psychopharmacology. In Kaplan and Sadock's Comprehensive Textbook of Psychiatry. 11th ed. Philadelphia: Lippincott Williams & Wilkins, 2024; 50–60.

Strawn JR, Ramsey LB, Croarkin PE. Pharmacogenetic testing and antidepressants in youth with depressive and anxiety disorders. J Am Acad Child Adolesc Psychiatry 2018;57(10); doi:10.1016/j.jaac.2018.07.733.

Strawn JR, Vaughn S, Ramsey LB. Pediatric psychopharmacology for depressive and anxiety disorders. Focus (Madison) 2022;20(2):184–90; doi:10.1176/appi.focus.20210036.

Vaughn SE, Strawn JR, Poweleit EA et al. The impact of marijuana on antidepressant treatment in adolescents: clinical and pharmacologic considerations. J Pers Med 2021;11(7):615; doi:10.3390/jpm11070615.

Weinberger AH, Zhu J, Lee J et al. Cannabis use among youth in the United States, 2004–2016: faster rate of increase among youth with depression. Drug Alcohol Depend 2020; 209:107894; doi:10.1016/j.drugalcdep.2020.107894.

List of Icons

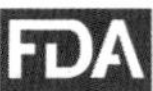 US FDA approved for pediatric use

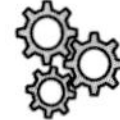 Class and mechanism of action

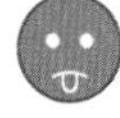 Notable side effects

 Life-threatening or dangerous side effects

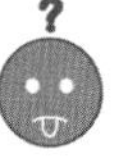 What to do about side effects

 Warnings and precautions

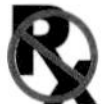 When not to prescribe

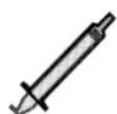 How to dose

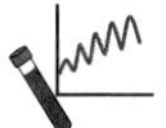 Pharmacokinetics

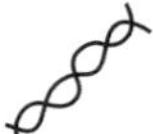 Pharmacogenetics

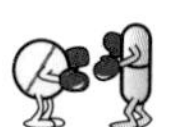 Drug interactions

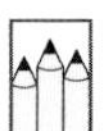 Dosing tips

 Onset of action

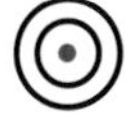 Primary target symptoms

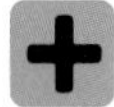 What is considered a positive result?

 What if it doesn't work?

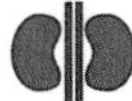 Renal impairment

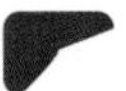
Hepatic impairment

Cardiac impairment

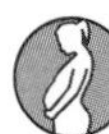
Pregnancy

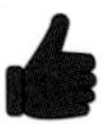
Potential advantages

Potential disadvantages

Pearls

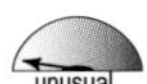

Unusual

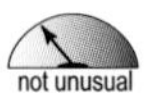

Not unusual

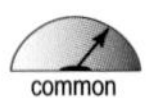

Common

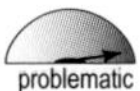

Problematic

ALPRAZOLAM

THERAPEUTICS

Brands

- Xanax
- Xanax XR

Generic

Yes

US FDA Approved for Pediatric Use

- None

Off-Label for Pediatric Use

- Approved in adults
- Generalized anxiety disorder (IR)
- Panic disorder (IR and XR)
- Other off-label uses
  - Other anxiety disorders
  - Anxiety associated with depression
  - Premenstrual dysphoric disorder
  - Irritable bowel syndrome and other somatic symptoms associated with anxiety disorders
  - Insomnia
  - Acute mania (adjunctive)
  - Acute psychosis (adjunctive)
  - Catatonia

Class and Mechanism of Action

- Neuroscience-based Nomenclature: GABA positive allosteric modulator (GABA-PAM)
- Benzodiazepine (anxiolytic)
- As positive allosteric modulators of GABA-A receptors, benzodiazepines (in the presence of GABA) increase the frequency of opening of the inhibitory chloride channels (although it does not increase the conductance of chloride across the individual channels or the time that the channel is open). This enhances the inhibitory effects of GABA.
- Inhibits neuronal activity presumably in amygdala-centered fear circuits to provide therapeutic benefits in anxiety disorders

SAFETY AND TOLERABILITY

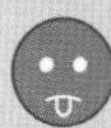

Notable Side Effects

- Sedation, fatigue, depression
- Dizziness, ataxia, slurred speech, weakness
- Forgetfulness, confusion
- Agitation and irritability
- Sialorrhea, dry mouth
- Rare hallucinations, mania
- Rare hypotension

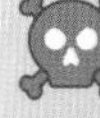

Life-Threatening or Dangerous Side Effects

- Respiratory depression, especially when taken with CNS depressants in overdose
- Rare hepatic dysfunction, renal dysfunction, blood dyscrasias

Growth and Maturation

- Not studied

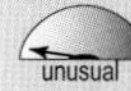

Weight Gain

- Reported but not expected

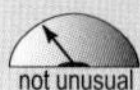

Sedation

- Occurs in significant minority
- Especially at initiation of treatment or when dose increases
- Tolerance often develops over time

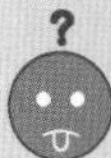

What to Do About Side Effects

- Wait
- Wait
- Wait
- Lower the dose
- Take largest dose at bedtime to avoid sedative effects during the day
- Switch to another agent
- Administer flumazenil if side effects are severe or life-threatening

How Drug Causes Side Effects

- Same mechanism for side effects as for therapeutic effects – namely due to excessive actions at benzodiazepine receptors
- Long-term adaptations in benzodiazepine receptors may explain the development of dependence, tolerance, and withdrawal
- Side effects are generally immediate, but immediate side effects often disappear in time

Warnings and Precautions

- Boxed warning regarding the increased risk of CNS depressant effects when benzodiazepines and opioid medications are used together, including specifically the risk of slowed or difficulty breathing and death

- If alternatives to the combined use of benzodiazepines and opioids are not available, clinicians should limit the dosage and duration of each drug to the minimum possible while still achieving therapeutic efficacy
- Patients and their caregivers should be warned to seek medical attention if unusual dizziness, lightheadedness, sedation, slowed or difficulty breathing, or unresponsiveness occur
- Dosage changes should be made in collaboration with prescriber
- Use with caution in patients with pulmonary disease; rare reports of death after initiation of benzodiazepines in patients with severe pulmonary impairment
- History of drug or alcohol abuse often creates greater risk for dependency
- Hypomania and mania have occurred in depressed patients taking alprazolam
- Use only with extreme caution if patient has obstructive sleep apnea
- Some depressed patients may experience a worsening of suicidal ideation
- Some patients may exhibit abnormal thinking or behavioral changes similar to those caused by other CNS depressants (i.e., either depressant actions or disinhibiting actions)

When Not to Prescribe

- If patient has angle-closure glaucoma
- If patient is taking ketoconazole or itraconazole (azole antifungal agents)
- If there is a proven allergy to alprazolam or any benzodiazepine

Long-Term Use

- Risk of dependence, particularly for treatment periods longer than 12 weeks and especially in patients with past or current polysubstance abuse

Habit Forming

- Alprazolam is a Schedule IV drug
- Patients may develop dependence and/or tolerance with long-term use

Overdose

- Fatalities have been reported both in monotherapy and in conjunction with alcohol; sedation, confusion, poor coordination, diminished reflexes, coma

DOSING AND USE

Usual Dosage Range

- Anxiety: alprazolam IR: 1–4 mg/day
- Panic: alprazolam IR: 5–6 mg/day
- Panic: alprazolam XR: 3–6 mg/day

Dosage Forms

- Alprazolam IR tablet 0.25 mg scored, 0.4 mg (Japan), 0.5 mg scored, 0.8 mg (Japan), 1 mg scored, 2 mg multiscored
- Alprazolam IR solution, concentrate 1 mg/mL
- Alprazolam XR tablet 0.5 mg, 1 mg, 2 mg, 3 mg

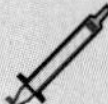

How to Dose

- For anxiety, alprazolam IR should be started at 0.75–1.5 mg/day divided into 3 doses; increase dose every 3–4 days until desired efficacy is reached; maximum dose generally 4 mg/day
- For panic, alprazolam IR should be started at 1.5 mg/day divided into 3 doses; increase 1 mg or less every 3–4 days until desired efficacy is reached, increasing by smaller amounts for dosage over 4 mg/day; may require as much as 10 mg/day for desired efficacy in difficult cases
- For panic, alprazolam XR should be started at 0.5–1 mg/day once daily in the morning; dose may be increased by 1 mg/day every 3–4 days until desired efficacy is reached; maximum dose generally 10 mg/day

Options for Administration

- Available as an extended-release formulation

Tests

- In patients with seizure disorders, concomitant medical illness, and/or those with multiple concomitant long-term medications, periodic liver tests and blood counts may be prudent

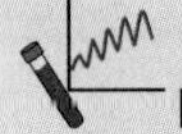

Pharmacokinetics

- Alprazolam is well absorbed after oral administration
- The onset of action is relatively rapid, with peak plasma concentrations occurring within 1 to 2 hours. Factors such as the formulation of the medication

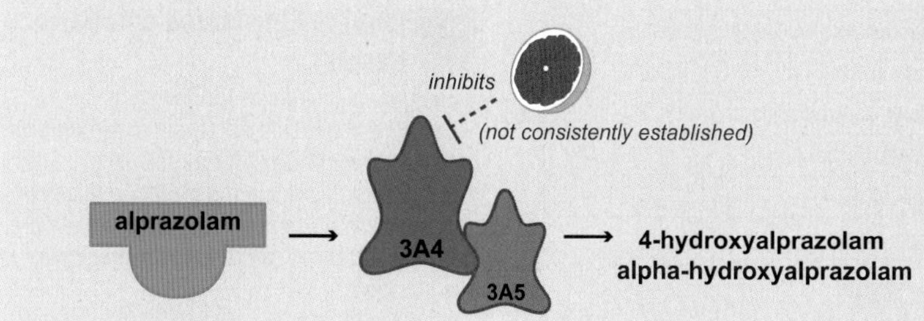

and individual variations can affect the absorption.

- Alprazolam is highly lipophilic, which allows it to distribute widely throughout the body, including the central nervous system; however, this also means that it leaves the CNS quickly
- Protein binding of alprazolam is about 80%
- Alprazolam undergoes extensive hepatic metabolism primarily via CYP3A4 (major) and to a lesser extent CYP3A5
- The major metabolites of alprazolam are 4-hydroxyalprazolam and α-hydroxyalprazolam. Of these, α-hydroxyalprazolam is the primary active metabolite
- Half-life of alprazolam in adults is 12–15 hours; there are limited data on its kinetics in youth

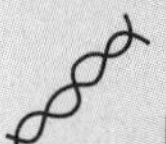

Pharmacogenetics

- No recommendations

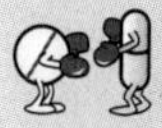

Drug Interactions

- Increased depressive effects when taken with other CNS depressants
- Inhibitors of CYP3A, such as nefazodone, fluvoxamine, fluoxetine, and even grapefruit juice, may decrease clearance of alprazolam and thereby raise alprazolam plasma levels and enhance sedative side effects; alprazolam dose may need to be lowered
- Thus, azole antifungal agents (such as ketoconazole and itraconazole), macrolide antibiotics, and protease inhibitors may also raise alprazolam plasma levels
- Inducers of CYP3A, such as carbamazepine, may increase clearance of alprazolam and lower alprazolam plasma levels and possibly reduce therapeutic effects

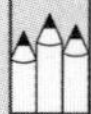

Dosing Tips

- For anxiety disorders, use lowest possible effective dose for the shortest possible period of time (a benzodiazepine sparing strategy). In adolescents, these medications may be administered prior to some anxiety-producing situations and can help to facilitate returning to school in patients with school refusal.
- Assess need for continuous treatment regularly
- Risk of dependence may increase with dose and duration of treatment and with more lipophilic benzodiazepines (e.g., alprazolam)
- For interdose symptoms of anxiety, can either increase dose or maintain same daily dose but divide into more frequent doses, or give as extended-release formulation
- Frequency of dosing in practice is often different than predicted from half-life, as duration for benzodiazepines is often related to redistribution (Stimpfl et al., 2023)
- Extended-release formulation only needs to be taken once or twice daily
- Do not break or chew XR tablets, as this will alter controlled-release properties
- Alprazolam and alprazolam XR are generally dosed about one-tenth the dosage of diazepam
- Alprazolam and alprazolam XR are generally dosed about twice the dosage of clonazepam

How to Switch

Use the accompanying equivalence table to convert from the alprazolam dose to the dose of the new benzodiazepine

Approximate equivalent dosage (mg)	
Alprazolam (Xanax)	0.5
Chlordiazepoxide (Librium)	25
Clonazepam (Klonopin)	0.25–0.5
Diazepam (Valium)	5
Lorazepam (Ativan)	1

How to Stop

- Seizures may rarely occur on withdrawal, especially if withdrawal is abrupt; greater risk for doses above 4 mg and in those with additional risks for seizures, including those with a history of seizures
- Taper by 0.5 mg every 3 days to reduce chances of withdrawal effects
- For difficult to taper cases, consider reducing dose much more slowly after reaching 3 mg/day, perhaps by as little as 0.25 mg per week or less (not for XR)
- Be sure to differentiate the reemergence of symptoms requiring reinstitution of treatment from withdrawal symptoms
- Benzodiazepine-dependent anxiety patients and insulin-dependent diabetics are not addicted to their medications. When benzodiazepine-dependent patients stop their medication, disease symptoms can reemerge, disease symptoms can worsen (rebound), and/or withdrawal symptoms can emerge

WHAT TO EXPECT

Onset of Action

- Some immediate relief with first dosing is common; can take several weeks with daily dosing for maximal therapeutic benefit

Duration of Action

- Duration of action varies for benzodiazepines, including alprazolam, in pediatric patients, but is generally considered to be from 10–12 hours

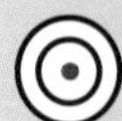

Primary Target Symptoms

- Panic attacks
- Anxiety

What Is Considered a Positive Result?

- The goal of treatment for anxiety is complete remission of current symptoms as well as prevention of future relapses
- If treatment works, it most often reduces or even eliminates symptoms, but is not a cure since symptoms can recur after medicine is stopped

How Long to Treat

- For short-term symptoms of anxiety – after a few weeks, discontinue use or use on an "as-needed" basis
- For long-term symptoms of anxiety, consider switching to an SSRI or SNRI for long-term maintenance
- If long-term maintenance with a benzodiazepine is necessary, continue treatment for 6 months after symptoms resolve, and then taper dose slowly

What If It Stops Working?

- If anxiety symptoms reemerge, consider an SSRI and re-trying psychotherapeutic approaches

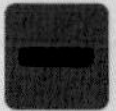

What If It Doesn't Work?

- Consider a trial of an SSRI
- When treating youth with anxiety disorders, many patients will have had significant anxiety for years prior to beginning treatment. As such, when anxiety is treated with alprazolam, their symptoms may be improved, but the patient has likely missed important developmental milestones (e.g., spending the night with friends, being able to ask questions in class). Developing these skills will take time. Beyond this, the family may have lived with the anxious child for years, and following treatment of the child, the family may need to readjust.
- Be mindful of family conflict contributing to the presentation; sometimes treating parental depression or anxiety disorders improves psychiatric and social function without any treatment of youth. Also, accommodation is common in families of youth with anxiety disorders and may need to be addressed specifically, as it can perpetuate symptoms.

TALKING TO PATIENTS AND CAREGIVERS

What to Tell Parents About Efficacy

- While the medicine helps by reducing symptoms and improving function, it is not a cure, and it is therefore necessary to keep taking the medication to sustain its therapeutic effects
- Since every treatment consideration depends on a risk/benefit analysis, parents should fully understand short- and long-term risks as well as benefits
- Often it is a good idea to tell parents whether the medication chosen is specifically approved for the disorder being treated, or whether it is being given for "unapproved" or "off-label" reasons based on good clinical practice, expert consensus, and/or prudent extrapolation of controlled data from adults

What to Tell Children and Adolescents About Efficacy

- We are trying to make you feel better
- It may be a good idea to give the medication a try; if it's not working very well, we can stop the medication and try something else
- Medications don't change who you are as a person; they give you the opportunity to be the best person you can be

What to Tell Parents About Side Effects

- Explain that mild side effects are expected at initiation or when increasing the dose and are usually transitory
- Predict side effects in advance (you will look clever and competent to the parents, unless you scare them with too much information and cause nocebo effects, in which case you won't look so clever when the patient develops lots of side effects and stops medication; use your judgment here); a balanced but honest presentation is an art rather than a science
- Ask parents to support the patient while side effects are occurring
- Parents should fully understand short- and long-term risks as well as benefits
- Explaining to the parents what to expect from medication treatment, and especially potential side effects, can help prevent early termination of medication

What to Tell Children and Adolescents About Side Effects

- Even if you get side effects, most of them get better or go away in a few days to a few weeks; however, we will likely not use this medication for a long time
- Explaining to child/adolescent what to expect from medication treatment, and especially potential side effects, can help prevent early termination of medication

What to Tell Teachers About the Medication (If Parents Consent)

- Alprazolam can make children/adolescents sleepy and make it difficult for children or adolescents to pay attention. In these situations, it is important to notify the clinician so that the dose can be decreased.
- Alprazolam may interfere with children's ability to engage in some activities at recess and in physical education class
- Encourage dialogue with parents/guardians about any behavior or mood changes

SPECIAL POPULATIONS

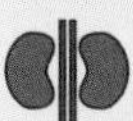

Renal Impairment

- Should be used with caution

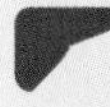

Hepatic Impairment

- Should begin with lower starting dose (0.5–0.75 mg/day in 2 or 3 divided doses)

Cardiac Impairment

- No data available

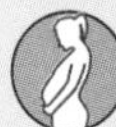

Pregnancy

- Possible increased risk of birth defects when benzodiazepines are taken during pregnancy
- Because of the potential risks, alprazolam is not generally recommended as treatment for anxiety during pregnancy, especially during the first trimester
- Drug should be tapered if discontinued
- Infants whose mothers received a benzodiazepine late in pregnancy may experience withdrawal effects

- Neonatal flaccidity has been reported in infants whose mothers took a benzodiazepine during pregnancy
- Seizures, even mild seizures, may cause harm to the embryo/fetus

Breast Feeding

- Some drug is found in breast milk
- Recommended either to discontinue drug or formula feed
- Effects on infant have been observed and include feeding difficulties, sedation, and weight loss

THE ART OF PSYCHOPHARMACOLOGY

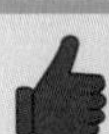

Potential Advantages

- Rapid onset of action
- Less sedation than some other benzodiazepines
- Availability of an XR formulation with longer duration of action

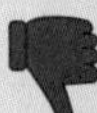

Potential Disadvantages

- Abuse especially risky in past or present substance users

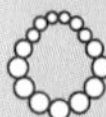

Pearls

- Despite trials of benzodiazepines in adults with anxiety disorders consistently demonstrating benefit, trials of benzodiazepines in pediatric patients have produced mixed results:
  - Small double-blind, placebo-controlled trials and meta-analyses do not reveal differences between benzodiazepines and placebo for the management of anxiety disorders. However, these studies were small and included very young children and high doses of short-acting benzodiazepines (e.g., alprazolam).
  - By contrast, for acute anxiety in children and adolescents, a meta-analysis of nearly 1,500 patients suggests that benzodiazepines are more effective than placebo in treating acute anxiety; in this meta-analysis, there was no significant difference in the risk of developing irritability or behavioral changes between benzodiazepine and control groups (Kuang et al., 2017)
  - In the pediatric benzodiazepine trials, the poor tolerability – particularly in younger patients – may be connected to age-related pharmacodynamic factors (Strawn and Stahl, 2023)
- The pharmacodynamics of the GABA receptor in children and adolescents differ from adults, with adult expression/function not being achieved until age 14–17½ years for subcortical regions and 18–22 years for cortical regions, although girls reach adult expression of GABA receptors slightly earlier than boys (Chugani et al., 2001)
- In adults with anxiety disorders, benzodiazepines may be a very useful adjunct to SSRIs and SNRIs in the treatment of numerous anxiety disorders; however, the evidence for this is limited in children and adolescents
- Grapefruit significantly affects the pharmacokinetics of most benzodiazepines (and other medications that are metabolized by CYP3A4). In fact, grapefruit increases peak benzodiazepine blood levels (Cmax) by almost 60%, increases the time to maximum concentration (Tmax) by 80%, and boosts absorption by up to 50%.
- Risk of seizure is greatest during the first 3 days after discontinuation of alprazolam, especially in those with prior seizures, head injuries, or withdrawal from drugs of abuse
- Clinical duration of action may be shorter than plasma half-life, leading to dosing more frequently than 2–3 times daily in some patients, especially for immediate-release alprazolam. This is primarily related to alprazolam's rapid redistribution.
- Adding fluvoxamine, fluoxetine, or nefazodone can increase alprazolam levels and make the patient very sleepy unless the alprazolam dose is lowered by half or more
- When using alprazolam to treat insomnia, remember that insomnia may be a symptom of some other primary disorder itself, and thus warrant evaluation for comorbid psychiatric and/or medical conditions
- Alprazolam XR may be less sedating than immediate-release alprazolam
- Alprazolam XR may be dosed less frequently than immediate-release alprazolam, and lead to less interdose breakthrough symptoms and less "clockwatching" in anxious patients
- Slower rises in plasma drug levels for alprazolam XR have the potential to reduce

euphoria/abuse liability, but this has not been proven
- If clonazepam can be considered a "long-acting alprazolam-like anxiolytic," then alprazolam XR can be considered "an even longer-acting clonazepam-like anxiolytic" with the potential of improved tolerability features in terms of less euphoria, abuse, dependence, and withdrawal problems, but this has not been proven
- Though not systematically studied, benzodiazepines have been used effectively to treat catatonia and are the initial recommended treatment

SUGGESTED READING

Chugani DC, Muzik O, Juhász C et al. Postnatal maturation of human GABAA receptors measured with positron emission tomography. Ann Neurol 2001;49(5):618–26.

Kuang H, Johnson JA, Mulqueen JM, Bloch MH. The efficacy of benzodiazepines as acute anxiolytics in children: a meta-analysis. Depress Anxiety 2017;34(10):888–96.

Nicotra CM, Strawn JS. Advances in pharmacotherapy for pediatric anxiety disorders. Child Adolesc Psychiatr Clin N Am 2023;32(3):573–87.

Sidorchuk A, Isomura K, Molero Y et al. Benzodiazepine prescribing for children, adolescents, and young adults from 2006 through 2013: a total population register-linkage study. PLoS Med 2018;15(8):e1002635.

Stimpfl JN, Mills JA, Strawn JR. Pharmacologic predictors of benzodiazepine response trajectory in anxiety disorders: a Bayesian hierarchical modeling meta-analysis. CNS Spectr 2023;28(1):53–60.

Strawn JR, Lu L, Peris TS, Levine A, Walkup JT. Research review: pediatric anxiety disorders – what have we learnt in the last 10 years? J Child Psychol Psychiatry 2021;62(2):114–39.

Strawn JR, Stahl SM. Case Studies: Stahl's Essential Psychopharmacology: Volume 4: Children and Adolescents. New York: Cambridge University Press, 2023.

THERAPEUTICS

Brands

- Elavil, other

Generic

Yes

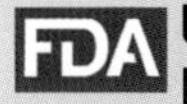

US FDA Approved for Pediatric Use

- Depression in adolescents

Off-Label for Pediatric Use

- Severe and treatment-resistant depression
- Anxiety
- Migraine prophylaxis
- Neuropathic pain/chronic pain

Class and Mechanism of Action

- Neuroscience-based Nomenclature: serotonin norepinephrine multi-modal (SN-MM)
- Tricyclic antidepressant (TCA)
- Serotonin and norepinephrine reuptake inhibitor
- Boosts neurotransmitters serotonin and norepinephrine
- Blocks serotonin reuptake pump (serotonin transporter), presumably increasing serotonergic neurotransmission
- Blocks norepinephrine reuptake pump (norepinephrine transporter), presumably increasing noradrenergic neurotransmission
- Presumably desensitizes both serotonin 1A receptors and beta adrenergic receptors
- Since dopamine is inactivated by norepinephrine reuptake in the frontal cortex, which largely lacks dopamine transporters, amitriptyline can increase dopamine neurotransmission in this part of the brain

SAFETY AND TOLERABILITY

Notable Side Effects

- Blurred vision, constipation, dry mouth
- Increased appetite, weight gain
- Dizziness, sedation, fatigue
- Nausea, diarrhea
- Sweating
- Urinary retention, heartburn, unusual taste in mouth
- Anxiety, nervousness, restlessness, weakness, headache
- Sexual dysfunction (impotence, change in libido)
- Rash, itching
- Note: patients with diagnosed or undiagnosed bipolar or psychotic disorders may be more vulnerable to CNS-activating actions of TCAs like amitriptyline; pay particular attention to signs of activation in children with developmental disorders, autism spectrum disorders, or brain injury, as they may not tolerate these side effects well
- Treatment-emergent activation syndrome (TEAS) includes agitation, anxiety, panic attacks, irritability, aggression, impulsivity, insomnia, and suicidality
- TEAS can represent side effects, but should not be confused with bipolar mania or the onset of suicidality and should be monitored and investigated with consideration of discontinuing or decreasing dose of amitriptyline or addition of another agent or switching to another agent to reduce these symptoms

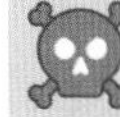

Life-Threatening or Dangerous Side Effects

- Paralytic ileus, hyperthermia (TCAs + anticholinergic agents)
- Lowered seizure threshold and rare seizures
- Orthostatic hypotension, arrhythmias, tachycardia
- QTc prolongation
- Some cases of sudden death have occurred in children taking TCAs
- Hepatic failure, extrapyramidal symptoms
- Increased intraocular pressure
- Rare induction of mania
- Rare suicidal ideation and behavior (suicidality) (short-term regulatory studies did not show any actual suicides in any age group and also did not show an increase in the risk of suicidality with antidepressants compared to placebo beyond age 24)

Growth and Maturation

- Growth should be monitored; long-term effects are unknown

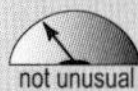

Weight Gain

- Limited experience in pediatric patients; in adults weight gain is not uncommon

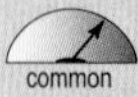

Sedation

- Many experience and/or can be significant in amount
- Tolerance to sedative effect may develop with long-term use

What to Do About Side Effects

- Wait, wait, wait: mild side effects are common, happen early, and usually improve with time, but treatment benefits can be delayed and often begin just as the side effects wear off
- Monitor side effects closely, especially when initiating treatment
- May wish to try dosing every other day to deal with side effects, or wash out for a week and try again at half dose or every other day
- May wish to give some drugs at night if not tolerated during the day
- For activation (jitteriness, anxiety, insomnia):
    - Consider a temporary dose reduction or a more gradual up-titration
    - Consider switching to another antidepressant
    - Optimize psychotherapeutic interventions
    - Activation and agitation may represent the induction of a bipolar state, especially a mixed dysphoric bipolar II condition sometimes associated with suicidal ideation, and may require the addition of lithium or an atypical antipsychotic, and/or discontinuation of amitriptyline
- Often best to try another monotherapy prior to resorting to augmentation strategies to treat side effects
- For insomnia: consider adding melatonin
- For GI upset: try giving medication with a meal. Giving antidepressants with food will, in general, decrease peak plasma concentrations and increase the time required for absorption (Strawn et al., 2021, 2023).
- Orthostatic symptoms are common in children and adolescents treated with TCAs, and the relative risk of orthostatic symptoms in a recent meta-analysis of youth treated with TCAs was 4.86 (Hazell and Mirzaie, 2013). Encouraging adequate hydration and salt intake can be helpful in the pediatric population.
- Tremor is common in pediatric patients treated with TCAs (RR 5.43) and is generally dose related
- Dry mouth is common in youth treated with TCAs (RR 3.35) (Hazell and Mirzaie, 2013). In adults, rates of dry mouth are higher in patients treated with TCAs compared to SSRIs, and TCAs reduce salivary flow by nearly 60%, whereas SSRIs reduce salivary flow by approximately 30% (Strawn et al., 2023). Interventions include lozenges, sprays, mouth rinses, gels, oils, and chewing gum, which broadly fall into two categories: saliva stimulants and saliva substitutes.
- For sweating with amitriptyline, consider topical agents. Topical agents have been used in pediatric populations with primary hyperhidrosis and include glycopyrronium tosylate (2.4%), a topical anticholinergic approved in the United States for primary axillary hyperhidrosis in patients ≥9 years (Hebert et al., 2020). Additionally, for antidepressant-related palmar–plantar hyperhidrosis, clinicians may consider aluminum salts (e.g., 12.5% aluminum chloride hexahydrate or 20% aluminum zirconium salts), which precipitate ions that obstruct eccrine ducts and in doing so block the movement of sweat to the skin surface.
- For sexual dysfunction:
    - Probably best to reduce dose or discontinue and try another agent

How Drug Causes Side Effects

- Theoretically due to increases in serotonin concentrations at serotonin receptors in parts of the brain and body other than those that cause therapeutic actions (e.g., unwanted actions of serotonin in sleep centers causing insomnia, unwanted actions of serotonin in the gut causing diarrhea)
- Increasing serotonin can cause diminished dopamine release and might contribute to emotional flattening, cognitive slowing, and apathy in some patients
- Anticholinergic activity may explain sedative effects, dry mouth, constipation, and blurred vision
- Sedative effects and weight gain may be due to antihistamine properties
- Blockade of alpha adrenergic 1 receptors may explain dizziness, sedation, and hypotension

- Cardiac arrhythmias and seizures, especially in overdose, may be caused by blockade of ion channels

Warnings and Precautions

- Consider distributing brochures provided by the FDA and the drug companies as well as the medication guides from the American Academy of Child & Adolescent Psychiatry (AACAP)
- Carefully consider monitoring patients regularly within the practical limits, particularly during the first several weeks of treatment
- Warn patients and their caregivers when possible about the possibility of activating side effects and advise them to report such symptoms immediately
- Carefully weigh the risks and benefits of pharmacological treatment against the risks and benefits of nontreatment with antidepressants and it is a good idea to document this in the patient's chart
- Add or initiate other antidepressants with caution for up to 2 weeks after discontinuing amitriptyline
- Use with caution in patients with history of seizures, urinary retention, angle-closure glaucoma, hyperthyroidism
- TCAs can increase QTc interval, especially at toxic doses, which can be attained not only by overdose but also by combining with drugs that inhibit TCA metabolism via CYP2D6
- Because TCAs can prolong QTc interval, use with caution in patients who have bradycardia or who are taking drugs that can induce bradycardia (e.g., beta blockers, calcium channel blockers, clonidine, digitalis)
- Because TCAs can prolong QTc interval, use with caution in patients who have hypokalemia and/or hypomagnesemia or who are taking drugs that can induce hypokalemia and/or hypomagnesemia (e.g., diuretics, stimulant laxatives, glucocorticoids, tetracosactide)
- As with any antidepressant, use with caution in patients with bipolar disorder unless treated with concomitant mood-stabilizing agent
- Monitor patients for activation and suicidal ideation and involve parents/guardians

When Not to Prescribe

- If patient is taking an MAO inhibitor
- If patient is recovering from myocardial infarction
- If patient is taking agents capable of significantly prolonging QTc interval (e.g., pimozide, thioridazine, selected antiarrhythmics, moxifloxacin, sparfloxacin)
- If there is a history of QTc prolongation or cardiac arrhythmia
- If patient is taking drugs that inhibit amitriptyline metabolism, including CYP2D6 inhibitors or CYP1A2 inhibitors
- If there is a proven allergy to amitriptyline or nortriptyline

Long-Term Use

- Growth should be monitored; long-term effects are unknown

Habit Forming

- No

Overdose

- Death may occur; convulsions, cardiac dysrhythmias, severe hypotension, CNS depression, coma, changes in ECG

DOSING AND USE

Usual Dosage Range

- Depression (ages 12 and older): 50 mg/day in divided doses
- Pain (ages 12 and older): 10 mg/day
- Ages 11 and younger: 1 mg/kg/day

Dosage Forms

- Tablet 10 mg, 25 mg, 50 mg, 75 mg, 100 mg, 150 mg

How to Dose

- Depression (ages 12 and older): titrate up to recommended dose of 10 mg three times per day and 20 mg at bedtime
- Pain (ages 12 and older): initial dose 10 mg/day; dose can be increased if pain control is not sufficient
- Ages 11 and younger: dosing is weight-based

Options for Administration

- Only available as a tablet

Tests

- Weight and BMI percentiles as well as blood pressure and heart rate during treatment
- Currently, the AACAP recommends ECGs prior to initiation of TCA therapy and after dose titration of TCAs
- Heart rate and blood pressure should be monitored in patients treated with TCAs
- Therapeutic drug monitoring is common in patients treated with TCAs, including amitriptyline
- Timing of serum samples: draw trough just before next dose (Hiemke et al., 2018), with once-daily bedtime dosing draw level 12 to 16 hours after dose
- Therapeutic reference range: amitriptyline + nortriptyline 80 to 200 ng/mL with alert levels generally >300 ng/mL (Hiemke et al., 2018)

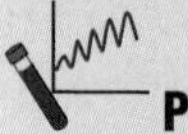

Pharmacokinetics

- Rapidly absorbed
- Protein binding is >90%
- CYP2C19 is the major enzyme responsible for demethylation and CYP2D6 is responsible for converting amitriptyline and its metabolite nortriptyline to hydroxy metabolites (Figure 1). Additionally, nortriptyline is an inhibitor of hydroxyamitriptyline.
- Bioavailability is 43 to 46% in adults
- Time to peak, serum: ~2 to 5 hours (Schulz et al., 1985)
- Plasma half-life is 10–28 hours in adults
- Food does not affect absorption

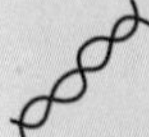

Pharmacogenetics

- The Clinical Pharmacogenetics Implementation Consortium provides recommendations for CYP2D6 and CYP2C19 for amitriptyline
- **CYP2D6 poor metabolizers:** Avoid tricyclic use due to the potential for side effects. Consider an alternative drug not metabolized by CYP2D6. If a TCA is warranted, consider a 50% reduction of recommended starting dose. Utilize therapeutic drug monitoring to guide dose adjustments.
- **CYP2D6 ultrarapid metabolizers:** Avoid tricyclic use due to potential lack of efficacy. Consider an alternative drug not metabolized by CYP2D6. If a TCA is warranted, consider titrating to a higher target dose (compared to normal

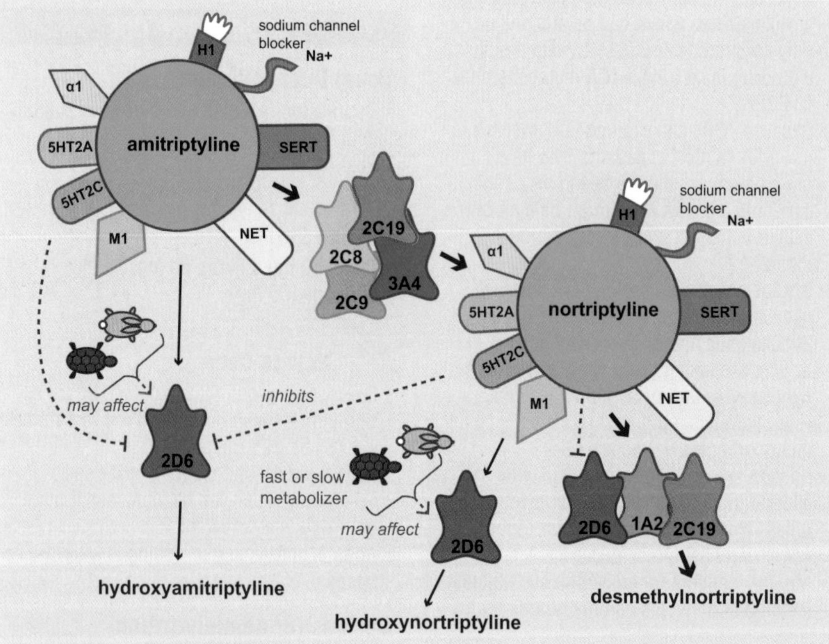

Figure 1 Amitriptyline (metabolism).

metabolizers). Utilize therapeutic drug monitoring to guide dose adjustments.

- **CYP2C19 rapid/ultrarapid metabolizers (optional):** Avoid tertiary amine use due to the potential for suboptimal response. Consider an alternative drug not metabolized by CYP2C19. TCAs without major CYP2C19 metabolism include the secondary amines nortriptyline and desipramine. If a tertiary amine is warranted, utilize therapeutic drug monitoring to guide dose adjustments.
- **CYP2C19 poor metabolizers:** Avoid tertiary amine use due to the potential for suboptimal response. Consider an alternative drug not metabolized by CYP2C19. TCAs without major CYP2C19 metabolism include secondary amines, nortriptyline, and desipramine. For tertiary amines, consider a 50% reduction of the recommended starting dose. Utilize therapeutic drug monitoring to guide dose adjustments.

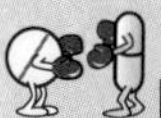

Drug Interactions

- Tramadol reported to increase the risk of seizures in patients taking an antidepressant
- Can cause a fatal "serotonin syndrome" when combined with MAO inhibitors, so do not use with MAO inhibitors or for at least 14 days after MAOIs are stopped
- Do not start an MAO inhibitor for at least 5 weeks after discontinuing amitriptyline
- Use of TCAs with anticholinergic drugs may result in paralytic ileus or hyperthermia
- Fluoxetine, paroxetine, bupropion, duloxetine, and other CYP2D6 inhibitors may increase TCA concentrations
- Fluvoxamine, a CYP1A2 inhibitor, decreases the conversion of amitriptyline to nortriptyline, and increases amitriptyline plasma concentrations
- Cimetidine may increase plasma concentrations of TCAs and cause anticholinergic symptoms
- Phenothiazines or haloperidol may raise TCA blood concentrations
- May alter effects of antihypertensive drugs
- Use of TCAs with sympathomimetic agents may increase sympathetic activity
- TCAs may inhibit hypotensive effects of clonidine

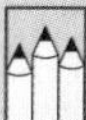

Dosing Tips

- Plasma levels are higher in lower-weight children; therefore, starting and target doses may be lower and longer intervals between dose increases may be needed (see How to Dose)
- Adolescents often need and receive adult doses, and dosing in most adolescent trials is bid. However, in younger patients, dosing may need to be tid.
- If given in a single dose, should generally be administered at bedtime because of its sedative properties
- If given in split doses, largest dose should generally be given at bedtime because of its sedative properties
- If patients experience nightmares, split dose and do not give large dose at bedtime
- Patients treated for chronic pain may require lower doses; however, trials of amitriptyline (1 mg/kg/day) for pediatric migraine have failed to separate from placebo (Powers et al., 2017)

How to Switch

- From another antidepressant to amitriptyline:
  - When tapering a prior antidepressant, see its entry in this manual for how to stop and how to taper off that specific drug
  - In situations when there are antidepressant-related side effects, try to stop the first agent before starting amitriptyline so that new side effects of amitriptyline can be distinguished from withdrawal effects of the first agent
  - If urgent, cross taper
- From amitriptyline to another antidepressant:
  - Generally, try to stop amitriptyline before starting another antidepressant
  - Taper to avoid withdrawal effects (dizziness, nausea, stomach cramps, sweating, tingling, dysesthesias)
  - Can reduce amitriptyline dose by 50% every 3 days, or slower if this rate still causes withdrawal symptoms
  - If necessary, can cross taper off amitriptyline this way while dosing up on another antidepressant simultaneously in urgent situations, being aware of all specific drug interactions to avoid

How to Stop

- Taper to avoid withdrawal effects (dizziness, nausea, sweating, tingling, dysesthesias) (Strawn et al., 2023)
- Even with gradual dose reduction, some withdrawal symptoms may appear within the first 2 weeks
- Many patients tolerate 50% dose reduction for 5–7 days, then another 50% reduction for 5–7 days, then discontinuation
- If withdrawal symptoms emerge during discontinuation, raise dose to stop symptoms and then restart withdrawal much more slowly

WHAT TO EXPECT

Onset of Action

- Some patients may experience increased energy or activation early after initiation of treatment
- Full onset of therapeutic actions in depression is usually delayed by 2–4 weeks

Duration of Action

- Effects are consistent over a 24-hour period
- May continue to work for many years to prevent relapse of symptoms

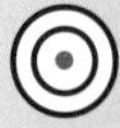

Primary Target Symptoms

- Depressed and/or irritable mood
- Anxiety (fear and worry are often target symptoms, but amitriptyline can occasionally and transiently increase these symptoms short term before improving them)
- Prior to initiation of treatment, it is helpful to develop a list of target symptoms of OCD (obsessive-compulsive disorder) and anxiety to monitor during treatment to better assess treatment response

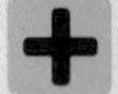

What Is Considered a Positive Result?

- The goal of treatment is complete remission of current symptoms as well as prevention of future relapses
- In practice, many patients have only a partial response where some symptoms are improved but others persist (especially insomnia, fatigue, and problems concentrating in depression), in which case higher doses of amitriptyline, adding a second agent, or switching to an agent with a different mechanism of action can be considered
- If treatment works, it most often reduces or even eliminates symptoms, but is not a cure since symptoms can recur after medicine is stopped
- The goal of treatment of chronic neuropathic pain is to reduce symptoms as much as possible, especially in combination with other treatments

How Long to Treat

- After symptoms are sufficiently reduced/eliminated, continue treating for 12 months for the first episode of depression. For patients with anxiety disorders, 9 months may be advisable (Hathaway et al., 2018).
- For second and subsequent episodes of depression, treatment may need to be longer. In general, in youth, relapse is most likely in the first 1–3 months after discontinuing an antidepressant (Emslie et al., 2004).
- Use in other anxiety disorders and chronic pain may also need to be indefinite, but long-term treatment is not well studied in these conditions

What If It Stops Working?

- Some patients who have an initial response may relapse even though they continue treatment, sometimes called "poop-out"
- Some patients may experience apparent lack of consistent efficacy due to activation syndrome or latent or underlying or newly evolved bipolar disorder, or major depressive episodes with mixed features, and require antidepressant discontinuation and a switch to a second generation antipsychotic

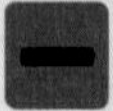

What If It Doesn't Work?

- Consider evaluation for another diagnosis (especially bipolar illness or depression with mixed features) or for a comorbid condition (e.g., medical illness, substance abuse)
- Be mindful of family conflict contributing to the presentation; sometimes treating parental depression can improve psychiatric and social function without any treatment of youth. Also, accommodation is common in families of youth with anxiety disorders and

may need to be addressed specifically, as it can perpetuate symptoms.
- Consider factors associated with poor response to SSRIs in treatment-resistant depression or anxiety disorders, such as severe symptoms, long-lasting symptoms, poor treatment adherence, prior nonresponse to other treatments, and the presence of comorbid disorders
- Consider other important potential factors such as ongoing conflicts, family psychopathology, and an adverse environment (e.g., poverty, chaos, violence, prior and ongoing psychological trauma, abuse, neglect). Additionally, when symptoms are prominent at school, consider the presence of a learning disorder.
- Institute trauma-informed care for appropriate children and adolescents
- A 2007 meta-analysis of published and unpublished trials in pediatric patients found that antidepressants had a number needed to treat (NNT) of 10 for depression, 6 for OCD, and 3 for anxiety disorders; thus, amitriptyline may not work in all children, so consider switching to another antidepressant (Bridge et al., 2007)
- Consider a dose adjustment
- Consider augmenting options:
  - Cognitive behavioral therapy (CBT), interpersonal psychotherapy for adolescents (IPT-A), light therapy, family therapy, and exercise especially in adolescents. For youth with OCD, it is important to ensure that cognitive behavioral therapy involves exposure, as these appear to be the vehicle for improvement.
  - For insomnia: sleep hygiene, CBT for insomnia, melatonin. It's probably best to avoid alpha 2 agonists in TCA-treated patients.
  - For anxiety: antihistamines or perhaps buspirone (although pediatric data are mixed)
  - Add lithium or atypical antipsychotics for bipolar depression, psychotic depression, treatment-resistant depression, or treatment-resistant anxiety disorders
  - TMS (transcranial magnetic stimulation) may have a role, although pediatric trials of TMS have been hampered by high sham response rates (Croarkin et al., 2021).

TALKING TO PATIENTS AND CAREGIVERS

What to Tell Parents About Efficacy

- Doesn't work right away; full therapeutic benefits may take 2–8 weeks, yet parents and teachers might see improvement before the patient does
- While the medicine helps by reducing symptoms and improving function, it is not a cure, and it is therefore necessary to keep taking the medication to sustain its therapeutic effects
- Since every treatment consideration depends on a risk/benefit analysis, parents should fully understand short- and long-term risks as well as benefits
- After successful treatment, continuation of amitriptyline may be necessary to prevent relapse, especially in those who have had more than one episode or a very severe episode
- Often a good idea to tell parents whether the medication chosen is specifically approved for the disorder being treated, or whether it is being given for "unapproved" or "off-label" reasons based on good clinical practice, expert consensus, and/or prudent extrapolation of controlled data from adults

What to Tell Children and Adolescents About Efficacy

- We are trying to make you feel better
- It may be a good idea to give the medication a try; if it's not working very well, we can stop the medication and try something else
- A good try takes 2 to 3 months or even longer
- If it does make you feel better, you cannot stop it right away or you may get sick again
- Medications don't change who you are as a person; they give you the opportunity to be the best person you can be

What to Tell Parents About Side Effects

- Explain that side effects are expected in many when starting and are most common in the first 2–3 weeks of starting or increasing the dose
- Tell parents many side effects go away and do so about the same time that therapeutic effects start

- Predict side effects in advance (you will look clever and competent to the parents, unless you scare them with too much information and cause nocebo effects, in which case you won't look so clever when the patient develops lots of side effects and stops medication; use your judgment here); a balanced but honest presentation is an art rather than a science
- Ask them to help monitor for increased suicidality and if present, report any such symptoms immediately
- Ask parents to support the patient while side effects are occurring
- Parents should fully understand short- and long-term risks as well as benefits
- Explaining to the parents what to expect from medication treatment, and especially potential side effects, can help prevent early termination of medication

What to Tell Children and Adolescents About Side Effects

- Even if you get side effects, most of them get better or go away in a few days to a few weeks
- Consider having a conversation about sexual side effects in some adolescents who can find these side effects confusing and especially burdensome
- Explaining to child/adolescent what to expect from medication treatment, and especially potential side effects, can help prevent early termination of medication
- Tell adolescents and children capable of understanding that some young patients, especially those who are depressed, may develop thoughts of hurting themselves, and if this happens, not to be alarmed but to tell their parents right away

What to Tell Teachers About the Medication (If Parents Consent)

- Amitriptyline can make children/adolescents tired
- If the patient is sleepy, ask whether the medication is keeping them up at night
- It is not abusable
- Encourage dialogue with parents/guardians about any behavior or mood changes

SPECIAL POPULATIONS

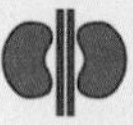

Renal Impairment

- Use with caution; may need to lower dose

Hepatic Impairment

- Use with caution; may need to lower dose

Cardiac Impairment

- ECG is recommended at baseline and after dose titrations
- TCAs have been reported to cause arrhythmias, prolongation of conduction time, orthostatic hypotension, sinus tachycardia
- TCAs produce QTc prolongation, which may be enhanced by the existence of bradycardia, hypokalemia, congenital or acquired long QTc interval, which should be evaluated prior to administering amitriptyline
- Use with caution if treating concomitantly with a medication likely to produce prolonged bradycardia, hypokalemia, slowing of intracardiac conduction, or prolongation of the QTc interval
- Avoid TCAs in patients with a known history of QTc prolongation
- Risk/benefit ratio may not justify use of TCAs in cardiac impairment

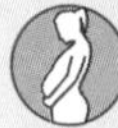

Pregnancy

- Controlled studies have not been conducted in pregnant women
- Amitriptyline crosses the placenta
- Adverse effects have been reported in infants whose mothers took a TCA (lethargy, withdrawal symptoms, fetal malformations)
- Must weigh the risk of treatment (first trimester fetal development, third trimester newborn delivery) to the child against the risk of no treatment (recurrence of depression, worsening of OCD, maternal health, infant bonding) to the mother and child
- For many patients this may mean continuing treatment during pregnancy

Breast Feeding

- Some drug is found in breast milk

- Recommended either to discontinue drug or formula feed
- Immediate postpartum period is a high-risk time for depression, especially in women who have had prior depressive episodes, so drug may need to be reinstituted late in the third trimester or shortly after childbirth to prevent a recurrence or exacerbation during the postpartum period
- Must weigh benefits of breast feeding with risks and benefits of antidepressant treatment versus nontreatment to both the infant and the mother
- For many patients this may mean continuing treatment during breast feeding

THE ART OF PSYCHOPHARMACOLOGY

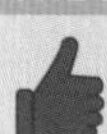

Potential Advantages

- In children and adolescents:
  - Patients with co-occurring pain syndromes
- All ages:
  - Patients with insomnia
  - Severe or treatment-resistant depression

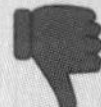

Potential Disadvantages

- In children:
  - Those who are already psychomotor agitated, angry, or irritable, and who do not have a psychiatric diagnosis
  - Those who may possibly have a mood disorder with mixed or bipolar features, especially those with these features and a family history of bipolar disorder
  - All randomized trials in youth with depression fail to show efficacy of TCAs
  - Patients with seizure disorders
- In adolescents:
  - Those who may possibly have a mood disorder with mixed or bipolar features, especially those with these features and a family history of bipolar disorder
  - All randomized trials in youth with depression fail to show efficacy of TCAs
  - Patients with seizure disorders
- All ages:
  - Cardiac patients
  - Patients with seizure disorders

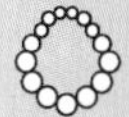

Pearls

- Clinical trials of amitriptyline in children and adolescents with depression have generally failed to demonstrate improvement in depression symptoms. In the first study, Kramer and Feiguine (1981) evaluated amitriptyline 200 mg versus placebo and found 80% of children receiving amitriptyline improved compared to 60% receiving placebo. In a second trial, 90% of youth receiving amitriptyline (5 mg/kg/day) and 90% of those receiving placebo had improved depressive symptoms (Kye et al., 1996). In the third trial of youth with depression, 77% of youth receiving amitriptyline and 79% of those receiving placebo improved (Birmaher et al., 1998).
- Because of the lack of efficacy in most pediatric trials of amitriptyline (and other TCAs), these agents are rarely used for depression in youth
- Alcohol should be avoided because of additive CNS effects
- Underweight patients may be more susceptible to adverse cardiovascular effects
- Children, patients with inadequate hydration, and patients with cardiac disease may be more susceptible to TCA-induced cardiotoxicity than healthy adults
- Patients on TCAs should be aware that they may experience symptoms such as photosensitivity or blue-green urine
- Patients who are poor CYP2D6 metabolizers may experience side effects at low or normal doses; in such cases, consider switching to another antidepressant not metabolized by CYP2D6

SUGGESTED READING

Birmaher B, Waterman GS, Ryan ND et al. Randomized, controlled trial of amitriptyline versus placebo for adolescents with "treatment-resistant" major depression. J Am Acad Child Adolesc Psychiatry 1998;37(5):527–35.

Bridge JA, Iyengar S, Salary CB et al. Clinical response and risk for reported suicidal ideation and suicide attempts in pediatric antidepressant treatment: a meta-analysis of randomized controlled trials. JAMA 2007;297(15):1683–96.

Cipriani A, Zhou X, Del Giovane C et al. Comparative efficacy and tolerability of antidepressants for major depressive disorder in children and adolescents: a network meta-analysis. Lancet 2016;388(10047):881–90.

Croarkin PE, Elmaadawi AZ, Aaronson ST et al. Left prefrontal transcranial magnetic stimulation for treatment-resistant depression in adolescents: a double-blind, randomized, sham-controlled trial. Neuropsychopharmacology 2021;46(2):462–9.

Emslie GJ, Heiligenstein JH, Hoog SL, et al. Fluoxetine treatment for prevention of relapse of depression in children and adolescents: a double-blind, placebo-controlled study. J Am Acad Child Adolesc Psychiatry 2004;43(11):1397–405.

Hathaway EE, Walkup JT, Strawn JR. Antidepressant treatment duration in pediatric depressive and anxiety disorders: how long is long enough? Curr Probl Pediatr Adolesc Health Care 2018;48(2):31–9.

Hazell P, Mirzaie M. Tricyclic drugs for depression in children and adolescents. Cochrane Database Syst Rev 2013;2013(6):CD002317. doi: 10.1002/14651858.CD002317.pub2.

Hebert AA, Glaser DA, Green L et al. Long-term efficacy and safety of topical glycopyrronium tosylate for the treatment of primary axillary hyperhidrosis: post hoc pediatric subgroup analysis from a 44-week open-label extension study. Pediatr Dermatol 2020;37(3):490–7.

Hicks JK, Sangkuhl K, Swen JJ et al. Clinical Pharmacogenetics Implementation Consortium guideline (CPIC) for CYP2D6 and CYP2C19 genotypes and dosing of tricyclic antidepressants: 2016 update. Clin Pharmacol Ther 2017;102(1):37–44.

Hiemke C, Bergemann N, Clement HW et al. Consensus guidelines for therapeutic drug monitoring in neuropsychopharmacology: update 2017. Pharma Copsychiatry 2018;51(1-02):9-62.

Kramer AD, Feiguine RJ. Clinical effects of amitriptyline in adolescent depression. A pilot study. J Am Acad Child Psychiatry 1981;20(3):636-44.

Kye CH, Waterman GS, Ryan ND et al. A randomized, controlled trial of amitriptyline in the acute treatment of adolescent major depression. J Am Acad Child Adolesc Psychiatry 1996;35(9):1139-44.

Powers SW, Coffey CS, Chamberlin LA, et al.; CHAMP Investigators. Trial of amitriptyline, topiramate, and placebo for pediatric migraine. N Engl J Med 2017;376(2):115–24.

Remington C, Ruth J, Hebert AA. Primary hyperhidrosis in children: a review of therapeutics. Pediatr Dermatol 2021;38(3):561–7.

Schulz P, Dick P, Blaschke TF, Hollister L. Discrepancies between pharmacokinetic studies of amitriptyline. Clin Pharmacokinet 1985;10(3):257-68.

Strawn JR, Poweleit EA, Uppugunduri CRS, Ramsey LB. Pediatric therapeutic drug monitoring for selective serotonin reuptake inhibitors. Front Pharmacol 2021;1(12):749692.

Strawn JR, Mills JA, Poweleit EA, Ramsey LB, Croarkin PE. Adverse effects of antidepressant medications and their management in children and adolescents. Pharmacotherapy 2023;43(7):647–90.

THERAPEUTICS

Brands

- Dexedrine Spansule
- ProCentra
- Xelstrym
- Zenzedi

Generic

Yes

FDA US FDA Approved for Pediatric Use

- Attention deficit hyperactivity disorder (Zenzedi, ages 3 to 16)
- Attention deficit hyperactivity disorder (ProCentra, ages 3 to 16)
- Attention deficit hyperactivity disorder (Dexedrine Spansule, ages 6 to 16)
- Attention deficit hyperactivity disorder (Xelstrym, ages 6 and older)
- Narcolepsy (Zenzedi, ages 6 and older)
- Narcolepsy (ProCentra, ages 6 and older)
- Narcolepsy (Dexedrine Spansule, ages 6 and older)

Off-Label for Pediatric Use

- Approved in adults
  - None
- Other off-label uses
  - Treatment-resistant depression (rarely used for this in children)
  - Stimulants are sometimes used to augment antidepressants
  - Stimulants also sometimes used to treat amotivational or lethargic states in the elderly with dementia but rarely in children for these symptoms

Class and Mechanism of Action

- Neuroscience-based Nomenclature: dopamine, norepinephrine reuptake inhibitor and releaser (DN-RIRe)
- Stimulant
- Increases norepinephrine and especially dopamine actions by blocking their reuptake and facilitating their release
- Enhancement of dopamine and norepinephrine actions in certain brain regions (e.g., dorsolateral prefrontal cortex) may improve attention, concentration, executive dysfunction, wakefulness, and cortical inhibitory control of striatum (i.e., theoretically "tunes" inefficient information processing in cortical–striatal pathways, improving "top-down" regulation of striatal and other subcortical drives)
- Enhancement of dopamine actions in other brain regions (e.g., basal ganglia) may decrease hyperactivity
- Enhancement of dopamine and norepinephrine in yet other brain regions (e.g., medial prefrontal cortex, hypothalamus) may improve depressive symptoms as well as nondepression-associated fatigue and sleepiness
- Hypothetically rebalances signal to noise ratios of cortical neurons: enhances focus on important tasks (signal), theoretically due to norepinephrine, and reduces awareness of background activity (noise), theoretically due to dopamine

SAFETY AND TOLERABILITY

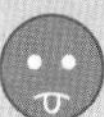

Notable Side Effects

- Anorexia and weight loss
- Nausea, abdominal pain
- Insomnia, headache, exacerbation of tics, tremor, dizziness, and possible irritability and anxiety. The risk of treatment-emergent irritability is higher with amphetamine-based stimulants compared to methylphenidate-based stimulants.
- Peripheral vasculopathy, including Raynaud's phenomenon
- Sexual dysfunction long term (impotence, libido changes) but can also improve sexual dysfunction short term

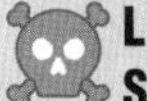

Life-Threatening or Dangerous Side Effects

- Psychosis
- Seizures
- Palpitations, tachycardia, hypertension
- Rare hypomania, mania, or suicidal ideation
- Cardiovascular adverse effects, death in patients with preexisting cardiac structural abnormalities often associated with a family history of cardiac disease

Growth and Maturation

- May temporarily slow normal growth in children (controversial): Multimodal Treatment of ADHD (MTA) showed children/adolescents grew more slowly but eventually reached their expected adult height

- Controversy exists because theoretically stimulants might suppress appetite and reduce caloric intake, which could affect potential growth; also, dopaminergic actions of stimulants might suppress growth hormone secretion and affect height development. However, expected adult height is likely attained with a delay if stimulants are continued, and slowing of growth is likely reversible with withdrawal of treatment.

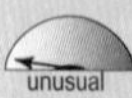

Weight Gain

- Patients may experience weight loss
- Weight gain is reported but not expected, rarely seen, controversial

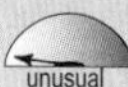

Sedation

- Activation much more common than sedation
- Sedation is reported but not expected, rarely seen, controversial

What to Do About Side Effects

- Wait, wait, wait: mild side effects are common, happen early, and usually improve with time, but treatment benefits can be delayed and often begin just as the side effects wear off
- Adjust dose
- Switch to a long-acting stimulant
- Switch to another agent
- For insomnia: avoid dosing in the midday, late afternoon, or evening
- However, insomnia is not always due to medication, but can be the result of relapse, rebound, and withdrawal effects from the daily dose, and in fact improves with additional late-day dosing of a short-acting stimulant
- Use beta blockers for peripheral autonomic side effects
- Often best to try another monotherapy prior to resorting to augmentation strategies to treat side effects, with the exception of an early-evening dose of a stimulant
- Monitor side effects closely
- For persistent insomnia: consider adding melatonin or an alpha 2 agonist, but only if not responsive to an early-evening dose of a stimulant
- For loss of appetite or loss of weight:
  - Give medication after breakfast
  - Switch to a nonstimulant
  - Eat a high-protein, high-carbohydrate breakfast prior to taking medication or within 10–15 minutes of ingesting medication; snack on high-protein, densely caloric foods throughout the school day and after school; eat dinner and then a second dinner or very heavy snack at bedtime
  - Add "liquid calories" (i.e., smoothies made with whole milk or ice cream, fruit, and protein powder; Boost or Ensure shakes)
  - Introduce "fourth meal" in the evening
  - Add cyproheptadine

How Drug Causes Side Effects

- Increases in norepinephrine peripherally can cause autonomic side effects, including tremor, tachycardia, hypertension, and cardiac arrhythmias
- Increases in norepinephrine and dopamine centrally can cause CNS side effects such as insomnia, agitation, psychosis (rarely)

Warnings and Precautions

- In children and adolescents:
  - Safety and efficacy of oral formulations not established in children under age 3; safety and efficacy of transdermal system not established in children under age 6
  - Use in young children should be reserved for the expert
  - Children who are not growing or gaining weight should stop treatment, at least temporarily
  - Usual dosing has been associated with sudden death in children with structural cardiac abnormalities
- Consider distributing brochures provided by the FDA and the drug companies
- All ages:
  - Stimulants used to treat ADHD are associated with peripheral vasculopathy, including Raynaud's phenomenon; careful observation for digital changes is necessary during treatment with ADHD stimulants
  - Carefully weigh the risks and benefits of pharmacological treatment against the risks and benefits of nonpharmacological

treatment, and it is a good idea to document this in the patient's chart
  - Use with caution in patients with any degree of hypertension, hyperthyroidism, or history of drug abuse
  - Many believe tics may be worsened by stimulants, but evidence does not support this association. A meta-analysis of 22 studies, including 2,385 individuals in treatment, found that the rate of new onset or worsening tics was 5.7% for those on stimulants versus 6.5% with placebo. In this analysis, there was no effect for type of stimulant, dose, duration of treatment, or age (Cohen et al., 2015). The presence of tics is not an absolute contraindication to use of stimulants.
  - May worsen symptoms of thought disorder and behavioral disturbance in psychotic patients
  - Stimulants have a high potential for abuse and must be used with caution in anyone with a current or past history of substance abuse or alcoholism, but stimulants for ADHD are less likely to be abused in terms of getting "high" and more likely to be used to stay awake, especially by college students. This misuse is the most common reason for diversion of prescription stimulants.
  - Youth are neither more nor less likely to develop alcohol and substance use disorders as a result of being treated with stimulant medication. In fact, current data suggest that treating ADHD in children and adolescents decreases the likelihood of developing a substance use disorder.
  - Adolescents and/or college students may divert/sell their medication to others for use in staying awake to study at the last minute, or to abuse; longer-acting preparations are harder to abuse than shorter-acting, immediate-release stimulants
  - Particular attention should be paid to the possibility of adolescents you are seeing for the first time feigning ADHD in order to obtain stimulants for nontherapeutic use or distribution to others; the drugs should in general be prescribed sparingly with documentation of appropriate use, and if there is any doubt about the accuracy of their complaints, refer them for psychological-educational or neuropsychological testing
  - Not an appropriate first-line treatment for depression or for normal fatigue
  - May lower the seizure threshold; as long as seizures are well controlled, it is generally safe to use stimulants
  - Emergence or worsening of activation and agitation may represent the induction of a bipolar state, especially a mixed dysphoric bipolar II condition sometimes associated with suicidal ideation, and may require the addition of lithium or an atypical antipsychotic, and/or discontinuation of D-amphetamine

When Not to Prescribe

- Treating ADHD comorbid with tics or Tourette syndrome is not contraindicated, but may be for the expert
- Patients with ADHD who are comorbid for motor or vocal tics of Tourette syndrome, or even with just a family history of Tourette syndrome, may experience worsening/onset of tics with stimulant treatment (controversial). Decision to use stimulants in such cases should weigh the potential benefits for ADHD against the risks of worsening tics and may require expert referral or consultation.
- Should generally not be administered with an MAOI, including within 14 days of MAOI use, except in heroic circumstances and by an expert
- If patient has arteriosclerosis, cardiovascular disease, or severe hypertension
- If patient has glaucoma
- If patient has structural cardiac abnormalities
- If there is a proven allergy to any sympathomimetic agent
- If the patient has an eating disorder other than binge-eating disorder, be very cautious

Long-Term Use

- Often used long-term for ADHD when ongoing monitoring documents continued efficacy
- Tolerance to therapeutic effects may develop in some patients
- Weight and height should be monitored during long-term treatment
- Periodic monitoring of weight, blood pressure

Habit Forming

- Paradoxically, stimulant abuse appears to be less likely in patients with ADHD than in those who do not have ADHD. In 2023, the FDA modified a boxed warning for stimulant medications, although they noted, "Our review found that nonmedical use has remained relatively stable over the past two decades, despite the increasing number of prescription stimulants dispensed." The new warning notes that stimulants have a "high potential for abuse and misuse, which can lead to the development of a substance use disorder, including addiction." The new warning also notes that stimulant medications "can be diverted for non-medical use into illicit channels or distribution." They recommend:
  - Counsel patients not to give any of their medicine to anyone else
  - Monitor for signs and symptoms of diversion, such as requesting refills more frequently than needed
  - Regularly assess and monitor for signs and symptoms of nonmedical use and addiction
  - Keep careful records of prescribing information, including quantity, frequency, and renewal requests, as required by state and federal laws
- Stimulant abuse in ADHD patients more likely if there is a preexisting history of alcohol/drug abuse
- Tolerance to stimulants is surprisingly rare in ADHD; tolerance should not be confused with reduction of therapeutic effects over time due to growth: as youth grow, dose usually must be increased; otherwise, the appearance of tolerance occurs when this in reality is underdosing
- Misuse may be more likely with immediate-release stimulants than with controlled-release stimulants

Overdose

- Rarely fatal; panic, hyperreflexia, rhabdomyolysis, rapid respiration, confusion, coma, hallucination, convulsion, arrhythmia, change in blood pressure, circulatory collapse

DOSING AND USE

Usual Dosage Range

- ADHD: 5–40 mg/day
- Narcolepsy: 5–60 mg/day

Dosage Forms

- Zenzedi (immediate-release tablet) 2.5 mg, 5 mg, 7.5 mg, 10 mg, 15 mg, 20 mg, 30 mg
- Dexedrine Spansule (extended-release capsule) 5 mg, 10 mg, 15 mg
- ProCentra (immediate-release oral solution) 5 mg/5 mL
- Xelstrym (transdermal patch) 4.5 mg/9 hr, 9 mg/9 hr, 13.5 mg/9 hr, 18 mg/9 hr

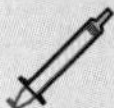

How to Dose in ADHD

- Ages 3 to 5: initial 2.5 mg/day; can increase by 2.5 mg each week; administered in divided doses (first dose on waking, additional dose(s) at intervals of 4–6 hours)
- Ages 6 and older (oral formulations): initial 5 mg once or twice daily; can increase by 5 mg each week; administered in divided doses (first dose on waking, additional dose(s) at intervals of 4–6 hours)
- Ages 6 to 17 (transdermal): initial 4.5 mg/9 hr; can increase by 4.5 mg each week; maximum recommended dose 18 mg/9 hr; should be applied 2 hours before an effect is needed and removed within 9 hours

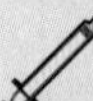

How to Dose in Narcolepsy

- Ages 6 to 12: initial 5 mg/day; can increase by 5 mg each week; administered in divided doses (all formulations; first dose on waking, additional dose(s) at intervals of 4–6 hours) or once a day (extended-release only)
- Ages 12 and older: initial 10 mg/day; can increase by 10 mg each week; administered in divided doses (all formulations; first dose on waking, additional dose(s) at intervals of 4–6 hours) or once a day (extended-release only)

Options for Administration

- Liquid formulation can be beneficial for patients with difficulty swallowing pills
- Extended-release capsule may have sufficient duration of action to eliminate the

need for lunchtime dosing in many but not all patients

Tests

- Before treatment, assess for presence of cardiac disease (history, family history, physical exam); consider whether electrocardiogram (ECG) is indicated
- Blood pressure should be monitored regularly, sitting and standing
- Monitor weight and height
- Current recommendations from the American Heart Association (AHA) are that it is reasonable but not mandatory to obtain an ECG prior to prescribing a stimulant to a child; the American Academy of Pediatrics (AAP) does not recommend an ECG prior to starting a stimulant for most children
- Document basic sleep patterns prior to starting a stimulant
- When necessary to rule out sleep apnea, nocturnal movements, or daytime sleepiness that may later be difficult to distinguish from side effects of stimulants, consider (rarely) a sleep study/ polysomnogram (e.g., obese adolescents)

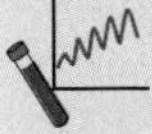

Pharmacokinetics

- Half-life approximately 9–11 hours
- Clinical duration of action often differs from pharmacokinetic half-life and can be longer for any formulation
- Substrate for CYP2D6
- Taking oral formulations with food may delay peak actions for 2–3 hours

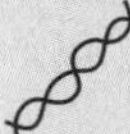

Pharmacogenetics

- No recommendations

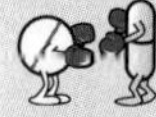

Drug Interactions

- May affect blood pressure and should be used cautiously with agents used to control blood pressure
- Gastrointestinal acidifying agents (guanethidine, reserpine, glutamic acid, ascorbic acid, fruit juices, etc.) and urinary acidifying agents (ammonium chloride, sodium phosphate, etc.) lower amphetamine plasma levels, so such agents can be useful to administer after an overdose but may also lower therapeutic efficacy of amphetamines
- Gastrointestinal alkalinizing agents (sodium bicarbonate, etc.) and urinary alkalinizing agents (acetazolamide, some thiazides) increase amphetamine plasma levels and potentiate amphetamine actions
- Desipramine and protriptyline can cause striking and sustained increases in brain concentrations of D-amphetamine and may also add to D-amphetamine cardiovascular effects
- Theoretically, other agents with norepinephrine reuptake blocking properties, such as venlafaxine, duloxetine, atomoxetine, milnacipran, and reboxetine, could also add to amphetamines' CNS and cardiovascular effects
- Amphetamines may counteract the sedative effects of antihistamines
- Haloperidol, chlorpromazine, and lithium may inhibit stimulatory effects of amphetamines
- Theoretically, amphetamines could inhibit the antipsychotic actions of antipsychotics
- Theoretically, amphetamines could inhibit the mood-stabilizing actions of atypical antipsychotics in some patients; however, stimulants can be safely combined with atypical antipsychotics by experts
- Combinations of amphetamines with mood stabilizers (lithium, anticonvulsants, atypical antipsychotics) are generally something for experts only when monitoring patients closely and when other options fail
- Absorption of phenobarbital, phenytoin, and ethosuximide is delayed by amphetamines
- Amphetamines inhibit adrenergic blockers and enhance adrenergic effects of norepinephrine
- Amphetamines may antagonize hypotensive effects of veratrum alkaloids and other antihypertensives
- Amphetamines increase the analgesic effects of meperidine
- Amphetamines contribute to excessive CNS stimulation if used with large doses of propoxyphene
- Amphetamines can raise plasma corticosteroid levels
- MAOIs slow metabolism of amphetamines and thus potentiate their actions, which can cause headache, hypertension, and rarely hypertensive crisis and malignant hyperthermia, sometimes with fatal results
- Use with MAOIs, including within 14 days of MAOI use, is not advised, but this can

sometimes be considered by experts who monitor depressed patients closely when other treatment options for depression fail

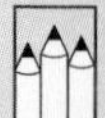

Dosing Tips

- Plasma levels are higher in lower-weight children; therefore, starting and target doses may be lower and longer intervals between dose increases may be needed (see How to Dose)
- The extended-release formulation can eliminate the hassle and pragmatic difficulties of lunchtime dosing at school, including storage problems, potential diversion, and the need for a medical professional to supervise dosing away from home
- If there are concerns about diversion or abuse, longer-acting stimulant preparations are much harder to abuse than immediate-release preparations
- Be aware that metabolism (and absorption) changes during puberty and entry into adolescence and becomes more like that of adults (i.e., slower than in children)
- If a child on a stable dose begins to lose tolerability with more side effects upon entering adolescence, this may signal the need for a dose reduction due to changing metabolism
- Immediate-release dextroamphetamine has a 4–6 hour duration of action
- Extended-release dextroamphetamine has up to an 8-hour duration of action
- Tablets contain tartrazine, which may cause allergic reactions, particularly in patients allergic to aspirin
- Transdermal system can be applied to the hip, upper arm, chest, upper back, or flank; change the site of application each day to minimize the risk of local skin reactions
- Avoid exposing transdermal system to external heat sources during wear because both the rate and extent of absorption are increased
- Dexedrine Spansule is controlled-release and should therefore not be chewed but rather should only be swallowed whole
- Avoid dosing late in the day because of the risk of insomnia
- Off-label uses are dosed the same as for ADHD
- Side effects are generally dose related

Drug Holidays

- Drug holidays were originally done in an attempt to avoid the possibility that stimulants may blunt height
- May be able to give drug holidays over the summer in order to reassess therapeutic utility and effects on growth and theoretically to allow catch-up from any growth suppression and assess any other side effects and the need to reinstitute stimulant treatment for the next school term
- However, most studies show that parental height is what determines a patient's final height, and that most children/adolescents taking stimulants reach their expected height, just more slowly than children/adolescents not exposed to stimulants
- May be possible to give weekend drug holidays and dose only during the school week for some ADHD patients, but there are risks as well:
  - Hyperactivity and impulsivity increase the chances of accidents (i.e., broken bones and head injuries) and illicit alcohol and drug abuse
  - Studies have shown that adolescents with ADHD who drive vehicles without their stimulants are much more likely to get into motor vehicle accidents and that the severity of the accident is much greater than would be expected
  - Hyperactive and impulsive children/adolescents tend to have more difficulties getting along with family members and friends, increasing the chances of developing low self-esteem and poor self-image
  - Social benefits can be lost over the summer if children/adolescents are taken off stimulants; social rejection by other children can lead to isolation and depression, increasing the chances of bullying, victimization, and further isolation and peer rejection
  - Inattention makes it harder for kids to learn the rules of life and pay attention to what is going on around them (e.g., noticing when a peer is not being a true friend, when someone is starting to get annoyed, when a car is coming toward you and you're in the middle of the street)

How to Switch

- When switching from one stimulant to another, the first one can be abruptly

stopped and the new one started the next morning. Side effects from abrupt discontinuation are not expected; however, some patients may experience marked fatigue and sleepiness for several days.
- See Appendix for approximate dosing equivalents when switching

How to Stop

- Taper not necessary, especially for patients who have only had short-term treatment or intermittent treatment
- However, if withdrawal symptoms develop, resume dosing the medication and then taper slowly over several days
- Withdrawal following chronic therapeutic use may unmask symptoms of the underlying disorder and may require follow-up and reinstitution of treatment
- Usually symptoms after discontinuation are return of symptoms of the underlying disorder rather than symptoms due to drug withdrawal
- Supervision during withdrawal is always recommended for any psychotropic medication

WHAT TO EXPECT

Onset of Action

- Some immediate effects can be seen with first dosing
- Takes a few days to attain therapeutic benefit generally

Duration of Action

- Immediate-release tablet: 4–5-hour duration
- Immediate-release solution: 4–6-hour duration
- Extended-release capsule: 6–8-hour duration
- Transdermal: peak at 6 hours

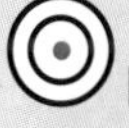

Primary Target Symptoms

- Concentration, attention span, distractibility
- Motor hyperactivity
- Impulsiveness
- Physical and mental fatigue
- Daytime sleepiness

What Is Considered a Positive Result?

- The goal of treatment of ADHD is reduction of symptoms of inattentiveness, motor hyperactivity, and/or impulsiveness that disrupt social, school, and/or occupational functioning
- Can also improve oppositional and disruptive behaviors associated with ADHD
- The goal of treatment is complete remission of symptoms
- If treatment works, it most often reduces or even eliminates symptoms, but is not a cure since symptoms often recur after medicine is stopped

How Long to Treat

- ADHD is typically a lifelong illness; if any symptoms improve, hyperactivity is more likely to improve than inattention
- Can tell parents there is some chance that their child can grow out of this in adulthood, but many adults continue to have symptoms of ADHD throughout adolescence and adulthood
- Continue treatment until all symptoms are under control or improvement is stable and then continue treatment as long as improvement persists
- Reevaluate the need for treatment periodically; some clinicians advise to periodically stop stimulants in patients who are not severely symptomatic to observe how the patient responds, but not routinely done by most clinicians
- Treatment for ADHD begun in childhood may need to be continued into adolescence and adulthood if continued benefit is documented

What If It Stops Working?

- Some patients who have an initial response may relapse even though they continue treatment, sometimes called "poop-out"
- Growth/developmental changes may contribute to apparent loss of efficacy as well as to new onset of side effects as metabolism slows and drug levels rise in transition from childhood to adolescence; dose adjustment (increase or decrease) should be considered
- Some patients may experience apparent lack of consistent efficacy due to activation of latent or underlying or newly evolved

bipolar disorder, major depressive episodes with mixed features of mania, new onset of major depression or an anxiety disorder (GAD, OCD, PD), and require stimulant discontinuation and a switch to the clinically appropriate medication(s)

What If It Doesn't Work?

- In practice, many patients have only a partial response, where some symptoms are improved but others persist, in which case higher doses of amphetamine, adding a second agent, or switching to an agent with a different mechanism of action can be considered
- Consider evaluation for another diagnosis or for a comorbid condition (e.g., medical illness, substance abuse). Also, when treating ADHD, consider the possibility of a learning disorder or learning weakness and consider school-based interventions.
- Consider the presence of nonadherence and counsel patient and parents
- Some ADHD patients and some depressed patients may experience lack of consistent efficacy due to activation of latent or underlying bipolar disorder and require either augmenting with a mood stabilizer or switching to a mood stabilizer
- Augmenting options:
  - Organizational skills training/executive function coaching
  - Exercise
  - Parent Management Training (PMT)
  - Coordinating with school for appropriate support
  - For the expert, can combine immediate-release formulation with a sustained-release formulation of D-amphetamine for ADHD
  - For the expert, can combine with modafinil, atomoxetine, or viloxazine for ADHD
  - For the expert, can occasionally combine with atypical antipsychotics in highly treatment-resistant cases of bipolar disorder or ADHD
  - For the expert, can combine with antidepressants to boost antidepressant efficacy in highly treatment-resistant cases of depression while carefully monitoring patient
  - Can combine with alpha 2 agonists such as guanfacine or clonidine
- Consider factors associated with poor response to any psychotropic medication in children and adolescents, such as severe symptoms, long-lasting symptoms, poor treatment adherence, prior nonresponse to other treatments, and the presence of comorbid psychiatric disorders or learning disorders
- Consider other important potential factors such as ongoing conflicts, family psychopathology, and an adverse environment (e.g., poverty, chaos, violence, prior and ongoing psychological trauma, abuse, bullying, less-than-ideal school placement, neglect)
- Institute trauma-informed care for appropriate children and adolescents

TALKING TO PATIENTS AND CAREGIVERS

What to Tell Parents About Efficacy

- Stimulant treatment for ADHD is one of the best studied of all medications in children and adolescents
- Often works right away once the dose is correct
- While the medicine helps ADHD by reducing symptoms and improving function, there are no cures for ADHD, and it is therefore necessary to keep taking the medication to sustain its therapeutic effects
- It does not work that day if the child/adolescent has not taken their medication in the morning
- For longer-acting stimulants, be careful not to give too late (i.e., after 11 am) because it can cause insomnia that night
- Does not stay in the body for a long time, so it stops working rapidly after you stop it
- Since every treatment consideration depends on a risk/benefit analysis, parents should fully understand short- and long-term risks as well as benefits compared to nontreatment of ADHD
- Although many stimulants are approved for ADHD, if using off-label, often a good idea to tell parents whether the medication chosen is specifically approved for the disorder being treated, or whether it is being given for "unapproved" or "off-label" reasons based on good clinical practice, expert consensus, and/or prudent extrapolation of controlled data from adults

- Best results are often obtained when medications are combined with behavioral therapy
- Stimulants wear off after a number of hours and symptoms may return. Therefore, parents may complain that the medication isn't working if their child/adolescent is using a stimulant that lasts 8 hours, because it may have worn off after the patient has come home from school (and that is when the parents are seeing the child/adolescent) in comparison to a stimulant that lasts 10–12 hours and may keep working after the child/adolescent comes home from school.
- The American Academy of Child & Adolescent Psychiatry (AACAP) has helpful handouts for parents

What to Tell Children and Adolescents About Efficacy

- Be specific about the symptoms being targeted: we are trying to help you remember things better, do your best at school, follow the rules, get into less trouble (as applicable)
- It may be a good idea to give the medication a try; if it's not working very well, we can stop the medication and try something else
- You can be part of a special plan to help us figure out if the medicine is helpful for you. Would you like to do that? (for the parents and prescriber, can consider here a trial both on and then off medication, and then on again to see if the effects are clear and thus worth continuing the medication)
- The medication can work right away but a good try can take a few months to find the right dose
- Even if it does make you feel better, it will wear off and no longer work shortly after you stop it
- This medicine does not last very long in your body, so even if it does work, it won't work if you don't take it that day
- The medication can help you decide what you want to do, like making good choices versus bad choices; the medicine does not make you do something you don't want to do
- Medications don't change who you are as a person; they give you the opportunity to be the best person you can be

What to Tell Parents About Side Effects

- Explain that side effects are expected in many when starting
- Tell parents many side effects of stimulants often go away in a few days to weeks, especially nausea and insomnia, but if they don't we will change the treatment
- Predict side effects in advance (you will look clever and competent to the parents, unless you scare them with too much information and cause nocebo effects, in which case you won't look so clever when the patient develops lots of side effects and stops medication; use your judgment here); a balanced but honest presentation is an art rather than a science
- Sometimes a trial off medication and then on again can clarify what the true therapeutic effects of the medication are
- Ask parents to support the patient while side effects are occurring
- Parents should fully understand short- and long-term risks as well as benefits
- Explaining to the parents what to expect from medication treatment, and especially what potential side effects to expect, can help prevent early termination

What to Tell Children and Adolescents About Side Effects

- When a medicine starts to work, your body can first experience this by giving you unpleasant sensations – just like if you take a cough medicine it may taste bad – these body sensations include loss of appetite and problems sleeping. So, just like with a cough medicine, the bad taste will often go away before the medicine begins to stop the cough – many medicines work like that. It's important for you to pay attention to what your body is telling you, and we'll go over some of the ways that can happen.
- Even if you get a side effect, it's not permanent (it won't last forever)
- Explaining to child/adolescent what to expect from medication treatment, and especially potential side effects, can help prevent early termination

What to Tell Teachers About the Medication (If Parents Consent)

- Stimulants can be very helpful in improving the symptoms of ADHD: namely, inattention, impulsivity, and hyperactivity
- It does not work if the child/adolescent has not taken their medication that morning
- If the patient is sleepy, ask whether the medication is keeping them up at night or if they are eating enough food
- If the patient won't eat lunch or snacks, ask whether the medication is making them lose their appetite
- Medically speaking, amphetamine is not a narcotic because doctors define narcotics as something that is sedating and sleep-inducing like opioids such as heroin and Oxycontin and not stimulants like amphetamine
- Amphetamine should be kept in school under lock and key or at the nurse's office or not brought to school at all because it can be diverted and misused by those who do not have ADHD. Some schools will suspend students who are caught with medications on their person or in their backpacks; most schools know the misuse or even abuse potential of stimulants.

SPECIAL POPULATIONS

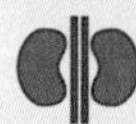

Renal Impairment

- No dose adjustment necessary for oral formulations
- Severe renal impairment (transdermal): maximum recommended dose is 13.5 mg/9 hr
- End stage renal disease (transdermal): maximum recommended dose is 9 mg/9 hr

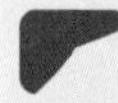

Hepatic Impairment

- Use with caution

Cardiac Impairment

- Use with caution, particularly in patients with recent myocardial infarction or other conditions that could be negatively affected by increased blood pressure
- Do not use in patients with structural cardiac abnormalities without consultation with a cardiologist

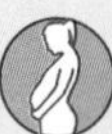

Pregnancy

- Controlled studies have not been conducted in pregnant women
- There is a greater risk of premature birth and low birth weight in infants whose mothers take D-amphetamine during pregnancy
- Infants whose mothers take D-amphetamine during pregnancy may experience withdrawal symptoms
- In animal studies, D-amphetamine caused delayed skeletal ossification and decreased postweaning weight gain in rats; no major malformations occurred in rat or rabbit studies
- Use in women of childbearing potential requires weighing potential benefits to the mother against potential risks to the fetus
- For ADHD patients, D-amphetamine should generally be discontinued before anticipated pregnancies
- National Pregnancy Registry for Psychiatric Medications: 1-866-961-2388 or https://womensmentalhealth.org/research/pregnancyregistry/

Breast Feeding

- Some drug is found in breast milk
- Recommended either to discontinue drug or formula feed
- If infant shows signs of irritability, drug may need to be discontinued

THE ART OF PSYCHOPHARMACOLOGY

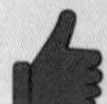

Potential Advantages

- In children:
  - Stimulants are probably the best studied psychotropic medications for use in children
  - Amphetamine is one of the best studied stimulants in children
- In adolescents:
  - Can improve school performance and grades, especially if ADHD has been unrecognized and untreated prior to adolescence
  - Can improve performance in high school and college students whose ADHD is compromising academic performance due to the increased demands of higher levels of study

- All ages:
  - May work in ADHD patients unresponsive to other stimulants
  - Established long-term efficacy of immediate-release and spansule formulations

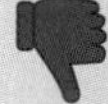

Potential Disadvantages

- Adolescents and especially college-age patients who divert their medication
- Patients with current substance abuse
- Patients with current manic or mixed symptoms associated with bipolar disorder or psychosis
- Patients with anorexia

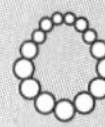

Pearls

- Half-life and duration of clinical action tend to be shorter in younger children than in adolescents and may require more frequent dosing or preferential use of long-acting preparations
- Drug abuse is no more likely and may even be lower (controversial) in ADHD adolescents treated with stimulants than in ADHD adolescents who are not treated with stimulants
- Stimulants have a moderate effect on decreasing ADHD symptoms and a moderate to large effect on decreasing aggression, oppositional behavior, and conduct problems in children with ADHD
- Meta-analyses suggest that when taking into account both efficacy and safety, methylphenidate is the best first-line stimulant in children and adolescents, whereas amphetamine is best in adults (Cortese et al., 2018)
- Stimulant dosing and titration are critical to optimizing response. Meta-analyses involving nearly 8,000 children/adolescents show that both methylphenidate and amphetamine salts have increased efficacy (but increased likelihood of discontinuation due to side effects) with higher doses (Farhat et al., 2022). In general, goal doses are often in the range of 0.8 mg/kg for methylphenidate and 0.5 mg/kg for amphetamine salts. However, these are rough guides that may not always be applicable depending on the formulation used and how completely (or incompletely) it's absorbed.
- Combinations of behavioral therapy or other nonmedication treatments along with stimulants may have better results than either treatment alone
- Some patients may benefit from an occasional addition of 5–10 mg of immediate-release D-amphetamine as an afternoon "booster" to their sustained-release Dexedrine spansules
- Rebound hyperactivity may occur in the afternoon and present with increased hyperactivity, restlessness, and irritability; if this occurs, can consider switching to a longer-acting agent or a nonstimulant or adding a short-acting stimulant
- On the other hand, too-high medication dosing may lead to cognitive rigidity, difficulty shifting attention, and seeming "spaced out" or "different"
- Many patients taking stimulants have early-morning ADHD symptoms and can be hard to get going, prepare for school, and be cooperative, especially for a few hours after awakening. In these patients, delayed-release/extended-release formulations may be especially helpful.
- Despite warnings, can be a useful adjunct to MAOIs for heroic treatment of highly refractory mood disorders when monitored with vigilance
- Can reverse sexual dysfunction caused by psychiatric illness and by some drugs such as SSRIs, including decreased libido, erectile dysfunction, delayed ejaculation, and anorgasmia
- Stimulants are a classic augmentation strategy for treatment-refractory depression, although this is most established in adults
- Interestingly, in some studies combining stimulants with alpha 2 agonists, decreased side effects are seen with the combination compared to either medication as monotherapy. This is likely because of complementary side effects.

SUGGESTED READING

Biederman J, Spencer TJ, Monuteaux MC, Faraone SV. A naturalistic 10-year prospective study of height and weight in children with attention-deficit hyperactivity disorder grown up: sex and treatment effects. J Pediatr 2010 Oct;157(4):635–40.

Cohen SC, Mulqueen JM, Ferracioli-Oda E et al. Meta-analysis: risk of tics associated with psychostimulant use in randomized, placebo-controlled trials. J Am Acad Child Adolesc Psychiatry 2015;54(9):728–36.

Cortese S, Adamo N, Del Giovane C et al. Comparative efficacy and tolerability of medications for attention-deficit hyperactivity disorder in children, adolescents, and adults: a systematic review and network meta-analysis. Lancet Psychiatry 2018;5(9):727–38.

Farhat LC, Flores JM, Behling E et al. The effects of stimulant dose and dosing strategy on treatment outcomes in attention-deficit/hyperactivity disorder in children and adolescents: a meta-analysis. Mol Psychiatry 2022;27(3):1562–72.

Jensen PS, Arnold LE, Swanson JM et al. 3-year follow-up of the NIMH MTA study. J Am Acad Child Adolesc Psychiatry 2007;46(8):989–1002.

The MTA Cooperative Group. A 14-month randomized clinical trial of treatment strategies for attention-deficit/hyperactivity disorder. The MTA Cooperative Group. Multimodal Treatment Study of Children with ADHD. Arch Gen Psychiatry 1999;56(12):1073–86.

Posner K, Melvin GA, Murray DW et al. Clinical presentation of attention-deficit/hyperactivity disorder in preschool children: the Preschoolers with Attention-Deficit/Hyperactivity Disorder Treatment Study (PATS). J Child Adolesc Psychopharmacol 2007;17(5):547–62.

Riddle MA, Yershova K, Lazzaretto D et al. The Preschool Attention-Deficit/Hyperactivity Disorder Treatment Study (PATS) 6-year follow-up. J Am Acad Child Adolesc Psychiatry 2013;52(3):264–78.

Swanson JM, Arnold LE, Molina BSG et al. Young adult outcomes in the follow-up of the multimodal treatment study of attention-deficit/hyperactivity disorder: symptom persistence, source discrepancy, and height suppression. J Child Psychol Psychiatry 2017;58(6):663–78.

Zhang L, Yao H, Li L et al. Risk of cardiovascular diseases associated with medications used in attention-deficit/hyperactivity disorder: a systematic review and meta-analysis. JAMA Netw Open 2022;5(11):e2243597.

THERAPEUTICS

Brands

- Adderall XR
- Adzenys XR-ODT
- Dyanavel XR
- Evekeo
- Evekeo ODT
- Mydayis

Generic

Yes

US FDA Approved for Pediatric Use

- Attention deficit hyperactivity disorder (Adderall, Evekeo, ages 3 and older)
- Attention deficit hyperactivity disorder (Dyanavel XR, ages 6 to 17)
- Attention deficit hyperactivity disorder (Adderall XR, Evekeo, Adzenys XR-ODT, ages 6 and older)
- Attention deficit hyperactivity disorder (Mydayis, ages 13 and older)
- Narcolepsy (Adderall, Evekeo, ages 6 and older)
- Exogenous obesity (Evekeo, ages 12 and older)

Off-Label for Pediatric Use

- Approved in adults
  - None
- Other off-label uses
  - Treatment-resistant depression (rarely used for this in children)
  - Stimulants are sometimes used to augment antidepressants
  - Stimulants also sometimes used to treat amotivational or lethargic states in the elderly with dementia but rarely in children for these symptoms

Class and Mechanism of Action

- Neuroscience-based Nomenclature: dopamine, norepinephrine reuptake inhibitor and releaser (DN-RIRe)
- Stimulant
- Increases norepinephrine and especially dopamine actions by blocking their reuptake and facilitating their release
- Enhancement of dopamine and norepinephrine actions in certain brain regions (e.g., dorsolateral prefrontal cortex) may improve attention, concentration, executive dysfunction, wakefulness, and cortical inhibitory control of striatum (i.e., theoretically "tunes" inefficient information processing in cortical–striatal pathways, improving "top-down" regulation of striatal and other subcortical drives)
- Enhancement of dopamine actions in other brain regions (e.g., basal ganglia) may decrease hyperactivity
- Enhancement of dopamine and norepinephrine in yet other brain regions (e.g., medial prefrontal cortex, hypothalamus) may improve depressive symptoms as well as nondepression-associated fatigue and sleepiness
- Hypothetically rebalances signal to noise ratios of cortical neurons: enhances focus on important tasks (signal), theoretically due to norepinephrine, and reduces awareness of background activity (noise), theoretically due to dopamine

SAFETY AND TOLERABILITY

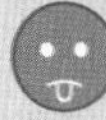

Notable Side Effects

- Anorexia and weight loss
- Nausea, abdominal pain
- Insomnia, headache, exacerbation of tics, tremor, dizziness, and possible irritability and anxiety. The risk of treatment-emergent irritability is higher with amphetamine-based stimulants compared to methylphenidate-based stimulants.
- Peripheral vasculopathy, including Raynaud's phenomenon
- Sexual dysfunction long term (impotence, libido changes) but can also improve sexual dysfunction short term

Life-Threatening or Dangerous Side Effects

- Psychosis
- Seizures
- Palpitations, tachycardia, hypertension
- Rare hypomania, mania, or suicidal ideation
- Cardiovascular adverse effects, death in patients with preexisting cardiac structural abnormalities often associated with a family history of cardiac disease

Growth and Maturation

- May temporarily slow normal growth in children (controversial): Multimodal Treatment of ADHD (MTA) showed children/

adolescents grew more slowly but eventually reached their expected adult height
- Controversy exists because theoretically stimulants might suppress appetite and reduce caloric intake, which could affect potential growth; also, dopaminergic actions of stimulants might suppress growth hormone secretion and affect height development. However, expected adult height is likely attained with a delay if stimulants are continued, and slowing of growth is likely reversible with withdrawal of treatment.

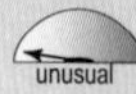

Weight Gain
- Patients may experience weight loss
- Weight gain is reported but not expected, rarely seen, controversial

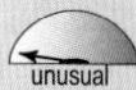

Sedation
- Activation much more common than sedation
- Sedation is reported but not expected, rarely seen, controversial

What to Do About Side Effects
- Wait, wait, wait: mild side effects are common, happen early, and usually improve with time, but treatment benefits can be delayed and often begin just as the side effects wear off
- Adjust dose
- Switch to a long-acting stimulant
- Switch to another agent
- For insomnia: avoid dosing in the midday, late afternoon, or evening
- However, insomnia is not always due to medication, but can be the result of relapse, rebound, and withdrawal effects from the daily dose, and in fact improves with additional late-day dosing of a short-acting stimulant
- Use beta blockers for peripheral autonomic side effects
- Often best to try another monotherapy prior to resorting to augmentation strategies to treat side effects, with the exception of an early-evening dose of a stimulant
- Monitor side effects closely, especially when initiating treatment
- For persistent insomnia: consider adding melatonin or an alpha 2 agonist
- For loss of appetite or loss of weight:
  - Give medication after breakfast
  - Switch to a nonstimulant
  - Eat a high-protein, high-carbohydrate breakfast prior to taking medication or within 10–15 minutes of ingesting medication; snack on high-protein, densely caloric foods throughout the school day and after school; eat dinner and then a second dinner or very heavy snack at bedtime
  - Add "liquid calories" (i.e., smoothies made with whole milk or ice cream, fruit, and protein powder; Boost or Ensure shakes)
  - Introduce "fourth meal" in the evening
  - Add cyproheptadine

How Drug Causes Side Effects
- Increases in norepinephrine peripherally can cause autonomic side effects, including tremor, tachycardia, hypertension, and cardiac arrhythmias
- Increases in norepinephrine and dopamine centrally can cause CNS side effects such as insomnia, agitation, psychosis (rarely)

Warnings and Precautions
- In children and adolescents:
  - Safety and efficacy not established in children under age 3
  - Use in young children should be reserved for the expert
  - Children who are not growing or gaining weight should stop treatment, at least temporarily
  - Usual dosing has been associated with sudden death in children with structural cardiac abnormalities
  - Consider distributing brochures provided by the FDA and the drug companies
- All ages:
  - Stimulants used to treat ADHD are associated with peripheral vasculopathy, including Raynaud's phenomenon; careful observation for digital changes is necessary during treatment with ADHD stimulants
  - Carefully weigh the risks and benefits of pharmacological treatment against the risks and benefits of nonpharmacological treatment and it is a good idea to document this in the patient's chart
  - Use with caution in patients with any degree of hypertension, hyperthyroidism, or history of drug abuse

- Many believe tics may be worsened by stimulants, but evidence does not support this association. A meta-analysis of 22 studies, including 2,385 individuals in treatment, found that the rate of new onset or worsening tics was 5.7% for those on stimulants versus 6.5% with placebo. In this analysis, there was no effect for type of stimulant, dose, duration of treatment, or age (Cohen et al., 2015). The presence of tics is not an absolute contraindication to use of stimulants.
- May worsen symptoms of thought disorder and behavioral disturbance in psychotic patients
- Stimulants have a high potential for abuse and must be used with caution in anyone with a current or past history of substance abuse or alcoholism, but stimulants for ADHD are less likely to be abused in terms of getting "high" and more likely to be used to stay awake, especially by college students. This misuse is the most common reason for diversion of prescription stimulants.
- Youth are neither more nor less likely to develop alcohol and substance use disorders as a result of being treated with stimulant medication. In fact, current data suggest that treating ADHD in children and adolescents decreases the likelihood of developing a substance use disorder.
- Adolescents and/or college students may divert/sell their medication to others for use in staying awake to study at the last minute, or to abuse; longer-acting preparations are harder to abuse than shorter-acting, immediate-release stimulants
- Particular attention should be paid to the possibility of adolescents you are seeing for the first time feigning ADHD in order to obtain stimulants for nontherapeutic use or distribution to others; the drugs should in general be prescribed sparingly with documentation of appropriate use, and if there is any doubt about the accuracy of their complaints, refer them for psychological-educational or neuropsychological testing
- Not an appropriate first-line treatment for depression or for normal fatigue
- May lower the seizure threshold; as long as seizures are well controlled, it is generally safe to use stimulants
- Emergence or worsening of activation and agitation may represent the induction of a bipolar state, especially a mixed dysphoric bipolar II condition sometimes associated with suicidal ideation, and may require the addition of lithium or an atypical antipsychotic, and/or discontinuation of D,L-amphetamine

When Not to Prescribe

- Treating ADHD comorbid with tics or Tourette syndrome is not contraindicated, but may be for the expert
- Patients with ADHD who are comorbid for motor or vocal tics of Tourette syndrome, or even with just a family history of Tourette syndrome, may experience worsening/onset of tics with stimulant treatment (controversial). Decision to use stimulants in such cases should weigh the potential benefits for ADHD against the risks of worsening tics, and may require expert referral or consultation.
- Should generally not be administered with an MAOI, including within 14 days of MAOI use, except in heroic circumstances and by an expert
- If patient has arteriosclerosis, cardiovascular disease, or severe hypertension
- If patient has glaucoma
- If patient has structural cardiac abnormalities
- If there is a proven allergy to any sympathomimetic agent
- If the patient has an eating disorder other than binge-eating disorder, be very cautious

Long-Term Use

- Often used long term for ADHD when ongoing monitoring documents continued efficacy
- Tolerance to therapeutic effects may develop in some patients
- Weight and height should be monitored during long-term treatment
- Periodic monitoring of blood pressure and heart rate

Habit Forming

- Paradoxically, stimulant abuse appears to be less likely in patients with ADHD than in those who do not have ADHD. In 2023, the FDA modified a boxed warning for

stimulant medications, although they noted, "Our review found that nonmedical use has remained relatively stable over the past two decades, despite the increasing number of prescription stimulants dispensed." The new warning notes that stimulants have a "high potential for abuse and misuse, which can lead to the development of a substance use disorder, including addiction." The new warning also notes that stimulant medications "can be diverted for non-medical use into illicit channels or distribution." They recommend:
  - Counsel patients not to give any of their medicine to anyone else
  - Monitor for signs and symptoms of diversion, such as requesting refills more frequently than needed
  - Regularly assess and monitor for signs and symptoms of nonmedical use and addiction
  - Keep careful records of prescribing information, including quantity, frequency, and renewal requests, as required by state and federal laws
- Stimulant abuse in ADHD patients more likely if there is a preexisting history of alcohol/drug abuse
- Tolerance to stimulants is surprisingly rare in ADHD; tolerance should not be confused with reduction of therapeutic effects over time due to growth: as youth grow, dose usually must be increased; otherwise, the appearance of tolerance occurs when this in reality is underdosing
- Misuse may be more likely with immediate-release stimulants than with controlled-release stimulants

Overdose

- Rarely fatal; panic, hyperreflexia, rhabdomyolysis, rapid respiration, confusion, coma, hallucination, convulsion, arrhythmia, change in blood pressure, circulatory collapse

DOSING AND USE

Usual Dosage Range

- Narcolepsy: 5–60 mg/day in divided doses
- ADHD: varies by formulation; see How to Dose section
- Exogenous obesity: 30 mg/day in divided doses

Dosage Forms

- Immediate-release tablet 5 mg double-scored, 7.5 mg double-scored, 10 mg double-scored, 12.5 mg double-scored, 15 mg double-scored, 20 mg double-scored, 30 mg double-scored
- Adderall XR (extended-release capsule) 5 mg, 10 mg, 15 mg, 20 mg, 25 mg, 30 mg
- Evekeo (immediate-release tablet) 5 mg scored, 10 mg double-scored
- Evekeo ODT (orally disintegrating tablet) 5 mg, 10 mg, 15 mg, 20 mg
- Adzenys XR-ODT (extended-release orally disintegrating tablet) 3.1 mg, 6.3 mg, 9.4 mg, 12.5 mg, 15.7 mg, 18.8 mg
- Mydayis (extended-release capsule) 12.5 mg, 25 mg, 37.5 mg, 50 mg
- Dyanavel XR (extended-release oral suspension) 2.5 mg/mL
- Dyanavel XR (extended-release tablet) 5 mg scored, 10 mg, 15 mg, 20 mg

How to Dose in ADHD

- Immediate-release Adderall or Evekeo (ages 3 to 5): initial 2.5 mg/day; can increase by 2.5 mg each week; administered in divided doses (first dose on waking, additional dose(s) at intervals of 4–6 hours)
- Immediate-release Adderall or Evekeo (ages 6 and older): initial 5 mg once or twice daily; can increase by 5 mg each week; maximum dose generally 40 mg/day; administered in divided doses (first dose on waking, additional dose(s) at intervals of 4–6 hours)
- Extended-release Adderall XR in ADHD (all ages): initial 10 mg/day in the morning; can increase by 5–10 mg/day at weekly intervals; maximum dose generally 60 mg/day; most adolescents and adults may require 40 mg/day
- Extended-release Dyanavel XR oral suspension and tablet (ages 6 to 17): initial 2.5 mg or 5 mg once in the morning; can increase by 2.5–10 mg/day every 4 to 7 days; maximum recommended dose 20 mg/day
- Extended-release Adzenys XR-ODT in ADHD (ages 6 to 12): initial 6.3 mg once in the morning; maximum dose 18.8 mg/day
- Extended-release Adzenys XR-ODT (ages 13 and older): initial 6.3 mg once in the morning; maximum dose 12.5 mg/day

- Extended-release Mydayis (ages 13 to 17): initial dose 12.5 mg immediately upon waking; can increase daily dose weekly by 12.5 mg; maximum recommended daily dose 25 mg; in adults maximum dose is 50 mg

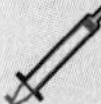

How to Dose in Narcolepsy

- Immediate-release Adderall or Evekeo (ages 6 to 12): initial 5 mg/day; can increase by 5 mg each week; administered in divided doses (first dose on waking, additional dose(s) at intervals of 4–6 hours)
- Immediate-release Adderall or Evekeo (ages 12 and older): initial 10 mg/day; can increase by 10 mg each week; administered in divided doses (first dose on waking, additional dose(s) at intervals of 4–6 hours)

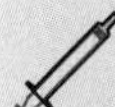

How to Dose in Exogenous Obesity

- Immediate-release Evekeo (ages 12 and older): usual daily dose 30 mg; taken in divided doses of 5–10 mg, 30–60 minutes before meals

Options for Administration

- Multiple formulation alternatives for patients with difficulty swallowing pills, including oral solution and orally disintegrating tablet
- Extended-release formulations have sufficient duration of action to eliminate the need for lunchtime dosing

Tests

- Before treatment, assess for presence of cardiac disease (history, family history, physical exam); consider whether electrocardiogram (ECG) is indicated
- Blood pressure and heart rate should be monitored regularly, sitting and standing
- Monitor weight and height
- Current recommendations from the American Heart Association (AHA) are that it is reasonable but not mandatory to obtain an ECG prior to prescribing a stimulant to a child; the American Academy of Pediatrics (AAP) does not recommend an ECG prior to starting a stimulant for most children
- Document basic sleep patterns prior to starting a stimulant
- When necessary to rule out sleep apnea, nocturnal movements, or daytime sleepiness that may later be difficult to distinguish from side effects of stimulants, consider (rarely) a sleep study/polysomnogram (e.g., obese adolescents)

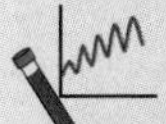

Pharmacokinetics

- For children ages 6–12, half-life for D-amphetamine is 9 hours and for L-amphetamine is 11 hours
- In adults, half-life for D-amphetamine is 10 hours and for L-amphetamine is 13 hours
- Clinical duration of action often differs from pharmacokinetic half-life and can be longer for any formulation
- Substrate for CYP2D6
- Taking with food may delay peak actions for 2–3 hours for most formulations; extended-release capsule and Dyanavel XR formulations can be taken with or without food

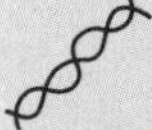

Pharmacogenetics

- No recommendations

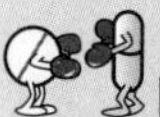

Drug Interactions

- May affect blood pressure and should be used cautiously with agents used to control blood pressure
- Gastrointestinal acidifying agents (guanethidine, reserpine, glutamic acid, ascorbic acid, fruit juices, etc.) and urinary acidifying agents (ammonium chloride, sodium phosphate, etc.) lower amphetamine plasma levels, so such agents can be useful to administer after an overdose but may also lower therapeutic efficacy of amphetamines
- Gastrointestinal alkalinizing agents (sodium bicarbonate, etc.) and urinary alkalinizing agents (acetazolamide, some thiazides) increase amphetamine plasma levels and potentiate amphetamine's actions
- Desipramine and protriptyline can cause striking and sustained increases in brain concentrations of amphetamine and may also add to amphetamine's cardiovascular effects
- Theoretically, other agents with norepinephrine reuptake blocking properties, such as venlafaxine, duloxetine, atomoxetine, milnacipran, and reboxetine, could also add to amphetamine's CNS and cardiovascular effects

- Amphetamines may counteract the sedative effects of antihistamines
- Haloperidol, chlorpromazine, and lithium may inhibit stimulatory effects of amphetamines
- Theoretically, amphetamines could inhibit the antipsychotic actions of antipsychotics
- Theoretically, amphetamines could inhibit the mood-stabilizing actions of atypical antipsychotics in some patients; however, stimulants can be safely combined with atypical antipsychotics by experts
- Combinations of amphetamines with mood stabilizers (lithium, anticonvulsants, atypical antipsychotics) are generally something for experts only, when monitoring patients closely and when other options fail
- Absorption of phenobarbital, phenytoin, and ethosuximide is delayed by amphetamines
- Amphetamines inhibit adrenergic blockers and enhance adrenergic effects of norepinephrine
- Amphetamines may antagonize hypotensive effects of veratrum alkaloids and other antihypertensives
- Amphetamines increase the analgesic effects of meperidine
- Amphetamines contribute to excessive CNS stimulation if used with large doses of propoxyphene
- Amphetamines can raise plasma corticosteroid levels
- MAOIs slow metabolism of amphetamines and thus potentiate their actions, which can cause headache, hypertension, and rarely hypertensive crisis and malignant hyperthermia, sometimes with fatal results
- Use with MAOIs, including within 14 days of MAOI use, is not advised, but this can sometimes be considered by experts who monitor depressed patients closely when other treatment options for depression fail

Dosing Tips

- Plasma levels are higher in lower-weight children; therefore, starting and target doses may be lower and longer intervals between dose increases may be needed (see How to Dose)
- The extended-release formulations can eliminate the hassle and pragmatic difficulties of lunchtime dosing at school, including storage problems, potential diversion, and the need for a medical professional to supervise dosing away from home
- If there are concerns about diversion or abuse, longer-acting stimulant preparations are much harder to abuse than immediate-release preparations
- Be aware that metabolism (and absorption) changes during puberty and entry into adolescence and becomes more like that of adults (i.e., slower than in children)
- If a child on a stable dose begins to lose tolerability with more side effects upon entering adolescence, this may signal the need for a dose reduction due to changing metabolism
- Immediate-release D,L-amphetamine has a 4–6-hour duration of action
- Extended-release tablets and oral suspensions have up to 12-hour duration of action
- Extended-release capsule has up to 16-hour duration of action (may occur with Vyvanse, Mydayis)
- Dyanavel XR oral suspension can be substituted with Dyanavel XR extended-release tablets on a mg-per-mg basis
- In all other cases, do not substitute amphetamine products on a mg-per-mg basis due to differing amphetamine base compositions and pharmacokinetic profiles (see Appendix)
- Most controlled-release formulations should not be chewed but rather should only be swallowed whole; however, Dyanavel XR extended-release tablets may be chewed or swallowed whole
- Adderall XR and Mydayis capsules can be opened up and sprinkled into applesauce, pudding, or yogurt
- Avoid dosing late in the day because of the risk of insomnia
- Off-label uses are dosed the same as for ADHD
- Side effects are generally dose related

Drug Holidays

- Drug holidays were originally done in an attempt to avoid the possibility that stimulants may blunt height
- May be able to give drug holidays over the summer in order to reassess therapeutic utility and effects on growth and theoretically to allow catch-up from any growth suppression and assess any

other side effects and the need to reinstitute stimulant treatment for the next school term
- However, most studies show that parental height is what determines a patient's final height, and that most children/adolescents taking stimulants reach their expected height, just more slowly than children/adolescents not exposed to stimulants
- May be possible to give weekend drug holidays and dose only during the school week for some ADHD patients, but there are risks as well:
  - Hyperactivity and impulsivity increase the chances of accidents (i.e., broken bones and head injuries) and illicit alcohol and drug abuse
  - Studies have shown that adolescents with ADHD who drive vehicles without their stimulants are much more likely to get into motor vehicle accidents and that the severity of the accident is much greater than would be expected
  - Hyperactive and impulsive children/adolescents tend to have more difficulties getting along with family members and friends, increasing the chances of developing low self-esteem and poor self-image
  - Social benefits can be lost over the summer if children/adolescents are taken off stimulants; social rejection by other children can lead to isolation and depression, increasing the chances of bullying, victimization, and further isolation and peer rejection
  - Inattention makes it harder for kids to learn the rules of life and pay attention to what is going on around them (e.g., noticing when a peer is not being a true friend, when someone is starting to get annoyed, when a car is coming toward you and you're in the middle of the street)

How to Switch
- When switching from one stimulant to another, the first one can be abruptly stopped and the new one started the next morning. Side effects from abrupt discontinuation are not expected; however, some patients may experience marked fatigue and sleepiness for several days.
- See Appendix for approximate dosing equivalents when switching

How to Stop
- Taper not necessary, especially for patients who have only had short-term treatment or intermittent treatment
- However, if withdrawal symptoms develop, resume dosing the medication and then taper slowly over several days
- Withdrawal following chronic therapeutic use may unmask symptoms of the underlying disorder and may require follow-up and reinstitution of treatment
- Usually symptoms after discontinuation are return of symptoms of the underlying disorder rather than symptoms due to drug withdrawal
- Supervision during withdrawal is always recommended for any psychotropic medication

WHAT TO EXPECT

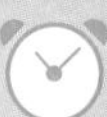

Onset of Action
- Some immediate effects can be seen with first dosing
- Takes a few days to attain therapeutic benefit generally

Duration of Action

Formulation	Generic / brand names	Duration
Immediate-release tablet	generic	4–6 hr
Immediate-release tablet	Evekeo	6 hr
Extended-release tablet	Adderall XR	8–12 hr, peak at 6–8 hr
Extended-release orally disintegrating tablet	Adzenys XR-ODT	8–12 hr, peak at 5 hr
Extended-release oral suspension	Dyanavel XR	10–12 hr, peak at 4 hr
Extended-release tablet	Dyanavel XR	10–12 hr, peak at 4 hr
Extended-release capsule	Mydayis	Up to 16 hr

- Immediate-release tablets: 4–6-hour duration
- Extended-release tablets and solutions: up to 12-hour duration

- Extended-release capsule: up to 16-hour duration

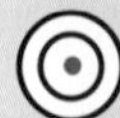

Primary Target Symptoms

- Concentration, attention span, distractibility
- Motor hyperactivity
- Impulsiveness
- Physical and mental fatigue
- Daytime sleepiness

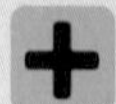

What Is Considered a Positive Result?

- The goal of treatment of ADHD is reduction of symptoms of inattentiveness, motor hyperactivity, and/or impulsiveness that disrupt social, school, and/or occupational functioning
- Can also improve oppositional and disruptive behaviors associated with ADHD
- The goal of treatment is complete remission of symptoms
- If treatment works, it most often reduces or even eliminates symptoms, but is not a cure since symptoms often recur after medicine is stopped

How Long to Treat

- ADHD is typically a lifelong illness; if any symptoms improve, hyperactivity is more likely to improve than inattention
- Can tell parents there is some chance that their child can grow out of this in adulthood, but many adults continue to have symptoms of ADHD throughout adolescence and adulthood
- Continue treatment until all symptoms are under control or improvement is stable and then continue treatment as long as improvement persists
- Reevaluate the need for treatment periodically; some clinicians advise to periodically stop stimulants in patients who are not severely symptomatic to observe how the patient responds, but not routinely done by most clinicians
- Treatment for ADHD begun in childhood may need to be continued into adolescence and adulthood if continued benefit is documented

What If It Stops Working?

- Some patients who have an initial response may relapse even though they continue treatment, sometimes called "poop-out"
- Growth/developmental changes may contribute to apparent loss of efficacy as well as to new onset of side effects as metabolism slows and drug levels rise in transition from childhood to adolescence; dose adjustment (increase or decrease) should be considered
- Some patients may experience apparent lack of consistent efficacy due to activation of latent or underlying or newly evolved bipolar disorder, major depressive episodes with mixed features of mania, new onset of major depression or an anxiety disorder (GAD, OCD, PD), and require stimulant discontinuation and a switch to the clinically appropriate medication(s)

What If It Doesn't Work?

- In practice, many patients have only a partial response where some symptoms are improved but others persist, in which case higher doses of amphetamine, adding a second agent, or switching to an agent with a different mechanism of action can be considered
- Consider evaluation for another diagnosis or for a comorbid condition (e.g., medical illness, substance abuse). Also, when treating ADHD, consider the possibility of a learning disorder or learning weakness and consider school-based interventions.
- Consider the presence of nonadherence and counsel patient and parents
- Some ADHD patients and some depressed patients may experience lack of consistent efficacy due to activation of latent or underlying bipolar disorder, and require either augmenting with a mood stabilizer or switching to a mood stabilizer
- Augmenting options:
  - Organizational skills training/executive function coaching
  - Exercise
  - Parent Management Training (PMT)
  - Coordinating with school for appropriate support
  - For the expert, can combine immediate-release formulation with a sustained-release formulation of D,L-amphetamine for ADHD
  - For the expert, can combine with modafinil, atomoxetine, or viloxazine for ADHD

- For the expert, can occasionally combine with atypical antipsychotics in highly treatment-resistant cases of bipolar disorder or ADHD
- For the expert, can combine with antidepressants to boost antidepressant efficacy in highly treatment-resistant cases of depression while carefully monitoring patient
- Can combine with alpha 2 agonists such as guanfacine or clonidine

- Consider factors associated with poor response to any psychotropic medication in children and adolescents, such as severe symptoms, long-lasting symptoms, poor treatment adherence, prior nonresponse to other treatments, and the presence of comorbid psychiatric disorders or learning disorders
- Consider other important potential factors such as ongoing conflicts, family psychopathology, and an adverse environment (e.g., poverty, chaos, violence, prior and ongoing psychological trauma, abuse, bullying, less-than-ideal school placement, neglect)
- Institute trauma-informed care for appropriate children and adolescents

TALKING TO PATIENTS AND CAREGIVERS

What to Tell Parents About Efficacy

- Stimulant treatment for ADHD is one of the best studied of all medications in children and adolescents
- Often works right away once the dose is correct
- While the medicine helps ADHD by reducing symptoms and improving function, there are no cures for ADHD, and it is therefore necessary to keep taking the medication to sustain its therapeutic effects
- It does not work that day if the child/adolescent has not taken their medication in the morning
- For longer-acting stimulants, be careful not to give too late (i.e., after 8 am) because it can cause insomnia that night
- Does not stay in the body for a long time, so it stops working rapidly after you stop it
- Since every treatment consideration depends on a risk/benefit analysis, parents should fully understand short- and long-term risks as well as benefits compared to nontreatment of ADHD
- Although many stimulants are approved for ADHD, if using off-label, often a good idea to tell parents whether the medication chosen is specifically approved for the disorder being treated, or whether it is being given for "unapproved" or "off-label" reasons based on good clinical practice, expert consensus, and/or prudent extrapolation of controlled data from adults
- Best results are often obtained when medications are combined with behavioral therapy
- Stimulants wear off after a number of hours and symptoms may return. Therefore, parents may complain that the medication isn't working if their child/adolescent is using a stimulant that lasts 8 hours, because it may have worn off after the patient has come home from school (and that is when the parents are seeing the child/adolescent) in comparison to a stimulant that lasts 10–12 hours and may keep working after the child/adolescent comes home from school.
- The American Academy of Child & Adolescent Psychiatry (AACAP) has helpful handouts for parents

What to Tell Children and Adolescents About Efficacy

- Be specific about the symptoms being targeted: we are trying to help you remember things better, do your best at school, follow the rules, get into less trouble (as applicable)
- It may be a good idea to give the medication a try; if it's not working very well, we can stop the medication and try something else
- You can be part of a special plan to help us figure out if the medicine is helpful for you. Would you like to do that? (for the parents and prescriber, can consider here a trial both on and then off medication, and then on again to see if the effects are clear and thus worth continuing the medication)
- The medication can work right away but a good try can take a few months to find the right dose
- Even if it does make you feel better, it will wear off and no longer work shortly after you stop it

- This medicine does not last very long in your body, so even if it does work, it won't work if you don't take it that day
- The medication can help you decide what you want to do, like making good choices versus bad choices; the medicine does not make you do something you don't want to do
- Medications don't change who you are as a person; they give you the opportunity to be the best person you can be

What to Tell Parents About Side Effects

- Explain that side effects are expected in many when starting
- Tell parents many side effects of stimulants often go away in a few days to weeks, especially nausea and insomnia, but if they don't we will change the treatment
- Predict side effects in advance (you will look clever and competent to the parents, unless you scare them with too much information and cause nocebo effects, in which case you won't look so clever when the patient develops lots of side effects and stops medication; use your judgment here); a balanced but honest presentation is an art rather than a science
- Sometimes a trial off medication and then on again can clarify what the true therapeutic effects of the medication are
- Ask parents to support the patient while side effects are occurring
- Parents should fully understand short- and long-term risks as well as benefits
- Explaining to the parents what to expect from medication treatment, and especially what potential side effects to expect, can help prevent early termination

What to Tell Children and Adolescents About Side Effects

- When a medicine starts to work, your body can first experience this by giving you unpleasant sensations – just like if you take a cough medicine it may taste bad – these body sensations include loss of appetite and problems sleeping. So, just like with a cough medicine, the bad taste will often go away before the medicine begins to stop the cough – many medicines work like that. It's important for you to pay attention to what your body is telling you, and we'll go over some of the ways that can happen.
- Even if you get a side effect, it's not permanent (it won't last forever)
- Explaining to child/adolescent what to expect from medication treatment, and especially potential side effects, can help prevent early termination

What to Tell Teachers About the Medication (If Parents Consent)

- Stimulants can be very helpful in improving the symptoms of ADHD: namely, inattention, impulsivity, and hyperactivity
- It does not work if the child/adolescent has not taken their medication that morning
- If the patient is sleepy, ask whether the medication is keeping them up at night or if they are eating enough food
- If the patient won't eat lunch or snacks, ask whether the medication is making them lose their appetite
- Medically speaking, amphetamine is not a narcotic, because doctors define a narcotic as something that is sedating and sleep-inducing, like opioids such as heroin and Oxycontin and not stimulants like amphetamine
- Amphetamine should be kept in school under lock and key or at the nurse's office or not brought to school at all because it can be diverted and misused by those who do not have ADHD. Some schools will suspend students who are caught with medications on their person or in their backpacks; most schools know the misuse or even abuse potential of stimulants.

SPECIAL POPULATIONS

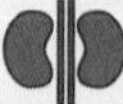

Renal Impairment

- No dose adjustment necessary

Hepatic Impairment

- No dose adjustment necessary

Cardiac Impairment

- Use with caution, particularly in patients with recent myocardial infarction or other conditions that could be negatively affected by increased blood pressure
- Do not use in patients with structural cardiac abnormalities without consultation with a cardiologist

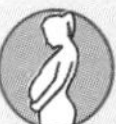

Pregnancy

- Controlled studies have not been conducted in pregnant women
- Infants whose mothers take D,L-amphetamine during pregnancy may experience withdrawal symptoms
- In rat and rabbit studies, D,L-amphetamine did not affect embryo-fetal development or survival throughout organogenesis at doses of approximately 1.5 and 8 times the maximum recommended human dose of 30 mg/day (child)
- In animal studies, D-amphetamine caused delayed skeletal ossification and decreased postweaning weight gain in rats; no major malformations occurred in rat or rabbit studies
- Use in women of childbearing potential requires weighing potential benefits to the mother against potential risks to the fetus
- For ADHD patients, D,L-amphetamine should generally be discontinued before anticipated pregnancies
- National Pregnancy Registry for Psychiatric Medications: 1-866-961-2388 or https://womensmentalhealth.org/research/pregnancyregistry/

Breast Feeding

- Some drug is found in breast milk
- Recommended either to discontinue drug or formula feed
- If infant shows signs of irritability, drug may need to be discontinued

THE ART OF PSYCHOPHARMACOLOGY

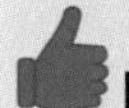

Potential Advantages

- In children:
  - Stimulants are probably the best studied psychotropic medications for use in children
  - Amphetamine is one of the best studied stimulants in children
- In adolescents:
  - Can improve school performance and grades, especially if ADHD has been unrecognized and untreated prior to adolescence
  - Can improve performance in high school and college students whose ADHD is compromising academic performance due to the increased demands of higher levels of study
- All ages:
  - May work in ADHD patients unresponsive to other stimulants, including pure D-amphetamine sulfate
  - Multiple options for drug delivery, peak actions, and duration of action

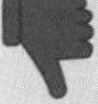

Potential Disadvantages

- Adolescents and especially college-age patients who divert their medication
- Patients with current substance abuse
- Patients with current manic or mixed symptoms associated with bipolar disorder or psychosis
- Patients with anorexia

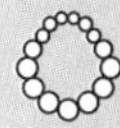

Pearls

- Half-life and duration of clinical action tend to be shorter in younger children than in adolescents and may require more frequent dosing or preferential use of long-acting preparations
- Drug abuse is no more likely and may even be lower (controversial) in ADHD adolescents treated with stimulants than in ADHD adolescents who are not treated with stimulants
- Stimulants have a moderate effect on decreasing ADHD symptoms and a moderate to large effect on decreasing aggression, oppositional behavior, and conduct problems in children with ADHD
- Meta-analyses suggest that when taking into account both efficacy and safety, methylphenidate is the best first-line stimulant in children and adolescents, whereas amphetamine is best in adults (Cortese et al., 2018)
- Stimulant dosing and titration are critical to optimizing response. Meta-analyses involving nearly 8,000 children/adolescents show that both methylphenidate and amphetamine salts have increased efficacy (but increased likelihood of discontinuation due to side effects) with higher doses (Farhat et al., 2022). In general, goal doses are often in the range of 0.8 mg/kg for methylphenidate and 0.5 mg/kg for amphetamine salts. However, these are rough guides that may not always be applicable depending on the formulation used and how completely (or incompletely) it's absorbed.

- Combinations of behavioral therapy or other nonmedication treatments along with stimulants may have better results than either treatment alone
- Formulation options with a duration of action up to 12 hours may be preferable for those ADHD patients who do homework in the evening, have after-school jobs or extracurricular activities, including sports, or whose symptoms affect their family and/or social life
- Some patients may benefit from an occasional addition of immediate-release D,L-amphetamine as an afternoon "booster" to their extended-release D,L-amphetamine
- Rebound hyperactivity may occur in the afternoon and present with increased hyperactivity, restlessness, and irritability; if this occurs, can consider switching to a longer-acting agent or a nonstimulant or adding a short-acting stimulant
- On the other hand, too-high medication dosing may lead to cognitive rigidity, difficulty shifting attention, and seeming "spaced out" or "different"
- Many patients taking stimulants have early-morning ADHD symptoms and can be hard to get going, prepare for school, and be cooperative, especially for a few hours after awakening. In these patients, delayed-release/extended-release formulations may be especially helpful.
- D-amphetamine may have more profound action on dopamine than norepinephrine, whereas L-amphetamine may have a more balanced action on both dopamine and norepinephrine; theoretically, this could lead to relatively more noradrenergic actions of the D,L-amphetamine than that of pure dextroamphetamine sulfate, but this is unproven and of no clear clinical significance
- Despite warnings, can be a useful adjunct to MAOIs for heroic treatment of highly refractory mood disorders when monitored with vigilance
- Can reverse sexual dysfunction caused by psychiatric illness and by some drugs such as SSRIs, including decreased libido, erectile dysfunction, delayed ejaculation, and anorgasmia
- Stimulants are a classic augmentation strategy for treatment-refractory depression, although this is most established in adults
- Interestingly, in some studies combining stimulants with alpha 2 agonists, decreased side effects are seen with the combination compared to either medication as monotherapy. This is likely because of complementary side effects.

SUGGESTED READING

Biederman J, Spencer TJ, Monuteaux MC, Faraone SV. A naturalistic 10-year prospective study of height and weight in children with attention-deficit hyperactivity disorder grown up: sex and treatment effects. J Pediatr 2010 Oct;157(4):635–40.

Cohen SC, Mulqueen JM, Ferracioli-Oda E et al. Meta-analysis: risk of tics associated with psychostimulant use in randomized, placebo-controlled trials. J Am Acad Child Adolesc Psychiatry 2015;54(9):728–36.

Cortese S, Adamo N, Del Giovane C et al. Comparative efficacy and tolerability of medications for attention-deficit hyperactivity disorder in children, adolescents, and adults: a systematic review and network meta-analysis. Lancet Psychiatry 2018;5(9):727–38.

Farhat LC, Flores JM, Behling E et al. The effects of stimulant dose and dosing strategy on treatment outcomes in attention-deficit/hyperactivity disorder in children and adolescents: a meta-analysis. Mol Psychiatry 2022;27(3):1562–72.

Jensen PS, Arnold LE, Swanson JM et al. 3-year follow-up of the NIMH MTA study. J Am Acad Child Adolesc Psychiatry 2007;46(8):989–1002.

The MTA Cooperative Group. A 14-month randomized clinical trial of treatment strategies for attention-deficit/hyperactivity disorder. The MTA Cooperative Group. Multimodal Treatment Study of Children with ADHD. Arch Gen Psychiatry 1999;56(12):1073–86.

Posner K, Melvin GA, Murray DW et al. Clinical presentation of attention-deficit/hyperactivity disorder in preschool children: the Preschoolers with Attention-Deficit/Hyperactivity Disorder Treatment Study (PATS). J Child Adolesc Psychopharmacol 2007;17(5):547–62.

Riddle MA, Yershova K, Lazzaretto D et al. The Preschool Attention-Deficit/Hyperactivity Disorder Treatment Study (PATS) 6-year follow-up. J Am Acad Child Adolesc Psychiatry 2013;52(3):264–78.

Swanson JM, Arnold LE, Molina BSG et al. Young adult outcomes in the follow-up of the multimodal treatment study of attention-deficit/hyperactivity disorder: symptom persistence, source discrepancy, and height suppression. J Child Psychol Psychiatry 2017;58(6):663–78.

Zhang L, Yao H, Li L et al. Risk of cardiovascular diseases associated with medications used in attention-deficit/hyperactivity disorder: a systematic review and meta-analysis. JAMA Netw Open 2022;5(11):e2243597.

ARIPIPRAZOLE

THERAPEUTICS

Brands

- Abilify
- Abilify Discmelt; Abilify MyCite
- Abilify Maintena
- Aristada
- Aristada Initio
- Asimtufii

Generic

Yes

US FDA Approved for Pediatric Use

- Schizophrenia (Abilify, ages 13 and older)
- Acute mania/mixed mania (Abilify, ages 10 and older, monotherapy and adjunct)
- Autism-related irritability (Abilify, ages 6–17)
- Tourette syndrome (Abilify, ages 6–18)

Off-Label for Pediatric Use

- Approved in adults
  - Schizophrenia (Abilify Maintena, Aristada, Aristada Initio, Asimtufii)
  - Maintaining stability in schizophrenia (Abilify)
  - Bipolar maintenance [monotherapy (Abilify, Abilify Maintena, Asimtufii) and adjunct (Abilify)]
  - Depression (adjunct) (Abilify)
  - Acute agitation associated with schizophrenia or bipolar disorder (IM; intramuscular) (Abilify)
- Other off-label uses
  - Bipolar depression
  - Other psychotic disorders
  - Behavioral disturbance / agitation in dementias
  - Behavioral disturbances in children and adolescents
  - Disorders associated with problems with impulse control
  - Posttraumatic stress disorder (PTSD)
  - Obsessive-compulsive disorder (adjunct to SSRIs)

Class and Mechanism of Action

- Neuroscience-based Nomenclature: dopamine, serotonin receptor partial agonist (DS-RPA)
- Dopamine partial agonist (atypical antipsychotic; second generation antipsychotic; sometimes called a third generation antipsychotic; also a mood stabilizer; sometimes called a dopamine stabilizer)
- As a partial agonist at dopamine D2 receptors, aripiprazole theoretically reduces dopamine output when dopamine concentrations are high, thus hypothetically improving positive symptoms (antipsychotic and antimanic actions), and increases dopamine output when dopamine concentrations are low, thus hypothetically improving mood, negative symptoms, and cognitive symptoms
- Interactions at a myriad of other neurotransmitter receptors may contribute to aripiprazole's efficacy
- Partial agonism at serotonin type 5HT1A receptors may be relevant at clinical doses, causing enhancement of dopamine release in certain brain regions, thus reducing motor side effects and possibly improving affective symptoms, negative symptoms, and cognitive symptoms
- Blocks serotonin 2A receptors, causing enhancement of dopamine release in certain brain regions and thus reducing motor side effects and possibly improving cognitive and affective symptoms
- Blockade of serotonin type 2C and 7 receptors as well as partial agonist actions at 5HT1A receptors may contribute to antidepressant actions

SAFETY AND TOLERABILITY

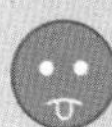

Notable Side Effects

- Drug-induced parkinsonism, akathisia, sedation, tremor, headache, dizziness, insomnia
- Nausea, vomiting, salivary hypersecretion
- Increased appetite, weight gain
- Orthostatic hypotension, occasionally during initial dosing
- Risk of drug-induced parkinsonism and dystonic reactions may be higher in children than it is in adults

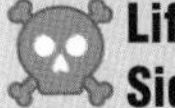

Life-Threatening or Dangerous Side Effects

- Hyperglycemia, in some cases extreme and associated with ketoacidosis or hyperosmolar coma or death, has been reported in patients taking atypical antipsychotics

- Rare neuroleptic malignant syndrome (NMS) may cause hyperpyrexia, muscle rigidity, delirium, and autonomic instability with elevated creatine phosphokinase, myoglobinuria (rhabdomyolysis), and acute renal failure
- Rare seizures
- As a class, antidepressants have been reported to increase the risk of suicidal thoughts and behaviors in children and young adults

Growth and Maturation

- Long-term effects are unknown

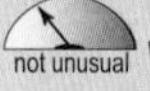

Weight Gain

- Less frequent and less severe than for most other antipsychotics
- However, may be more risk of weight gain in children than in adults. Current practice often includes adding metformin in pediatric patients who experience early weight gain (or are at high risk of antipsychotic weight gain, i.e., greater than 85th percentile for BMI).

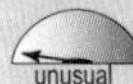

Sedation

- Reported in a few patients but not expected
- May be more likely to be sedating in children than in adults
- Can be activating

What to Do About Side Effects

- Wait, wait, wait: mild side effects are common, happen early, and usually improve with time, but treatment benefits can be delayed
- Monitor side effects closely, especially when initiating treatment
- Children and adolescents with autism spectrum disorders may be particularly sensitive to side effects, so start with low doses and titrate slowly
- Because aripiprazole has a very long half-life, may wish to try dosing every other day to deal with side effects at least in the short term, or wash out for a week and try again at half dose or every other day
- Usually best to give at night to reduce daytime side effects
- Often best to try another monotherapy trial of a different antipsychotic prior to resorting to augmentation strategies to treat side effects
- Exercise and diet programs and medical management for high BMI percentiles, diabetes, dyslipidemia. Also, randomized controlled trials in youth suggest that omega-3 fatty acids can reduce SGA-related hypertriglyceridemia.
- Reduce the dose, particularly for drug-induced parkinsonism, akathisia, sedation, and tremor
- For motor side effects: consider reducing dose or switching to another agent. Augmenting with diphenhydramine or benztropine is less preferred in youth.
- For akathisia: reduce the dose or add a beta blocker; if these are ineffective, raising the dose of the beta blocker may be helpful. Using a 5HT2A antagonist such as mirtazapine or cyproheptadine to treat drug-induced akathisia is less common in children and adolescents compared to adults.
- For activation (agitation, restlessness, insomnia):
  - Administer dose in the morning
  - Consider a temporary dose reduction or a more gradual up-titration
  - Consider adding a benzodiazepine short term (caution in children and adolescents)
  - Consider switching to another antipsychotic
  - Agitation due to undertreatment and inadequate dosing of the targeted disorder can be difficult to distinguish from drug-induced akathisia and activation; one approach for managing agitation/activation/akathisia when the specific side effect is difficult to distinguish is to raise the dose of aripiprazole; can also consider using the Barnes akathisia rating scale
  - If the patient improves after increasing the dose of aripiprazole, the symptoms are more likely to be due to inadequate dosing of the targeted disorder
  - If the patient worsens after increasing the dose of aripiprazole, the symptoms are more likely to be drug induced and require further dose reduction, adding an agent to improve tolerability or switching to another antipsychotic

How Drug Causes Side Effects

- Blocking alpha 1 adrenergic receptors can cause dizziness, hypotension, and syncope.

However, these effects may be less commonly seen as side effects in pediatric patients compared to adults.
- Partial agonist actions at dopamine D2 receptors in the striatum can cause drug-induced parkinsonism, akathisia, and activation symptoms
- Partial agonist actions at serotonin 5HT1A receptors can cause nausea, occasional vomiting
- Mechanism of weight gain and increased incidence of diabetes and dyslipidemia with atypical antipsychotics is unknown, and risks vary based on the particular agent

Warnings and Precautions

- Consider distributing brochures provided by the FDA and the drug companies or have the pharmacy do this for the parents
- When aripiprazole is used to treat depressive mood disorders off-label in children, either as a monotherapy or an augmenting agent to an SSRI/SNRI, it is a good idea to warn patients and their caregivers about the possibility of activating side effects and suicidality as for any antidepressant in this age group and advise them to report such symptoms immediately
- Carefully weigh the risks and benefits of pharmacological treatment against the risks and benefits of nontreatment with an antipsychotic and it is a good idea to document this in the patient's chart
- Use with caution in patients with conditions that predispose to hypotension (dehydration, overheating)
- Atypical antipsychotics have the potential for cognitive and motor impairment, especially related to sedation
- Atypical antipsychotics can cause body temperature dysregulation; use caution in patients who may experience conditions that increase body temperature (e.g., strenuous exercise, saunas, extreme heat, dehydration, or concomitant anticholinergic medication)
- Add or initiate other antipsychotics with caution for a few weeks after discontinuing aripiprazole; aripiprazole has a long half-life and can take a few weeks to wash out entirely
- As with any antipsychotic, use with caution in patients with history of seizures

When Not to Prescribe

- If there is a proven allergy to aripiprazole
- For behavioral control in the absence of a psychiatric diagnosis

Long-Term Use

- In adults, oral aripiprazole is approved to delay relapse in long-term treatment of schizophrenia and for long-term maintenance in bipolar disorder
- Often used for long-term maintenance in various behavioral disorders

Habit Forming

- No

Overdose

- No fatalities have been reported; sedation, vomiting

DOSING AND USE

Usual Dosage Range

- 5–15 mg/day for aggression or irritability due to autism
- 5–20 mg/day for Tourette syndrome depending on weight
- 10–30 mg/day for schizophrenia and mania

Dosage Forms

- Tablet 2 mg, 5 mg, 10 mg, 15 mg, 20 mg, 30 mg
- Orally disintegrating tablet 10 mg, 15 mg
- Oral solution 1 mg/mL
- Injection 9.75 mg/1.3 mL
- Long-acting injectable (LAI) (Abilify Maintena) 300 mg, 400 mg
- LAI (Aristada) 441 mg, 662 mg, 882 mg, 1064 mg
- Single-dose injection (Initio) 675 mg
- LAI (Asimtufii) 720 mg, 960 mg

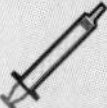

How to Dose

- Autism: initial dose 2 mg/day; can increase by 5 mg/day at intervals of no less than 1 week; maximum dose 30 mg/day
- Bipolar mania: initial dose 10 mg/day; can increase by 5 mg/day at intervals of no less than 1 week; maximum dose 30 mg/day
- Depression (adjunct): initial dose 2–5 mg/day; can increase by 5 mg/day at intervals

of no less than 1 week; maximum dose 15 mg/day
- OCD (adjunct): initial dose 2–5 mg/day; can increase by 5 mg/day at intervals of no less than every 8–12 weeks; maximum dose 15 mg/day
- Tourette syndrome (patients weighing less than 50 kg): initial dose 2 mg/day; after 2 days increase to 5 mg/day; after 1 additional week can increase to 10 mg/day if needed
- Tourette syndrome (patients weighing more than 50 kg): initial dose 2 mg/day; after 2 days increase to 5 mg/day; after 5 additional days can increase to 10 mg/day; can increase by 5 mg/day at intervals of no less than 1 week; maximum dose 20 mg/day
- Schizophrenia, mania: initial dose 2 mg/day; after 2 days increase to 5 mg/day; after 2 more days increase to 10 mg/day; subsequent increases can occur in 5-mg increments; maximum approved dose 30 mg/day

Options for Administration

- Oral solution: solution doses can be substituted for tablet doses on a mg-per-mg basis up to 25 mg; patients receiving 30 mg tablet should receive 25 mg solution
- Long-acting injectable formulations not approved in children/adolescents and few studies; probably best not to use long-acting injectables in children at all, and only with caution off-label in adolescents who are older and have adult body weights

Tests

- Before starting aripiprazole:
  - Plan to monitor weight and metabolic parameters more closely than in adults since children and adolescents may be more prone to metabolic side effects than adults
  - Weigh all patients and monitor weight gain against that expected for normal growth, using the pediatric height/weight chart to monitor. In particular, monitor BMI percentiles.
  - Get baseline personal and family history of diabetes, obesity, dyslipidemia, hypertension, and cardiovascular disease
  - Obtain blood pressure, fasting plasma glucose (or hemoglobin A1C), and a lipid profile
- After starting aripiprazole:
  - BMI percentile monthly for 3 months, then quarterly
  - Consider monitoring fasting triglycerides in patients at high risk for metabolic complications
  - Blood pressure, fasting plasma glucose (or hemoglobin A1C), lipid profile within 3 months and then annually
  - Treat or refer for treatment and consider switching to another atypical antipsychotic for patients who become overweight, obese, pre-diabetic, diabetic, or dyslipidemic while receiving an atypical antipsychotic
  - Even in patients without known diabetes, be vigilant for the rare but life-threatening onset of diabetic ketoacidosis, which always requires immediate treatment, by monitoring for the rapid onset of polyuria, polydipsia, weight loss, nausea, vomiting, dehydration, rapid respiration, weakness, and clouding of sensorium, even coma
  - Patients with low white blood cell count (WBC) or history of drug-induced leukopenia/neutropenia should have complete blood count (CBC) monitored frequently during the first few months and aripiprazole should be discontinued at the first sign of decline of WBC in the absence of other causative factors
  - Patients should be monitored periodically for the development of abnormal movements using neurological exam and the Abnormal Involuntary Movement Scale (AIMS)

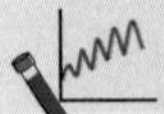

Pharmacokinetics

- Metabolized primarily by CYP3A4 and CYP2D6 (Figure 1). The major metabolite is dehydroaripiprazole, which contributes to total drug activity. CYP2D6 poor metabolizers undergo approximately an 80% increase in aripiprazole plasma concentrations and a 30% decrease in dehydroaripiprazole plasma concentrations (package insert). Finally, dehydroaripiprazole is eliminated through oxidation, possibly involving CYP3A4 (Caccia).
- Like aripiprazole, more than 99% of dehydroaripiprazole is bound to plasma protein (Swainston Harrison and Perry, 2004)

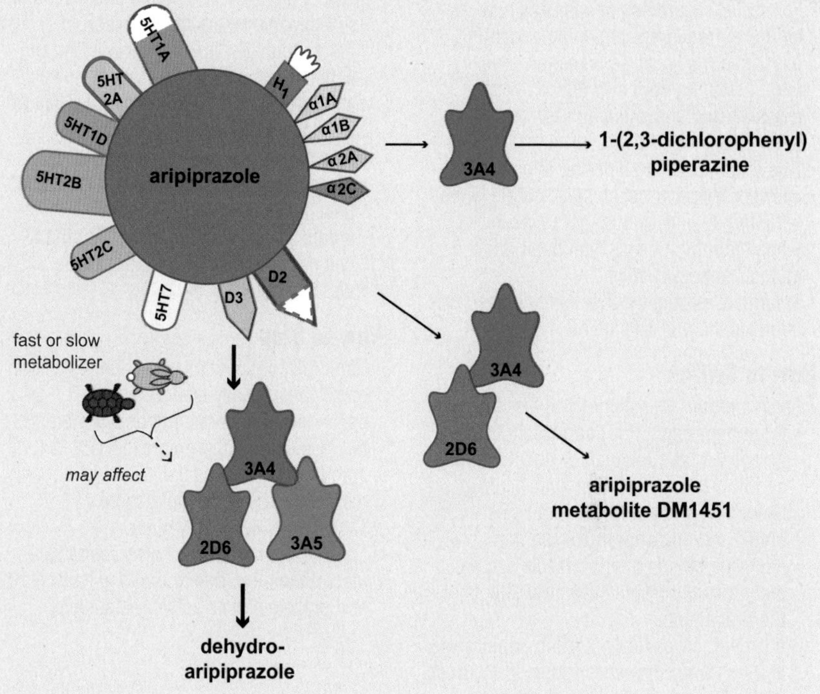

Figure 1 Metabolism of aripiprazole.

- Mean elimination half-life in adults is 75 hours (aripiprazole) and 94 hours (major metabolite dehydroaripiprazole). However, in CYP2D6 poor metabolizers, the mean elimination half-life for aripiprazole is about 146 hours (package insert).
- In clinical trials of patients ages 10 to 17, the body-weight-corrected aripiprazole clearance was similar to that of adults, and peak concentrations occurred, on average, 2 hours after administration (compared to 3–5 hours in adults)
- Food does not affect absorption

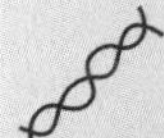

Pharmacogenetics

- CYP2D6 poor metabolizers undergo approximately an 80% increase in aripiprazole plasma concentrations and a 30% decrease in dehydroaripiprazole plasma concentrations (package insert)
- **CYP2D6 poor metabolizers:** FDA recommends using "half the usual dose"

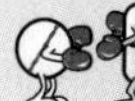

Drug Interactions

- Ketoconazole and possibly other CYP3A4 inhibitors such as fluvoxamine and fluoxetine may increase plasma levels of aripiprazole
- Carbamazepine and possibly other inducers of CYP3A4 may decrease plasma levels of aripiprazole
- Inhibitors of CYP2D6 such as paroxetine, fluoxetine, and duloxetine may increase plasma levels of aripiprazole
- Aripiprazole may enhance the effects of some antihypertensive drugs

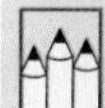

Dosing Tips

- Children should generally be dosed at the lower end of the dosage spectrum when drug is initiated
- Consider administering 1–5 mg as the oral solution for children and adolescents

- For some, regardless of age, less may be more: frequently, patients not acutely psychotic may need to be dosed lower (e.g., 2–10 mg/day) in order to avoid akathisia and activation and for maximum tolerability
- Due to its very long half-life, aripiprazole will take longer to reach steady state when initiating dosing, and longer to wash out when stopping dosing than most other atypical antipsychotics
- Treatment should be suspended if absolute neutrophil count falls below 1,000/mm^3

How to Switch

- From another antipsychotic to aripiprazole:
  - When tapering a prior antipsychotic, see its entry in this manual for how to stop and how to taper off that specific drug
  - Generally, try to stop the first agent before starting aripiprazole so that new side effects of aripiprazole can be distinguished from withdrawal effects of the first agent
  - If urgent, cross taper starting aripiprazole at 2 to 10 mg/day while reducing the dose of the first agent for a few days, then further reduce or discontinue the first antipsychotic while increasing the dose of aripiprazole as necessary and as tolerated
- From aripiprazole to another antipsychotic:
  - Aripiprazole tapers itself, so abrupt discontinuation leads to drug levels and active metabolite levels floating down slowly over 2–6 weeks while tapering up the dose of the new antipsychotic
  - Aripiprazole has higher affinity for D2 receptors than many other antipsychotics have for D2 receptors, so the antipsychotic with the lower D2 affinity will not act fully until aripiprazole is washed out

How to Stop

- Rapid discontinuation of any antipsychotic could theoretically lead to rebound psychosis and worsening of symptoms, but less likely with aripiprazole due to its long half-life and the half-life of its active metabolite, dehydroaripiprazole
- Taper rarely necessary since aripiprazole tapers itself after immediate discontinuation, due to the long half-life of aripiprazole and its active metabolites

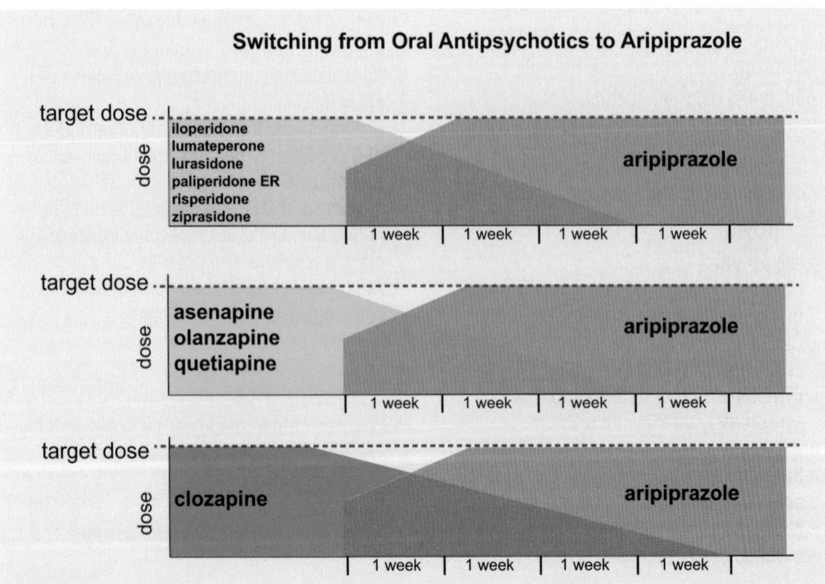

WHAT TO EXPECT

Onset of Action

- Psychotic and manic symptoms can improve within 1 week of oral dosing, but it may take several weeks for full effect on behavior as well as on cognition and affective stabilization
- If it is not working within 6–8 weeks, it may require a dosage increase or it may not work at all
- Acute intramuscular dosing for agitation can have onset within minutes to an hour, but not well studied or specifically approved for children/adolescents

Duration of Action

- Effects of oral medication are consistent over a 24-hour period
- Oral medication may continue to work for many years to prevent relapse of symptoms

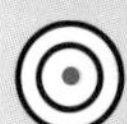

Primary Target Symptoms

- Positive symptoms of psychosis
- Negative symptoms of psychosis
- Manic symptoms
- Unstable mood and depression
- Obsessions and/or compulsions
- Aggressive symptoms
- Agitation
- Irritability and behavioral symptoms (in autism)
- Motor and vocal tics (Tourette syndrome)
- Prior to initiation of treatment, it is helpful to develop a list of target symptoms of the underlying disorder specific for the patient being treated for monitoring to better assess treatment response

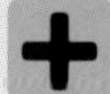

What Is Considered a Positive Result?

- In schizophrenia:
  - Most often reduces positive symptoms but does not eliminate them
  - Can improve negative symptoms, as well as aggressive, cognitive, and affective symptoms but less so than for positive symptoms
  - Can improve acute agitation
  - In children or adolescents with a first episode of psychosis, initial response may be greater than for recurrent episodes of psychosis in adults
- In bipolar disorder:
  - Many patients may experience a reduction of symptoms of mania by half or more
  - Can improve agitation in bipolar mania
  - Can reduce and/or eliminate depressive symptoms
- In depression:
  - Full elimination of depressed mood, anxiety, and other symptoms of depression is the goal
- In OCD:
  - Reduction of obsessions and/or compulsions
- In autism:
  - Can decrease irritability, social withdrawal, stereotypy, and inappropriate speech
- In Tourette syndrome:
  - Can reduce both motor and vocal tics

How Long to Treat

- In schizophrenia and bipolar disorder:
  - Continue treatment until reaching a plateau of improvement
  - After reaching a satisfactory plateau, continue treatment for at least a year after first episode of psychosis or mania
  - For second and subsequent episodes of psychosis or mania, treatment may need to be indefinite
- In depression:
  - If it is the first episode, continue for 6–12 months after reaching full remission
  - If it is the second episode, continue for 12–24 months after reaching full remission
  - If it is the third or greater episode, continue treatment indefinitely
- In OCD:
  - Continue for 6–12 months after reaching symptom remission
  - Can do a trial of medication discontinuation after a year to see if continued treatment at the same dose is necessary
  - Treatment may have to be indefinite
- In autism:
  - Treat as long as aripiprazole improves irritability in autism; however, it may be prudent to periodically discontinue the medication if symptoms are well controlled to see if continued medication treatment is necessary, as irritability can change as the patient with autism goes through neurodevelopmental changes and medication may become unnecessary
- In Tourette syndrome:

- Treatment may need to be long term and indefinite, as aripiprazole reduces motor and vocal tics but is not a cure
- Can do a trial of medication discontinuation after a year to see if continued treatment at the same dose is necessary

What If It Stops Working?

- Check for nonadherence, possibly by checking plasma drug level, and consider switching to another antipsychotic with fewer side effects
- Some patients who have an initial response may relapse even though they continue treatment, sometimes called "poop-out"
- Growth/developmental changes may contribute to apparent loss of efficacy as well as to new onset of side effects as metabolism slows and drug levels rise in transition from childhood to adolescence; dose adjustment (increase or decrease) should be considered
- Screen for the development of a new comorbid disorder, especially substance use
- Screen for adverse changes in the home or school environment

What If It Doesn't Work?

- Consider evaluation for another diagnosis (especially bipolar illness or depression with mixed features) or for a comorbid condition (e.g., medical illness, substance use)
- Consider other important potential factors such as ongoing conflicts, family psychopathology, and an adverse environment (e.g., inadequate school placement or educational services, bullying, poverty, chaos, violence, prior and ongoing psychological trauma, abuse, neglect)
- Institute trauma-informed care for appropriate children and adolescents
- For schizophrenia or bipolar disorder:
  - Try one of the other atypical antipsychotics
  - If no first-line atypical antipsychotic is effective, consider higher doses or augmentation with valproate, lithium, or lamotrigine
  - Consider initiating psychotherapy. In adolescents with bipolar disorder (and those with affective symptoms who are at risk of developing bipolar disorder), family-focused psychotherapy can be particularly helpful (Miklowitz et al., 2020).
  - Consider presence of concomitant drug abuse
- For autism and Tourette syndrome, consider another atypical antipsychotic, especially risperidone
- For off-label treatment of treatment-resistant depression in adolescents/children, aripiprazole is given off-label as an augmenting agent to SSRIs/SNRIs, so probably best to discontinue aripiprazole rather than add another drug and switch to another antidepressant and/or to another augmenting agent

TALKING TO PATIENTS AND CAREGIVERS

What to Tell Parents About Efficacy

- For acute symptoms, it can work right away
- Intramuscular aripiprazole can be given by a healthcare professional on an as needed basis for some symptoms like agitation; oral aripiprazole can be given by a parent under supervision by a healthcare professional off-label on an as needed basis as well
- Oral aripiprazole is given every day
- Explain which use aripiprazole is being chosen for, how to tell if the drug is working by targeting specific symptoms, and why this is being done
- Once the child/adolescent calms down, at some point after one dose or after several days of dosing or after long-term dosing, we should all assess whether the medication should be continued
- While the medicine helps by reducing symptoms and improving function, it is not a cure, and it therefore may be necessary to keep taking the medication long term to sustain its therapeutic effects
- Since every treatment consideration depends on a risk/benefit analysis, parents should fully understand short- and long-term risks as well as benefits
- There are several studies and a lot of clinical experience in giving aripiprazole to children and adolescents
- Often a good idea to tell parents whether the medication chosen is specifically

approved for the disorder being treated, or whether it is being given for "unapproved" or "off-label" reasons based on good clinical practice, expert consensus, and/or prudent extrapolation of controlled data from adults

What to Tell Children and Adolescents About Efficacy

- Be specific about the symptoms being targeted: we are trying to help you ...
- Give the medication a try; if it's not working very well, we can stop the medication and try something else
- A good try often takes many months
- If it does make you feel better, you cannot stop it right away or you may get sick again
- Medications don't change who you are as a person; they give you the opportunity to be the best person you can be

What to Tell Parents About Side Effects

- Explain that side effects are expected in many when starting
- Tell parents many side effects go away and do so about the same time that therapeutic effects start
- Predict side effects in advance (you will look clever and competent to the parents, unless you scare them with too much information and cause nocebo effects, in which case you won't look so clever when the patient develops lots of side effects and stops medication; use your judgment here); a balanced but honest presentation is an art rather than a science
- Ask parents to support the patient while side effects are occurring
- Parents should fully understand short- and long-term risks as well as benefits
- Explaining to the parents what to expect from medication treatment, and especially what potential side effects to expect, can help prevent early termination of medication

What to Tell Children and Adolescents About Side Effects

- Even if you get side effects, most of them get better or go away in a few weeks
- If you have side effects that are bothering you, tell your parents and your parents should tell me
- Consider having a conversation about sexual side effects in some adolescents who can find these side effects confusing and especially burdensome
- Explaining to child/adolescent what to expect from medication treatment, and especially potential side effects, can help prevent early termination of medication

What to Tell Teachers About the Medication (If Parents Consent)

- Aripiprazole can make children/adolescents restless
- Aripiprazole can make children/adolescents sedated
- It is not abusable
- Encourage dialogue with parents/guardians about any behavior or mood changes
- Notify the clinician of increased restlessness or akathisia symptoms, which may be apparent in the school setting

SPECIAL POPULATIONS

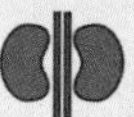

Renal Impairment

- Dose adjustment not necessary

Hepatic Impairment

- Dose adjustment not necessary

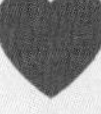

Cardiac Impairment

- Use in patients with cardiac impairment has not been studied; however, the risk of orthostatic hypotension in pediatric patients is less than in adults, as children rely less on peripheral vasoconstriction to regulate blood pressure

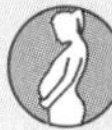

Pregnancy

- Controlled studies have not been conducted in pregnant women
- There is a risk of abnormal muscle movements and withdrawal symptoms in newborns whose mothers took an antipsychotic during the third trimester; symptoms may include agitation, abnormally increased or decreased muscle tone, tremor, sleepiness, severe difficulty breathing, and difficulty feeding
- In animal studies, aripiprazole demonstrated developmental toxicity, including possible

teratogenic effects, at doses higher than the maximum recommended human dose
- Psychotic symptoms may worsen during pregnancy, and some form of treatment may be necessary
- Aripiprazole may be preferable to anticonvulsant mood stabilizers if treatment is required during pregnancy
- National Pregnancy Registry for Atypical Antipsychotics: 1-866-961-2388 or http://womensmentalhealth.org/clinical-and-research-programs/pregnancyregistry/

Breast Feeding
- Some drug is found in breast milk
- Recommended either to discontinue drug or formula feed
- Infants of women who choose to breast feed while on aripiprazole should be monitored for possible adverse effects

THE ART OF PSYCHOPHARMACOLOGY

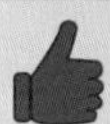

Potential Advantages
- In children:
  - Approved for manic/mixed episodes, irritability associated with autism, and Tourette syndrome
- In adolescents:
  - Approved for schizophrenia, manic/mixed episodes, irritability associated with autism, and Tourette syndrome
  - Off-label for those who may possibly have major depressive episodes with mixed features, especially those with these features and a family history of bipolar disorder
- All ages:
  - Use of the intramuscular injection for patients requiring rapid onset of antipsychotic action without dosage titration orally or if an acute treatment is necessary (off-label in children and adolescents)

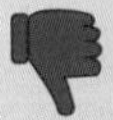

Potential Disadvantages
- In children:
  - Those who are already psychomotor agitated, angry, or irritable, and who do not have a psychiatric diagnosis
  - May be more difficult to dose
  - May be more susceptible to side effects
  - Those who have unacceptable weight gain
- In adolescents:
  - May be more susceptible to side effects
  - Those who have unacceptable weight gain
- All ages:
  - Patients in whom sedation is desired (many other antipsychotics are more sedating)

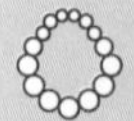

Pearls
- May have less weight gain in children/adolescents than some other atypical antipsychotics, but children/adolescents may have more weight gain on aripiprazole than adults on aripiprazole. In children and adolescents, weight gain may not consistently be dose related.
- Aripiprazole is commonly used in combination with antidepressant medications; however, consider lower doses of aripiprazole when combining with fluoxetine or paroxetine, which are strong inhibitors of CYP2D6. Combining fluoxetine or paroxetine with aripiprazole results in higher aripiprazole exposure.
- High affinity of aripiprazole for D2 receptors means that combining with D2 antagonist antipsychotics could reverse their actions
- Thus, this may interfere with the efficacy of the second antipsychotic with lower D2 affinity combined with aripiprazole with higher affinity, in which case it often does not make sense to combine aripiprazole with other antipsychotics, and this may need to be taken into consideration as well when switching and cross-titrating with another antipsychotic
- Thus, this may also reverse some side effects of some other antipsychotics, and it is anecdotally observed that low doses of aripiprazole may do this in some patients without interfering with efficacy of the other antipsychotic while reducing its side effects
- One well-known example of this is the case of hyperprolactinemia with or without galactorrhea, when administration of even low-dose aripiprazole (1–5 mg) off-label can reverse the hyperprolactinemia/galactorrhea of other antipsychotics, also proving that aripiprazole interferes with the D2 actions of other antipsychotics. Of note, in adults aripiprazole is associated with dose-dependent prolactin level reductions, and at least one prospective trial in children

and adolescents suggests similar effects in youth (Koch et al., 2023).

- Partial agonist actions do not mean partial efficacy for psychosis, but anecdotally, aripiprazole may be better positioned as a first-line antipsychotic for first episode or early-onset psychosis due to a good tolerability profile with good efficacy in many adolescents as well as adults
- However, for the most treatment-resistant patients with psychosis or mania, aripiprazole may not anecdotally be as effective as some other antipsychotics such as clozapine or even olanzapine

SUGGESTED READING

Caccia S. Pharmacokinetics and metabolism update for some recent antipsychotics. Expert Opin Drug Metab Toxicol 2011;7(7):829–46.

Correll CU, Kohegyi E, Zhao C et al. Oral aripiprazole as maintenance treatment in adolescent schizophrenia: results from a 52-week, randomized, placebo-controlled withdrawal study. J Am Acad Child Adolesc Psychiatry 2017;56(9):784–92.

Earle JF. An introduction to the psychopharmacology of children and adolescents with autism spectrum disorder. J Child Adolesc Psychiatr Nurs 2016;29(2):62–71.

Ellul P, Delorme R, Cortese S. Metformin for weight gain associated with second-generation antipsychotics in children and adolescents: a systematic review and meta-analysis. CNS Drugs 2018;32(12):1103–12.

Fung LK, Mahajan R, Nozzolillo A et al. Pharmacologic treatment of severe irritability and problem behaviors in autism: a systematic review and meta-analysis. Pediatrics 2016;137 suppl 2: S124-35.

Jukic MM, Smith RL, Haslemo T, Molden E, Ingelman-Sundberg M. Effect of CYP2D6 genotype on exposure and efficacy of risperidone and aripiprazole: a retrospective, cohort study. Lancet Psychiatry 2019;6(5):418–26.

Koch MT, Carlson HE, Kazimi MM, Correll CU. Antipsychotic-related prolactin levels and sexual dysfunction in mentally ill youth: a 3-month cohort-study. J Am Acad Child Adolesc Psychiatry 2023 ;62(9):1021–50.

Lytle S, McVoy M, Sajatovic M. Long-acting injectable antipsychotics in children and adolescents. J Child Adolesc Psychopharmacol 2017;27(1):2–9.

Miklowitz DJ, Schneck CD, Walshaw PD et al. Effects of family-focused therapy vs enhanced usual care for symptomatic youths at high risk for bipolar disorder: a randomized clinical trial. JAMA Psychiatry 2020;77(5):455–63.

Pillay J, Boylan K, Carrey N et al. First- and Second-Generation Antipsychotics in Children and Young Adults: Systematic Review Update [Internet]. Rockville, MD: Agency for Healthcare Research and Quality (US); 2017 Mar. Report No.: 17-EHC001-EF. AHRQ Comparative Effectiveness Reviews.

Rossow KM, Vaughn SE, Strawn JR, Van Driest SL, Ramsey LB. The need for a refined understanding of CYP2D6 in second-generation antipsychotic outcomes in children and adolescents. Pharmacogenomics 2021;22(8):447–50.

Salazar de Pablo G, Pastor Jordá C, Vaquerizo-Serrano J et al. Systematic review and meta-analysis: efficacy of pharmacological interventions for irritability and emotional dysregulation in autism spectrum disorder and predictors of response. J Am Acad Child Adolesc Psychiatry 2023;62(2):151–68.

Swainston Harrison T, Perry CM. Aripiprazole: a review of its use in schizophrenia and schizoaffective disorder. Drugs 2004;64(15):1715–36.

Wang S, Wei YZ, Yang JH et al. The efficacy and safety of aripiprazole for tic disorders in children and adolescents: a systematic review and meta-analysis. Psychiatry Res 2017;254:24–32.

THERAPEUTICS

Brands

- Saphris (sublingual)
- Secuado (transdermal)

Generic

Yes

US FDA Approved for Pediatric Use

- Acute mania/mixed mania (Saphris, ages 10 and older, monotherapy)

Off-Label for Pediatric Use

- Approved in adults
  - Schizophrenia (Saphris, Secuado)
  - Bipolar maintenance (Saphris)
  - Acute mania / mixed mania (Saphris, adjunct)
- Other off-label uses
  - Other psychotic disorder
  - Treatment-resistant depression (adjunct)
  - Behavioral disturbances in children and adolescents
  - Disorders associated with problems with impulse control
  - Posttraumatic stress disorder

Class and Mechanism of Action

- Neuroscience-based Nomenclature: dopamine, serotonin, norepinephrine receptor antagonist (DSN-RAn)
- Atypical antipsychotic (serotonin-dopamine antagonist; second generation antipsychotic; also a mood stabilizer)
- Blocks dopamine 2 receptors, reducing positive symptoms of psychosis and stabilizing affective symptoms
- Blockade of serotonin type 2A receptors may also contribute at clinical doses to the enhancement of dopamine release in certain brain regions, thus theoretically reducing motor side effects
- Interactions at a myriad of other neurotransmitter receptors may contribute to asenapine's efficacy
- Serotonin 2C, serotonin 7, and alpha 2 antagonist properties may contribute to antidepressant actions
- Partial agonist at 5HT1A receptors, which may be beneficial for mood, anxiety, and cognition in a number of disorders

SAFETY AND TOLERABILITY

Notable Side Effects

- Sedation, dizziness, fatigue
- Oral hypoesthesia, dysgeusia
- Nausea, increased appetite, weight gain
- Akathisia, extrapyramidal symptoms (EPS, also called drug-induced parkinsonism)
- May increase risk for diabetes and dyslipidemia
- Risk of drug-induced parkinsonism and dystonic reactions may be higher in children than it is in adults
- Risk of withdrawal dyskinesias
- Application site reactions have been reported: oral ulcers, blisters, peeling/sloughing, inflammation

Life-Threatening or Dangerous Side Effects

- Type 1 hypersensitivity reactions (anaphylaxis, angioedema, low blood pressure, rapid heart rate, swollen tongue, difficulty breathing, wheezing, rash)
- Hyperglycemia, in some cases extreme and associated with ketoacidosis or hyperosmolar coma or death, has been reported in patients taking atypical antipsychotics
- Rare neuroleptic malignant syndrome (NMS) may cause hyperpyrexia, muscle rigidity, delirium, and autonomic instability with elevated creatine phosphokinase, myoglobinuria (rhabdomyolysis), and acute renal failure
- Rare seizures
- As a class, antipsychotics are associated with an increased risk of death and cerebrovascular events in elderly patients with dementia; not approved for treatment of dementia-related psychosis

Growth and Maturation

- Long-term effects are unknown

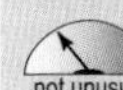

Weight Gain

- Occurs in a significant minority
- May be more risk of weight gain and metabolic effects in children than in adults

Sedation

- Many patients experience and/or can be significant in amount
- May be more likely to be sedating in children than in adults especially upon initiation of treatment

What to Do About Side Effects

- Wait, wait, wait: mild side effects are common, happen early, and usually improve with time, but treatment benefits can be delayed
- Monitor side effects closely, especially when initiating treatment
- Often best to try another monotherapy trial of a different antipsychotic prior to resorting to augmentation strategies to treat side effects
- Exercise and diet programs and medical management for high BMI percentiles, diabetes, dyslipidemia. Also, randomized controlled trials in youth suggest that omega-3 fatty acids can reduce SGA-related hypertriglyceridemia.
- Reduce the dose, particularly for drug-induced parkinsonism, akathisia, sedation, and tremor
- For drug-induced parkinsonism: consider reducing dose or switching to another agent. Augmenting with diphenhydramine or benztropine is less preferred in youth.
- For akathisia: reduce the dose or add a beta blocker. If these are ineffective, raising the dose of the beta blocker may be helpful.
- Using a 5HT2A antagonist such as mirtazapine or cyproheptadine to treat drug-induced akathisia is less common in children and adolescents compared to adults
- For activation (agitation, restlessness, insomnia):
  - Administer dose in the morning
  - Consider a temporary dose reduction or a more gradual up-titration
  - Consider adding a 5HT2A antagonist such as trazodone or mirtazapine rather than a benzodiazepine or Z-drug hypnotic
  - Consider adding a benzodiazepine short term (caution in children and adolescents)
  - Consider switching to another antipsychotic
  - Agitation due to undertreatment and inadequate dosing of the targeted disorder can be difficult to distinguish from drug-induced akathisia and activation; one approach for managing agitation/activation/akathisia when the specific side effect is difficult to distinguish is to raise the dose of asenapine; can also consider using the Barnes akathisia rating scale
  - If the patient improves after increasing the dose of asenapine, the symptoms are more likely to be due to inadequate dosing of the targeted disorder
  - If the patient worsens after increasing the dose of asenapine, the symptoms are more likely to be drug induced and require further dose reduction, adding an agent to improve tolerability or switching to another antipsychotic

How Drug Causes Side Effects

- By blocking alpha 1 adrenergic receptors, it can cause dizziness, sedation, and hypotension
- By blocking dopamine 2 receptors in the striatum, it can cause motor side effects, akathisia, and activation symptoms
- By blocking dopamine 2 receptors in the pituitary, it can theoretically cause elevations in prolactin
- Mechanism of any possible weight gain is unknown but may relate to effects at 5HT2C receptors
- Mechanism of any possible increased incidence of diabetes or dyslipidemia is unknown

Warnings and Precautions

- Carefully weigh the risks and benefits of pharmacological treatment against the risks and benefits of nontreatment with an antipsychotic and it is a good idea to document this in the patient's chart
- Use with caution in patients with conditions that predispose to hypotension (dehydration, overheating)
- Atypical antipsychotics have the potential for cognitive and motor impairment, especially related to sedation
- Atypical antipsychotics can cause body temperature dysregulation; use caution in patients who may experience conditions that increase body temperature (e.g., strenuous exercise, saunas, extreme heat,

dehydration, or concomitant anticholinergic medication)
- As with any antipsychotic, use with caution in patients with history of seizures

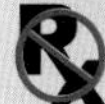

When Not to Prescribe
- In patients with severe hepatic impairment
- If there is a proven allergy to asenapine

Long-Term Use
- In adults, approved for long-term maintenance in bipolar disorder

Habit Forming
- No

Overdose
- Agitation, confusion

DOSING AND USE

Usual Dosage Range
- Bipolar mania: 5–20 mg/day in 2 divided doses
- Schizophrenia, sublingual (not approved): 5–20 mg/day in 2 divided doses
- Schizophrenia, transdermal (not approved): 3.8 mg/24 hours

Dosage Forms
- Sublingual tablet 2.5 mg, 5 mg, 10 mg
- Transdermal system 3.8 mg/24 hours, 5.7 mg/24 hours, 7.6 mg/24 hours

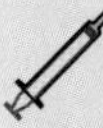

How to Dose
- Must be administered sublingually; patients may not eat or drink for 10 minutes following administration or medicine will wash away and not be absorbed
- Bipolar mania: initial 5 mg/day in 2 divided doses; after 3 days can increase to 10 mg/day in 2 divided doses; after 3 more days can increase to 20 mg/day in 2 divided doses

Options for Administration
- Sublingual dosage form only

Tests
- Before starting asenapine:
  - Plan to monitor weight and metabolic parameters more closely than in adults since children and adolescents may be more prone to metabolic side effects than adults
  - Weigh all patients and monitor weight gain against that expected for normal growth, using the pediatric height/weight chart to monitor. In particular, monitor BMI percentiles.
  - Get baseline personal and family history of diabetes, obesity, dyslipidemia, hypertension, and cardiovascular disease
  - Obtain blood pressure, fasting plasma glucose (or hemoglobin A1C), and a lipid profile
- After starting asenapine:
  - BMI percentile monthly for 3 months, then quarterly
  - Consider monitoring fasting triglycerides monthly in patients at high risk for metabolic complications
  - Blood pressure, fasting plasma glucose (or hemoglobin A1C), lipid profile within 3 months and then annually
  - Treat or refer for treatment and consider switching to another atypical antipsychotic for patients who become overweight, obese, pre-diabetic, diabetic, or dyslipidemic while receiving an atypical antipsychotic
  - Even in patients without known diabetes, be vigilant for the rare but life-threatening onset of diabetic ketoacidosis, which always requires immediate treatment, by monitoring for the rapid onset of polyuria, polydipsia, weight loss, nausea, vomiting, dehydration, rapid respiration, weakness, and clouding of sensorium, even coma
  - Patients with low white blood cell count (WBC) or history of drug-induced leukopenia/neutropenia should have complete blood count (CBC) monitored frequently during the first few months and asenapine should be discontinued at the first sign of decline of WBC in the absence of other causative factors
  - Patients should be monitored periodically for the development of abnormal movements using neurological exam and the Abnormal Involuntary Movement Scale (AIMS)

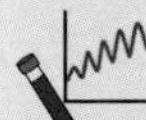

Pharmacokinetics
- Asenapine has a moderate volume of distribution, indicating that it distributes throughout the body tissues
- Asenapine is primarily metabolized by CYP1A2, CYP3A4, and CYP2D6 (Figure 1)

- It is highly protein-bound, primarily to albumin (approximately 95%)
- In children and adolescents, absorption is rapid (Tmax ~1 hour) (Figure 2) with an apparent terminal half-life between 16 and 32 hours in children and adolescents ages 10–17 years; this is similar to the half-life observed in adults (13–39 hours)
- In children and adolescents, steady state is attained within 8 days
- Peak concentrations tend to be about 30% higher in younger patients (age 10–11) compared to older adolescents (Dogterom et al., 2018)
- Optimal bioavailability is with sublingual administration (~35%); if food or liquid is consumed within 10 minutes of administration, bioavailability decreases to 28%; bioavailability decreases to 2% if swallowed

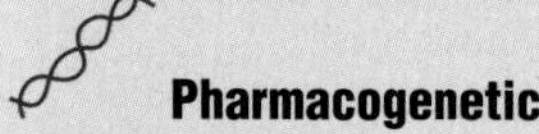

Pharmacogenetics

- No recommendations

Drug Interactions

- May increase effect of antihypertensive agents
- CYP1A2 inhibitors (e.g., fluvoxamine) can raise asenapine levels
- Via CYP2D6 inhibition, asenapine could theoretically interfere with the analgesic effects of codeine and increase the plasma levels of some beta blockers and of atomoxetine
- Via CYP2D6 inhibition, asenapine could theoretically increase concentrations of thioridazine and cause dangerous cardiac arrhythmias

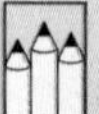

Dosing Tips

- Asenapine is not absorbed after swallowing (less than 2% bioavailable orally) and thus must be administered sublingually (35% bioavailable), as swallowing renders asenapine inactive
- Youth should be instructed to place the tablet under the tongue and allow it to dissolve completely, which will occur in seconds; the tablet should not be divided, crushed, chewed, or swallowed
- Patients may not eat or drink for 10 minutes following sublingual administration so that the drug in the oral cavity can be absorbed locally and not washed into the stomach (where it would not be absorbed)

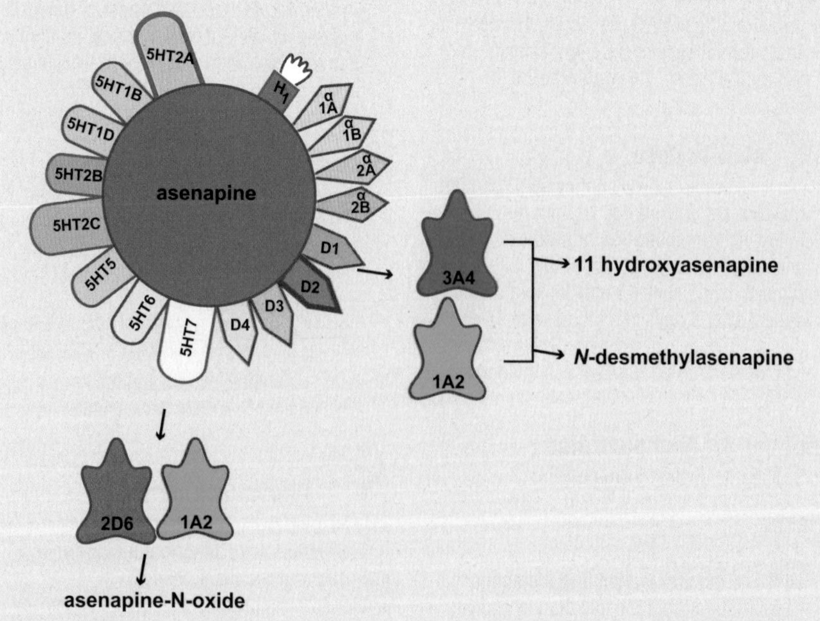

Figure 1 Asenapine metabolism.

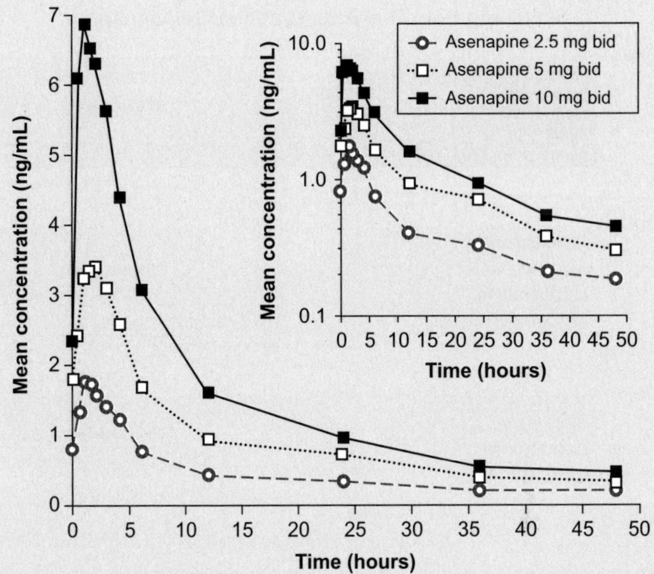

Figure 2 Mean asenapine plasma concentration–time profiles in children and adolescents ages 10–17. Reproduced from Dogterom et al., 2018.

- Pediatric patients may be more sensitive to dystonia with initial dosing if the recommended titration schedule is not followed
- Once-daily use seems theoretically possible because of the half-life of asenapine, but this has not been extensively studied and may be limited by the need to expose the limited sublingual surface area to a limited amount of sublingual drug dosage
- Some patients may respond to doses greater than 20 mg/day, but no single administration should be greater than 10 mg, thus necessitating 3 or 4 separate daily doses
- May be one of the most rapid onset antipsychotics available that is not an injection
- Due to rapid onset of action (can be within minutes), can be used as a rapid-acting "prn" or "as needed" dose for agitation or transient worsening of psychosis or mania instead of an injection
- Treatment should be suspended if absolute neutrophil count falls below 1,000/mm^3

How to Switch

- From another antipsychotic to asenapine:
  - When tapering a prior antipsychotic, see its entry in this manual for how to stop and how to taper off that specific drug
  - Generally, try to stop the first agent before starting asenapine so that new side effects of asenapine can be distinguished from withdrawal effects of the first agent
  - If urgent, cross taper off the other antipsychotic while asenapine is started at a low dose, with dose adjustments down of the other antipsychotic, and up for asenapine every 3 to 7 days
  - However, sedation may be more severe if cross tapering until the original antipsychotic washes out and the patient becomes tolerant to asenapine
- From asenapine to another antipsychotic:
  - Generally, try to stop asenapine before starting the new antipsychotic so that new side effects of the next drug can be distinguished from any withdrawal effects from asenapine
  - If urgent, cross taper off asenapine by cutting the dose in half, as the new antipsychotic is also started with dose adjustments down of asenapine and up for the new antipsychotic
  - Be vigilant to increased sedation when asenapine is combined with another antipsychotic

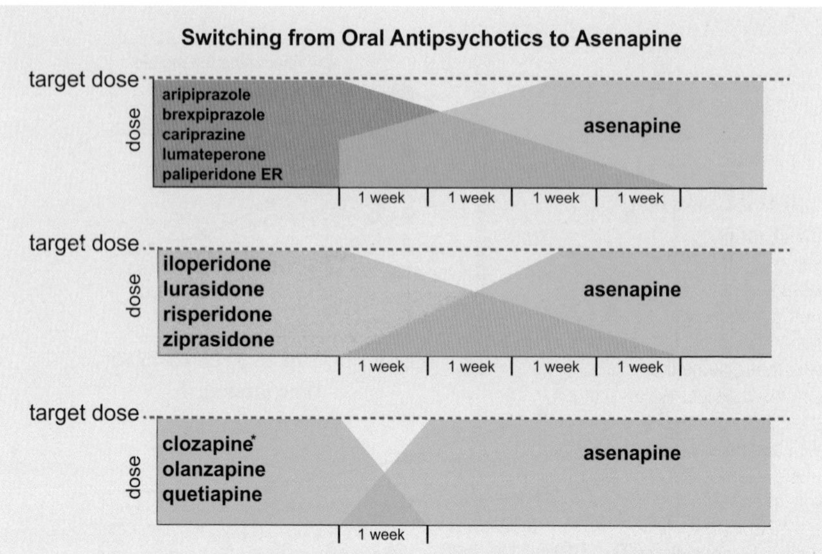

How to Stop

- Slow down-titration of oral formulation (over 6–8 weeks), especially when simultaneously beginning a new antipsychotic while switching (i.e., cross-titration)
- Rapid oral discontinuation may lead to rebound psychosis and worsening of symptoms
- Rapid oral discontinuation may lead to withdrawal dyskinesias, which are generally reversible in the pediatric population. Of note, withdrawal dyskinesias are more common in pediatric patients than in adults.

WHAT TO EXPECT

Onset of Action

- Psychotic and manic symptoms can improve within 1 week, but it may take several weeks for full effect on behavior as well as on cognition and affective stabilization
- If it is not working within 6–8 weeks, it may require a dosage increase or it may not work at all

Duration of Action

- Effects are consistent over a 24-hour period
- May continue to work for many years to prevent relapse of symptoms

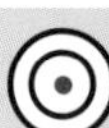

Primary Target Symptoms

- Manic symptoms
- Positive symptoms of psychosis
- Negative symptoms of psychosis
- Prior to initiation of treatment, it is helpful to develop a list of target symptoms of the underlying disorder specific for the patient being treated for monitoring to better assess treatment response

What Is Considered a Positive Result?

- In bipolar disorder:
  - Many patients may experience a reduction of symptoms by half or more
- In schizophrenia:
  - Most often reduces positive symptoms but does not eliminate them
  - Can improve negative symptoms, as well as aggressive, cognitive, and affective symptoms, but less so than for positive symptoms
  - In children or adolescents with a first episode of psychosis, initial response may be greater than for recurrent episodes of psychosis in adults

How Long to Treat

- In schizophrenia and bipolar disorder:
  - Continue treatment until reaching a plateau of improvement

- After reaching a satisfactory plateau, continue treatment for at least a year after first episode of psychosis or mania
- For second and subsequent episodes of psychosis or mania, treatment may need to be indefinite

What If It Stops Working?

- Check for nonadherence and consider switching to another antipsychotic with fewer side effects
- Some patients who have an initial response may relapse even though they continue treatment, sometimes called "poop-out"
- Growth/developmental changes may contribute to apparent loss of efficacy as well as to new onset of side effects as metabolism slows and drug levels rise in transition from childhood to adolescence; dose adjustment (increase or decrease) should be considered
- Screen for the development of a new comorbid disorder, especially substance use
- Screen for adverse changes in the home or school environment

What If It Doesn't Work?

- Consider evaluation for another diagnosis (especially bipolar illness or depression with mixed features) or for a comorbid condition (e.g., medical illness, substance use)
- Consider other important potential factors such as ongoing conflicts, family psychopathology, and an adverse environment (e.g., inadequate school placement or educational services, bullying, poverty, chaos, violence, prior and ongoing psychological trauma, abuse, neglect)
- Institute trauma-informed care for appropriate children and adolescents
- For schizophrenia or bipolar disorder:
  - Try one of the other atypical antipsychotics
  - If no first-line atypical antipsychotic is effective, consider higher doses or augmentation with valproate, lithium, or lamotrigine
  - Consider initiating psychotherapy. In adolescents with bipolar disorder (and those with affective symptoms who are at risk of developing bipolar disorder), family-focused psychotherapy can be particularly helpful (Miklowitz et al., 2020).
  - Consider presence of concomitant drug abuse

TALKING TO PATIENTS AND CAREGIVERS

What to Tell Parents About Efficacy

- For acute symptoms, it can work right away
- Asenapine is usually given every day
- Some parents use an extra dose on an as needed basis for symptoms that are transiently worse
- Explain which use asenapine is being chosen for, how to tell if the drug is working by targeting specific symptoms, and why this is being done
- Once the child/adolescent calms down, at some point after one dose or after several days of dosing or after long-term dosing, we should all assess whether the medication should be continued
- While the medicine helps by reducing symptoms and improving function, it is not a cure, and it therefore may be necessary to keep taking the medication long term to sustain its therapeutic effects
- Since every treatment consideration depends on a risk/benefit analysis, parents should fully understand short- and long-term risks as well as benefits
- Often a good idea to tell parents whether the medication chosen is specifically approved for the disorder being treated, or whether it is being given for "unapproved" or "off-label" reasons based on good clinical practice, expert consensus, and/or prudent extrapolation of controlled data from adults

What to Tell Children and Adolescents About Efficacy

- Be specific about the symptoms being targeted: we are trying to help you …
- Give the medication a try; if it's not working very well, we can stop the medication and try something else
- A good try often takes several weeks
- If it does make you feel better, you cannot stop it right away or you may get sick again
- Medications don't change who you are as a person; they give you the opportunity to be the best person you can be

What to Tell Parents About Side Effects

- Explain that side effects are expected in many when starting
- Tell parents many side effects go away and do so about the same time that therapeutic effects start
- Predict side effects in advance (you will look clever and competent to the parents, unless you scare them with too much information and cause nocebo effects, in which case you won't look so clever when the patient develops lots of side effects and stops medication; use your judgment here); a balanced but honest presentation is an art rather than a science
- Ask parents to support the patient while side effects are occurring
- Parents should fully understand short- and long-term risks as well as benefits
- Explaining to the parents what to expect from medication treatment, and especially what potential side effects to expect, can help prevent early termination of medication

What to Tell Children and Adolescents About Side Effects

- Even if you get side effects, most of them get better or go away in a few weeks
- If you have side effects that are bothering you, tell your parents and your parents should tell me
- Consider having a conversation about sexual side effects in some adolescents who can find these side effects confusing and especially burdensome
- Explaining to child/adolescent what to expect from medication treatment, and especially potential side effects, can help prevent early termination of medication

What to Tell Teachers About the Medication (If Parents Consent)

- Asenapine can make children/adolescents sedated
- It is not abusable
- Encourage dialogue with parents/guardians about any behavior or mood changes
- Notify the clinician of increased restlessness or akathisia symptoms, which may be apparent in the school setting

SPECIAL POPULATIONS

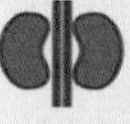

Renal Impairment

- Dose adjustment not generally necessary

Hepatic Impairment

- No dose adjustment necessary for mild to moderate impairment
- Contraindicated in patients with severe hepatic impairment

Cardiac Impairment

- Use in patients with cardiac impairment has not been studied; however, the risk of orthostatic hypotension in pediatric patients is less than in adults, as children rely less on peripheral vasoconstriction to regulate blood pressure

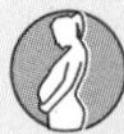

Pregnancy

- Controlled studies have not been conducted in pregnant women
- There is a risk of abnormal muscle movements and withdrawal symptoms in newborns whose mothers took an antipsychotic during the third trimester; symptoms may include agitation, abnormally increased or decreased muscle tone, tremor, sleepiness, severe difficulty breathing, and difficulty feeding
- In animal studies, asenapine increased post-implantation loss and decreased pup weight and survival at doses similar to or less than recommended clinical doses; there was no increase in the incidence of structural abnormalities
- Psychotic symptoms may worsen during pregnancy, and some form of treatment may be necessary
- National Pregnancy Registry for Atypical Antipsychotics: 1-866-961-2388 or http://womensmentalhealth.org/clinical-and-research-programs/pregnancyregistry/

Breast Feeding

- Some drug is present in breast milk
- Recommended either to discontinue drug or formula feed
- Infants of women who choose to breast feed while on asenapine should be monitored for possible adverse effects; sedation, failure to thrive, jitteriness, tremor, and abnormal muscle movements have been reported

THE ART OF PSYCHOPHARMACOLOGY

Potential Advantages

- In children and adolescents:
  - Approved for manic/mixed episodes
  - For patients who have trouble swallowing pills
- All ages:
  - Patients requiring rapid onset of antipsychotic action without dosage titration

Potential Disadvantages

- In children and adolescents:
  - Efficacy for schizophrenia was not demonstrated in an 8-week, placebo-controlled, double-blind trial in adolescent patients ages 12 to 17 years
  - May be more susceptible to side effects, including weight gain and sedation
- All ages:
  - Patients who are less likely to be adherent

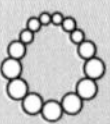

Pearls

- Asenapine's chemical structure is related to the antidepressant mirtazapine, and it shares many of the same pharmacological binding properties of mirtazapine plus many others
- Not approved for depression, but binding properties suggest potential use in treatment-resistant and bipolar depression
- Sublingual administration may require prescribing asenapine to reliable, adherent patients, or those who have someone who can supervise drug administration
- Since there is very rapid onset of action after sublingual administration, can use as a prn treatment of short-term symptom worsening, like an injection without a needle, if the patient cooperates sufficiently for sublingual administration
- Patients with inadequate responses to atypical antipsychotics may benefit from determination of plasma drug levels and, if low, a dosage increase even beyond the usual prescribing limits

SUGGESTED READING

Dogterom P, Riesenberg R, de Greef R et al. Asenapine pharmacokinetics and tolerability in a pediatric population. Drug Des Devel Ther 2018;12:2677–93.

Findling RL, Landbloom RL, Szegedi A et al. Asenapine for the acute treatment of pediatric manic or mixed episode of bipolar I disorder. J Am Acad Child Adolesc Psychiatry 2015;54(12):1032–41.

Findling RL, Landbloom RL, Mackle M et al. Long-term safety of asenapine in pediatric patients diagnosed with bipolar I disorder: a 50-week open-label, flexible-dose trial. Paediatr Drugs 2016;18(5):367–78.

Miklowitz DJ, Schneck CD, Walshaw PD et al. Effects of family-focused therapy vs enhanced usual care for symptomatic youths at high risk for bipolar disorder: a randomized clinical trial. JAMA Psychiatry 2020 1;77(5):455–63.

Pagsberg AK, Tarp S, Glintborg D et al. Acute antipsychotic treatment of children and adolescents with schizophrenia-spectrum disorders: a systematic review and network meta-analysis. J Am Acad Child Adolesc Psychiatry 2017;56(3):191–202.

Pillay J, Boylan K, Carrey N et al. First- and Second-Generation Antipsychotics in Children and Young Adults: Systematic Review Update [Internet]. Rockville, MD: Agency for Healthcare Research and Quality (US); 2017 Mar. Report No.: 17-EHC001-EF. AHRQ Comparative Effectiveness Reviews.

THERAPEUTICS

Brands

- Strattera

Generic

Yes

US FDA Approved for Pediatric Use

- Attention deficit hyperactivity disorder (Strattera, ages 6 and older)

Off-Label for Pediatric Use

- Approved in adults
  - None
- Other off-label uses
  - Treatment-resistant depression

Class and Mechanism of Action

- Neuroscience-based Nomenclature: norepinephrine reuptake inhibitor (N-RI)
- Selective norepinephrine reuptake inhibitor (NRI)
- Boosts neurotransmitter norepinephrine/ noradrenaline and may also increase dopamine in the prefrontal cortex
- Blocks norepinephrine reuptake pumps, also known as norepinephrine transporters
- Presumably this increases noradrenergic neurotransmission
- Since dopamine is inactivated by norepinephrine reuptake in the frontal cortex, which largely lacks dopamine transporters, atomoxetine can also increase dopamine neurotransmission in this part of the brain

SAFETY AND TOLERABILITY

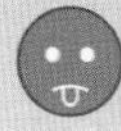

Notable Side Effects

- Fatigue, sleepiness, headache, irritability
- Decreased appetite, nausea, vomiting, abdominal pain
- Increased heart rate (6–9 beats/min)
- Increased blood pressure (2–4 mmHg)

Life-Threatening or Dangerous Side Effects

- Rare priapism
- Severe liver damage (rare)
- Rare hypomania, mania, or suicidal ideation
- Cardiovascular adverse effects, sudden death in patients with preexisting cardiac structural abnormalities often associated with a family history of cardiac disease

Growth and Maturation

- Changes not reported

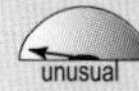

Weight Gain

- Patients may experience weight loss, but typically less than with stimulants because there is generally less appetite suppression
- Weight gain is reported but not expected, rarely seen

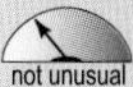

Sedation

- Occurs in significant minority, particularly in children
- Insomnia may occur

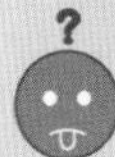

What to Do About Side Effects

- Wait, wait, wait: mild side effects are common, happen early, and usually improve with time, but treatment benefits can be delayed and often begin just as the side effects wear off
- Monitor side effects closely, especially when initiating treatment
- Lower the dose
- If giving once daily, can change to split dose twice daily
- If atomoxetine is sedating, take at night to reduce daytime drowsiness
- Often best to try another monotherapy prior to resorting to augmentation strategies to treat side effects
- Activation and agitation may represent the induction of a bipolar state, especially a mixed dysphoric bipolar II condition sometimes associated with suicidal ideation, and may require the addition of lithium or an atypical antipsychotic and/or discontinuation of atomoxetine

How Drug Causes Side Effects

- Norepinephrine increases in parts of the brain and body and at receptors other than those that cause therapeutic actions (e.g., unwanted actions of norepinephrine on acetylcholine release causing decreased appetite, increased heart rate and blood pressure, dry mouth, urinary retention)

- Lack of enhancing dopamine activity in limbic areas theoretically explains atomoxetine's lack of abuse potential

Warnings and Precautions

- In children and adolescents:
  - Safety and efficacy not established in children under age 6
  - Use in young children should be reserved for the expert
  - Children who are not growing or gaining weight should stop treatment, at least temporarily
  - Usual dosing has been associated with sudden death in children with structural cardiac abnormalities
  - Consider distributing brochures provided by the FDA and the drug companies
  - Warn patients and their caregivers about the possibility of activating side effects and advise them to report such symptoms immediately
- All ages:
  - Carefully weigh the risks and benefits of pharmacological treatment against the risks and benefits of nonpharmacological treatment and it is a good idea to document this in the patient's chart
  - Use with caution in patients with hypertension, tachycardia, cardiovascular disease, or cerebrovascular disease
  - Use with caution if at all in patients with bipolar disorder
  - Use with caution in patients with urinary retention, benign prostatic hypertrophy
  - Rare reports of hepatotoxicity; although causality has not been established, atomoxetine should be discontinued in patients who develop jaundice or other evidence of significant liver dysfunction
  - Use with caution with antihypertensive drugs
  - Monitor patients for activation of suicidal ideation
  - Emergence or worsening of activation and agitation may represent the induction of a bipolar state, especially a mixed dysphoric bipolar II condition sometimes associated with suicidal ideation, and may require the addition of lithium or an atypical antipsychotic and/or discontinuation of atomoxetine

When Not to Prescribe

- If patient is taking an MAO inhibitor (except as noted under Drug Interactions)
- If patient has pheochromocytoma or history of pheochromocytoma
- If patient has a severe cardiovascular disorder that might deteriorate with clinically important increases in heart rate and blood pressure
- If patient has structural cardiac abnormalities
- If patient has angle-closure glaucoma
- If there is a proven allergy to atomoxetine

Long-Term Use

- Safe
- Long-term use may be associated with growth suppression in children (controversial), so weight and height should be monitored during long-term treatment; for patients who are not growing or gaining weight satisfactorily, interruption of treatment should be considered

Habit Forming

- No

Overdose

- No fatalities have been reported as monotherapy; sedation, agitation, hyperactivity, abnormal behavior, gastrointestinal symptoms

DOSING AND USE

Usual Dosage Range

- 0.5–1.2 mg/kg/day in children up to 70 kg; 40–100 mg/day in children over 70 kg and adults

Dosage Forms

- Capsule 10 mg, 18 mg, 25 mg, 40 mg, 60 mg, 80 mg, 100 mg

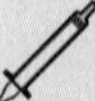

How to Dose

- For children 70 kg or less: initial dose 0.5 mg/kg per day; after 7 days can increase to 1.2 mg/kg per day either once in the morning or divided; maximum dose 1.4 mg/kg per day or 100 mg/day, whichever is less
- For children over 70 kg and adults: initial dose 40 mg/day; after 7 days can increase to 80 mg/day once in the morning or divided;

after 2–4 weeks can increase to 100 mg/day if necessary; maximum daily dose 100 mg

Options for Administration

- Oral formulation only

Tests

- Blood pressure (sitting and standing) and pulse should be measured at baseline and monitored following dose increases and periodically during treatment
- Monitor weight and height

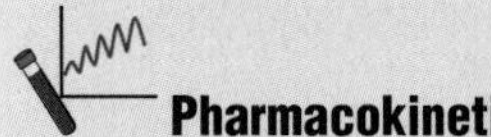

Pharmacokinetics

- Well absorbed after oral administration, with peak plasma concentrations typically occurring 1 to 2 hours after dosing. However, food can delay the absorption, resulting in a slight decrease in the peak plasma concentration and a delay in the time to reach peak levels.
- Atomoxetine has a moderate volume of distribution, indicating that it distributes throughout the body. It is highly bound to plasma proteins (98%), primarily to albumin.
- Extensively metabolized in the liver by CYP2D6. The major metabolite formed is 4-hydroxyatomoxetine (O-desmethylatomoxetine), which is also pharmacologically active but has lower potency compared to the parent compound. Other minor metabolites include *N*-desmethylatomoxetine and glucuronide conjugates (Figure 1).
- The elimination half-life of atomoxetine is approximately 4 to 5 hours in normal CYP2D6 metabolizers and approximately 20 hours in poor metabolizers (individuals with deficient CYP2D6 function). The drug and its metabolites are primarily excreted in the urine, with less than 3% being eliminated unchanged. In CYP2D6 poor metabolizers, the elimination half-life of the 4-hydroxyatomoxetine metabolite is also prolonged.

Pharmacogenetics

- Because atomoxetine is extensively metabolized by CYP2D6, variants impacting CYP2D6 may alter drug exposure (Figure 2)

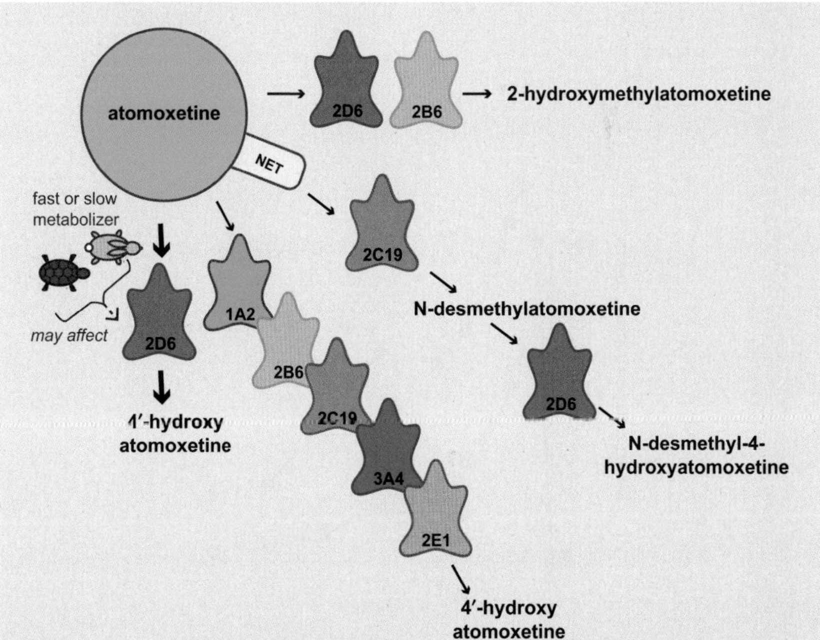

Figure 1 Atomoxetine metabolism is heavily influenced by CYP2D6 and variants of CYP2D6 may significantly affect exposure (i.e., blood concentrations over time). Therefore, alternative titration and goal doses are recommended by CPIC based on CYP2D6 phenotypes.

- **CYP2D6 ultrarapid metabolizers:** Unlikely that patient will achieve adequate serum concentrations with standard dosing
  - Clinical Pharmacogenetics Implementation Consortium (CPIC) recommended dosing: initiate with a dose of 0.5 mg/kg/day and increase to 1.2 mg/kg/day after 3 days. If there is no clinical response and no adverse events after 2 weeks, consider obtaining a peak plasma concentration (1 to 2 hours after dose is administered). If peak plasma concentration is <200 ng/mL, consider a proportional increase in dose to approach 400 ng/mL.
- **CYP2D6 intermediate metabolizers:** Patient may be at increased risk of atomoxetine-related adverse effects
  - CPIC recommended dosing: initiate with a dose of 0.5 mg/kg/day. If there is no clinical response or adverse events after 2 weeks, consider obtaining a plasma concentration 2–4 hours after dosing. If plasma concentration is <200 ng/mL, consider a proportional dose increase to achieve a concentration to approach 400 ng/mL. If unacceptable side effects are present at any time, consider a reduction in dose.
- **CYP2D6 poor metabolizers:** Patient may be at increased risk of atomoxetine-related adverse effects
  - CPIC recommended dosing: initiate with a dose of 0.5 mg/kg/day. If there is no clinical response or adverse events after 2 weeks, consider obtaining a plasma concentration 4 hours after dosing. If plasma concentration is <200 ng/mL, consider a proportional dose increase to achieve a concentration to approach 400 ng/mL. If unacceptable side effects are present at any time, consider a reduction in dose.

Drug Interactions

- Tramadol increases the risk of seizures in patients taking an antidepressant
- Plasma concentrations of atomoxetine may be increased by drugs that inhibit CYP2D6 (e.g., paroxetine, fluoxetine), so atomoxetine dose should be reduced by half if these agents are coadministered
- Coadministration of atomoxetine and oral or IV albuterol may lead to increases in heart rate and blood pressure

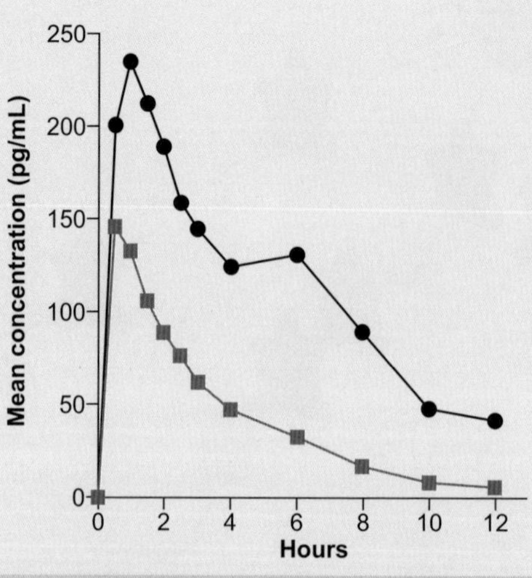

Figure 2 Atomoxetine concentration over time based on CYP2D6 metabolism.

- Coadministration with methylphenidate does not increase cardiovascular side effects beyond those seen with methylphenidate alone
- Use with caution with MAO inhibitors, including 14 days after MAOIs are stopped (for the expert)

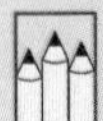

Dosing Tips

- Be aware that metabolism changes during puberty and entry into adolescence and becomes more like adults (i.e., slower than in children)
- If a child on a stable dose begins to lose tolerability with more side effects upon entering adolescence, this may signal the need for a dose reduction due to changing metabolism
- Can be given once a day in the morning
- Efficacy with once-daily dosing despite a half-life of 5 hours suggests therapeutic effects persist beyond direct pharmacological effects, unlike stimulants whose effects are generally closely correlated with plasma drug levels
- Once-daily dosing may increase gastrointestinal side effects
- Lower starting dose allows detection of those patients who may be especially sensitive to side effects such as tachycardia and increased blood pressure
- Patients especially sensitive to the side effects of atomoxetine may include those individuals deficient in the enzyme that metabolizes atomoxetine, CYP2D6 (i.e., 7% of Caucasians and 2% of African Americans)
- In such individuals, drug should be titrated slowly to tolerability and effectiveness
- Other individuals may require up to 1.8 mg/kg total daily dose

How to Switch

- Generally, try to stop the first agent before starting a new drug so that side effects from the new medication can be distinguished from withdrawal effects of the first agent
- Side effects from abrupt discontinuation are not expected
- If urgent, can usually cross taper from a stimulant to a nonstimulant, or vice versa, by decreasing the first medication perhaps by a quarter to half, and starting the new medication at a low dose

How to Stop

- Side effects from abrupt discontinuation are not expected
- However, if withdrawal symptoms develop, resume dosing the medication and then taper slowly over several days
- Withdrawal following chronic therapeutic use may unmask symptoms of the underlying disorder and may require follow-up and reinstitution of treatment
- Usually symptoms after discontinuation of atomoxetine are return of symptoms of the underlying disorder rather than symptoms due to drug withdrawal
- Supervision during withdrawal is always recommended for any psychotropic medication

WHAT TO EXPECT

Onset of Action

- Onset of therapeutic actions in ADHD can be seen as early as the first week of dosing
- Therapeutic actions may continue to improve for 8–12 weeks. Atomoxetine response may take longer to show improvement compared to other nonstimulant medications (e.g., viloxazine, guanfacine, clonidine).

Duration of Action

- Effects are consistent over a 24-hour period

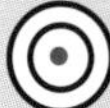

Primary Target Symptoms

- Concentration, attention span, distractibility
- Motor hyperactivity
- Impulsiveness
- Depressed mood

What Is Considered a Positive Result?

- The goal of treatment of ADHD is reduction of symptoms of inattentiveness, motor hyperactivity, and/or impulsiveness that disrupt social, school, and/or occupational functioning
- The goal of treatment is complete remission of symptoms
- If treatment works, it most often reduces or even eliminates symptoms, but is not a cure

since symptoms often recur after medicine is stopped

How Long to Treat

- ADHD is typically a lifelong illness; if any symptoms improve, hyperactivity is more likely to improve than inattention
- Can tell parents there is some chance that their child can grow out of this in adulthood, but many adults continue to have symptoms of ADHD throughout adolescence and adulthood
- Continue treatment until all symptoms are under control or improvement is stable and then continue treatment as long as improvement persists
- Reevaluate the need for treatment periodically; some clinicians advise to periodically taper ADHD medication in patients who are not severely symptomatic to observe how the patient responds, but not routinely done by most clinicians
- Treatment for ADHD begun in childhood may need to be continued into adolescence and adulthood if continued benefit is documented

What If It Stops Working?

- Some patients who have an initial response may relapse even though they continue treatment, sometimes called "poop-out"
- Growth/developmental changes may contribute to apparent loss of efficacy as well as to new onset of side effects as metabolism slows and drug levels rise in transition from childhood to adolescence; dose adjustment (increase or decrease) should be considered
- Some patients may experience apparent lack of consistent efficacy due to activation of latent or underlying or newly evolved bipolar disorder, major depressive episodes with mixed features of mania, or new onset of major depression or an anxiety disorder (GAD, OCD, PD), and require medication discontinuation and a switch to the clinically appropriate medication(s)

What If It Doesn't Work?

- In practice, many patients have only a partial response where some symptoms are improved but others persist, in which case higher doses of atomoxetine, adding a second agent, or switching to an agent with a different mechanism of action can be considered
- Consider evaluation for another diagnosis or for a comorbid condition (e.g., medical illness, substance abuse). Also, when treating ADHD, consider the possibility of a learning disorder or learning weakness and consider school-based interventions.
- Consider nonadherence and counsel patient and parents
- Some ADHD patients and some depressed patients may experience lack of consistent efficacy due to activation of latent or underlying bipolar disorder, and require either augmenting with a mood stabilizer or switching to a mood stabilizer
- Augmenting options:
  - Cognitive behavioral therapy (CBT)
  - Parent Management Training (PMT)
  - Behavioral modification
  - Coordinating with school for appropriate support
  - Best to attempt other monotherapies prior to augmenting
  - Augmentation with a stimulant is commonly used for treatment-resistant ADHD symptoms, especially inattention and hyperactivity
  - Augmentation with an alpha 2 agonist can be used for treatment-resistant ADHD symptoms, especially oppositional and aggressive/impulsive behaviors
  - Triple therapy with a stimulant, alpha 2 agonist, and viloxazine for especially treatment-resistant cases is for the expert
  - SSRIs, SNRIs, or mirtazapine for treatment-resistant depression (use combinations of antidepressants with atomoxetine with caution, as this may theoretically activate bipolar disorder and suicidal ideation)
  - For the expert, can combine with modafinil, methylphenidate, or amphetamine for ADHD
  - For the expert, can occasionally combine with mood stabilizers or atypical antipsychotics in highly treatment-resistant cases of bipolar disorder including bipolar disorder comorbid with ADHD
- Consider factors associated with poor response to any psychotropic medication in children and adolescents, such as severe symptoms, long-lasting symptoms, poor treatment adherence, prior nonresponse

to other treatments, and the presence of comorbid psychiatric disorders or learning disorders
- Consider other important potential factors such as ongoing conflicts, family psychopathology, and an adverse environment (e.g., poverty, chaos, violence, prior and ongoing psychological trauma, abuse, bullying, less than ideal school placement, neglect)
- Institute trauma-informed care for appropriate children and adolescents

TALKING TO PATIENTS AND CAREGIVERS

What to Tell Parents About Efficacy

- It doesn't work right away; full therapeutic benefits may take 4–8 weeks
- This medicine generally takes longer to start working than stimulants for ADHD
- It is not a stimulant
- While the medicine helps ADHD by reducing symptoms and improving function, there are no cures for ADHD, and it is therefore necessary to keep taking the medication to sustain its therapeutic effects
- Since every treatment consideration depends on a risk/benefit analysis, parents should fully understand short- and long-term risks as well as benefits compared to nontreatment of ADHD
- Often a good idea to tell parents whether the medication chosen is specifically approved for the disorder being treated, or whether it is being given for "unapproved" or "off-label" reasons based on good clinical practice, expert consensus, and/or prudent extrapolation of controlled data from adults
- Best results are often obtained when medications are combined with behavioral therapy
- The American Academy of Child & Adolescent Psychiatry (AACAP) has helpful handouts for parents

What to Tell Children and Adolescents About Efficacy

- Be specific about the symptoms being targeted: we are trying to help you remember things better, do your best at school, follow the rules, get into less trouble (as applicable)
- It may be a good idea to give the medication a try; if it's not working very well, we can stop the medication and try something else
- You can be part of a special plan to help us figure out if the medicine is helpful for you. Would you like to do that? (for the parents and prescriber, can consider here a trial both on and then off medication, and then on again to see if the effects are clear and thus worth continuing the medication)
- A good try takes 2 to 3 months
- Even if it does make you feel better, it will wear off and no longer work shortly after you stop it
- The medication can help you decide what you want to do, like making good choices versus bad choices; the medicine does not make you do something you don't want to do
- Medications don't change who you are as a person; they give you the opportunity to be the best person you can be

What to Tell Parents About Side Effects

- Explain that side effects are expected in many when starting
- Tell parents many side effects go away and do so about the same time that therapeutic effects start
- Predict side effects in advance (you will look clever and competent to the parents, unless you scare them with too much information and cause nocebo effects, in which case you won't look so clever when the patient develops lots of side effects and stops medication; use your judgment here); a balanced but honest presentation is an art rather than a science
- Tell them this medication works like some antidepressants, and all antidepressants have a warning in children and adolescents for increased suicidality (i.e., suicidal thoughts and behavior), but the FDA studies did not show any actual suicides in any age group nor risk beyond age 24, and this was observed in children and adolescents with depression, not ADHD
- Ask them to help monitor for these symptoms and if present, report any such symptoms immediately
- Ask parents to support the patient while side effects are occurring
- Parents should fully understand short- and long-term risks as well as benefits
- Explaining to the parents what to expect from medication treatment, and especially

what potential side effects to expect, can help prevent early termination

What to Tell Children and Adolescents About Side Effects

- When a medicine starts to work, your body can first experience this by giving you unpleasant sensations – just like if you take a cough medicine it may taste bad – these body sensations include loss of appetite and problems sleeping. So, just like with a cough medicine, the bad taste will often go away before the medicine begins to stop the cough – many medicines work like that. It's important for you to pay attention to what your body is telling you, and we'll go over some of the ways that can happen.
- Even if you get a side effect, it's not permanent (it won't last forever)
- Explaining to child/adolescent what to expect from medication treatment, and especially potential side effects, can help prevent early termination
- Tell adolescents and children capable of understanding that some young patients, especially those who are depressed, may develop thoughts of hurting themselves, and if this happens, not to be alarmed but to tell their parents right away

What to Tell Teachers About the Medication (If Parents Consent)

- Atomoxetine can be helpful in improving the symptoms of ADHD: namely, inattention, impulsivity, and hyperactivity
- Some students will experience side effects from the medications that you may notice in or outside the classroom; many of these side effects can be modified
- If the patient is sleepy, ask whether the medication is keeping them up at night or if they are eating enough food

SPECIAL POPULATIONS

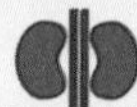

Renal Impairment

- Dose adjustment not generally necessary

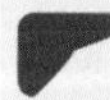

Hepatic Impairment

- For patients with moderate liver impairment, dose should be reduced to 50% of normal dose
- For patients with severe liver impairment, dose should be reduced to 25% of normal dose

Cardiac Impairment

- Use with caution because atomoxetine can increase heart rate and blood pressure
- Do not use in patients with structural cardiac abnormalities

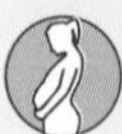

Pregnancy

- Controlled studies have not been conducted in pregnant women
- Some animal studies have shown adverse effects
- Use in women of childbearing potential requires weighing potential benefits to the mother against potential risks to the fetus
- For women of childbearing potential, atomoxetine should generally be discontinued before anticipated pregnancies

Breast Feeding

- Unknown if atomoxetine is secreted in human breast milk, but all psychotropics assumed to be secreted in breast milk
- Recommend either to discontinue drug or formula feed

THE ART OF PSYCHOPHARMACOLOGY

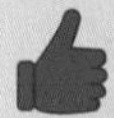

Potential Advantages

- In children:
  - For patients whose parents do not want them to take a stimulant or who cannot tolerate or do not respond to stimulants
- In adolescents:
  - For patients who have a history of diverting or abusing stimulants
  - Can improve school performance and grades, especially if ADHD has been unrecognized and untreated prior to adolescence
  - Can improve performance in high school and college students whose ADHD is compromising academic performance due to the increased demands of higher levels of study

- All ages:
  - No known abuse potential; not a controlled substance
  - No withdrawal reactions

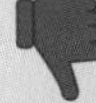

Potential Disadvantages

- In children:
  - Those who are psychomotor agitated, angry, or irritable, and who do not have a psychiatric diagnosis
  - Possible activation of suicidality/bipolar disorder
- In adolescents:
  - Those who may possibly have an untreated mood or anxiety disorder or who refuse treatment for them
  - Possible activation of suicidality/bipolar disorder
- All ages:
  - May not act as rapidly as stimulants when initiating treatment in some patients
  - May take months to realize full extent of improvement
  - Those who need to take drugs that are CYP2D6 inhibitors or those who are poor metabolizers of CYP2D6 and do not tolerate atomoxetine

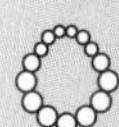

Pearls

- Probably a second-line treatment for children who cannot tolerate stimulants
- Anecdotally, may be more effective for symptoms of inattention than for symptoms of hyperactivity or impulsivity in some patients
- Can be a first-line treatment for adolescents who wish to avoid a trial of a stimulant
- Unlike stimulants, atomoxetine is not abusable and has little or no value to friends of adolescent patients who may otherwise divert stimulant medications, especially when responsible for self-administration of medication in college settings
- Despite its name as a selective norepinephrine reuptake inhibitor, atomoxetine enhances both dopamine and norepinephrine in the frontal cortex, presumably accounting for its therapeutic actions on attention and concentration
- Since dopamine is inactivated by norepinephrine reuptake in the frontal cortex, which largely lacks dopamine transporters, atomoxetine can increase dopamine as well as norepinephrine in this part of the brain, presumably causing therapeutic actions in ADHD
- Since dopamine is inactivated by dopamine reuptake in the nucleus accumbens, which largely lacks norepinephrine transporters, atomoxetine does not increase dopamine in this part of the brain, presumably explaining why atomoxetine lacks abuse potential
- Atomoxetine's known mechanism of action as a selective norepinephrine reuptake inhibitor suggests its efficacy as an antidepressant
- Pro-noradrenergic actions may be theoretically useful for the treatment of chronic pain
- Atomoxetine's mechanism of action and its potential antidepressant actions suggest it has the potential to destabilize latent or undiagnosed bipolar disorder, similar to the known actions of proven antidepressants
- Unlike stimulants, atomoxetine may not exacerbate tics in Tourette syndrome patients with comorbid ADHD
- Not well documented to improve oppositional/aggressive behaviors like some other ADHD medications

SUGGESTED READING

Catalá-López F, Hutton B, Nuñez-Beltrán A et al. The pharmacological and non-pharmacological treatment of attention deficit hyperactivity disorder in children and adolescents: a systematic review with network meta-analyses of randomised trials. PLoS One. 2017;12(7):e0180355.

Gayleard JL, Mychailyszyn MP. Atomoxetine treatment for children and adolescents with Attention-Deficit/ Hyperactivity Disorder (ADHD): a comprehensive meta-analysis of outcomes on parent-rated core symptomatology. Atten Defic Hyperact Disord 2017;9(3):149–60.

Kemper AR, Maslow GR, Hill S et al. Attention Deficit Hyperactivity Disorder: Diagnosis and Treatment in Children and Adolescents. Comparative Effectiveness Review No. 203. AHRQ Publication No. 18-EHC005-EF. Rockville, MD: Agency for Healthcare Research and Quality; January 2018.

Kim SH, Byeon JY, Kim YH et al. Physiologically based pharmacokinetic modeling of atomoxetine with regard to CYP2D6 genotypes. Sci Rep 2018;8(1):12405.

Pliszka S ; AACAP Work Group on Quality Issues. Practice parameter for the assessment and treatment of children and adolescents with attention-deficit/hyperactivity disorder. J Am Acad Child Adolesc Psychiatry 2007;46(7):894–921.

Stiefel G, Besag FM. Cardiovascular effects of methylphenidate, amphetamines, and atomoxetine in the treatment of attention-deficit hyperactivity disorder. Drug Saf 2010;33(10):821–42.

Trzepacz PT, Williams DW, Feldman PD et al. CYP2D6 metabolizer status and atomoxetine dosing in children and adolescents with ADHD. Eur Neuropsychopharmacol 2008;18(2):79–86.

THERAPEUTICS

Brands
- Rexulti

Generic
No

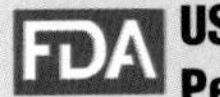

US FDA Approved for Pediatric Use
- Schizophrenia (ages 13 and older)

Off-Label for Pediatric Use
- Approved in adults
  - Treatment-resistant depression (adjunct)
  - Treatment of agitation associated with dementia due to Alzheimer's disease
- Other off-label uses
  - Acute mania / mixed mania
  - Other psychotic disorders
  - Bipolar maintenance
  - Bipolar depression
  - Behavioral disturbances in children and adolescents
  - Disorders associated with problems with impulse control
  - Posttraumatic stress disorder

Class and Mechanism of Action
- Neuroscience-based Nomenclature: dopamine, serotonin receptor partial agonist (DS-RPA)
- Dopamine partial agonist (atypical antipsychotic; second generation antipsychotic; sometimes called a third generation antipsychotic; also a mood stabilizer; sometimes called a dopamine stabilizer)
- As a partial agonist at dopamine D2 receptors, brexpiprazole theoretically reduces dopamine output when dopamine concentrations are high, thus hypothetically improving positive symptoms (antipsychotic and antimanic actions), and increases dopamine output when dopamine concentrations are low, thus hypothetically improving mood, negative symptoms, and cognitive symptoms
- Interactions at a myriad of other neurotransmitter receptors may contribute to brexpiprazole's efficacy
- Partial agonist at 5HT1A receptors, which may be beneficial for mood, anxiety, and cognition in a number of disorders
- Blocks serotonin 2A receptors, causing enhancement of dopamine release in certain brain regions and thus reducing motor side effects and possibly improving cognitive and affective symptoms
- Blockade of alpha 1B receptors may reduce arousal symptoms in posttraumatic stress disorder and in agitation associated with dementia as well as motor side effects such as akathisia
- Blockade of alpha 2C receptors may contribute to antidepressant actions
- Actions at dopamine 3 receptors could theoretically contribute to brexpiprazole's efficacy
- Blocks serotonin 7 receptors, which may be beneficial for mood, cognitive impairment, and negative symptoms in schizophrenia, and also in bipolar disorder and major depressive disorder

SAFETY AND TOLERABILITY

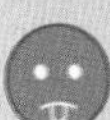

Notable Side Effects
- Akathisia (dose dependent), restlessness (dose dependent), anxiety
- Weight gain
- Sedation, headache
- Risk of drug-induced parkinsonism and dystonic reactions may be higher in children than it is in adults

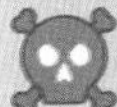

Life-Threatening or Dangerous Side Effects
- Hyperglycemia, in some cases extreme and associated with ketoacidosis or hyperosmolar coma or death, has been reported in patients taking atypical antipsychotics
- Rare neuroleptic malignant syndrome (NMS) may cause hyperpyrexia, muscle rigidity, delirium, and autonomic instability with elevated creatine phosphokinase, myoglobinuria (rhabdomyolysis), and acute renal failure
- Rare seizures
- As a class, antidepressants have been reported to increase the risk of suicidal thoughts and behaviors in children and young adults

Growth and Maturation
- Long-term effects are unknown

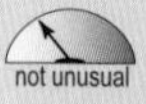

Weight Gain

- Occurs in a significant minority
- However, may be more risk of weight gain in children than in adults. Current practice often includes adding metformin in pediatric patients who experience early weight gain (or are at high risk of antipsychotic weight gain, i.e., greater than 85th percentile for BMI).

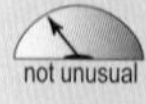

Sedation

- Occurs in a significant minority
- May be more likely to be sedating in children than in adults

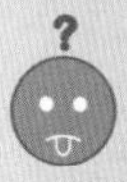

What to Do About Side Effects

- Wait, wait, wait: mild side effects are common, happen early, and usually improve with time, but treatment benefits can be delayed
- Monitor side effects closely, especially when initiating treatment
- Usually best to give at night to reduce daytime side effects
- Often best to try another monotherapy trial of a different antipsychotic prior to resorting to augmentation strategies to treat side effects
- Exercise and diet programs and medical management for high BMI percentiles, diabetes, dyslipidemia. Also, randomized controlled trials in youth suggest that omega-3 fatty acids can reduce SGA-related hypertriglyceridemia.
- Reduce the dose, particularly for drug-induced parkinsonism, akathisia, sedation, and tremor
- For motor side effects: consider reducing dose or switching to another agent. Augmenting with diphenhydramine or benztropine is less preferred in youth.
- For akathisia: reduce the dose or add a beta blocker; if these are ineffective, raising the dose of the beta blocker may be helpful. Using a 5HT2A antagonist such as mirtazapine or cyproheptadine to treat drug-induced akathisia is less common in children and adolescents compared to adults.
- For activation: (agitation, restlessness, insomnia)
  - Administer dose in the morning
  - Consider a temporary dose reduction or a more gradual up-titration
  - Consider adding a benzodiazepine short term (caution in children and adolescents)
  - Consider switching to another antipsychotic
  - Agitation due to undertreatment and inadequate dosing of the targeted disorder can be difficult to distinguish from drug-induced akathisia and activation; one approach for managing agitation/activation/akathisia when the specific side effect is difficult to distinguish is to raise the dose of brexpiprazole; can also consider using the Barnes akathisia rating scale
  - If the patient improves after increasing the dose of brexpiprazole, the symptoms are more likely to be due to inadequate dosing of the targeted disorder
  - If the patient worsens after increasing the dose of brexpiprazole, the symptoms are more likely to be drug induced and require further dose reduction, adding an agent to improve tolerability or switching to another antipsychotic

How Drug Causes Side Effects

- Blocking alpha 1 adrenergic receptors can cause dizziness, hypotension, and syncope. However, these effects may be less commonly seen as side effects in pediatric patients compared to adults.
- Partial agonist actions at dopamine D2 receptors in the striatum can cause drug-induced parkinsonism, akathisia, and activation symptoms
- Partial agonist actions at serotonin 5HT1A receptors can cause nausea, occasional vomiting
- Mechanism of weight gain and increased incidence of diabetes and dyslipidemia with atypical antipsychotics is unknown, and risks vary based on the particular agent

Warnings and Precautions

- If brexpiprazole is used to treat depressive mood disorders off-label in children, either as a monotherapy or an augmenting agent to an SSRI/SNRI, it is a good idea to warn patients and their caregivers about the possibility of activating side effects and suicidality as for any antidepressant in this age group and advise them to report such symptoms immediately

- Carefully weigh the risks and benefits of pharmacological treatment against the risks and benefits of nontreatment with an antipsychotic, and it is a good idea to document this in the patient's chart
- Use with caution in patients with conditions that predispose to hypotension (dehydration, overheating)
- Atypical antipsychotics have the potential for cognitive and motor impairment, especially related to sedation
- Atypical antipsychotics can cause body temperature dysregulation; use caution in patients who may experience conditions that increase body temperature (e.g., strenuous exercise, saunas, extreme heat, dehydration, or concomitant anticholinergic medication)
- Add or initiate other antipsychotics with caution for a few weeks after discontinuing brexpiprazole; brexpiprazole has a long half-life and can take a few weeks to wash out entirely
- As with any antipsychotic, use with caution in patients with history of seizures

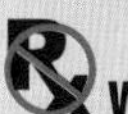

When Not to Prescribe

- If there is a proven allergy to brexpiprazole

Long-Term Use

- Safety and efficacy demonstrated in schizophrenia in adults in a maintenance study lasting over 1 year
- Should periodically reevaluate long-term usefulness in individual patients, but treatment may need to continue for many years

Habit Forming

- No

Overdose

- Limited experience

DOSING AND USE

Usual Dosage Range

- Schizophrenia: 2–4 mg once daily
- Depression: 2 mg once daily

Dosage Forms

- Tablet 0.25 mg, 0.5 mg, 1 mg, 2 mg, 3 mg, 4 mg

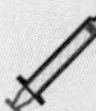

How to Dose

- Schizophrenia (ages 13 to 17): initial 0.5 mg once daily for days 1–4; increase to 1 mg once daily for days 5–7; increase to 2 mg once daily on day 8; weekly dose increases can be made in 1 mg increments; maximum dose 4 mg once daily

Options for Administration

- Oral tablet options only

Tests

- Before starting brexpiprazole:
  - Plan to monitor weight and metabolic parameters more closely than in adults since children and adolescents may be more prone to metabolic side effects than adults
  - Weigh all patients and monitor weight gain against that expected for normal growth, using the pediatric height/weight chart to monitor. In particular, monitor BMI percentiles.
  - Get baseline personal and family history of diabetes, obesity, dyslipidemia, hypertension, and cardiovascular disease
  - Obtain blood pressure, fasting plasma glucose (or hemoglobin A1C), and a lipid profile
- After starting brexpiprazole:
  - BMI percentile monthly for 3 months, then quarterly
  - Consider monitoring fasting triglycerides in patients at high risk for metabolic complications
  - Blood pressure, fasting plasma glucose (or hemoglobin A1C), lipid profile within 3 months and then annually
  - Treat or refer for treatment and consider switching to another atypical antipsychotic for patients who become overweight, obese, pre-diabetic, diabetic, or dyslipidemic while receiving an atypical antipsychotic
  - Even in patients without known diabetes, be vigilant for the rare but life-threatening onset of diabetic ketoacidosis, which always requires immediate treatment, by monitoring for the rapid onset of polyuria, polydipsia, weight loss, nausea, vomiting, dehydration, rapid respiration, weakness, and clouding of sensorium, even coma
  - Patients with low white blood cell count (WBC) or history of drug-

induced leukopenia/neutropenia should have complete blood count (CBC) monitored frequently during the first few months, and brexpiprazole should be discontinued at the first sign of decline of WBC in the absence of other causative factors
- Patients should be monitored periodically for the development of abnormal movements using neurological exam and the Abnormal Involuntary Movement Scale (AIMS)

Pharmacokinetics

- Brexpiprazole is well absorbed and reaches peak plasma concentrations within 2–4 hours (Figure 1)
- Food does not have a significant effect on the bioavailability of brexpiprazole, so it can be taken with or without food
- Brexpiprazole exhibits high protein binding, primarily to albumin, with approximately 99% bound in the plasma. The drug has a large volume of distribution, indicating extensive distribution into tissues throughout the body.
- Brexpiprazole is metabolized by multiple cytochrome enzymes, although the primary cytochrome is CYP3A4, with additional contributions from CYP2D6 and CYP2C19. The major active metabolite (DM-3411) exhibits similar pharmacological activity to brexpiprazole (Figure 2).
- Mean half-life 91 hours (brexpiprazole) and 86 hours (major metabolite DM-3411)

Pharmacogenetics

- The Clinical Pharmacogenetics Implementation Consortium (CPIC) does not provide dosing recommendations for brexpiprazole based on pharmacokinetic genes. However, in patients receiving a strong/moderate CYP3A4 inhibitor who are known CYP2D6 poor metabolizers, brexpiprazole should be administered at one-quarter the usual dose.

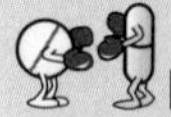

Drug Interactions

- In patients receiving a strong/moderate CYP3A4 inhibitor (e.g., ketoconazole),

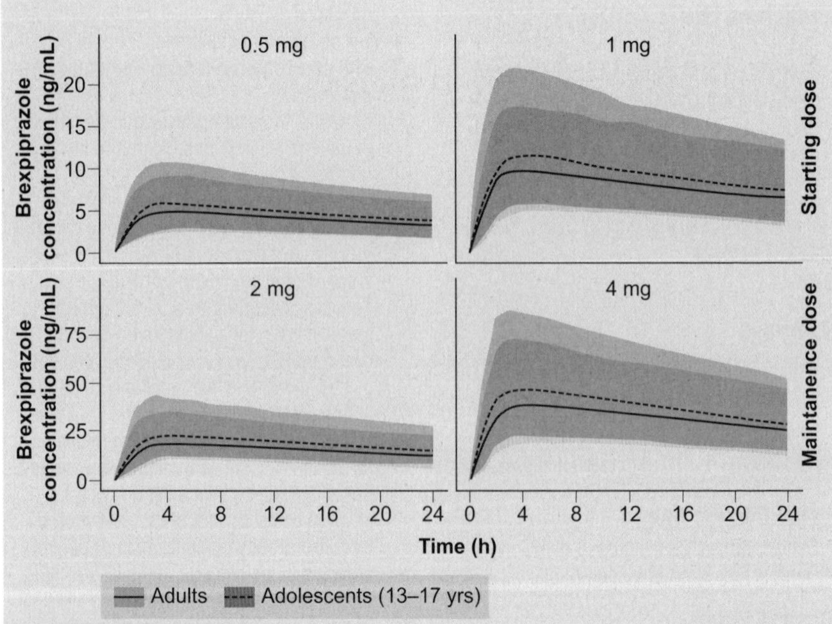

Figure 1 Brexpiprazole concentration–time curves for multiple doses of brexpiprazole in adolescents and adults.

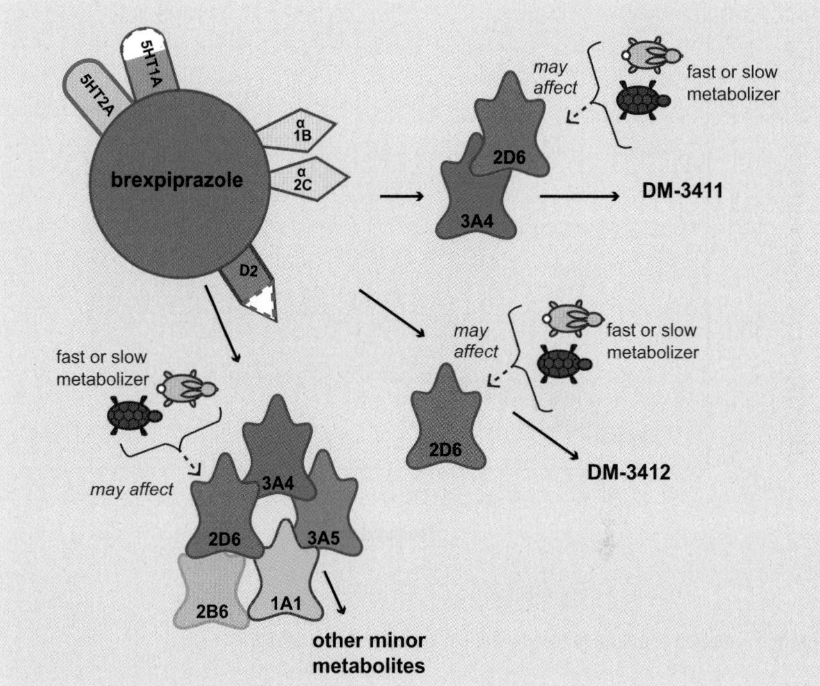

Figure 2 Metabolism of brexpiprazole.

brexpiprazole should be administered at half the usual dose

- In patients receiving a strong CYP3A4 inducer (e.g., carbamazepine), brexpiprazole should be administered at double the usual dose
- In patients with schizophrenia who are receiving a strong/moderate CYP2D6 inhibitor (e.g., quinidine) or who are known CYP2D6 poor metabolizers, brexpiprazole should be administered at half the usual dose
- However, clinical trials in major depressive disorder took into account the potential concomitant administration of strong CYP2D6 inhibitors (e.g., paroxetine, fluoxetine), so the dose of brexpiprazole does not need to be adjusted in these cases
- In patients receiving both a strong/moderate CYP3A4 inhibitor and a strong/moderate CYP2D6 inhibitor, brexpiprazole should be administered at one-quarter the usual dose
- In patients receiving a strong/moderate CYP3A4 inhibitor who are known CYP2D6 poor metabolizers, brexpiprazole should be administered at one-quarter the usual dose

Dosing Tips

- Children should generally be dosed at the lower end of the dosage spectrum when drug is initiated. Additionally, because the recommended titration is slower in adolescents compared to adults, adolescents will take longer to reach steady state (Figure 3).
- Can be taken with or without food
- For some, regardless of age, less may be more: frequently, patients not acutely psychotic may need to be dosed lower in order to avoid akathisia and activation and for maximum tolerability
- Due to its very long half-life, brexpiprazole will take longer to reach steady state when initiating dosing, and longer to wash out when stopping dosing, than most other atypical antipsychotics
- Treatment should be suspended if absolute neutrophil count falls below 1,000/mm^3

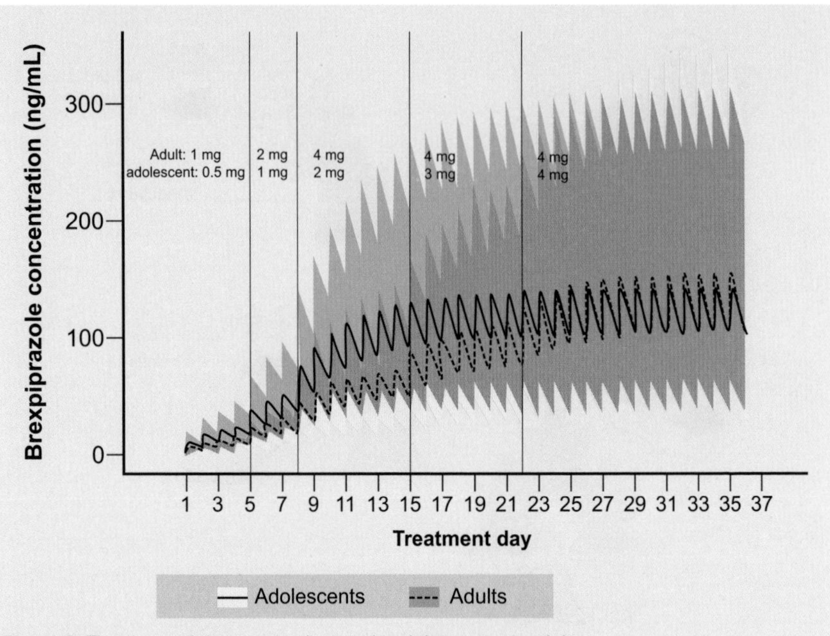

Figure 3 Titration and time to steady state in adolescents vs. adults.

How to Switch

- From another antipsychotic to brexpiprazole:
  - When tapering a prior antipsychotic, see its entry in this manual for how to stop and how to taper off that specific drug
  - Generally, try to stop the first agent before starting brexpiprazole so that new side effects of brexpiprazole can be distinguished from withdrawal effects of the first agent
  - If urgent, cross taper starting brexpiprazole while reducing the dose of the first agent for a few days, then further reduce or discontinue the first antipsychotic while increasing the dose of brexpiprazole as necessary and as tolerated
- From brexpiprazole to another antipsychotic:
  - Brexpiprazole tapers itself, so abrupt discontinuation leads to drug levels and active metabolite levels floating down slowly over 2–6 weeks while tapering up the dose of the new antipsychotic
  - Brexpiprazole has higher affinity for D2 receptors than many other antipsychotics have for D2 receptors, so the antipsychotic with the lower D2 affinity will not act fully until brexpiprazole is washed out

How to Stop

- Rapid discontinuation of any antipsychotic could theoretically lead to rebound psychosis and worsening of symptoms, but less likely with brexpiprazole due to its long half-life
- Taper rarely necessary since brexpiprazole tapers itself after immediate discontinuation, due to the long half-life of brexpiprazole and its active metabolites

Switching from Oral Antipsychotics to Brexpiprazole

target dose
dose
aripiprazole
cariprazine
brexpiprazole
1 week | 1 week | 1 week | 1 week

target dose
dose
iloperidone
lumateperone
lurasidone
paliperidone ER
risperidone
ziprasidone
brexpiprazole
1 week | 1 week | 1 week | 1 week

target dose
dose
asenapine
olanzapine
quetiapine
brexpiprazole
1 week | 1 week | 1 week | 1 week

target dose
dose
clozapine
brexpiprazole
1 week | 1 week | 1 week | 1 week

WHAT TO EXPECT

Onset of Action

- Psychotic and manic symptoms can improve within 1 week, but it may take several weeks for full effect on behavior as well as on cognition and affective stabilization
- If it is not working within 6–8 weeks, it may require a dosage increase or it may not work at all

Duration of Action

- Effects are consistent over a 24-hour period
- May continue to work for many years to prevent relapse of symptoms

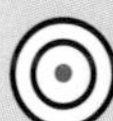

Primary Target Symptoms

- Positive symptoms of psychosis
- Negative symptoms of psychosis
- Manic symptoms
- Unstable mood and depression
- Aggressive symptoms
- Prior to initiation of treatment, it is helpful to develop a list of target symptoms of the underlying disorder specific for the patient being treated for monitoring to better assess treatment response

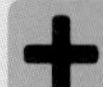

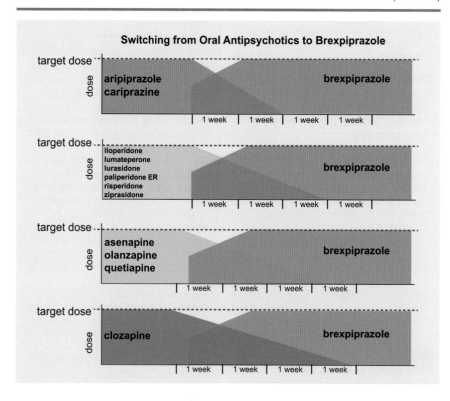

What Is Considered a Positive Result?

- In schizophrenia:
  - Most often reduces positive symptoms but does not eliminate them
  - Can improve negative symptoms, as well as aggressive, cognitive, and affective symptoms but less so than for positive symptoms
  - In children or adolescents with a first episode of psychosis, initial response may be greater than for recurrent episodes of psychosis in adults

How Long to Treat

- In schizophrenia:
  - Continue treatment until reaching a plateau of improvement
  - After reaching a satisfactory plateau, continue treatment for at least a year after first episode of psychosis

  - For second and subsequent episodes of psychosis, treatment may need to be indefinite

What If It Stops Working?

- Check for nonadherence, possibly by checking plasma drug level, and consider switching to another antipsychotic with fewer side effects
- Some patients who have an initial response may relapse even though they continue treatment, sometimes called "poop-out"
- Growth/developmental changes may contribute to apparent loss of efficacy as well as to new onset of side effects as metabolism slows and drug levels rise in transition from childhood to adolescence; dose adjustment (increase or decrease) should be considered
- Screen for the development of a new comorbid disorder, especially substance use
- Screen for adverse changes in the home or school environment

What If It Doesn't Work?

- Consider evaluation for another diagnosis (especially bipolar illness or depression with mixed features) or for a comorbid condition (e.g., medical illness, substance use)
- Consider other important potential factors such as ongoing conflicts, family psychopathology, and an adverse environment (e.g., inadequate school placement or educational services, bullying, poverty, chaos, violence, prior and ongoing psychological trauma, abuse, neglect)
- Institute trauma-informed care for appropriate children and adolescents
- For schizophrenia:
  - Try one of the other atypical antipsychotics
  - If no first-line atypical antipsychotic is effective, consider higher doses or augmentation with valproate, lithium, or lamotrigine
  - Consider initiating psychotherapy. In adolescents with bipolar disorder (and those with affective symptoms who are at risk of developing bipolar disorder), family-focused psychotherapy can be particularly helpful (Miklowitz et al., 2020).
  - Consider presence of concomitant drug abuse

TALKING TO PATIENTS AND CAREGIVERS

What to Tell Parents About Efficacy

- For acute symptoms, it can work right away
- Oral brexpiprazole is given every day
- Explain which use brexpiprazole is being chosen for, how to tell if the drug is working by targeting specific symptoms, and why this is being done
- Once the child/adolescent calms down, at some point after one dose or after several days of dosing or after long-term dosing, we should all assess whether the medication should be continued
- While the medicine helps by reducing symptoms and improving function, it is not a cure, and it therefore may be necessary to keep taking the medication long term to sustain its therapeutic effects
- Since every treatment consideration depends on a risk/benefit analysis, parents should fully understand short- and long-term risks as well as benefits
- There are several studies and a lot of clinical experience giving brexpiprazole to children and adolescents
- Often a good idea to tell parents whether the medication chosen is specifically approved for the disorder being treated, or whether it is being given for "unapproved" or "off-label" reasons based on good clinical practice, expert consensus, and/or prudent extrapolation of controlled data from adults

What to Tell Children and Adolescents About Efficacy

- Be specific about the symptoms being targeted: we are trying to help you …
- Give the medication a try; if it's not working very well, we can stop the medication and try something else
- A good try often takes several weeks
- If it does make you feel better, you cannot stop it right away or you may get sick again
- Medications don't change who you are as a person; they give you the opportunity to be the best person you can be

What to Tell Parents About Side Effects

- Explain that side effects are expected in many when starting

- Tell parents many side effects go away and do so about the same time that therapeutic effects start
- Predict side effects in advance (you will look clever and competent to the parents, unless you scare them with too much information and cause nocebo effects, in which case you won't look so clever when the patient develops lots of side effects and stops medication; use your judgment here); a balanced but honest presentation is an art rather than a science
- Ask parents to support the patient while side effects are occurring
- Parents should fully understand short- and long-term risks as well as benefits
- Explaining to the parents what to expect from medication treatment, and especially what potential side effects to expect, can help prevent early termination of medication

What to Tell Children and Adolescents About Side Effects

- Even if you get side effects, most of them get better or go away in a few weeks
- If you have side effects that are bothering you, tell your parents and your parents should tell me
- Consider having a conversation about sexual side effects in some adolescents who can find these side effects confusing and especially burdensome
- Explaining to child/adolescent what to expect from medication treatment, and especially potential side effects, can help prevent early termination of medication

What to Tell Teachers About the Medication (If Parents Consent)

- Brexpiprazole can make children/adolescents restless
- Brexpiprazole can make children/adolescents sedated
- It is not abusable
- Encourage dialogue with parents/guardians about any behavior or mood changes
- Notify the clinician of increased restlessness or akathisia symptoms, which may be apparent in the school setting

SPECIAL POPULATIONS

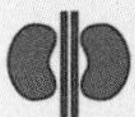

Renal Impairment

Moderate, severe, or end-stage (CrCl < 60 mL/minute): maximum recommended dose for depression is 2 mg once daily and for schizophrenia is 3 mg once daily

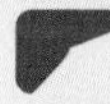

Hepatic Impairment

- Moderate to severe (Child–Pugh score ≥ 7): maximum recommended dose for depression is 2 mg once daily and for schizophrenia is 3 mg once daily

Cardiac Impairment

Use in patients with cardiac impairment has not been studied; however, the risk of orthostatic hypotension in pediatric patients is less than in adults, as children rely less on peripheral vasoconstriction to regulate blood pressure. In adolescents treated with brexpiprazole, approximately 11% experience orthostatic hypotension (registration trial).

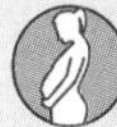

Pregnancy

- Controlled studies have not been conducted in pregnant women
- In animal studies, brexpiprazole did not demonstrate teratogenicity
- There is a risk of abnormal muscle movements and withdrawal symptoms in newborns whose mothers took an antipsychotic during the third trimester; symptoms may include agitation, abnormally increased or decreased muscle tone, tremor, sleepiness, severe difficulty breathing, and difficulty feeding
- Psychotic symptoms may worsen during pregnancy, and some form of treatment may be necessary
- Brexpiprazole may be preferable to anticonvulsant mood stabilizers if treatment is required during pregnancy
- National Pregnancy Registry for Atypical Antipsychotics: 1-866-961-2388 or http://womensmentalhealth.org/clinical-and-research-programs/pregnancyregistry/

Breast Feeding

- Unknown if brexpiprazole is secreted in human breast milk, but all psychotropics assumed to be secreted in breast milk

- Recommended either to discontinue drug or bottle feed
- Infants of women who choose to breast feed while on brexpiprazole should be monitored for possible adverse effects

THE ART OF PSYCHOPHARMACOLOGY

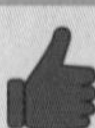

Potential Advantages

- Approved in adolescents (ages 13 to 17) for schizophrenia

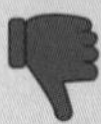

Potential Disadvantages

- In children:
  - Those who are already psychomotor agitated, angry, or irritable, and who do not have a psychiatric diagnosis
  - May be more susceptible to side effects
  - Those who have unacceptable weight gain
- In adolescents:
  - May be more susceptible to side effects
  - Those who have unacceptable weight gain
- All ages:
  - Patients in whom sedation is desired (many other antipsychotics are more sedating)

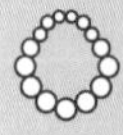

Pearls

- May have less weight gain in children/adolescents than some other atypical antipsychotics, but children/adolescents may have more weight gain on brexpiprazole than adults on brexpiprazole
- Approved in adults as an adjunct treatment for depression (e.g., to SSRIs, SNRIs), but not studied in children or adolescents
- Animal data suggest that brexpiprazole may improve cognitive impairment in schizophrenia
- In adults, brexpiprazole has shown evidence of efficacy especially in combination with sertraline for posttraumatic stress disorder
- Not approved for mania, but almost all atypical antipsychotics approved for acute treatment of schizophrenia have proven effective in the acute treatment of mania as well
- Pharmacological differences from aripiprazole suggest less akathisia with brexpiprazole, but no head-to-head trials
- Compared to aripiprazole, brexpiprazole has more potent binding of several receptor sites relative to dopamine 2 receptor binding, namely, 5HT1A, 5HT2A, and alpha 1 receptors; however, the clinical significance of these differences is still under investigation
- Partial agonist actions do not mean partial efficacy for psychosis, but anecdotally, brexpiprazole may be better positioned as a first-line antipsychotic for first episode or early-onset psychosis due to a good tolerability profile with good efficacy in many children/adolescents as well as adults
- However, for the most treatment-resistant patients with psychosis or mania, brexpiprazole may not anecdotally be as effective as some other antipsychotics such as clozapine or even olanzapine

SUGGESTED READING

ClinicalTrials.gov [Internet]. Bethesda (MD): National Library of Medicine (US). Identifier NCT03292848, Trial to assess the pharmacokinetics, safety, tolerability of oral brexpiprazole in children (6 to <13 years old) with central nervous system disorders; 2017 Oct 10 [cited 2022 Mar 25]. Available from: https://clinicaltrials.gov/ct2/show/NCT03292848?term=brexpiprazole&age=0&draw=2&rank=3

ClinicalTrials.gov [Internet]. Bethesda (MD): National Library of Medicine (US). Identifier NCT02411695, Study to assess the safety, tolerability and pharmacokinetics of oral brexpiprazole (OPC- 34712) in adolescents with schizophrenia; 2015 Mar [cited 2022 Mar 25]. Available from: https://clinicaltrials.gov/ct2/show/NCT02411695?term=brexpiprazole&age=0&draw=2&rank=6

Koch MT, Carlson HE, Kazimi MM, Correll CU. Antipsychotic-related prolactin levels and sexual dysfunction in mentally ill youth: a 3-month cohort-study. J Am Acad Child Adolesc Psychiatry 2023 ;62(9):1021–50.

Miklowitz DJ, Schneck CD, Walshaw PD et al. Effects of family-focused therapy vs enhanced usual care for symptomatic youths at high risk for bipolar disorder: a randomized clinical trial. JAMA Psychiatry 2020 1;77(5):455–63.

Pillay J, Boylan K, Carrey N et al. First- and Second-Generation Antipsychotics in Children and Young Adults: Systematic Review Update [Internet]. Rockville, MD: Agency for Healthcare Research and Quality (US); 2017 Mar. Report No.: 17-EHC001-EF. AHRQ Comparative Effectiveness Reviews.

THERAPEUTICS

Brands

- Aplenzin
- Wellbutrin
- Wellbutrin SR
- Wellbutrin XL
- Zyban

Generic

Yes

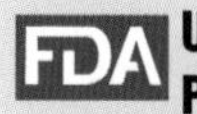

US FDA Approved for Pediatric Use

- None

Off-Label for Pediatric Use

- Approved in adults
  - Major depressive disorder (bupropion, bupropion SR, and bupropion XL)
  - Seasonal affective disorder (bupropion XL)
  - Nicotine addiction (bupropion SR)
- Other off-label uses
  - Bipolar depression
  - Attention deficit hyperactivity disorder (ADHD)
  - Sexual dysfunction

Class and Mechanism of Action

- Neuroscience-based Nomenclature: dopamine reuptake inhibitor and releaser (D-RIRe)
- NDRI (norepinephrine dopamine reuptake inhibitor); often classified as a drug for depression (i.e., antidepressant), but it is not just an antidepressant; smoking cessation treatment
- Bupropion presumably increases noradrenergic neurotransmission by blocking the norepinephrine reuptake pump (transporter), which results in desensitization of beta adrenergic receptors
- Since dopamine is inactivated by norepinephrine reuptake in the frontal cortex, which largely lacks dopamine transporters, bupropion can increase dopamine neurotransmission in this part of the brain
- Bupropion blocks the dopamine reuptake pump (dopamine transporter), presumably increasing dopaminergic neurotransmission

SAFETY AND TOLERABILITY

Notable Side Effects

- Dry mouth, constipation, nausea
- Insomnia, dizziness, headache, agitation, anxiety, tremor
- Sweating
- Weight loss, anorexia
- Myalgia, abdominal pain, tinnitus, rash
- Hypertension

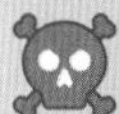

Life-Threatening or Dangerous Side Effects

- Rare seizures (higher incidence for immediate-release than for sustained-release; risk increases with doses above the recommended maximums; risk increases for patients with predisposing factors)
- Anaphylactoid/anaphylactic reactions and Stevens–Johnson syndrome have been reported
- Rare induction of mania
- Rare suicidal ideation and behavior (suicidality) (short-term regulatory studies did not show any actual suicides in any age group and also did not show an increase in the risk of suicidality with antidepressants compared to placebo beyond age 24)

Growth and Maturation

- Growth should be monitored; long-term effects are unknown

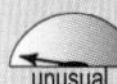

Weight Gain

- Reported but not expected
- May cause weight loss

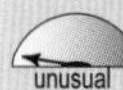

Sedation

- Reported but not expected

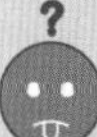

What to Do About Side Effects

- Wait, wait, wait: mild side effects are common, happen early, and usually improve with time, but treatment benefits can be delayed and often begin just as the side effects wear off
- Monitor side effects closely, especially when initiating treatment
- May wish to try dosing every other day to deal with side effects, or wash out for

a week and try again at half dose or every other day
- Keep dose as low as possible
- Take no later than mid-afternoon to avoid insomnia
- For activation (jitteriness, anxiety, insomnia):
  - Administer dose in the morning
  - Consider a temporary dose reduction or a more gradual up-titration
  - Consider switching to another antidepressant
  - Optimize psychotherapeutic interventions
  - Activation and agitation may represent the induction of a bipolar state, especially a mixed dysphoric bipolar II condition sometimes associated with suicidal ideation, and may require the addition of lithium or an atypical antipsychotic and/or discontinuation of bupropion
- Often best to try another monotherapy prior to resorting to augmentation strategies to treat side effects
- For insomnia: consider adding melatonin

How Drug Causes Side Effects

- Side effects are probably caused in part by actions of norepinephrine and dopamine in brain areas with undesired effects (e.g., insomnia, tremor, agitation, headache, dizziness)
- Side effects are probably also caused in part by actions of norepinephrine in the periphery with undesired effects (e.g., sympathetic and parasympathetic effects such as dry mouth, constipation, nausea, anorexia, sweating)

Warnings and Precautions

- Consider distributing brochures provided by the FDA and the drug companies as well as the medication guides from the American Academy of Child & Adolescent Psychiatry (AACAP)
- Carefully consider monitoring patients regularly within the practical limits, particularly during the first several weeks of treatment
- Warn patients and their caregivers when possible about the possibility of activating side effects and advise them to report such symptoms immediately
- Carefully weigh the risks and benefits of pharmacological treatment against the risks and benefits of nontreatment with antidepressants and it is a good idea to document this in the patient's chart
- Use cautiously with other drugs that increase seizure risk (TCAs, lithium, phenothiazines, thioxanthenes, some antipsychotics) or in patients with history of seizure
- Bupropion should be used with caution in patients taking levodopa or amantadine, as these agents can potentially enhance dopamine neurotransmission and be activating
- Do not use if patient has severe insomnia
- As with any antidepressant, use with caution in patients with bipolar disorder unless treated with concomitant mood-stabilizing agent
- Monitor patients for activation and suicidal ideation and involve parents/guardians
- Discontinuing smoking may lead to pharmacokinetic or pharmacodynamic changes in other drugs the patient is taking, which could potentially require dose adjustment

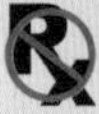

When Not to Prescribe

- Zyban or Aplenzin in combination with each other or with any formulation of bupropion
- If patient has history of seizures
- If patient is anorexic or bulimic, either currently or in the past, but see Pearls
- If patient is abruptly discontinuing alcohol, sedative use, or anticonvulsant medication
- If patient has had recent head injury
- If patient has a nervous system tumor
- If patient is taking an MAO inhibitor (except as noted under Drug Interactions)
- If patient is taking thioridazine
- Not generally recommended in patients taking tricyclic antidepressants (see Drug Interactions)
- If there is a proven allergy to bupropion

Long-Term Use

- Growth should be monitored; long-term effects are unknown

Habit Forming

- Not typically, but can be abused by individuals who crush and then snort or inject it

Overdose

- Rarely lethal; seizures, cardiac disturbances, hallucinations, loss of consciousness

DOSING AND USE

Usual Dosage Range

- Children may require lower doses initially, with a maximum dose of 300 mg/day
- Adolescent dosage may follow adult pattern:
  - Bupropion: 225–450 mg in 3 divided doses (maximum single dose 150 mg)
  - Bupropion SR: 200–400 mg in 2 divided doses (maximum single dose 200 mg)
  - Bupropion XL: 150–450 mg once daily (maximum single dose 450 mg)
  - Bupropion hydrobromide: 174–522 mg once daily (maximum single dose 522 mg)

Dosage Forms

- Bupropion: tablet 75 mg, 100 mg
- Bupropion SR (sustained-release): tablet 100 mg, 150 mg, 200 mg
- Bupropion XL (extended-release): tablet 150 mg, 300 mg, 450 mg
- Bupropion hydrobromide (extended-release): tablet 174 mg, 378 mg, 522 mg

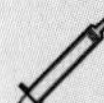

How to Dose

- Children may require lower doses initially; maximum dose 300 mg/day
- Dosage may follow adult pattern for adolescents:
  - Depression: for bupropion immediate-release, dosing should be in divided doses, starting at 75 mg twice daily, increasing to 100 mg twice daily, then to 100 mg 3 times daily; maximum dose 450 mg per day
  - Depression: for bupropion SR, initial dose 100 mg twice a day, increase to 150 mg twice a day after at least 3 days; wait 4 weeks or longer to ensure drug effects before increasing dose; maximum dose 400 mg total per day
  - Depression: for bupropion XL, initial dose 150 mg once daily in the morning; can increase to 300 mg once daily after 4 days; maximum single dose 450 mg once daily
  - Depression: for bupropion hydrobromide, initial dose 174 mg once daily in the morning; can increase to 522 mg administered as a single dose
  - Nicotine addiction: for bupropion SR, initial dose 150 mg/day once a day, increase to 150 mg twice a day after at least 3 days; maximum dose 300 mg/day; bupropion treatment should begin 1–2 weeks before smoking is discontinued

Options for Administration

- Generally, do not use immediate-release formulations for children/adolescents
- Best to use XL once-daily formulation; however, for dose titration or split doses for better tolerability, can use twice-a-day SR formulation

Tests

- Recommended to assess blood pressure at baseline and periodically during treatment
- Monitor weight and height against that expected for normal growth

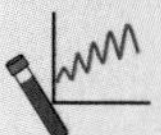

Pharmacokinetics

- Inhibits CYP2D6 and the primary enzyme involved in metabolism of bupropion to hydroxybupropion is CYP2B6 (Figure 1)
- Elimination half-life 10–14 hours in adults. In adolescents, the elimination half-life for the SR formulation is approximately 12 hours, while the half-life for the SR formulation is 16.5 hours.
- In adolescents, the time to maximum concentration (Tmax) is 3.4 hours for the SR formulation and 5 hours for the XL formulation (Figure 2)
- The maximum concentrations (Cmax) at steady state are higher for the XL formulation compared to the SR formulation in adolescents (Figure 2)
- In children and adolescents (ages 11–16), like in adults, bupropion pharmacokinetics are linear
- Relative to the SR formulation, the XL formulation produces more sustained levels of both parent compound and metabolites. For clinicians, this means that once-daily dosing of the XL formulation produces fewer fluctuations in plasma levels and more consistent exposure to bupropion and its metabolites (Daviss et al., 2006).
- Food does not affect absorption

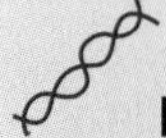

Pharmacogenetics

- Bupropion and its metabolites (erythrohydrobupropion, threohydrobupropion, hydroxybupropion)

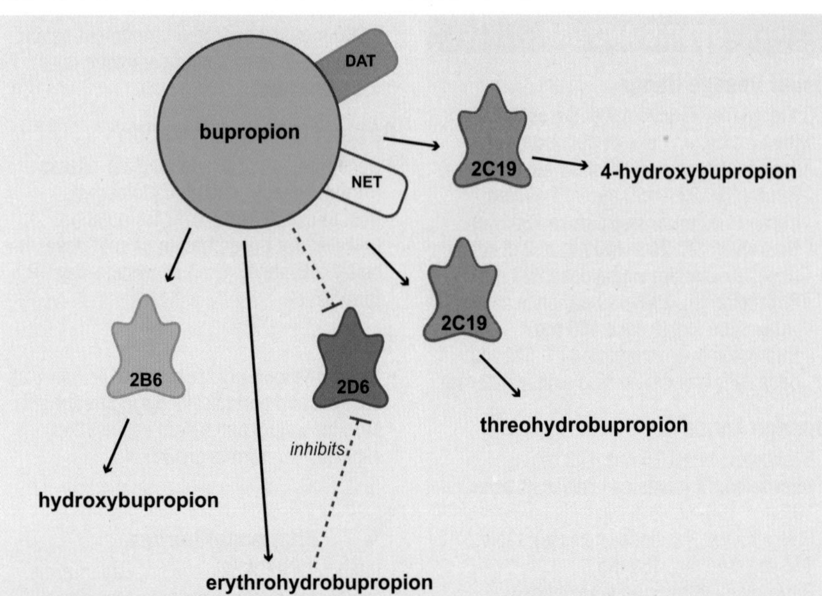

Figure 1 Metabolism of bupropion. Bupropion as well as its metabolite, erythrohydrobupriopion, inhibit CYP2D6.

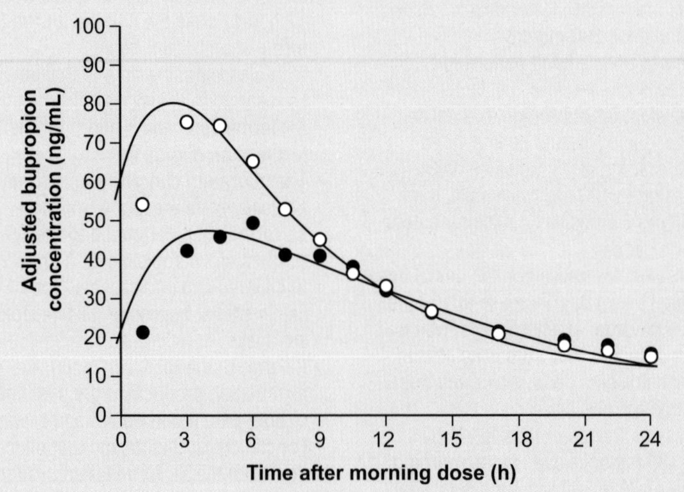

Figure 2 Concentration–time curves for bupropion SR and bupropion XL in adolescents. Open circles represent bupropion SR and closed circles represent concentrations in patients treated with the XL formulation. Adapted from Daviss et al., 2006.

are CYP2D6 inhibitors. Therefore, coadministration of bupropion with drugs that are metabolized by CYP2D6 can increase the exposure of drugs that are substrates of CYP2D6.

- The FDA-approved drug label for bupropion acknowledges that bupropion inhibits CYP2D6 and can affect the concentrations of CYP2D6 metabolized mediations, and recommends, "when used concomitantly with WELLBUTRIN, it may be necessary to decrease the dose of these CYP2D6 substrates, particularly for drugs with a narrow therapeutic index." However, while there are recommendations for several compounds containing bupropion (e.g., bupropion–dextromethorphan), there are no specific recommendations from the FDA to adjust the dose of bupropion in patients based on CYP2D6 or CYP2B6.

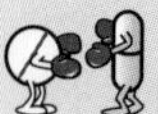

Drug Interactions

- Tramadol reported to increase the risk of seizures in adults taking an antidepressant
- Can increase tricyclic antidepressant levels; use with caution with tricyclic antidepressants or when switching from a TCA to bupropion
- Use with caution with MAO inhibitors, including 14 days after MAOIs are stopped (for the expert)
- There is increased risk of hypertensive reaction if bupropion is used in conjunction with MAO inhibitors or other drugs that increase norepinephrine
- There may be an increased risk of hypertension if bupropion is combined with nicotine replacement therapy
- Via CYP2D6 inhibition, bupropion could interfere with the analgesic actions of codeine and increase the plasma levels of some beta blockers, atomoxetine, and some other antidepressants like fluoxetine
- Via CYP2D6 inhibition, bupropion could theoretically increase concentrations of thioridazine and cause dangerous cardiac arrhythmias
- False-positive urine immunoassay screening tests for amphetamines have been reported in patients taking bupropion due to a lack of specificity of the screening tests. False-positive results may be expected for several days following the discontinuation of bupropion

Dosing Tips

- Adolescents often need and receive adult doses
- XL formulation has replaced immediate-release and SR formulations as the preferred option and should be administered once daily in the morning
- XL is best dosed once a day, whereas SR is best dosed twice daily, and immediate-release is best dosed 3 times daily. When using the SR formulation, giving the second dose no later than 5 pm may help to reduce bupropion-related insomnia.
- Dosing higher than 450 mg/day (400 mg/day SR) increases seizure risk
- Patients who do not respond to 450 mg/day should discontinue use or get blood levels of bupropion and its major active metabolite hydroxy-bupropion
- If levels of parent drug and active metabolite are low despite dosing at 450 mg/day, experts can prudently increase dosing beyond the therapeutic range while monitoring closely, informing the patient of the potential risk of seizures and weighing risk/benefit ratios in difficult-to-treat patients
- For smoking cessation, may be used in conjunction with nicotine replacement therapy
- Do not break or chew SR or XL tablets, as this will alter controlled-release properties
- The more anxious and agitated the patient, the lower the starting dose, the slower the titration
- If intolerable anxiety, insomnia, agitation, akathisia, or activation occurs either upon dosing initiation or discontinuation, consider the possibility of activated bipolar disorder and switch to an atypical antipsychotic or a mood stabilizer
- These symptoms may also indicate the need to evaluate for a mixed features episode and thus discontinuing bupropion and considering an atypical antipsychotic or lithium

How to Switch

- From another antidepressant to bupropion:
  - When tapering a prior antidepressant, see its entry in this manual for how to stop and how to taper off that specific drug
  - In situations when there are antidepressant-related side effects, try to stop the first agent before starting bupropion so that new side effects of bupropion can be distinguished from withdrawal effects of the first agent
  - If urgent, cross taper
- From bupropion to another antidepressant:
  - Generally, try to stop bupropion before starting another antidepressant. Bupropion may be more easily stopped compared to SSRIs in pediatric patients.
  - There are no well-documented tolerance, dependence, or withdrawal reactions

How to Stop

- Tapering can be considered, but no well-documented tolerance, dependence, or withdrawal reactions

WHAT TO EXPECT

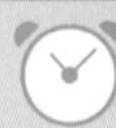

Onset of Action

- Some patients may experience increased energy or activation early after initiation of treatment
- Full onset of therapeutic actions is usually delayed by 2–4 weeks
- If it is not working within 6–8 weeks, it may require a dosage increase or it may not work at all

Duration of Action

- Effects are consistent over a 24-hour period
- May continue to work for many years to prevent relapse of symptoms

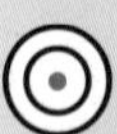

Primary Target Symptoms

- Depressed and/or irritable mood
- Hypersomnia
- Cravings associated with nicotine withdrawal
- Inattention/distractibility
- Prior to initiation of treatment, it is helpful to develop a list of target symptoms of depression and to monitor during treatment to better assess treatment response

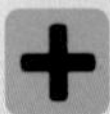

What Is Considered a Positive Result?

- The goal of treatment is complete remission of current symptoms as well as prevention of future relapses
- In practice, many patients have only a partial response where some symptoms are improved but others persist (especially insomnia, fatigue, and problems concentrating in depression), in which case higher doses of bupropion, adding a second agent, or switching to an agent with a different mechanism of action can be considered
- If treatment works, it most often reduces or even eliminates symptoms, but is not a cure since symptoms can recur after medicine is stopped

How Long to Treat

- For adolescents with depression, generally, 9–12 months of antidepressant treatment is recommended (Hathaway et al., 2018)
- For anxiety disorders, 6–9 months of antidepressant treatment may be sufficient, though many clinicians extend treatment to 12 months based on extrapolation of data from adults with anxiety disorders (Hathaway et al., 2018; Strawn et al., 2021)
- Extended treatment periods may decrease the risk of long-term morbidity and recurrence; however, the goal of treatment is ultimately remission, rather than duration of antidepressant pharmacotherapy (Hathaway et al., 2018)
- In terms of the length of antidepressant treatment, evidence-based guidelines represent a starting point; appropriate treatment duration varies, and patient-specific response, psychological factors, and timing of discontinuation must be considered for individual pediatric patients (Hathaway et al., 2018)

What If It Stops Working?

- Some patients who have an initial response may relapse even though they continue treatment, sometimes called "poop-out"
- Some patients may experience apparent lack of consistent efficacy due to activation syndrome or latent or underlying or newly evolved bipolar disorder, or major depressive episodes with mixed features of mania, and require antidepressant discontinuation and a switch to a second generation antipsychotic

What If It Doesn't Work?

- Consider evaluation for another diagnosis (especially bipolar illness or depression with mixed features) or for a comorbid condition (e.g., medical illness, substance abuse)
- When treating youth with anxiety disorders, many patients will have had significant anxiety for years prior to beginning treatment. As such, when anxiety is treated with an SSRI, their symptoms may be improved, but the patient has likely missed important developmental milestones (e.g., spending the night with friends, being able to ask questions in class). Developing these skills will take time. Beyond this, the family

may have lived with the anxious child for years and following treatment of the child, the family may need to readjust.

- Be mindful of family conflict contributing to the presentation; sometimes treating parental depression or anxiety disorders improves psychiatric and social function without any treatment of youth. Also, accommodation is common in families of youth with anxiety disorders and may need to be addressed specifically, as it can perpetuate symptoms.
- Consider factors associated with poor response to antidepressants in treatment-resistant depression or anxiety disorders, such as severe symptoms, long-lasting symptoms, poor treatment adherence, prior nonresponse to other treatments, and the presence of comorbid disorders
- Consider other important potential factors such as ongoing conflicts, family psychopathology, and an adverse environment (e.g., poverty, chaos, violence, prior and ongoing psychological trauma, abuse, neglect)
- Institute trauma-informed care for appropriate children and adolescents
- A 2007 meta-analysis of published and unpublished trials in pediatric patients found that antidepressants had a number needed to treat (NNT) of 10 for depression, 6 for OCD, and 3 for anxiety disorders (Bridge et al., 2007); thus, bupropion may not work in all children, so consider switching to another antidepressant
- Consider a dose adjustment
- Consider augmenting options:
  - Cognitive behavioral therapy (CBT), interpersonal psychotherapy for adolescents (IPT-A), light therapy, family therapy, and exercise especially in adolescents
  - For partial response (depression): use caution when adding medications to bupropion, especially in children since there are not sufficient studies of augmentation in children or adolescents; however, for the expert, consider SSRIs, SNRIs, aripiprazole, or other atypical antipsychotics such as quetiapine; use combinations of antidepressants with caution, as this may activate bipolar disorder and suicidal ideation
  - For insomnia: sleep hygiene, CBT for insomnia, melatonin, or alpha 2 agonists
  - For anxiety: buspirone, antihistamines
  - Add lithium or atypical antipsychotics for bipolar depression, psychotic depression, treatment-resistant depression, or treatment-resistant anxiety disorders
  - TMS (transcranial magnetic stimulation) may have a role although pediatric trials of TMS have been hampered by high sham response rates (Croarkin et al., 2021)
  - ECT (case studies show effectiveness; cognitive side effects are similar to those in adults; reserve for treatment-resistant cases)
- Can be added to SSRIs to reverse SSRI-induced sexual dysfunction, SSRI-induced apathy

TALKING TO PATIENTS AND CAREGIVERS

What to Tell Parents About Efficacy

- Doesn't work right away; full therapeutic benefits may take up to 8 weeks, yet parents and teachers might see improvement before the patient does
- While the medicine helps by reducing symptoms and improving function, it is not a cure, and it is therefore necessary to keep taking the medication to sustain its therapeutic effects
- Since every treatment consideration depends on a risk/benefit analysis, parents should fully understand short- and long-term risks as well as benefits
- After successful treatment, continuation of bupropion may be necessary to prevent relapse, especially in those who have had more than one episode or a very severe episode. In general, when treating depression in children and adolescents, medications are continued for 12 months after symptoms have resolved, while for anxiety disorders, clinicians have generally treated for 6–9 months (Hathaway et al., 2018).
- Often a good idea to tell parents whether the medication chosen is specifically approved for the disorder being treated, or whether it is being given for "unapproved" or "off-label" reasons based on good clinical practice, expert consensus, and/or prudent extrapolation of controlled data from adults

What to Tell Children and Adolescents About Efficacy

- We are trying to make you feel better
- It may be a good idea to give the medication a try; if it's not working very well, we can stop the medication and try something else
- A good try takes 2 to 3 months or even longer
- If it does make you feel better, you cannot stop it right away or you may feel sad or worried again
- Medications don't change who you are as a person; they give you the opportunity to be the best person you can be

What to Tell Parents About Side Effects

- Explain that side effects are expected in many when starting and are most common in the first 2–3 weeks of starting or increasing the dose
- Tell parents many side effects go away and do so about the same time that therapeutic effects start
- Predict side effects in advance (you will look clever and competent to the parents, unless you scare them with too much information and cause nocebo effects, in which case you won't look so clever when the patient develops lots of side effects and stops medication; use your judgment here); a balanced but honest presentation is an art rather than a science
- Ask them to help monitor for increased suicidality and if present, report any such symptoms immediately
- Ask parents to support the patient while side effects are occurring
- Parents should fully understand short- and long-term risks as well as benefits
- Explaining to the parents what to expect from medication treatment, and especially potential side effects, can help prevent early termination of medication

What to Tell Children and Adolescents About Side Effects

- Even if you get side effects, most of them get better or go away in a few days to a few weeks
- Consider having a conversation about sexual side effects in some adolescents who can find these side effects confusing and especially burdensome
- Explaining to child/adolescent what to expect from medication treatment, and especially potential side effects, can help prevent early termination of medication
- Tell adolescents and children capable of understanding that some young patients, especially those who are depressed, may develop thoughts of hurting themselves, and if this happens, not to be alarmed but to tell their parents right away

What to Tell Teachers About the Medication (If Parents Consent)

- Bupropion can make children/adolescents jittery or restless and may cause tremor, which may impact tasks requiring fine motor skills
- It may decrease appetite
- If the patient is sleepy, ask whether the medication is keeping them up at night
- It is not abusable
- Encourage dialogue with parents/guardians about any behavior or mood changes

SPECIAL POPULATIONS

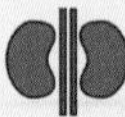

Renal Impairment

- Lower initial dose, perhaps give less frequently
- Drug concentration may be increased
- Patient should be monitored closely

Hepatic Impairment

- Lower initial dose, perhaps give less frequently
- Patient should be monitored closely
- In severe hepatic cirrhosis, bupropion XL should be administered at no more than 150 mg every other day

Cardiac Impairment

- Limited available data
- Evidence of rise in supine blood pressure
- Use with caution

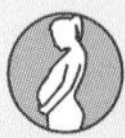

Pregnancy

- Controlled studies have not been conducted in pregnant women
- Epidemiological studies do not indicate increased risk of congenital malformations overall or of cardiovascular malformations

- In animal studies, no clear evidence of teratogenicity has been observed; however, slightly increased incidences of fetal malformations and skeletal variations were observed in rabbit studies at doses approximately equal to and greater than the maximum recommended human doses, and greater and decreased fetal weights were observed in rat studies at doses greater than the maximum recommended human doses
- Pregnant women wishing to stop smoking may consider behavioral therapy before pharmacotherapy
- Not generally recommended for use during pregnancy, especially during first trimester
- Must weigh the risk of treatment (first trimester fetal development, third trimester newborn delivery) to the child against the risk of no treatment (recurrence of depression, maternal health, infant bonding) to the mother and child
- For many patients, this may mean continuing treatment during pregnancy

Breast Feeding

- Some drug is found in breast milk
- If child becomes irritable or sedated, breast feeding or drug may need to be discontinued
- Immediate postpartum period is a high-risk time for depression, especially in women who have had prior depressive episodes, so drug may need to be reinstituted late in the third trimester or shortly after childbirth to prevent a recurrence during the postpartum period
- Must weigh benefits of breast feeding with risks and benefits of antidepressant treatment versus nontreatment to both the infant and the mother
- For many patients, this may mean continuing treatment during breast feeding

THE ART OF PSYCHOPHARMACOLOGY

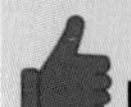

Potential Advantages

- In children and adolescents:
  - Might be useful for those not responding to SSRIs/SNRIs
  - Might be useful as an adjunct for treatment-resistant depression, particularly to address anergia, fatigue, and amotivation
  - Can be used off-label for ADHD and may be helpful in patients with co-occurring depression and ADHD
  - May be preferred for those who wish to avoid sexual dysfunction or sedation
- All ages:
  - Patients with atypical depression (hypersomnia, increased appetite)
  - Bipolar depression
  - Patients concerned about sexual dysfunction
  - Patients concerned about weight gain
  - Patients with seizure disorders

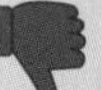

Potential Disadvantages

- In children and adolescents:
  - Those who are already psychomotor agitated, angry, or irritable, and who do not have a psychiatric diagnosis
  - Those who may possibly have a mood disorder with mixed or bipolar features, especially those with these features and a family history of bipolar disorder
- All ages:
  - Patients experiencing weight loss associated with their depression
  - Patients who are excessively activated

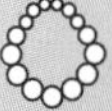

Pearls

- May be effective if SSRIs have failed or for SSRI "poop-out"
- Reduces hypersomnia and fatigue and may improve motivation
- Approved to help reduce craving during smoking cessation in adults, and some small studies suggest that it may have beneficial effects in adolescents with co-occurring substance use disorders and ADHD
- In network meta-analyses, bupropion is more effective than placebo in reducing ADHD symptoms (Cortese et al., 2018)
- May rarely cause sexual dysfunction and may be effective adjunctively in reducing sexual side effects in adults (Luft et al., 2018)
- May exacerbate tics
- Bupropion may not be as effective in pediatric anxiety disorders as SSRIs
- Extreme caution in eating disorders due to increased risk of seizures is related to past observations when bupropion immediate-release was dosed at especially high levels

to low body weight patients with active anorexia nervosa

- Current practice suggests that patients of normal BMI without additional risk factors for seizures can benefit from bupropion, especially if given prudent doses of the XL formulation; such treatment should be administered by experts, and patients should be monitored closely and informed of the potential risks
- As bromide salts have anticonvulsant properties, hydrobromide salts of bupropion could theoretically reduce risk of seizures, but this has not been proven

SUGGESTED READING

Bridge JA, Iyengar S, Salary CB et al. Clinical response and risk for reported suicidal ideation and suicide attempts in pediatric antidepressant treatment: a meta-analysis of randomized controlled trials. JAMA 2007;297(15):1683–96.

Cipriani A, Zhou X, Del Giovane C et al. Comparative efficacy and tolerability of antidepressants for major depressive disorder in children and adolescents: a network meta-analysis. Lancet 2016;388:881–90.

Cortese S, Adamo N, Del Giovane C et al. Comparative efficacy and tolerability of medications for attention-deficit hyperactivity disorder in children, adolescents, and adults: a systematic review and network meta-analysis. Lancet Psychiatry 2018;5(9):727–38.

Croarkin PE, Elmaadawi AZ, Aaronson ST et al. Left prefrontal transcranial magnetic stimulation for treatment-resistant depression in adolescents: a double-blind, randomized, sham-controlled trial. Neuropsychopharmacology 2021;46(2):462–9.

Daviss WB, Perel JM, Rudolph GR et al. Steady-state pharmaco- kinetics of bupropion SR in juvenile patients. J Am Acad Child Adolesc Psychiatry 2005;44:349Y357.

Daviss WB, Perel JM, Birmaher B et al. Steady-state clinical pharmacokinetics of bupropion extended-release in youths. J Am Acad Child Adolesc Psychiatry 2006;45(12):1503–9.

Hathaway EE, Walkup JT, Strawn JR. Antidepressant treatment duration in pediatric depressive and anxiety disorders: how long is long enough? Curr Probl Pediatr Adolesc Health Care 2018;48(2):31–9.

Luft MJ, Lamy M, DelBello MP, McNamara RK, Strawn JR. Antidepressant-induced activation in children and adolescents: risk, recognition and management. Curr Probl Pediatr Adolesc Health Care 2018;48(2):50–62.

Strawn JR, Lu L, Peris TS, Levine A, Walkup JR. Research review: pediatric anxiety disorders – what have we learnt in the last 10 years? J Child Psychol Psychiatry 2021;62(2):114–39.

Strawn JR, Mills JA, Poweleit EA, Ramsey LB, Croarkin PE. Adverse effects of antidepressant medications and their management in children and adolescents. Pharmacotherapy 2023;43(7):675–90.

THERAPEUTICS

Brands
- BuSpar

Generic
Yes

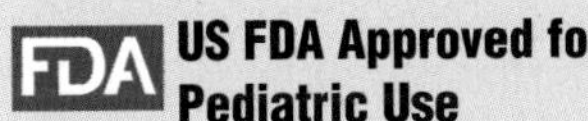

US FDA Approved for Pediatric Use
- None

Off-Label for Pediatric Use
- Approved in adults
  - Management of anxiety disorders
  - Short-term treatment of symptoms of anxiety
- Other off-label uses
  - Mixed anxiety and depression
  - Treatment-resistant depression (adjunctive)

Class and Mechanism of Action
- Neuroscience-based Nomenclature: serotonin receptor partial agonist (S-RPA)
- Anxiolytic (azapirone; serotonin 1A partial agonist; serotonin stabilizer)
- Binds to serotonin type 1A receptors
- Partial agonist actions postsynaptically may theoretically diminish serotonergic activity and contribute to anxiolytic actions
- Partial agonist actions at presynaptic somatodendritic serotonin autoreceptors may theoretically enhance serotonergic activity and contribute to antidepressant actions

SAFETY AND TOLERABILITY

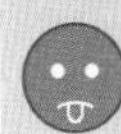

Notable Side Effects
- In the two double-blind, placebo-controlled trials of buspirone in youth, lightheadedness was the only adverse event that occurred more frequently in buspirone-treated patients than placebo-treated patients (10% vs. 2%, $p < 0.001$) (Strawn et al., 2018)

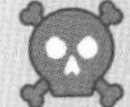

Life-Threatening or Dangerous Side Effects
- Side-effect profile is mild

Growth and Maturation
- Not studied

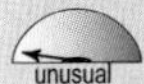

Weight Gain
- Reported but not expected

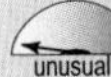

Sedation
- Reported but not expected

What to Do About Side Effects
- Wait, wait, wait: mild side effects are common, happen early, and usually improve with time, but treatment benefits can be delayed and often begin just as the side effects wear off
- Monitor side effects closely, especially when initiating treatment
- Give total daily dose divided into 3, 4, or more doses
- Often best to try another monotherapy prior to resorting to augmentation strategies to treat side effects
- For activation (jitteriness, anxiety, insomnia):
  - Consider a temporary dose reduction or a more gradual up-titration
  - Consider switching to an SSRI or potentially an SNRI (other than venlafaxine)
  - Optimize psychotherapeutic interventions
  - Activation and agitation may represent the induction of a bipolar state, especially a mixed dysphoric bipolar II condition sometimes associated with suicidal ideation, and may require the addition of lithium, or an atypical antipsychotic, and/or discontinuation of buspirone
- For GI upset: try giving medication with a meal (absorption is affected by food, so administration with or without food should be consistent)

How Drug Causes Side Effects
- Serotonin partial agonist actions in parts of the brain and body and at receptors other than those that cause therapeutic actions

Warnings and Precautions
- Although the side-effect profile of buspirone is mild, patients may experience dizziness or lightheadedness

When Not to Prescribe

- If patient is taking an MAO inhibitor (except as noted under Drug Interactions)
- If there is a proven allergy to buspirone

Long-Term Use

- Not studied

Habit Forming

- No

Overdose

- No deaths reported in monotherapy; sedation, dizziness, small pupils, nausea, vomiting

DOSING AND USE

Usual Dosage Range

- 10–30 mg/day divided in two doses

Dosage Forms

- Tablet 5 mg scored, 7.5 mg, 10 mg scored, 15 mg multiscored, 30 mg multiscored

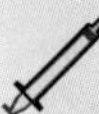

How to Dose

- Initial dose 5 mg/day twice daily; increase in 5 mg/day increments every 2–3 days until desired efficacy is reached

Options for Administration

- Tablets are scored so they can be bisected (5 mg, 10 mg, 15 mg, and 30 mg tablets) or trisected (15 mg, 30 mg tablets)

Tests

- None for healthy individuals

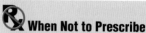

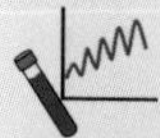

Pharmacokinetics

- Buspirone is well absorbed from the gastrointestinal tract, but its bioavailability is relatively low and highly variable, ranging from 5% to 60% due to extensive first-pass metabolism in the liver
- Buspirone's absorption in children, adolescents, and adults was rapid, with peak plasma concentrations generally attained around 1–1½ hours following administration (Salazar et al., 2001; Strawn et al., 2018)
- Food can delay the absorption of buspirone, but it does not significantly affect the overall extent of absorption
- Buspirone has a moderate protein binding of approximately 95%. It is widely distributed throughout the body, including the CNS, and crosses the blood–brain barrier. The drug has a relatively large volume of distribution, indicating extensive tissue distribution.
- Buspirone undergoes extensive hepatic metabolism, primarily via CYP3A4 (Figure 1)
- Buspirone is primarily metabolized into an active metabolite called 1-pyrimidinylpiperazine (1-PP). 1-PP is thought to contribute to buspirone's pharmacological effects, as it has affinity for serotonin receptors.
- As the dose of buspirone is titrated from 7.5 mg bid to 30 mg bid in children and adolescents, the total exposure for buspirone increased in a ratio greater than the dose increment in all groups, consistent with the current labeling for buspirone that indicates nonlinear pharmacokinetics (Salazar et al., 2001)

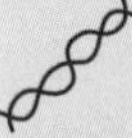

Pharmacogenetics

- No recommendations

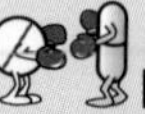

Drug Interactions

- Use with caution with MAO inhibitors, including 14 days after MAOIs are stopped (for the expert)
- CYP3A4 inhibitors (e.g., fluxotine, fluvoxamine, nefazodone) may reduce clearance of buspirone and raise its plasma levels, so the dose of buspirone may need to be lowered when given concomitantly with these agents
- CYP3A4 inducers (e.g., carbamazepine) may increase clearance of buspirone, so the dose of buspirone may need to be raised
- Buspirone may increase plasma concentrations of haloperidol
- Buspirone may raise levels of nordiazepam, the active metabolite of diazepam, which may result in increased symptoms of dizziness, headache, or nausea

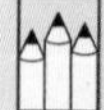

Dosing Tips

- Requires dosing 2–3 times a day for full effect
- Absorption is affected by food, so administration with or without food should be consistent

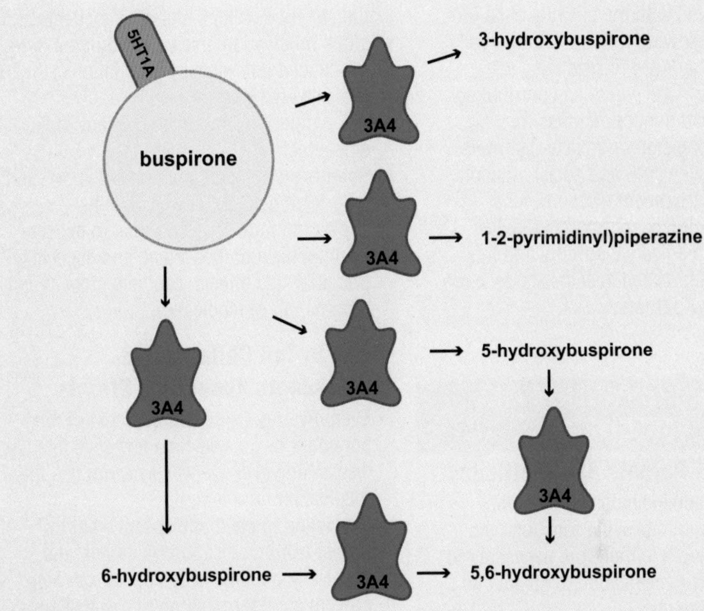

Figure 1 Buspirone metabolism.

How to Switch

- Taper generally not necessary

How to Stop

- Taper generally not necessary

WHAT TO EXPECT

Onset of Action

- Full onset of therapeutic actions is usually delayed by 2–4 weeks
- If it is not working within 6–8 weeks, it may require a dosage increase or it may not work at all

Duration of Action

- Effects are consistent over a 24-hour period

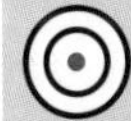

Primary Target Symptoms

- Anxiety

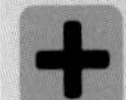

What Is Considered a Positive Result?

- The goal of treatment for anxiety is complete remission of current symptoms as well as prevention of future relapses
- If treatment works, it most often reduces or even eliminates symptoms, but is not a cure since symptoms can recur after medicine is stopped

How Long to Treat

- In general, for antidepressant therapy in anxious youth, treatment should be 9–12 months. A similar time frame for buspirone is reasonable.

What If It Stops Working?

- If anxiety symptoms reemerge, consider an SSRI, and re-trying psychotherapeutic approaches

What If It Doesn't Work?

- Consider a trial of an SSRI
- When treating youth with anxiety disorders, many patients will have had significant anxiety for years prior to beginning treatment. As such, when anxiety is treated with buspirone, their symptoms may be improved, but the patient has likely missed important developmental milestones (e.g., spending the night with friends, being able to ask questions in class). Developing these skills will take time. Beyond this, the family

may have lived with the anxious child for years and following treatment of the child, the family may need to readjust.
- Be mindful of family conflict contributing to the presentation; sometimes treating parental depression or anxiety disorders improves psychiatric and social function without any treatment of youth. Also, accommodation is common in families of youth with anxiety disorders and may need to be addressed specifically, as it can perpetuate symptoms.

TALKING TO PATIENTS AND CAREGIVERS

What to Tell Parents About Efficacy

- While the medicine helps by reducing symptoms and improving function, it is not a cure, and it is therefore necessary to keep taking the medication to sustain its therapeutic effects
- Since every treatment consideration depends on a risk/benefit analysis, parents should fully understand short- and long-term risks as well as benefits
- Often a good idea to tell parents whether the medication chosen is specifically approved for the disorder being treated, or whether it is being given for "unapproved" or "off-label" reasons based on good clinical practice, expert consensus, and/or prudent extrapolation of controlled data from adults

What to Tell Children and Adolescents About Efficacy

- We are trying to make you feel better
- It may be a good idea to give the medication a try; if it's not working very well, we can stop the medication and try something else
- Medications don't change who you are as a person; they give you the opportunity to be the best person you can be

What to Tell Parents About Side Effects

- Explain that mild side effects are expected at initiation or when increasing the dose and are usually transitory
- Predict side effects in advance (you will look clever and competent to the parents, unless you scare them with too much information and cause nocebo effects, in which case you won't look so clever when the patient develops lots of side effects and stops medication; use your judgment here); a balanced but honest presentation is an art rather than a science
- Ask parents to support the patient while side effects are occurring
- Parents should fully understand short- and long-term risks as well as benefits
- Explaining to the parents what to expect from medication treatment, and especially potential side effects, can help prevent early termination of medication

What to Tell Children and Adolescents About Side Effects

- Even if you get side effects, most of them get better or go away in a few days to a few weeks; however, we will likely not use this medication for a long time
- Explaining to child/adolescent what to expect from medication treatment, and especially potential side effects, can help prevent early termination of medication

What to Tell Teachers About the Medication (If Parents Consent)

- Buspirone can make children/adolescents lightheaded or dizzy
- It is not abusable
- Encourage dialogue with parents/guardians about any behavior or mood changes

SPECIAL POPULATIONS

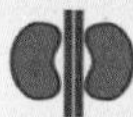

Renal Impairment

- Use with caution
- Not recommended for patients with severe renal impairment

Hepatic Impairment

- Use with caution
- Not recommended for patients with severe hepatic impairment

Cardiac Impairment

- Not systematically evaluated in patients with cardiac impairment

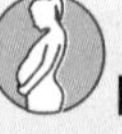

Pregnancy

- Controlled studies have not been conducted in pregnant women

- Animal studies have not shown adverse effects
- Not generally recommended for use during pregnancy
- National Pregnancy Registry for Psychiatric Medications: 1-866-961-2388 or https://womensmentalhealth.org/research/pregnancyregistry/

Breast Feeding

- Some drug is found in breast milk
- Trace amounts may be present in nursing children whose mothers are on buspirone
- If child becomes irritable or sedated, breast feeding or drug may need to be discontinued

THE ART OF PSYCHOPHARMACOLOGY

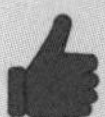

Potential Advantages

- Favorable safety and tolerability profile
- Lack of sexual dysfunction or weight gain

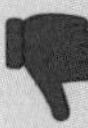

Potential Disadvantages

- Likely much less effective than SSRIs for anxiety

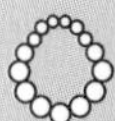

Pearls

- Buspirone is generally well tolerated in pediatric patients with anxiety disorders and has a side-effect profile that is consistent with the known tolerability profile of buspirone in adults (Goldberg and Finnerty 1979; Lader and Scotto 1998)
- Buspirone is associated with discontinuation rates similar to SSRIs and SNRIs in pediatric patients with anxiety disorders (Dobson et al., 2019); however, pediatric trials of buspirone suffered from a high placebo response rate and were underpowered to detect small treatment effects for buspirone in youth with GAD

SUGGESTED READING

Dobson ET, Bloch MH, Strawn JR. Efficacy and tolerability of pharmacotherapy for pediatric anxiety disorders: a network meta-analysis. J Clin Psychiatry 2019;80(1):17r12064.

Goldberg HL, Finnerty RJ. The comparative efficacy of buspirone and diazepam in the treatment of anxiety. Am J Psychiatry 1979;136(9):1184–7.

Lader M, Scotto JC. A multicentre double-blind comparison of hydroxyzine, buspirone and placebo in patients with generalized anxiety disorder. Psychopharmacology (Berl) 1998;139(4):402–6.

Nicotra CM, Strawn JR. Advances in pharmacotherapy for pediatric anxiety disorders. Child Adolesc Psychiatr Clin N Am 2023;32(3):573–87.

Salazar DE, Frackiewicz EJ, Dockens R et al. Pharmacokinetics and tolerability of buspirone during oral administration to children and adolescents with anxiety disorder and normal healthy adults. J Clin Pharmacol 2001;41(12):1351–8.

Strawn JR, Mills JA, Cornwall GJ et al. Buspirone in children and adolescents with anxiety: a review and Bayesian analysis of abandoned randomized controlled trials. J Child Adolesc Psychopharmacol 2018;28(1):2–9.

CARBAMAZEPINE

THERAPEUTICS

Brands

- Carbatrol
- Equetro
- Tegretol

Generic

Yes

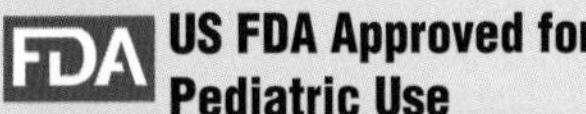

US FDA Approved for Pediatric Use

- Partial seizures with complex symptomatology
- Generalized tonic-clonic seizures (grand mal)
- Mixed seizure patterns

Off-Label for Pediatric Use

- Approved in adults
  - Pain associated with true trigeminal neuralgia
  - Acute mania/mixed mania (Equetro)
- Other off-label uses
  - Glossopharyngeal neuralgia
  - Bipolar depression
  - Bipolar maintenance
  - Psychosis, schizophrenia (adjunctive)

Class and Mechanism of Action

- Anticonvulsant, voltage-sensitive sodium channel modulator
- Acts as a use-dependent blocker of voltage-sensitive sodium channels
- Interacts with the open channel conformation of voltage-sensitive sodium channels
- Interacts at a specific site of the alpha pore-forming subunit of voltage-sensitive sodium channels
- Inhibits release of glutamate

SAFETY AND TOLERABILITY

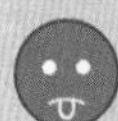

Notable Side Effects

- Sedation, dizziness, unsteadiness, confusion
- Nausea, vomiting, constipation, dry mouth
- Blurred vision
- Benign leukopenia (transient; in up to 10%)
- Rash

Life-Threatening or Dangerous Side Effects

- Rare aplastic anemia, agranulocytosis (unusual bleeding or bruising, mouth sores, infections, fever, sore throat)
- Rare severe dermatological reactions (purpura, Stevens–Johnson syndrome)
- Rare anaphylaxis and angioedema
- Rare cardiac problems
- Rare induction of psychosis or mania
- Syndrome of inappropriate antidiuretic hormone secretion (SIADH) with hyponatremia
- Increased frequency of generalized convulsions (in patients with atypical absence seizures)
- Rare activation of suicidal ideation and behavior (suicidality)

Growth and Maturation

- Not studied

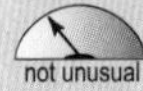

Weight Gain

- Occurs in significant minority

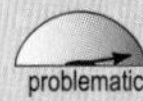

Sedation

- Frequent and can be significant in amount
- Some patients may not tolerate it
- Dose related
- Can wear off with time, but commonly does not wear off at high doses
- CNS side effects significantly lower with controlled-release formulation (e.g., Equetro, Carbatrol)

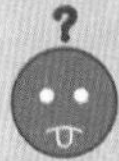

What to Do About Side Effects

- Wait
- Wait
- Wait
- Take with food or split dose to avoid gastrointestinal effects
- Extended-release carbamazepine can be sprinkled on soft food
- Take at night to reduce daytime sedation
- Switch to another agent or to extended-release carbamazepine

How Drug Causes Side Effects

- CNS side effects theoretically due to excessive actions at voltage-sensitive sodium channels

- Major metabolite (carbamazepine-10, 11 epoxide) may be the cause of many side effects
- Mild anticholinergic effects may contribute to sedation, blurred vision

Warnings and Precautions

- Patients should be monitored carefully for signs of unusual bleeding or bruising, mouth sores, infections, fever, or sore throat, as the risk of aplastic anemia and agranulocytosis with carbamazepine use is 5–8 times greater than in the general population (risk in the untreated general population is 6 patients per 1 million per year for agranulocytosis and 2 patients per 1 million per year for aplastic anemia)
- Because carbamazepine has a tricyclic chemical structure, use with caution with MAO inhibitors, including 14 days after MAOIs are stopped (for the expert)
- May exacerbate angle-closure glaucoma
- Because carbamazepine can lower plasma levels of hormonal contraceptives, it may also reduce their effectiveness
- Use with caution in patients with mixed seizure disorders that include atypical absence seizures because carbamazepine has been associated with increased frequency of generalized convulsions in such patients
- Individuals with the HLA-B*1502 allele are at increased risk of developing Stevens–Johnson syndrome and toxic epidermal necrolysis
- Warn patients and their caregivers about the possibility of activation of suicidal ideation and advise them to report such side effects immediately

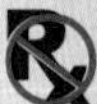

When Not to Prescribe

- If patient has history of bone marrow suppression
- If patient tests positive for the HLA-B*1502 allele
- If there is a proven allergy to carbamazepine
- Suspension: in patients with hereditary problems with fructose intolerance

Long-Term Use

- May lower sex drive
- Monitoring of liver, kidney, thyroid functions, blood counts, and sodium may be required

Habit Forming

- No

Overdose

- Can be fatal (lowest known fatal dose in adults is 3.2 g, in adolescents is 4 g, and in children is 1.6 g); nausea, vomiting, involuntary movements, arrhythmia, urinary retention, trouble breathing, sedation, coma

DOSING AND USE

Usual Dosage Range

- 400–1,200 mg/day
- Under age 6: 10–20 mg/kg per day

Dosage Forms

- Tablet 100 mg, 200 mg, 300 mg, 400 mg
- Chewable tablet 100 mg, 200 mg
- Extended-release tablet 100 mg, 200 mg, 400 mg
- Extended-release capsule 100 mg, 200 mg, 300 mg
- Oral solution 100 mg/5 mL

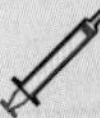

How to Dose

- Therapeutic range of total carbamazepine in plasma is considered the same for children and adults
- For bipolar disorder and seizures (ages 13 and older): initial 200 mg twice daily (tablet) or 1 teaspoon (100 mg) 4 times a day (suspension); each week increase by up to 200 mg/day in divided doses (2 doses for extended-release formulation, 3–4 doses for other tablets); maximum dose generally 1,200 mg/day for adults and 1,000 mg/day for children under age 15; maintenance dose generally 800–1,200 mg/day for adults; some patients may require up to 1,600 mg/day
- Seizures, ages 6–12: initial dose 100 mg twice daily (tablets) or 0.5 teaspoon (50 mg) 4 times a day (suspension); each week increase by up to 100 mg/day in divided doses (2 doses for extended-release formulation, 3–4 doses for all other formulations); maximum dose generally 1,000 mg/day; maintenance dose generally 400–800 mg/day
- Seizures, ages 5 and younger: initial 10–20 mg/kg per day in divided doses (2–3 doses for tablet formulations, 4 doses for

suspension); increase weekly as needed; maximum dose generally 35 mg/kg/day
- Trigeminal neuralgia: initial 100 mg twice daily (tablet) or 0.5 teaspoon (50 mg) 4 times a day; each week increase by up to 200 mg/day in divided doses (100 mg every 12 hours for tablet formulations, 50 mg 4 times a day for suspension formulation); maximum dose generally 1,200 mg/day
- Lower initial dose and slower titration should be used for carbamazepine suspension

Options for Administration

- Extended-release capsule contents can be sprinkled on food

Tests

- Before starting: blood count and liver, kidney, and thyroid function tests
- During treatment: blood count every 2–4 weeks for 2 months, then every 3–6 months throughout treatment
- During treatment: liver, kidney, and thyroid function tests every 6–12 months
- Consider monitoring sodium levels because of possibility of hyponatremia
- Before starting: individuals with ancestry across broad areas of Asia should consider screening for the presence of the HLAB*1502 allele; those with HLA-B*1502 should not be treated with carbamazepine

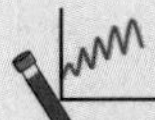

Pharmacokinetics

- Bioavailability of carbamazepine in children is about 75–85%, and it is approximately 75–85% bound to plasma proteins
- Is not only a substrate for CYP3A4, but also an inducer of CYP3A4. Maximal autoinduction usually occurs 2–3 weeks after starting. Because of the autoinduction, the ultimate maintenance dose can't be started as the initial dose. Additional autoinduction occurs with subsequent increases in dose (Figure 1).
- Carbamazepine is extensively metabolized primarily by CYP3A4 and CYP2C8. These metabolic processes lead to the formation of several active and inactive metabolites, including the active metabolite carbamazepine-10,11 epoxide (Figure 2).
- Elimination of carbamazepine and its metabolites primarily occurs through the kidneys
- Initial half-life 26–65 hours (35–40 hours for extended-release formulation); half-life decreases to 12–17 hours with repeated doses
- Half-life of active metabolite is approximately 34 hours
- Thus, carbamazepine induces its own metabolism, often requiring an upward dosage adjustment
- Is also an inducer of CYP2C9 and weakly of 1A2 and 2C19

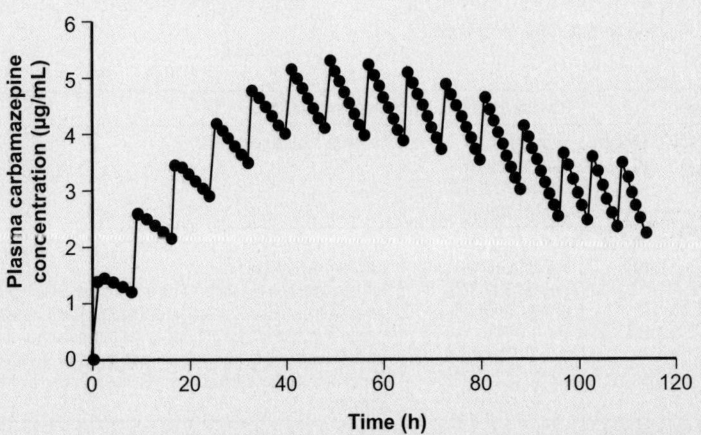

Figure 1 Carbamazepine concentration–time curve showing autoinduction of CYP3A4. As autoinduction occurs. Maximimal autoinduction generally occurs 2-3 weeks after beginning carbamazepine.

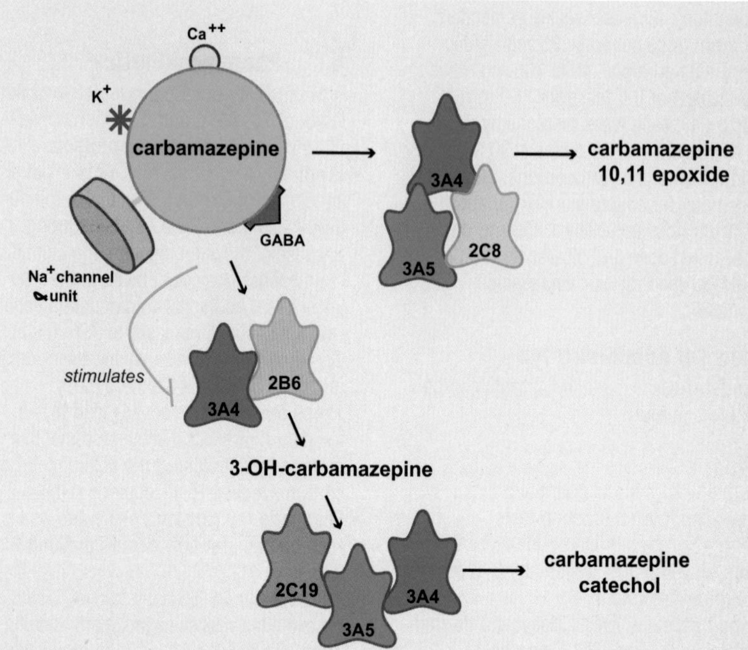

Figure 2 Carbamazepine metabolism. Carbamazepine is a strong inducer of CYP3A4.

- Food does not affect absorption

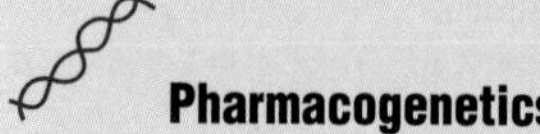

Pharmacogenetics

- Before starting: individuals with ancestry across broad areas of Asia should consider screening for the presence of the HLAB*1502 allele. See accompanying table.

Drug Interactions

- Enzyme-inducing antiepileptic drugs (carbamazepine itself as well as phenobarbital, phenytoin, and primidone) may increase the clearance of carbamazepine and lower its plasma levels

Genotype	Risk implication	Recommendation
HLAB*1502 negative and HLA-A*3101 negative	Normal risk of carbamazepine-induced SJS/TEN, DRESS, and MPE	Standard dosing guidelines
HLAB*1502 negative and HLA-A*3101 positive	Greater risk of carbamazepine-induced SJS/TEN, DRESS, and MPE	Carbamazepine-naïve patients for whom alternative agents are available: do not use Carbamazepine-naïve patients for whom alternative agents are not available: consider using carbamazepine with increased monitoring; discontinue at first sign of cutaneous reactions For patients who have previously used carbamazepine for >3 months without cutaneous adverse reactions, cautiously consider
HLAB*1502 positive and any HLA-A*3101	Greater risk of carbamazepine-induced SJS/TEN	Carbamazepine-naïve patients: do not use For patients previously treated with carbamazepine for >3 months without cutaneous reactions, cautiously consider

Abbreviations: DRESS: Drug Reaction with Eosinophilia and Systemic Symptoms; MPE: maculopapular exanthema; SJS/TENS: Stevens–Johnson syndrome/toxic epidermal necrolysis

- CYP3A4 inducers, such as carbamazepine itself, can lower the plasma levels of carbamazepine
- CYP3A4 inhibitors (nefazodone, fluvoxamine, fluoxetine, and others) can increase plasma levels of carbamazepine
- Carbamazepine can increase plasma levels of clomipramine, phenytoin, primidone
- Carbamazepine decreases plasma levels of acetaminophen, clozapine, some benzodiazepines, dicumarol, doxycycline, theophylline, warfarin, rivaroxaban, apixaban, dabigatran, edoxaban, and haloperidol as well as other anticonvulsants such as phensuximide, methsuximide, ethosuximide, phenytoin, tiagabine, topiramate, lamotrigine, and valproate
- Carbamazepine can decrease plasma levels of hormonal contraceptives and reduce their efficacy
- Combined use of carbamazepine with other anticonvulsants may lead to altered thyroid function
- Combined use of carbamazepine and lithium may increase risk of neurotoxic effects
- Depressive effects are increased by other CNS depressants (alcohol, MAOIs, other anticonvulsants, etc.)
- Combined use of carbamazepine suspension with liquid formulations of chlorpromazine has been shown to result in excretion of an orange rubbery precipitate; because of this, combined use of carbamazepine suspension with any liquid medicine is not recommended

Dosing Tips

- Higher peak levels occur with the suspension formulation than with the same dose of the tablet formulation, so suspension should generally be started at a lower dose and titrated slowly
- Take carbamazepine with food to avoid gastrointestinal effects
- Slow-dose titration may delay onset of therapeutic action but enhance tolerability to sedating side effects
- Controlled-release formulations (e.g., Equetro, Carbatrol) can significantly reduce sedation and other CNS side effects
- Should titrate slowly in the presence of other sedating agents, such as other anticonvulsants, in order to best tolerate additive sedative side effects
- Can sometimes minimize the impact of carbamazepine upon the bone marrow by dosing slowly and monitoring closely when initiating treatment; initial trend to leukopenia/neutropenia may reverse with continued conservative dosing over time and allow subsequent dosage increases with careful monitoring
- Carbamazepine often requires a dosage adjustment upward with time, as the drug induces its own metabolism, thus lowering its own plasma levels over the first several weeks to months of treatment (Figure 2)
- Do not break or chew carbamazepine extended-release tablets, as this will alter controlled-release properties

How to Switch

- From another medication to carbamazepine:
  - When tapering a prior medication, see its entry in this manual for how to stop and how to taper off that specific drug
  - Generally, try to stop the first agent before starting carbamazepine so that new side effects of carbamazepine can be distinguished from withdrawal effects of the first agent
  - If urgent, cross taper
- Off carbamazepine to another medication:
  - Generally, try to stop carbamazepine before starting the new medication so that new side effects of the next drug can be distinguished from any withdrawal effects from carbamazepine
  - Taper; may need to adjust dosage of concurrent medications as carbamazepine is being discontinued
  - If urgent, cross taper

How to Stop

- Taper; may need to adjust dosage of concurrent medications as carbamazepine is being discontinued
- Rapid discontinuation may increase the risk of relapse in bipolar disorder
- Epilepsy patients may seize upon withdrawal, especially if withdrawal is abrupt
- Discontinuation symptoms uncommon

WHAT TO EXPECT

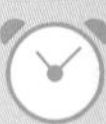

Onset of Action

- For acute mania, effects should occur within a few weeks
- May take several weeks to months to optimize an effect on mood stabilization
- Should reduce seizures by 2 weeks

Duration of Action

- Effects are consistent over a 24-hour period
- May continue to work for many years to prevent relapse of symptoms

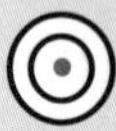

Primary Target Symptoms

- Incidence of seizures
- Unstable mood, especially mania
- Pain

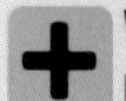

What Is Considered a Positive Result?

- The goal of treatment is complete remission of symptoms (e.g., seizures, mania, pain)

How Long to Treat

- Continue treatment until all symptoms are gone or until improvement is stable and then continue treating indefinitely as long as improvement persists
- Continue treatment indefinitely to avoid the recurrence of mania and seizures
- Treatment of chronic neuropathic pain most often reduces but does not eliminate pain and is not a cure since symptoms usually recur after medicine stopped

What If It Stops Working?

- Check for nonadherence, possibly by checking plasma drug level, and consider switching to another agent with fewer side effects
- Screen for the development of a new comorbid disorder, especially substance abuse
- Screen for adverse changes in the home or school environment

What If It Doesn't Work?

- Consider evaluation for another diagnosis or for a comorbid condition (e.g., medical illness, substance abuse)
- Consider other important potential factors such as ongoing conflicts, family psychopathology, and an adverse environment (e.g., poverty, chaos, violence, prior and ongoing psychological trauma, abuse, neglect)
- Institute trauma-informed care for appropriate children and adolescents
- Many patients have only a partial response where some symptoms are improved but others persist or continue to wax and wane without stabilization of mood
- Consider increasing dose or switching to another agent with demonstrated efficacy in bipolar disorder (one of the atypical antipsychotics or lithium)
- Consider initiating rehabilitation and psychotherapy such as cognitive remediation, although these may be less well standardized for children/adolescents than for adults
- Consider presence of concomitant drug abuse
- Consider augmentation with lithium, an atypical antipsychotic, or an antidepressant (with caution because antidepressants can destabilize mood in some patients, including induction of rapid cycling or suicidal ideation; in particular, consider bupropion; also SSRIs, SNRIs, others; generally, avoid TCAs, MAOIs)
- Consider augmentation with lamotrigine (carbamazepine can decrease lamotrigine levels)

TALKING TO PATIENTS AND CAREGIVERS

What to Tell Parents About Efficacy

- For acute symptoms, it can work right away
- Explain which use carbamazepine is being chosen for, how to tell if the drug is working by targeting specific symptoms, and why this is being done
- Once the child/adolescent calms down, at some point after one dose or after several days of dosing or after long-term dosing, we should all assess whether the medication should be continued
- While the medicine helps by reducing symptoms and improving function, it is not a cure, and it therefore may be necessary to keep taking the medication long term to sustain its therapeutic effects
- Since every treatment consideration depends on a risk/benefit analysis, parents should fully understand short- and long-term risks as well as benefits

- Often a good idea to tell parents whether the medication chosen is specifically approved for the disorder being treated, or whether it is being given for "unapproved" or "off-label" reasons based on good clinical practice, expert consensus, and/ or prudent extrapolation of controlled data from adults

What to Tell Children and Adolescents About Efficacy

- Be specific about the symptoms being targeted: we are trying to help you ...
- Give the medication a try; if it's not working very well, we can stop the medication and try something else
- A good try often takes 2 to 3 months
- If it does make you feel better, you cannot stop it right away or you may get sick again
- Medications don't change who you are as a person; they give you the opportunity to be the best person you can be

What to Tell Parents About Side Effects

- Explain that side effects are expected in many when starting
- Tell parents many side effects go away and do so about the same time that therapeutic effects start
- Predict side effects in advance (you will look clever and competent to the parents, unless you scare them with too much information and cause nocebo effects, in which case you won't look so clever when the patient develops lots of side effects and stops medication; use your judgment here); a balanced but honest presentation is an art rather than a science
- Ask parents to support the patient while side effects are occurring
- Parents should fully understand short- and long-term risks as well as benefits
- Explaining to the parents what to expect from medication treatment, and especially what potential side effects to expect, can help prevent early termination of medication

What to Tell Children and Adolescents About Side Effects

- Even if you get a side effect, we can usually reduce it over time
- If you have side effects that are bothering you, tell your parents and your parents should tell me
- Consider having a conversation about sexual side effects in some adolescents who can find these side effects confusing and especially burdensome
- Explaining to child/adolescent what to expect from medication treatment, and especially potential side effects, can help prevent early termination of medication

What to Tell Teachers About the Medication (If Parents Consent)

- Carbamazepine can make children/ adolescents sedated
- It is not abusable
- Encourage dialogue with parents/guardians about any behavior or mood changes

SPECIAL POPULATIONS

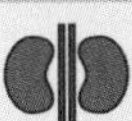

Renal Impairment

- Carbamazepine is renally secreted, so the dose may need to be lowered

Hepatic Impairment

- Drug should be used with caution
- Rare cases of hepatic failure have occurred

Cardiac Impairment

- Drug should be used with caution

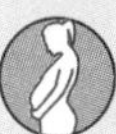

Pregnancy

- Use during first trimester may raise risk of neural tube defects (e.g., spina bifida) or other congenital anomalies; risk increases with polypharmacy
- Use in women of childbearing potential requires weighing potential benefits to the mother against the risks to the fetus; education regarding contraception should be provided
- If drug is continued, perform tests to detect birth defects
- If drug is continued, start on folate 1 mg/ day early in pregnancy to reduce risk of neural tube defects
- Antiepileptic Drug Pregnancy Registry: (888) 233-2334 or www.aedpregnancyregistry.org
- Use of anticonvulsants in combination may cause a higher prevalence of teratogenic effects than anticonvulsant monotherapy

- Taper drug if discontinuing
- Seizures, even mild seizures, may cause harm to the embryo/fetus
- For bipolar patients, carbamazepine should generally be discontinued before anticipated pregnancies
- Recurrent bipolar illness during pregnancy can be quite disruptive
- For bipolar patients, given the risk of relapse in the postpartum period, some form of mood stabilizer treatment may need to be restarted immediately after delivery if patient is unmedicated during pregnancy
- Atypical antipsychotics may be preferable to lithium or anticonvulsants such as carbamazepine if treatment of bipolar disorder is required during pregnancy
- Bipolar symptoms may recur or worsen during pregnancy, and some form of treatment may be necessary

Breast Feeding

- Some drug is found in breast milk
- Recommended either to discontinue drug or formula feed
- If drug is continued while breast feeding, infant should be monitored for possible adverse effects, including hematological effects
- If infant shows signs of irritability or sedation, drug may need to be discontinued
- Some cases of neonatal seizures, respiratory depression, vomiting, and diarrhea have been reported in infants whose mothers received carbamazepine during pregnancy
- Bipolar disorder may recur during the postpartum period, particularly if there is a history of prior postpartum episodes of either depression or psychosis
- Relapse rates may be lower in women who receive prophylactic treatment for postpartum episodes of bipolar disorder
- Atypical antipsychotics and anticonvulsants such as valproate may be safer than carbamazepine during the postpartum period when breast feeding

THE ART OF PSYCHOPHARMACOLOGY

Potential Advantages

- Treatment-resistant bipolar and psychotic disorders

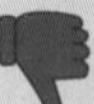

Potential Disadvantages

- Patients who do not wish to or cannot comply with blood testing and close monitoring
- Patients who cannot tolerate sedation
- Pregnant patients

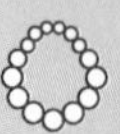

Pearls

- Carbamazepine was the first anticonvulsant widely used for the treatment of bipolar disorder and is now formally approved for acute mania and mixed mania in adults
- An extended-release formulation has better evidence of efficacy and improved tolerability in bipolar disorder than does immediate-release carbamazepine
- Dosage frequency as well as sedation, diplopia, confusion, and ataxia may be reduced with extended-release carbamazepine
- Risk of serious side effects is greatest in the first few months of treatment
- Common side effects such as sedation often abate after a few months
- May be effective in patients who fail to respond to lithium or other mood stabilizers
- May be effective for the depressed phase of bipolar disorder and for maintenance in bipolar disorder
- Can be complicated to use with concomitant medications

SUGGESTED READING

Findling RL, Ginsberg LD. The safety and effectiveness of open-label extended-release carbamazepine in the treatment of children and adolescents with bipolar I disorder suffering from a manic or mixed episode. Neuropsychiatr Dis Treat 2014;10:1589–97.

Phillips EJ, Sukasem C, Whirl-Carrillo M et al. Clinical Pharmacogenetics Implementation Consortium guideline for HLA genotype and use of carbamazepine and oxcarbazepine: 2017 update. Clin Pharmacol Ther 2018 103(4):574–81.

THERAPEUTICS

Brands
- Thorazine

Generic
Yes

US FDA Approved for Pediatric Use
- Severe behavioral problems associated with oppositional defiant disorder or other disruptive behavioral disorders, or for attention deficit hyperactivity disorder (ADHD) in pediatric patients who show excessive motor activity with accompanying conduct disorders (oral, intramuscular for acute, severe agitation in hospitalized patients)
- Nausea/vomiting (oral, rectal, intramuscular, intravenous)
- Tetanus (intramuscular, adjunct)
- Intractable hiccups (adolescents, oral, intramuscular, intravenous)
- Acute intermittent porphyria (adolescents, oral, intramuscular)

Off-Label for Pediatric Use
- Approved in adults
  - Schizophrenia (oral)
  - Acute psychosis (intramuscular)
- Other off-label uses
  - Agitation or delirium in hospitalized patients without underlying psychiatric illness (oral, intramuscular, intravenous)
  - Bipolar disorder
  - Migraine
  - Neonatal abstinence syndrome

Class and Mechanism of Action
- Neuroscience-based Nomenclature: dopamine and serotonin receptor antagonist (DS-RAn)
- Conventional antipsychotic (neuroleptic, phenothiazine, dopamine 2 antagonist, antiemetic)
- Blocks dopamine 2 receptors, reducing positive symptoms of psychosis and improving other behaviors
- Combination of dopamine D2, histamine H1, and cholinergic M1 blockade in the vomiting center may reduce nausea and vomiting

SAFETY AND TOLERABILITY

Notable Side Effects
- Akathisia
- Drug-induced parkinsonism
- Dry mouth, constipation, blurred vision, urinary retention
- Dizziness, sedation
- Weight gain
- Decreased sweating
- Hypotension
- Galactorrhea, amenorrhea
- Sexual dysfunction
- Impaired memory
- Tardive dyskinesia (risk is higher in children than in adults)
- Risk of potentially irreversible, involuntary dyskinetic movements may increase with cumulative dose and treatment duration
- Rare tachycardia, syncope

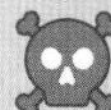

Life-Threatening or Dangerous Side Effects
- Rare neuroleptic malignant syndrome (NMS) may cause hyperpyrexia, muscle rigidity, delirium, and autonomic instability with elevated creatine phosphokinase, myoglobinuria (rhabdomyolysis), and acute renal failure
- Rare seizures
- Rare jaundice, agranulocytosis
- Rare priapism

Growth and Maturation
- Long-term effects are unknown

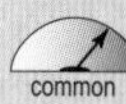

Weight Gain
- Many experience and/or can be significant in amount

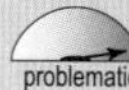

Sedation
- Frequent and can be significant in amount
- Tolerance to sedation can develop over time

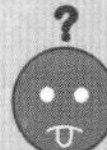

What to Do About Side Effects
- Wait, wait, wait: mild side effects are common, happen early, and usually improve with time, but treatment benefits can be delayed
- Monitor side effects closely, especially when initiating treatment

- May wish to give at night if not tolerated during the day and doesn't disrupt sleep
- Often best to try another monotherapy trial of a different antipsychotic prior to resorting to augmentation strategies to treat side effects
- Exercise and diet programs and medical management for high BMI percentiles, diabetes, dyslipidemia. Also, randomized controlled trials in youth suggest that omega-3 fatty acids can reduce SGA-related hypertriglyceridemia.
- Reduce the dose, particularly for drug-induced parkinsonism, akathisia, sedation, and tremor
- For drug-induced parkinsonism: consider reducing dose or switching to another agent. Augmenting with diphenhydramine or benztropine is less preferred in youth.
- For akathisia: reduce the dose or add a beta blocker. If these are ineffective, raising the dose of the beta blocker may be helpful.
- Using a 5HT2A antagonist such as mirtazapine or cyproheptadine to treat drug-induced akathisia is less common in children and adolescents compared to adults
- Agitation due to undertreatment and inadequate dosing of the targeted disorder can be difficult to distinguish from drug-induced akathisia and activation; one approach for managing agitation/activation/akathisia when the specific side effect is difficult to distinguish is to raise the dose of chlorpromazine
- If the patient improves after increasing the dose of chlorpromazine, the symptoms are more likely to be due to inadequate dosing of the targeted disorder
- If the patient worsens after increasing the dose of chlorpromazine, the symptoms are more likely to be drug induced and require further dose reduction, adding an agent to improve tolerability or switching to another antipsychotic

How Drug Causes Side Effects

- By blocking dopamine 2 receptors in the striatum, it can cause motor side effects, akathisia, and activation symptoms
- By blocking dopamine 2 receptors in the pituitary, it can cause elevations in prolactin
- By blocking dopamine 2 receptors excessively in the mesocortical and mesolimbic dopamine pathways, especially at high doses, it can cause worsening of negative and cognitive symptoms (neuroleptic-induced deficit syndrome)
- Blocking muscarinic cholinergic receptors can cause dry mouth, blurred vision, urinary retention, constipation, and paralytic ileus
- Antihistaminic actions may cause sedation, weight gain
- Blocking alpha 1 adrenergic receptors can cause dizziness, hypotension, and syncope
- Mechanism of any possible increased incidence of diabetes or dyslipidemia is unknown

Warnings and Precautions

- Carefully weigh the risks and benefits of pharmacological treatment against the risks and benefits of nontreatment with an antipsychotic and it is a good idea to document this in the patient's chart
- If signs of neuroleptic malignant syndrome develop, treatment should be immediately discontinued
- Use cautiously in patients with alcohol withdrawal or convulsive disorders because of possible lowering of seizure threshold
- Use with caution in patients with respiratory disorders, glaucoma, or urinary retention
- Use with caution in patients with hematological disease
- Avoid extreme heat exposure
- Avoid undue exposure to sunlight
- Antiemetic effect of chlorpromazine may mask signs of other disorders or overdose; suppression of cough reflex may cause asphyxia

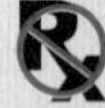

When Not to Prescribe

- If patient is in a comatose state
- If patient is taking metrizamide or large doses of CNS depressants
- If patient has a sulfite hypersensitivity (injectable preparations)
- If there is a proven allergy to chlorpromazine
- If there is a known sensitivity to any phenothiazine
- Do not use if patient shows signs of Reye's syndrome

Long-Term Use

- Should periodically reevaluate long-term usefulness in individual patients, but treatment may need to continue for many years

Habit Forming

- No

Overdose

- Drug-induced parkinsonism, sedation, hypotension, coma, respiratory depression

DOSING AND USE

Usual Dosage Range

- For severe psychosis:
  - Adolescents: consider initiating at 50 mg qHS and titrating to 100 mg in 7–10 days (or faster in hospitalized adolescents); may titrate to a maximum dose of 200 mg qHS
- For severe behavioral problems:
  - Children, oral: initially 0.55 mg/kg every 4 to 6 hours, as needed
  - Children, intramuscular: 0.55 mg/kg every 6 to 8 hours, as needed
- For nausea/vomiting:
  - Children: 0.55 mg/kg every 6 to 8 hours
  - Adolescents: 10–25 mg orally every 4 to 6 hours, as needed

Dosage Forms

- Tablet 10 mg, 25 mg, 50 mg, 100 mg, 200 mg
- Capsule 30 mg, 75 mg, 150 mg (not in United States)
- Ampul 25 mg/mL; 1 mL, 2 mL
- Vial 25 mg/mL; 10 mL
- Liquid 10 mg/5 mL (discontinued in United States)
- Suppository 25 mg, 100 mg (discontinued in United States)

How to Dose

- For severe behavioral problems:
  - Children, oral: initially 0.55 mg/kg every 4 to 6 hours, as needed; increase gradually every 3 to 4 days as needed to control symptoms. If hospitalized, high dosages (i.e., 50 to 100 mg/day or up to 200 mg/day in older children) may be required to treat severe disturbances or psychotic conditions. Continue the titrated effective dose for at least 2 weeks, then gradually reduce the dosage to the lowest effective dose that controls symptoms.
  - Children, intramuscular: 0.55 mg/kg every 6 to 8 hours, as needed; maximum daily dose 40 mg/day (children less than 5 years or 22.7 kg) or 75 mg/day (children ages 5 to 12 or 22.7 to 45.5 kg); convert to oral therapy as soon as possible
- For nausea/vomiting:
  - Children, oral: 0.55 mg/kg every 6 to 8 hours, as needed
  - Children (at least 6 months old), intramuscular: initially 0.55 mg/kg; repeat every 6 to 8 hours as needed; duration of action may be up to 12 hours; switch to oral therapy as soon as possible; maximum daily dose 40 mg/day (children less than 5 years or 22.7 kg) or 75 mg/day (children ages 5 to 12 or 22.7 to 45.5 kg)
  - Adolescents, oral: 10–25 mg every 4 to 6 hours, as needed
  - Adolescents, intramuscular: initially 12.5–25 mg; if no hypotension occurs, repeat 25–50 mg every 3 to 4 hours as needed; switch to oral therapy after vomiting stops
- For nausea/vomiting during surgical procedures:
  - Children (at least 6 months old), intramuscular: initially 0.25 mg/kg; if no hypotension occurs, may repeat once, 30 minutes after initial dose
  - Children (greater than 6 months old), intravenous: 1 mg after dosage dilution to 1 mg/mL with NS; administer IV over at least 2 minutes (i.e., rate should not exceed 0.5 mg/minute); may repeat at 2-minute intervals as needed; total dosage administered via fractional IV injections must not exceed 0.25 mg/kg
  - Adolescents, intramuscular: initially 12.5 mg; if no hypotension occurs, may repeat once, 30 minutes after initial dose
  - Adolescents, intravenous: 2 mg after dosage dilution to a concentration of 1 mg/mL with 0.9% sodium chloride injection; administer IV over at least 2 minutes; may repeat at 2-minute intervals as needed; total dosage administered via fractional IV injections must not exceed 25 mg
- For tetanus:
  - Children (at least 6 months old), intramuscular or intermittent intravenous dosage: 0.55 mg/kg IV or IM every 6 to 8 hours. If the IV route is used, follow manufacturer directions for dosage dilution to 1 mg/mL with NS and administer dose via IV infusion at a rate

no faster than 0.5 mg/minute. Maximum daily dose 40 mg/day (children less than 5 years or 22.7 kg) or 75 mg/day (children ages 5 to 12 or 22.7 to 45.5 kg).
  - Adolescents, intramuscular or intermittent intravenous dosage: 25 to 50 mg IM or IV every 6 to 8 hours; usually given in conjunction with barbiturates. If the IV route is used, follow manufacturer directions for dosage dilution to 1 mg/mL with 0.9% sodium chloride for injection and administer dose via IV infusion at a rate no faster than 1 mg/minute.
- For intractable hiccups:
  - Adolescents, oral: 25–50 mg 3–4 times per day; if symptoms persist for 2 to 3 days, parenteral therapy is indicated
  - Adolescents, intramuscular: if after 2 to 3 days there is no response to oral therapy, a single dose of 25 to 50 mg IM may be administered
  - Adolescents, continuous IV infusion dosage: may be used if symptoms persist despite IM dosing; patient should remain flat during the entire infusion, with blood pressure closely monitored. Add 25 to 50 mg of chlorpromazine injection to 500 to 1,000 mL of 0.9% sodium chloride for injection; administer slowly IV at a rate specified by the prescriber. Do not exceed an IV rate of 1 mg/minute. Discontinue treatment when the infusion is completed.
- Intermittent porphyria:
  - Adolescents, oral: 25–50 mg 3–4 times per day; treatment usually continues for several weeks
  - Adolescents, intramuscular: 25 mg 3–4 times per day until the patient can take oral therapy

Options for Administration

- Tablet may be crushed prior to administration

Tests

- Before starting chlorpromazine:
  - Plan to monitor weight and metabolic parameters more closely than in adults since children and adolescents may be more prone to these side effects than adults
  - Weigh all patients and monitor weight gain against that expected for normal growth, using the pediatric height/weight chart to monitor
  - Get baseline personal and family history of diabetes, obesity, dyslipidemia, hypertension, and cardiovascular disease
  - Obtain blood pressure, fasting plasma glucose (or hemoglobin A1C), and a lipid profile
- After starting chlorpromazine:
  - Monitor weight and BMI percentile
  - Consider monitoring fasting triglycerides in patients at high risk for metabolic complications
  - Patients with low white blood cell count (WBC) or history of drug-induced leukopenia/neutropenia should have complete blood count (CBC) monitored frequently during the first few months and chlorpromazine should be discontinued at the first sign of decline of WBC in the absence of other causative factors
  - Patients should be monitored periodically for the development of abnormal movements using neurological exam and the Abnormal Involuntary Movement Scale (AIMS)
  - Monitoring elevated prolactin levels is of dubious clinical benefit
  - Phenothiazines may cause false-positive phenylketonuria results

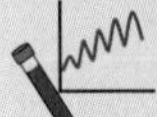

Pharmacokinetics

- The metabolism of chlorpromazine occurs primarily in the liver, where it undergoes extensive hepatic metabolism. The major metabolic pathways involve oxidation and conjugation reactions mediated by various enzymes, including cytochrome P450 enzymes, such as CYP2D6 and CYP1A2 (Figure 1). Chlorpromazine also inhibits CYP2D6 and to a lesser extent, inhibits CYP1A2.
- Chlorpromazine has a relatively high volume of distribution, which means it distributes extensively into body tissues. It crosses the blood–brain barrier and accumulates in the central nervous system, contributing to its therapeutic effects.
- Chlorpromazine is highly protein-bound (around 90%), primarily to albumin
- Elimination half-life of chlorpromazine in pediatric patients is approximately 20–30 hours (in adults it is approximately 8–33 hours)

inhibits
2D6
1A2
chlorpromazine
5HT2A
5HT2C
M1 M3 M4 M5
H1
α1
D1 D2 D3 D4
5HT6 5HT7
2D6 → 7-hydroxylchlorpromazine
1A2
3A4
chlorpromazine-5-sulfoxide
stimulates
1A2
mono-n-desmethylchlorpromazine
1A2 → di-n-desmethylchlorpromazine

Figure 1 Metabolism of chlorpromazine.

- The drug and its metabolites are primarily excreted in the urine, with a small portion eliminated in feces

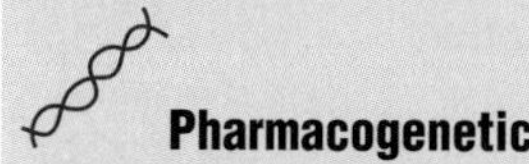

Pharmacogenetics

- No recommendations

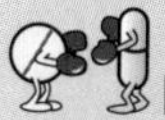

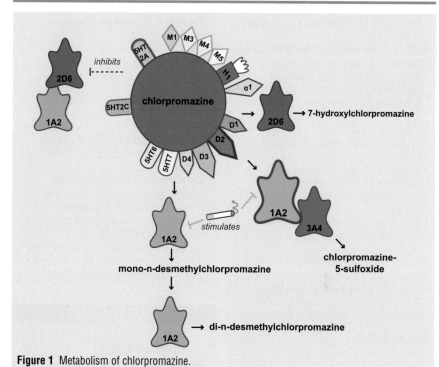

Drug Interactions

- May decrease the effects of levodopa, dopamine agonists
- May increase the effects of antihypertensive drugs except for guanethidine, whose antihypertensive actions chlorpromazine may antagonize
- Additive effects may occur if used with CNS depressants
- Some pressor agents (e.g., epinephrine) may interact with chlorpromazine to lower blood pressure
- Alcohol and diuretics may increase the risk of hypotension
- Reduces effects of anticoagulants
- May reduce phenytoin metabolism and increase phenytoin levels
- Plasma levels of chlorpromazine and propranolol may increase if used concomitantly
- Some patients taking a neuroleptic and lithium have developed an encephalopathic syndrome similar to neuroleptic malignant syndrome

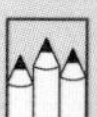

Dosing Tips

- Start at a low dose
- For "as needed" prn use, determine dose over time after several administrations by raising the dose to achieve what is the best-acting and best-tolerated single oral dose for short-term relief of target symptoms
- For daily dosing, total daily dose will be lower if the patient is taking another antipsychotic concomitantly, especially another sedating antipsychotic
- Few studies of administering chlorpromazine as an "as needed" prn medication on top of another daily antipsychotic in children or adolescents, so caution is needed until the individual

patient's tolerability to such a combination is determined
- Legacy use of low doses of chlorpromazine have been administered historically to provide short-term relief of daytime agitation and anxiety and to enhance sedative hypnotic actions in psychotic as well as in nonpsychotic patients, including children and adolescents, but other treatment options such as benzodiazepines or atypical antipsychotics are now preferred
- Can be taken with or without food
- Anti-nausea effects are delayed when administered rectally, with a duration of 3–4 days
- Ampuls and vials contain sulfites that may cause allergic reactions, particularly in patients with asthma
- One of the few antipsychotics available as a suppository, although this formulation has been discontinued in the United States
- Treatment should be suspended if absolute neutrophil count falls below 1,000/mm^3

How to Switch

- From another antipsychotic to chlorpromazine:
  - When tapering a prior antipsychotic, see its entry in this manual for how to stop and how to taper off that specific drug
  - Generally, try to stop the first agent before starting chlorpromazine so that new side effects of chlorpromazine can be distinguished from withdrawal effects of the first agent
  - If urgent, cross taper off the other antipsychotic while chlorpromazine is started at a low dose, with dose adjustments down of the other antipsychotic, and up for chlorpromazine, every 3 to 7 days
- Off chlorpromazine to another antipsychotic:
  - Generally, try to stop chlorpromazine before starting the new antipsychotic so that new side effects of the next drug can be distinguished from any withdrawal effects from chlorpromazine
  - If urgent, cross taper off chlorpromazine by cutting the dose in half as the new antipsychotic is also started with dose adjustments down of chlorpromazine and up for the new antipsychotic while monitoring for anticholinergic rebound symptoms from the withdrawal of chlorpromazine

How to Stop

- Slow down-titration of oral formulation (over 6–8 weeks), especially when simultaneously beginning a new antipsychotic while switching (i.e., cross-titration)
- Rapid oral discontinuation may lead to rebound psychosis and worsening of symptoms
- Rapid oral discontinuation may lead to withdrawal dyskinesias, sometimes reversible, as well as anticholinergic rebound symptoms, especially in children following long-term daily use
- If antiparkinsonian agents are being used, they should be continued for a few weeks after chlorpromazine is discontinued

WHAT TO EXPECT

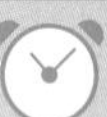

Onset of Action

- Actions on nausea and vomiting are immediate
- Actions on behavioral symptoms including positive symptoms of psychosis can be proportionate to sedation and can occur simultaneously with the onset of sedation

Duration of Action

- Can last up to 24 hours, depending upon how agitated or psychotic the behavior is that is being targeted and upon how much sedation a given dose causes, with more sedation having longer duration of action than when there is little or no sedation

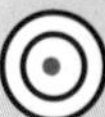

Primary Target Symptoms

- Motor and autonomic hyperactivity
- Psychosis and agitation
- Violent or aggressive behavior
- Nausea/vomiting

What Is Considered a Positive Result?

- For severe behavior problems:
  - Immediate and short-term (a few hours) relief of symptoms if given during an acute exacerbation on an "as needed" prn basis (most common use)

- Longer-term improvement in disruptive and psychotic behaviors if used daily

How Long to Treat

- For severe behavior problems:
  - Can be used on an "as needed" prn basis for as long as acute exacerbations of target symptoms are present and not responding to an increased dose of the daily antipsychotic

What If It Stops Working?

- For "as needed" prn use, if it doesn't work, likely the dose is too low, so cautiously raise the dose
- Rare cases become disinhibited from sedating agents, in which case select a different agent that is less sedating
- Check for nonadherence if giving it daily, possibly by checking plasma drug level and consider switching to another antipsychotic with fewer side effects
- Some patients who have an initial response may relapse even though they continue treatment, sometimes called "poop-out"
- Growth/developmental changes may contribute to apparent loss of efficacy as well as to new onset of side effects as metabolism slows and drug levels rise in transition from childhood to adolescence; dose adjustment (increase or decrease) should be considered
- Screen for the development of a new comorbid disorder, especially substance use
- Screen for adverse changes in the home or school environment

What If It Doesn't Work?

- Consider evaluation for another diagnosis (especially bipolar illness or depression with mixed features) or for a comorbid condition (e.g., medical illness, substance use)
- Consider other important potential factors such as ongoing conflicts, family psychopathology, and an adverse environment (e.g., poverty, chaos, violence, prior and ongoing psychological trauma, abuse, neglect)
- Institute trauma-informed care for appropriate children and adolescents
- For severe behavior problems:
  - Raise the dose
  - Try one of the atypical antipsychotics
  - Consider nonadherence and switch to another antipsychotic with fewer side effects
  - Consider initiating rehabilitation and psychotherapy such as cognitive remediation
  - Consider presence of concomitant drug use

TALKING TO PATIENTS AND CAREGIVERS

What to Tell Parents About Efficacy

- For acute symptoms, it can work right away
- Explain which use chlorpromazine is being chosen for, how to tell if the drug is working by targeting specific symptoms, and why this is being done
- Once the child/adolescent calms down, at some point after one dose or after several days of dosing or after long-term dosing, we should all assess whether the medication should be continued, added to a different medication, or switched to a different medication
- While the medicine helps by reducing symptoms and improving function, it is not a cure, and it therefore may be necessary to keep taking the medication long term to sustain its therapeutic effects
- Since every treatment consideration depends on a risk/benefit analysis, parents should fully understand short- and long-term risks as well as benefits
- Often a good idea to tell parents whether the medication chosen is specifically approved for the disorder being treated, or whether it is being given for "unapproved" or "off-label" reasons based on good clinical practice, expert consensus, and/or prudent extrapolation of controlled data from adults
- Usually, chlorpromazine is being used for urgent worsening of symptoms, but a second generation atypical antipsychotic is being used for everyday symptoms

What to Tell Children and Adolescents About Efficacy

- Be specific about the symptoms being targeted: we are trying to help you ...
- Give the medication a try; if it's not working very well, we can stop the medication and try something else

- A good try often takes several weeks
- Medications don't change who you are as a person; they give you the opportunity to be the best person you can be

What to Tell Parents About Side Effects

- Explain that side effects are expected in many when starting, especially sedation
- In fact, causing sedation in order to stop targeted symptoms is the reason chlorpromazine is being given
- Tell parents many side effects from everyday use go away and do so about the same time that therapeutic effects start
- Predict side effects in advance (you will look clever and competent to the parents, unless you scare them with too much information and cause nocebo effects, in which case you won't look so clever when the patient develops lots of side effects and stops medication; use your judgment here); a balanced but honest presentation is an art rather than a science
- Ask parents to support the patient while side effects are occurring
- Parents should fully understand short- and long-term risks as well as benefits
- Explaining to the parents what to expect from medication treatment, and especially what potential side effects to expect, can help prevent early termination of medication

What to Tell Children and Adolescents About Side Effects

- Even if you get a side effect, we can usually reduce it over time
- If you have side effects that are bothering you, tell your parents and your parents should tell me
- Consider having a conversation about sexual side effects in some adolescents who can find these side effects confusing and especially burdensome
- Explaining to child/adolescent what to expect from medication treatment, and especially potential side effects, can help prevent early termination of medication

What to Tell Teachers About the Medication (If Parents Consent)

- Chlorpromazine can make children/adolescents restless and have tremor and stiffness
- Chlorpromazine can make children/adolescents sedated
- It is not abusable
- Encourage dialogue with parents/guardians about any behavior or mood changes
- Notify the clinician of increased restlessness or akathisia symptoms, which may be apparent in the school setting

SPECIAL POPULATIONS

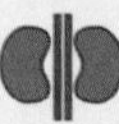

Renal Impairment

- Dose adjustment not needed; not removed by hemodialysis

Hepatic Impairment

- Use with caution; patients who develop jaundice secondary to chlorpromazine use should have therapy discontinued

Cardiac Impairment

- Cardiovascular toxicity can occur, especially orthostatic hypotension

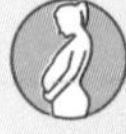

Pregnancy

- Controlled studies have not been conducted in pregnant women
- There is a risk of abnormal muscle movements and withdrawal symptoms in newborns whose mothers took an antipsychotic during the third trimester; symptoms may include agitation, abnormally increased or decreased muscle tone, tremor, sleepiness, severe difficulty breathing, and difficulty feeding
- Reports of extrapyramidal symptoms, jaundice, hyperreflexia, hyporeflexia in infants whose mothers took a phenothiazine during pregnancy
- Some animal studies have shown adverse effects
- Chlorpromazine should generally not be used during the first trimester
- Chlorpromazine should be used during pregnancy only if clearly needed
- Psychotic symptoms may worsen during pregnancy, and some form of treatment may be necessary
- Atypical antipsychotics may be preferable to conventional antipsychotics or

anticonvulsant mood stabilizers if treatment is required during pregnancy

Breast Feeding

- Some drug is found in breast milk
- Effects on infant have been observed (dystonia, tardive dyskinesia, sedation)
- Recommended either to discontinue drug or formula feed

THE ART OF PSYCHOPHARMACOLOGY

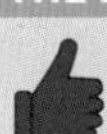

Potential Advantages

- In children and adolescents:
    - Approved for severe behavior problems
- All ages:
    - Intramuscular formulation for emergency use
    - Patients who require sedation for behavioral control

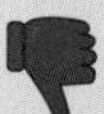

Potential Disadvantages

- In children and adolescents:
    - May be more susceptible to side effects
- All ages:
    - Patients who wish to avoid sedation
    - Patients who wish to avoid anticholinergic side effects, especially patients on clozapine

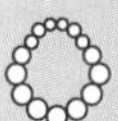

Pearls

- Chlorpromazine has a broad spectrum of efficacy, but risk of tardive dyskinesia and the availability of alternative treatments make its utilization now for psychosis as a short-term and second-line treatment option
- Adding chlorpromazine as the choice for patients who require sedation or behavioral control, either as a daily or as a prn (as needed) treatment should be avoided in order to reduce the chances of potentially fatal paralytic ileus in patients on concomitant anticholinergics, including antipsychotic drugs with anticholinergic properties such as clozapine
- Chlorpromazine is a low-potency phenothiazine
- Sedative actions of low-potency phenothiazines are an important aspect of their therapeutic actions in some patients and side-effect profile in others
- Low-potency phenothiazines like chlorpromazine have a greater risk of cardiovascular side effects

SUGGESTED READING

Heng Vong C, Bajard A, Thiesse P et al. Deep sedation in pediatric imaging: efficacy and safety of intravenous chlorpromazine. Pediatr Radiol 2012;42(5):552–61.

Kanis JM, Timm NL. Chlorpromazine for the treatment of migraine in a pediatric emergency department. Headache 2014;54(2):335–42.

Pantuck EJ, Pantuck CB, Anderson KE, Conney AH, Kappas A. Cigarette smoking and chlorpromazine disposition and actions. Clin Pharmacol Ther 1982;31(4):533–8.

Terndrup TE, Dire DJ, Madden CM et al. A prospective analysis of intramuscular meperidine, promethazine, and chlorpromazine in pediatric emergency department patients. Ann Emerg Med 1991;20(1):31–5.

Weiss G, Minde K, Douglas V, Werry J, Sykes D. Comparison of the effects of chlorpromazine, dextroamphetamine and methylphenidate on the behaviour and intellectual functioning of hyperactive children. Can Med Assoc J 1971;104(1):20–5.

THERAPEUTICS

Brands
- Celexa

Generic
Yes

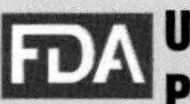

US FDA Approved for Pediatric Use
- None

Off-Label for Pediatric Use
- Approved in adults
  - Depression
- Other off-label uses
  - Separation anxiety disorder
  - Obsessive-compulsive disorder (OCD)
  - Social anxiety disorder
  - Panic disorder (PD)
  - Generalized anxiety disorder (GAD)
  - Premenstrual dysphoric disorder (PMDD)
  - Posttraumatic stress disorder (PTSD)

Class and Mechanism of Action
- Neuroscience-based Nomenclature: serotonin reuptake inhibitor (S-RI)
- SSRI (selective serotonin reuptake inhibitor); often classified as a drug for depression (i.e., antidepressant), but it is not just an antidepressant
- Citalopram presumably increases serotonergic neurotransmission by blocking the serotonin reuptake pump (transporter, SERT), which results in the desensitization of serotonin receptors, especially serotonin 1A receptors. Citalopram also binds allosterically at the SERT, which increases its binding at the active site.
- In adolescents with anxiety disorders, the S-enantiomer of citalopram (escitalopram) increases the connections between the amygdala and regions of the brain that dampen the activity of the amygdala (i.e., prefrontal cortex) (Lu et al., 2021). These changes in brain circuits in adolescents predict more clinical improvement (Lu et al., 2021).
- Citalopram also has mild antagonist actions at histamine H1 receptors, and this may contribute to some sedation and weight gain in pediatric patients
- Citalopram's inactive R-enantiomer may interfere with the therapeutic actions of the active S-enantiomer at serotonin reuptake pumps

SAFETY AND TOLERABILITY

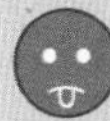

Notable Side Effects
- Several central nervous system side effects (insomnia but also sedation, especially if not sleeping at night, agitation, headache, dizziness)
- Note: patients with diagnosed or undiagnosed bipolar or psychotic disorders may be more vulnerable to CNS-activating actions of SSRIs like citalopram; pay particular attention to signs of activation in children with developmental disorders or autism spectrum disorders. In fact, two trials of citalopram in children with autism spectrum disorder observed more side effects compared to placebo and that these included higher rates of CNS-related activating adverse events (King et al., 2009; Simonoff et al., 2022).
- Treatment-emergent activation syndrome (TEAS) includes agitation, anxiety, panic attacks, irritability, impulsivity, and insomnia. For citalopram/escitalopram in pediatric patients, the risk of activation is greater in slower CYP2C19 metabolizers and has been associated with greater blood levels of citalopram/escitalopram.
- TEAS can represent side effects but should not be confused with bipolar mania or the onset of suicidality and should be monitored and investigated with consideration of discontinuing or decreasing the dose of citalopram or addition of another agent or switching to another agent to reduce these symptoms
- Gastrointestinal (nausea, diarrhea, constipation, dry mouth)
- Sexual dysfunction (boys: delayed ejaculation, erectile dysfunction; boys and girls: decreased sexual desire, anorgasmia)
- Autonomic (sweating)
- Bruising and rare bleeding
- Syndrome of inappropriate antidiuretic hormone secretion (SIADH)

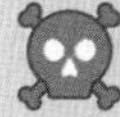

Life-Threatening or Dangerous Side Effects
- Rare seizures
- Rare induction of mania
- Rare suicidal ideation and behavior (suicidality) (short-term regulatory studies did not show any actual suicides in any age group and also did not show an increase in

the risk of suicidality with antidepressants compared to placebo beyond age 24)

Growth and Maturation

- In adolescents, citalopram may increase visceral fat mass and have unclear effects on bone mineralization

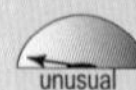

Weight Gain

- Weight gain is dose related and more common in adolescents who are slower CYP2C19 metabolizers

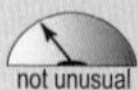

Sedation

- Occurs in significant minority of patients and may be more apparent at higher doses

What to Do About Side Effects

- Wait, wait, wait: mild side effects are common, happen early, and usually improve with time, but treatment benefits can be delayed and often begin just as the side effects wear off. However, some side effects may emerge later such as weight gain.
- Monitor side effects closely, especially when initiating treatment
- May wish to give in the evening or at bedtime, particularly if the medication is associated with sedation
- For activation (jitteriness, anxiety, insomnia):
  - Activation with citalopram is dose related and also is more likely in slower CYP2C19 metabolizers. Consider a temporary dose reduction or a more gradual up-titration
  - Administer dose in the morning
  - Consider switching to another SSRI or potentially an SNRI (other than venlafaxine)
  - Optimize psychotherapeutic interventions
  - Activation and agitation may represent the induction of a bipolar state, especially a mixed dysphoric bipolar II condition sometimes associated with suicidal ideation, and may require the addition of lithium or an atypical antipsychotic, and/or discontinuation of citalopram
- Often best to try another monotherapy prior to resorting to augmentation strategies to treat side effects
- For insomnia: consider adding melatonin
- For GI upset: try giving medication with a meal
- For sexual dysfunction:
  - Probably best to reduce dose or discontinue and try another agent
  - Consider adding daytime exercise, bupropion, or buspirone
- For emotional flattening, apathy: consider adding bupropion (with caution as little experience in children)

How Drug Causes Side Effects

- Theoretically due to increases in serotonin concentrations at serotonin receptors in parts of the brain and body other than those that cause therapeutic actions (e.g., unwanted actions of serotonin in sleep centers causing insomnia, unwanted actions of serotonin in the gut causing diarrhea)
- Increasing serotonin can cause diminished dopamine release and might contribute to emotional flattening, cognitive slowing, and apathy in some patients
- Citalopram's unique mild antihistamine properties may contribute to sedation and fatigue in some patients

Warnings and Precautions

- Consider distributing the brochures provided by the FDA and the drug companies as well as the medication guides from the American Academy of Child & Adolescent Psychiatry (AACAP)
- Carefully consider monitoring patients regularly within the practical limits, particularly during the first several weeks of treatment
- Warn patients and their caregivers when possible about the possibility of activating side effects and advise them to report such symptoms
- Carefully weigh the risks and benefits of pharmacological treatment against the risks and benefits of nontreatment with antidepressants and make sure to document this in the patient's chart
- As with any antidepressant, use with caution in patients with history of seizure
- As with any antidepressant, use with caution in patients with bipolar disorder unless treated with concomitant mood-stabilizing agent
- Monitor patients for activation and suicidal ideation and involve parents/guardians

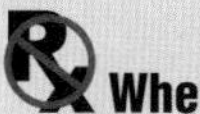

When Not to Prescribe

- If patient is taking an MAO inhibitor
- If patient is taking thioridazine or pimozide
- If there is a proven allergy to citalopram or escitalopram

Long-Term Use

- Weight gain has been observed in citalopram-treated youth, so growth should be monitored; long-term effects are unknown

Habit Forming

- No

Overdose

- Rare fatalities have been reported with citalopram overdose, both alone and in combination with other drugs
- Symptoms may include vomiting, sedation, heart rhythm disturbances, dizziness, sweating, nausea, tremor, and rarely amnesia, confusion, coma, convulsions

DOSING AND USE

Usual Dosage Range

- Depression and OCD: 10–40 mg/day

Dosage Forms

- Tablet 10 mg, 20 mg scored, 40 mg scored
- Solution 10 mg/5 mL

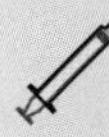

How to Dose

- In children (depression and anxiety disorders): initial dose 10 mg/day; after 1–2 weeks can increase to 20 mg/day and after another 2 weeks, can increase to 30–40 mg/day
- Because citalopram concentrations vary so significantly in adolescents based on their CYP2C19 activity, clinicians could consider adjusting the dose based on CYP2C19 activity

Options for Administration

- Liquid formulation can be beneficial for patients requiring very slow titration and in those who cannot swallow tablets

Tests

- None for healthy individuals; however, EKG may be reasonable at doses >20 mg/day or in patients with a history of long QT-syndrome

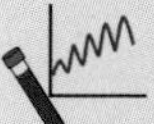

Pharmacokinetics

- Parent drug has 23–45-hour half-life in adults. In pediatric patients (ages 7–11), concentrations over time are 30% higher than in adolescents and adults. Similarly, peak concentrations are higher in pediatric patients compared to adults (Figure 1).
- The time to peak concentrations for citalopram is shorter in pediatric patients (2.9±0.8 hr) compared to adults (3.8±0.5 hr) and the clearance is faster in pediatric patients (18.3±4.2 L/hr) compared to adults (25.4±8 L/hr). However, clearance and half-life are significantly influenced by pharmacogenetic factors (see Pharmacogenetics).
- Substrate for CYP2C19 and 3A4 as well as CYP2D6 (Figure 2)
- Citalopram has moderate protein binding (80%).
- Very weak inhibitor of CYP2D6
- Food does not alter absorption
- In adults (and likely in pediatric populations), R-citalopram is metabolized more slowly than escitalopram which results in a higher plasma concentration of the R-enantiomer compared to the S-enantiomer (Kreilgaard et al., 2008). This has generally been observed to be a 1:4 ratio of the two enantiomers.

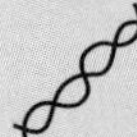

Pharmacogenetics

- Because citalopram and escitalopram are extensively metabolized by CYP2C19, variants impacting CYP2C19 activity may alter drug exposure. CYP2C19 poor metabolizers, including children and adolescents, have increased concentrations and reduced clearance, which may increase the risk of adverse drug reactions, including increased drug discontinuation or switching.
- **CYP2C19 ultrarapid metabolizers:** CPIC recommends clinicians consider a clinically appropriate alternative antidepressant not predominantly metabolized by CYP2C19. If citalopram or escitalopram are clinically appropriate, and adequate efficacy is not

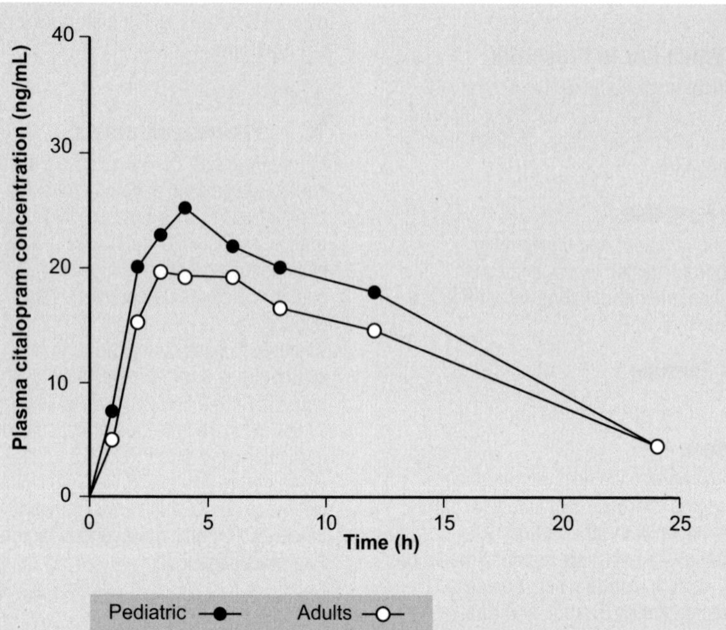

Figure 1 Plasma concentrations of citalopram after a single dose of 20 mg citalopram. Source: FDA Clinical Pharmacology/Biopharmaceutics Review, 2002.

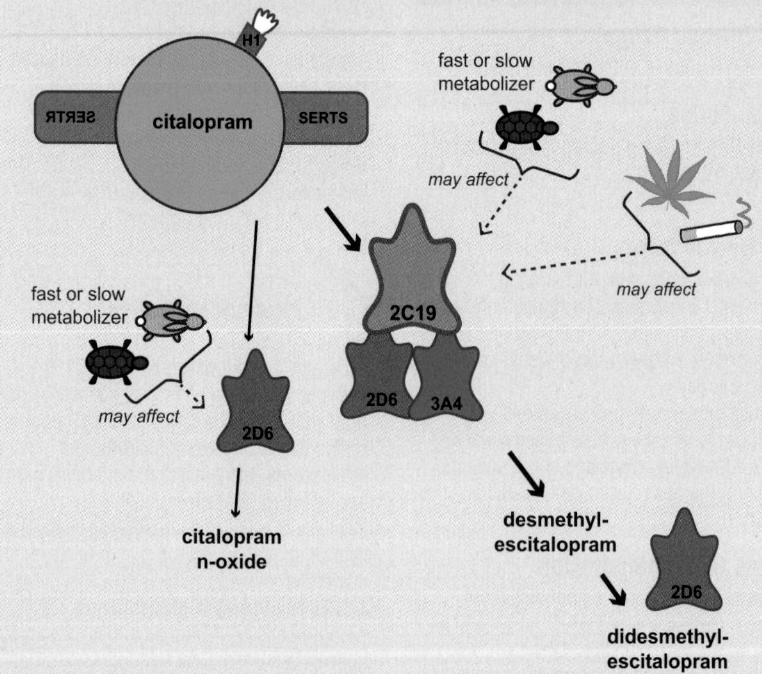

Figure 2 Citalopram metabolism. The metbaolism of citalopram (and escitalopram) is heavily dependent on CYP2C19 and variation in CYP2C19 activity influences concentrations of citalopram (and escitalopram) in children and adolescents.

achieved at standard maintenance dosing, consider titrating to a higher maintenance dose.

- **CYP2C19 normal metabolizers:** CPIC recommends that clinicians initiate therapy with recommended starting dose. If patient does not adequately respond to recommended maintenance dosing, consider titrating to a higher maintenance dose or switching to a clinically appropriate alternative antidepressant not predominantly metabolized by CYP2C19.
- **CYP2C19 intermediate metabolizers:** CPIC recommends (moderate) that clinicians initiate the standard starting dose but consider a slower titration and lower maintenance dose than normal metabolizers
- **CYP2C19 poor metabolizers:** CPIC recommends that clinicians consider an antidepressant not predominantly metabolized by CYP2C19. If citalopram or escitalopram are clinically appropriate, consider a lower starting dose, slower titration, and 50% reduction of the standard maintenance dose as compared to normal metabolizers.
- Additionally, per the FDA warning, citalopram 20 mg/day is the maximum recommended dose in CYP2C19 poor metabolizers due to the risk of QT prolongation. FDA product labeling additionally cautions that citalopram dose should be limited to 20 mg/day in patients with hepatic impairment and in those taking a CYP2C19 inhibitor.

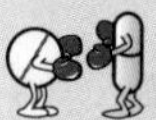

Drug Interactions

- Tramadol increases the risk of seizures in adults taking an antidepressant
- Can increase tricyclic antidepressant levels; use with caution with tricyclic antidepressants
- Can cause a fatal "serotonin syndrome" when combined with MAO inhibitors, so do not use with MAO inhibitors or for at least 14 days after MAOIs are stopped
- Do not start an MAO inhibitor for at least 5 half-lives (5 to 7 days for most drugs) after discontinuing citalopram
- Can theoretically cause weakness, hyperreflexia, and incoordination when combined with sumatriptan, or possibly with other triptans, requiring careful monitoring of patient
- Possible increased risk of bleeding
- Should not be dosed above 20 mg/day in patients taking a CYP2C19 inhibitor (e.g., cimetidine) due to risk of QT prolongation

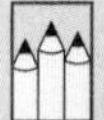

Dosing Tips

- Starting and target doses may be lower and longer intervals between dose increases may be needed (see How to Dose)
- Adolescents often need and receive adult doses
- If a child on a stable dose begins to lose tolerability with more side effects upon entering adolescence, this may signal the need for a dose reduction; however, clinicians should also enquire about changes in smoking – including cannabis – which have been shown to increase citalopram concentrations (Vaughn et al., 2021)
- Given once daily, with or without food, any time of day tolerated
- Citalopram should no longer be prescribed at doses greater than 40 mg/day because it can cause abnormal changes in the electrical activity of the heart
- Some controversy with FDA dosage limit of 40 mg/day, and higher doses may be prescribed by experts, particularly in patients who may be ultrarapid CYP2C19 metabolizers. However, at high doses of citalopram, EKG is recommended.
- The more anxious and agitated the patient, the lower the starting dose, the slower the titration
- If intolerable anxiety, insomnia, agitation, akathisia, or activation occurs either upon dosing initiation or discontinuation, consider an alternative SSRI. Importantly, the risk of activation with one SSRI does not predict the likelihood of activation with another SSRI.

How to Switch

- From another antidepressant to citalopram:
  - When tapering a prior antidepressant, see its entry in this manual for how to stop and how to taper off that specific drug
  - Generally, try to stop the first agent before starting citalopram so that new side effects of citalopram can be distinguished from withdrawal effects of the first agent
  - If necessary, can cross taper off the prior antidepressant and dose up on citalopram simultaneously in urgent situations, being aware of all specific drug interactions to avoid

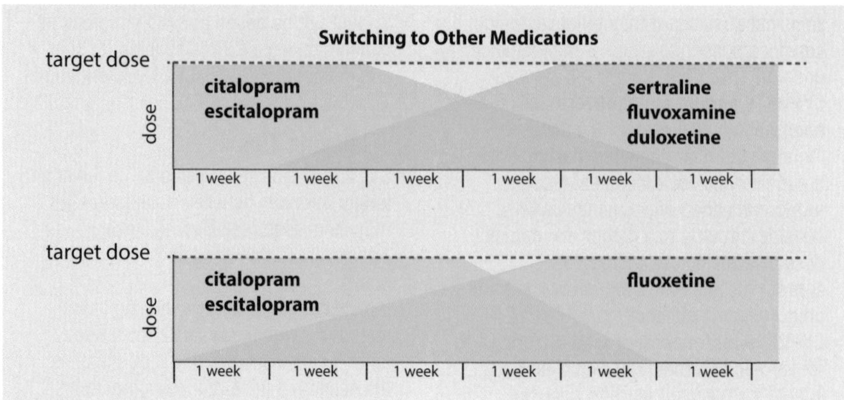

- Off citalopram to another antidepressant:
  - In situations when there are antidepressant-related side effects, try to stop citalopram before starting another antidepressant
  - Stopping citalopram often means tapering off since discontinuing many SSRIs can cause withdrawal symptoms
  - Can reduce citalopram dose by 50% every 3 to 7 days, or slower if this rate still causes withdrawal symptoms
  - If necessary, can cross taper off citalopram this way while dosing up on another antidepressant simultaneously in urgent situations, being aware of all specific drug interactions to avoid

How to Stop

- Taper may not be necessary; however, tapering to avoid potential withdrawal reactions is generally prudent
- Many patients tolerate 50% dose reduction for 3 days, then another 50% reduction for 3 days, then discontinuation. More recently, however, hyperbolic discontinuation of SSRIs has been recommended in which the dose of the SSRI is halved every 4 weeks, and this may be a preferable strategy in youth (Strawn et al., 2023). Also, when SSRIs are stopped, the risk of relapse is highest during the first 8 weeks after discontinuation.
- If withdrawal symptoms emerge during discontinuation, raise dose to stop symptoms and then restart withdrawal much more slowly, such as reducing citalopram by 5 mg every 3 to 7 days

WHAT TO EXPECT

Onset of Action

- Some patients may experience increased energy or activation early after initiation of treatment
- Full onset of therapeutic actions is usually delayed by 2–4 weeks
- If it is not working within 6–8 weeks, it may require a dosage increase or it may not work at all

Duration of Action

- Effects are consistent over a 24-hour period
- May continue to work for many years to prevent relapse of symptoms

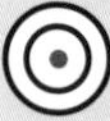

Primary Target Symptoms

- Depressed and/or irritable mood
- Anxiety (fear and worry are often target symptoms, but citalopram can occasionally and transiently increase these symptoms short term before improving them)
- Sleep disturbance, both hypersomnia and insomnia (eventually, but can actually cause insomnia, especially short term)
- Prior to initiation of treatment, it is helpful to develop a list of target symptoms of depression and/or anxiety to monitor during treatment to better assess treatment response

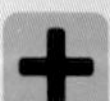

What Is Considered a Positive Result?

- The goal of treatment is complete remission of current symptoms as well as prevention of future relapses

- In practice, many patients have only a partial response where some symptoms are improved but others persist (especially insomnia, fatigue, and problems concentrating in depression), in which case higher doses of citalopram, adding a second agent, or switching to an agent with a different mechanism of action can be considered
- If treatment works, it most often reduces or even eliminates symptoms, but is not a cure since symptoms can recur after medicine is stopped

How Long to Treat

- For adolescents with depression, generally, 9–12 months of antidepressant treatment is recommended (Hathaway et al., 2018)
- For anxiety disorders, 6–9 months of antidepressant treatment may be sufficient, though many clinicians extend treatment to 12 months based on extrapolation of data from adults with anxiety disorders (Hathaway et al., 2018; Strawn et al., 2023)
- Extended treatment periods may decrease the risk of long-term morbidity and recurrence; however, the goal of treatment is ultimately remission, rather than duration of antidepressant pharmacotherapy (Hathaway et al., 2018)
- In terms of the length of antidepressant treatment, evidence-based guidelines represent a starting point; appropriate treatment duration varies, and patient-specific response, psychological factors, and timing of discontinuation must be considered for individual pediatric patients (Hathaway et al., 2018)

What If It Stops Working?

- Some patients who have an initial response may relapse even though they continue treatment, sometimes called "poop-out"
- Some patients may experience apparent lack of consistent efficacy due to activation syndrome or latent or underlying or newly evolved bipolar disorder, or major depressive episodes with mixed features, and require antidepressant discontinuation and a switch to a second generation antipsychotic

What If It Doesn't Work?

- Consider evaluation for another diagnosis (especially bipolar illness or depression with mixed features) or for a comorbid condition (e.g., medical illness, substance abuse)
- When treating youth with anxiety disorders, many patients will have had significant anxiety for years prior to beginning treatment. As such, when anxiety is treated with an SSRI, their symptoms may be improved, but the patient has likely missed important developmental milestones (e.g., spending the night with friends, being able to ask questions in class). Developing these skills will take time. Beyond this, the family may have lived with the anxious child for years and following treatment of the child, the family may need to readjust.
- Be mindful of family conflict contributing to the presentation; sometimes treating parental depression or anxiety disorders improves psychiatric and social function without any treatment of youth. Also, accommodation is common in families of youth with anxiety disorders and may need to be addressed specifically, as it can perpetuate symptoms.
- Consider factors associated with poor response to SSRIs in treatment-resistant depression or anxiety disorders, such as severe symptoms, long-lasting symptoms, poor treatment adherence, prior nonresponse to other treatments, and the presence of comorbid disorders
- Consider other important potential factors such as ongoing conflicts, family psychopathology, and an adverse environment (e.g., poverty, chaos, violence, prior and ongoing psychological trauma, abuse, neglect). Additionally, when symptoms are prominent at school, consider the presence of a learning disorder.
- Institute trauma-informed care for appropriate children and adolescents
- A 2007 meta-analysis of published and unpublished trials in pediatric patients found that antidepressants had a number needed to treat (NNT) of 10 for depression, 6 for OCD, and 3 for anxiety disorders; thus, citalopram may not work in all children, so consider switching to another antidepressant (Bridge et al., 2007)
- Consider a dose adjustment
- Consider augmenting options:
  - Cognitive behavioral therapy (CBT), interpersonal psychotherapy for

adolescents (IPT-A), light therapy, family therapy, and exercise especially in adolescents
  - For partial response (depression): use caution when adding medications to citalopram, especially in children since there are not sufficient studies of augmentation in children or adolescents; however, for the expert, consider bupropion, aripiprazole, or other atypical antipsychotics such as quetiapine; use combinations of antidepressants with caution, as this may activate bipolar disorder and suicidal ideation
  - For insomnia: sleep hygiene, CBT for insomnia, melatonin, or alpha 2 agonists
  - For anxiety: buspirone, antihistamines
  - Add lithium or atypical antipsychotics for bipolar depression, psychotic depression, treatment-resistant depression, or treatment-resistant anxiety disorders. However, with citalopram, use caution when adding atypical antipsychotics associated with a risk of QT prolongation.
  - TMS (transcranial magnetic stimulation) may have a role, although pediatric trials of TMS have been hampered by high sham response rates (Croarkin et al., 2021)
  - ECT (case studies show effectiveness; cognitive side effects are similar to those in adults; reserve for treatment-resistant cases)

TALKING TO PATIENTS AND CAREGIVERS

What to Tell Parents About Efficacy

- Doesn't work right away; full therapeutic benefits may take up to 8 weeks, yet parents and teachers might see improvement before the patient does
- While the medicine helps by reducing symptoms and improving function, it is not a cure, and it is therefore necessary to keep taking the medication to sustain its therapeutic effects
- Since every treatment consideration depends on a risk/benefit analysis, parents should fully understand short- and long-term risks as well as benefits
- After successful treatment, continuation of citalopram may be necessary to prevent relapse, especially in those who have had more than one episode or a very severe episode. In general, when treating depression in children and adolescents, medications are continued for 12 months after symptoms have resolved, while for anxiety disorders, clinicians have generally treated for 6–9 months (Hathaway et al., 2018).
- Often a good idea to tell parents whether the medication chosen is specifically approved for the disorder being treated, or if it is "unapproved" or "off-label" but nevertheless good clinical practice and based upon prudent extrapolation of controlled data from adults and from experience in children and adolescents instead of formal FDA approval

What to Tell Children and Adolescents About Efficacy

- We are trying to make you feel better
- It may be a good idea to give the medication a try; if it's not working very well, we can stop the medication and try something else
- A good try takes 2 to 3 months or even longer
- If it does make you feel better, you cannot stop it right away or you may feel sad or worried again
- Medications don't change who you are as a person; they give you the opportunity to be the best person you can be

What to Tell Parents About Side Effects

- Explain that side effects are expected in many when starting and are most common in the first 2–3 weeks of starting or increasing the dose
- Some SSRI side effects emerge early and resolve quickly (e.g., activation, gastrointestinal symptoms). In contrast, other side effects are late-emerging (e.g., weight gain) or persistent (e.g., sexual dysfunction). Discussing the temporal course of the side effects and distinguishing between persistent and transient side effects is critical. Ensuring that patients are aware not only of side effects but the tendency of some side effects to be transient is important and should be part of discussions with patients and their families. For many, knowing that a side effect is likely transient, as opposed to persistent,

may significantly influence the patient and family's anxiety or fears related to medication (Strawn et al., 2023).
- Tell parents many side effects go away and do so about the same time that therapeutic effects start
- Predict side effects in advance (you will look clever and competent to the parents unless you scare them with too much information and cause nocebo effects, in which case you won't look so clever when the patient develops lots of side effects and stops medication; use your judgment here); a balanced but honest presentation is an art rather than a science
- Ask them to help monitor for increased suicidality and if present, report any such symptoms immediately
- Ask parents to support the patient while side effects are occurring
- Parents should fully understand short- and long-term risks as well as benefits
- Explaining to the parents what to expect from medication treatment, and especially potential side effects, can help prevent early termination of medication

What to Tell Children and Adolescents About Side Effects

- Even if you get side effects, most of them get better or go away in a few days to a few weeks
- Consider having a conversation about sexual side effects in some adolescents who can find these side effects confusing and especially burdensome
- Explaining to child/adolescent what to expect from medication treatment, and especially potential side effects, can help prevent early termination of medication
- Tell adolescents and children capable of understanding that some young patients, especially those who are depressed, may develop thoughts of hurting themselves, and if this happens, not to be alarmed but to tell their parents right away

What to Tell Teachers About the Medication (If Parents Consent)

- It is not abusable
- Encourage dialogue with parents/guardians about any behavior or mood changes

SPECIAL POPULATIONS

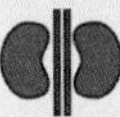

Renal Impairment

- No dose adjustment for mild to moderate impairment
- Use cautiously in patients with severe impairment

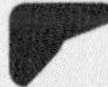

Hepatic Impairment

- Should not be used at doses greater than 20 mg/day
- May need to dose cautiously at the lower end of the dose range in some patients for maximal tolerability

Cardiac Impairment

- May cause abnormal changes in the electrical activity of the heart at doses greater than 40 mg/day
- In a study using US claims data, the crude incident rate of adverse cardiac events in pediatric patients taking citalopram was 15.5/10,000 person-years (Czaja et al., 2013)

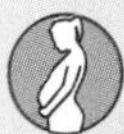

Pregnancy

- Controlled studies have not been conducted in pregnant women
- Not generally recommended for use during pregnancy, especially during first trimester
- Nonetheless, continuous treatment during pregnancy may be necessary and has not been proven to be harmful to the fetus
- At delivery there may be more bleeding in the mother and transient irritability or sedation in the newborn
- Must weigh the risk of treatment (first trimester fetal development, third trimester newborn delivery) to the child against the risk of no treatment (recurrence of depression, maternal health, infant bonding) to the mother and child
- For many patients, this may mean continuing treatment during pregnancy
- Exposure to SSRIs early in pregnancy may be associated with increased risk of septal heart defects (absolute risk is small)
- SSRI use beyond the 20th week of pregnancy may be associated with increased risk of pulmonary hypertension in newborns, although this is not proven

- Exposure to SSRIs late in pregnancy may be associated with increased risk of gestational hypertension and preeclampsia
- Neonates exposed to SSRIs or SNRIs late in the third trimester have developed complications requiring prolonged hospitalization, respiratory support, and tube feeding; reported symptoms are consistent with either a direct toxic effect of SSRIs and SNRIs or, possibly, a drug discontinuation syndrome, and include respiratory distress, cyanosis, apnea, seizures, temperature instability, feeding difficulty, vomiting, hypoglycemia, hypotonia, hypertonia, hyperreflexia, tremor, jitteriness, irritability, and constant crying

Breast Feeding

- Some drug is found in breast milk
- Trace amounts may be present in nursing children whose mothers are on citalopram
- If child becomes irritable or sedated, breast feeding or drug may need to be discontinued
- Immediate postpartum period is a high-risk time for depression, especially in women who have had prior depressive episodes, so drug may need to be reinstituted late in the third trimester or shortly after childbirth to prevent a recurrence during the postpartum period
- Must weigh benefits of breast feeding with risks and benefits of antidepressant treatment versus nontreatment to both the infant and the mother
- For many patients, this may mean continuing treatment during breast feeding

THE ART OF PSYCHOPHARMACOLOGY

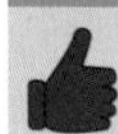

Potential Advantages

- In children:
  - May be better tolerated than some other SSRIs
  - Not specifically approved, but preliminary data suggest citalopram may be safe and effective in children and adolescents with OCD and with depression
- In adolescents:
  - May be better tolerated than some other SSRIs
  - Not specifically approved, but preliminary data suggest citalopram may be safe and effective in children and adolescents with OCD and with depression
- All ages:
  - Patients taking concomitant medications (few drug interactions)
  - Patients requiring faster onset of action
  - In general, citalopram may be better tolerated than some other SSRIs, with fewer drug interactions than most

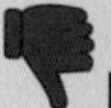

Potential Disadvantages

- In children and adolescents:
  - Those who are already psychomotor agitated, angry, or irritable, and who do not have a psychiatric diagnosis
  - Those who may possibly have a mood disorder with mixed or bipolar features, especially those with these features and a family history of bipolar disorder
- All ages:
  - May require dosage titration to attain optimal efficacy
  - Can be sedating in some patients

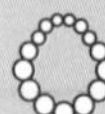

Pearls

- SSRIs show greater efficacy in pediatric anxiety disorders compared to depression
- In anxious youth, SSRIs produce faster and greater improvement compared to SNRIs (Strawn et al., 2018)
- Can cause cognitive and affective "flattening"
- Documentation of efficacy in anxiety disorders is less comprehensive than for escitalopram and other SSRIs
- Some evidence suggests that citalopram treatment during only the luteal phase may be more effective than continuous treatment for patients with PMDD

SUGGESTED READING

Alaghband-Rad J, Hakimshooshtary M. A randomized controlled clinical trial of citalopram versus fluoxetine in children and adolescents with obsessive-compulsive disorder (OCD). Eur Child Adolesc Psychiatry 2009;18(3):131–5.

Aldrich SL, Poweleit EA, Prows CA et al. Influence of CYP2C19 metabolizer status on escitalopram/citalopram tolerability and response in youth with anxiety and depressive disorders. Front Pharmacol 2019;10:99.

Bousman CA, Stevenson JM, Ramsey LB et al. Clinical Pharmacogenetics Implementation Consortium (CPIC) guideline for CYP2D6, CYP2C19, CYP2B6, SLC6A4, and HTR2A genotypes and serotonin reuptake inhibitor antidepressants. Clin Pharmacol Ther 2023;114(1):51–68.

Bridge JA, Iyengar S, Salary CB et al. Clinical response and risk for reported suicidal ideation and suicide attempts in pediatric antidepressant treatment: a meta-analysis of randomized controlled trials. JAMA 2007;297(15):1683–96.

Croarkin PE, Elmaadawi AZ, Aaronson ST et al. Left prefrontal transcranial magnetic stimulation for treatment-resistant depression in adolescents: a double-blind, randomized, sham-controlled trial. Neuropsychopharmacology 2021;46(2):462–9.

Czaja AS, Valuck RJ, Anderson HD. Comparative safety of selective serotonin reuptake inhibitors among pediatric users with respect to adverse cardiac events. Pharmacoepidemiol Drug Saf 2013;22(6):607–14.

Hathaway EE, Walkup JT, Strawn JR. Antidepressant treatment duration in pediatric depressive and anxiety disorders: how long is long enough? Curr Probl Pediatr Adolesc Health Care 2018;48(2):31–9.

King BH, Hollander E, Sikich L et al. Lack of efficacy of citalopram in children with autism spectrum disorders and high levels of repetitive behavior: citalopram ineffective in children with autism. Arch Gen Psychiatry 2009;66(6):583–90.

Kreilgaard M, Smith DG, Brennum LT, Sánchez C. Prediction of clinical response based on pharmacokinetic/pharmacodynamic models of 5-hydroxytryptamine reuptake inhibitors in mice. Br J Pharmacol 2008;155(2):276–84.

Lu L, Mills JA, Li Hailong et al. Acute neurofunctional effects of escitalopram in pediatric anxiety: a double-blind, placebo-controlled trial. J Am Acad Child Adolesc Psychiatry 2021;60(10):1309-18.

Matthäus F, Haddjeri N, Sánchez C et al. The allosteric citalopram binding site differentially interferes with neuronal firing rate and SERT trafficking in serotonergic neurons. Eur Neuropsychopharmacol 2016;26(11):1806–17.

Sangkuhl K, Klein TE, Altman RB. PharmGKB summary: citalopram pharmacokinetics pathway. Pharmacogenet Genomics 2011;21(11):769–72.

Simonoff E, Mowlem F, Pearson et al. Citalopram did not significantly improve anxiety in children with autism spectrum disorder undergoing treatment for core symptoms: secondary analysis of a trial to reduce repetitive behaviors. J Child Adolesc Psychopharmacol 2022;32(4):233–41.

Strawn JR, Mills JA, Sauley BA, Welge JA. The impact of antidepressant dose and class on treatment response in pediatric anxiety disorders: a meta-analysis. J Am Acad Child Adolesc Psychiatry 2018;57(4):235–44.e2.

Strawn JR, Mills JA, Poweleit EA, Ramsey LB, Croarkin PE. Adverse effects of antidepressant medications and their management in children and adolescents. Pharmacotherapy 2023;43(7):675–90.

Vaughn SE, Strawn JR, Poweleit EA, Sarangdhar M, Ramsey LB. The impact of marijuana on antidepressant treatment in adolescents: clinical and pharmacologic considerations. J Pers Med 2021;11(7):615.

THERAPEUTICS

Brands

- Anafranil

Generic

Yes

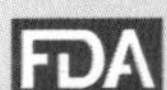

US FDA Approved for Pediatric Use

- Obsessive-compulsive disorder (OCD) (ages 10 and older)

Off-Label for Pediatric Use

- Depression
- Severe and treatment-resistant depression
- Anxiety
- Neuropathic pain/chronic pain

Class and Mechanism of Action

- Neuroscience-based Nomenclature: serotonin reuptake inhibitor (S-RI)
- Tricyclic antidepressant (TCA)
- Clomipramine is a potent serotonin reuptake inhibitor, but its metabolite desmethylclomipramine has minimal serotonergic activity and potent noradrenergic activity. At steady state the ratio of clomipramine to desmethylclomipramine is roughly 1:2–3 because clomipramine has a half-life of 12–36 hours and desmethylclomipramine has a half-life of approximately 72 hours. Thus, after oral administration, much of the therapeutic effect of clomipramine's serotonergic activity is lost and replaced by the noradrenergic activity of desmethylclomipramine.
- Clomipramine presumably increases serotonergic neurotransmission by blocking the serotonin reuptake pump (transporter), which results in desensitization of serotonin receptors, especially serotonin 1A receptors
- Clomipramine presumably increases noradrenergic neurotransmission by blocking the norepinephrine reuptake pump (transporter), which results in desensitization of beta adrenergic receptors
- Since dopamine is inactivated by norepinephrine reuptake in the frontal cortex, which largely lacks dopamine transporters, clomipramine can increase dopamine neurotransmission in this part of the brain

SAFETY AND TOLERABILITY

Notable Side Effects

- Blurred vision, constipation, dry mouth
- Weight loss
- Dizziness, sedation, fatigue
- Nausea, diarrhea
- Sweating
- Urinary retention, heartburn, unusual taste in mouth
- Anxiety, nervousness, restlessness, weakness, headache
- Sexual dysfunction (impotence, change in libido)
- Rash, itching
- Note: patients with diagnosed or undiagnosed bipolar or psychotic disorders may be more vulnerable to CNS-activating actions of TCAs like clomipramine; pay particular attention to signs of activation in children with developmental disorders, autism spectrum disorders, or brain injury as they may not tolerate these side effects well
- Treatment-emergent activation syndrome (TEAS) includes agitation, anxiety, panic attacks, irritability, aggression, impulsivity, insomnia, and suicidality
- TEAS can represent side effects, but should not be confused with bipolar mania or the onset of suicidality and should be monitored and investigated with consideration of discontinuing or decreasing dose of clomipramine or addition of another agent or switching to another agent to reduce these symptoms

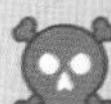

Life-Threatening or Dangerous Side Effects

- Paralytic ileus, hyperthermia (TCAs + anticholinergic agents)
- Lowered seizure threshold and rare seizures
- Orthostatic hypotension, arrhythmias, tachycardia
- QTc prolongation
- Some cases of sudden death have occurred in children taking TCAs
- Hepatic failure, extrapyramidal symptoms
- Increased intraocular pressure
- Rare induction of mania
- Rare suicidal ideation and behavior (suicidality) (short-term regulatory studies

did not show any actual suicides in any age group and also did not show an increase in the risk of suicidality with antidepressants compared to placebo beyond age 24)

Growth and Maturation

- Growth should be monitored; long-term effects are unknown

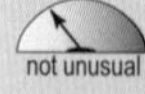

Weight Gain

- Unlike in adults, in whom 20% experience weight gain while taking clomipramine, only 2% of youth experience weight gain

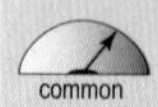

Sedation

- Many experience and/or can be significant in amount
- Tolerance to sedative effect may develop with long-term use

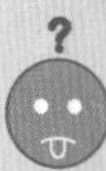

What to Do About Side Effects

- Wait, wait, wait: mild side effects are common, happen early, and usually improve with time, but treatment benefits can be delayed and often begin just as the side effects wear off
- Monitor side effects closely, especially when initiating treatment
- May wish to try dosing every other day to deal with side effects, or wash out for a week and try again at half dose or every other day
- May wish to give some drugs at night if not tolerated during the day
- For activation (jitteriness, anxiety, insomnia):
  - Consider a temporary dose reduction or a more gradual up-titration
  - Consider switching to another antidepressant
  - Optimize psychotherapeutic interventions
  - Activation and agitation may represent the induction of a bipolar state, especially a mixed dysphoric bipolar II condition sometimes associated with suicidal ideation, and may require the addition of lithium or an atypical antipsychotic and/or discontinuation of clomipramine
- Often best to try another monotherapy prior to resorting to augmentation strategies to treat side effects
- For insomnia: consider adding melatonin
- For GI upset: try giving medication with a meal. However, clomipramine is associated with nearly twice the rate of vomiting in youth compared to adults. Giving antidepressants with food will, in general, decrease peak plasma concentrations and increase the time required for absorption (Strawn et al., 2021, 2023).
- For sexual dysfunction: probably best to reduce dose or discontinue and try another agent

How Drug Causes Side Effects

- Theoretically due to increases in serotonin concentrations at serotonin receptors in parts of the brain and body other than those that cause therapeutic actions (e.g., unwanted actions of serotonin in sleep centers causing insomnia, unwanted actions of serotonin in the gut causing diarrhea)
- Increasing serotonin can cause diminished dopamine release and might contribute to emotional flattening, cognitive slowing, and apathy in some patients
- Anticholinergic activity may explain sedative effects, dry mouth, constipation, and blurred vision
- Sedative effects and weight gain may be due to antihistamine properties
- Blockade of alpha adrenergic 1 receptors may explain dizziness, sedation, and hypotension
- Cardiac arrhythmias and seizures, especially in overdose, may be caused by blockade of ion channels

Warnings and Precautions

- Consider distributing brochures provided by the FDA and the drug companies as well as the medication guides from the American Academy of Child & Adolescent Psychiatry (AACAP)
- Carefully consider monitoring patients regularly within the practical limits, particularly during the first several weeks of treatment
- Warn patients and their caregivers when possible about the possibility of activating side effects and advise them to report such symptoms immediately
- Carefully weigh the risks and benefits of pharmacological treatment against the risks and benefits of nontreatment with

antidepressants and it is a good idea to document this in the patient's chart
- Add or initiate other antidepressants with caution for up to 2 weeks after discontinuing clomipramine
- Use with caution in patients with history of seizures, urinary retention, angle-closure glaucoma, hyperthyroidism
- TCAs can increase QTc interval, especially at toxic doses, which can be attained not only by overdose but also by combining with drugs that inhibit TCA metabolism via CYP2D6
- Because TCAs can prolong QTc interval, use with caution in patients who have bradycardia or who are taking drugs that can induce bradycardia (e.g., beta blockers, calcium channel blockers, clonidine, digitalis)
- Because TCAs can prolong QTc interval, use with caution in patients who have hypokalemia and/or hypomagnesemia or who are taking drugs that can induce hypokalemia and/or hypomagnesemia (e.g., diuretics, stimulant laxatives, glucocorticoids, tetracosactide)
- As with any antidepressant, use with caution in patients with bipolar disorder unless treated with concomitant mood-stabilizing agent
- Monitor patients for activation and suicidal ideation and involve parents/guardians

When Not to Prescribe
- If patient is taking an MAO inhibitor
- If patient is recovering from myocardial infarction
- If patient is taking agents capable of significantly prolonging QTc interval (e.g., pimozide, thioridazine, selected antiarrhythmics, moxifloxacin, sparfloxacin)
- If there is a history of QTc prolongation or cardiac arrhythmia
- If patient is taking drugs that inhibit clomipramine metabolism, including CYP2D6 inhibitors or CYP1A2 inhibitors, except by an expert (see Pearls)
- If there is a proven allergy to clomipramine

Long-Term Use
- Growth should be monitored; long-term effects are unknown

Habit Forming
- No

Overdose
- Death may occur; convulsions, cardiac dysrhythmias, severe hypotension, CNS depression, coma, changes in ECG

DOSING AND USE

Usual Dosage Range
- Generally dosed the same as in adults: 100–250 mg/day

Dosage Forms
- Capsule 25 mg, 50 mg, 75 mg

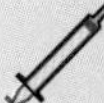

How to Dose
- Generally dosed the same as in adults: initial dose 25 mg/day; dose should be titrated to a maximum of 100 mg/day after 2 weeks, after which dose can then be titrated over several weeks up to a maximum of 250 mg/day; during titration, dose should be divided and given with meals in order to minimize gastrointestinal side effects; after titration, the total daily dose may be given once daily at bedtime to minimize daytime sedation

Options for Administration
- Cutting capsules for fractional dosing or to add contents to food for patients with trouble swallowing is generally not recommended

Tests
- Monitoring of plasma drug levels is potentially available at specialty laboratories for the expert. Many clinicians treating adolescents with OCD will use the therapeutic ranges commonly reported for adults:
  - Clomipramine: 70–200 ng/mL
  - Desmethylclomipramine (norclomipramine): 150–300 ng/mL
  - Total: clomipramine + desmethylclomipramine: 220–500 ng/mL
- Weight and BMI percentiles as well as blood pressure and heart rate during treatment
- Currently, the AACAP recommends ECGs prior to initiation of TCA therapy and after dose titration of TCAs

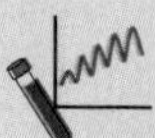

Pharmacokinetics

- Substrate for CYP2D6 and 1A2; is also a substrate for CYP2C19 and 3A4
- Metabolized to an active metabolite, desmethylclomipramine, a predominantly norepinephrine reuptake inhibitor, by demethylation via CYP1A2 as well as CYP2C19 and CYP3A4 (see Figure 1)
- Inhibits CYP2D6
- Half-life of clomipramine is approximately 12–36 hours in youth, but the half-life of its metabolite, desmethylclomipramine, is approximately 72 hours
- Time to peak plasma concentration 2 to 6 hours
- At steady state the ratio of clomipramine to desmethylclomipramine is roughly 1:2–3 because of this difference in half-life between clomipramine and desmethylclomipramine
- Food does not affect absorption

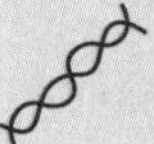

Pharmacogenetics

- The Clinical Pharmacogenetics Implementation Consortium (CPIC) provides optional recommendations for CYP2D6 and CYP2C19 for clomipramine:
  - **CYP2D6 poor metabolizers (optional):** Avoid tricyclic use due to the potential for side effects. Consider an alternative drug not metabolized by CYP2D6. If a TCA is warranted, consider a 50% reduction of recommended starting dose. Utilize therapeutic drug monitoring to guide dose adjustments.
  - **CYP2D6 ultrarapid metabolizers (optional):** Avoid tricyclic use due to potential lack of efficacy. Consider an alternative drug not metabolized by CYP2D6. If a TCA is warranted, consider titrating to a higher target dose (compared to normal metabolizers). Utilize therapeutic drug monitoring to guide dose adjustments.
  - **CYP2C19 rapid/ultrarapid metabolizers (optional):** Avoid tertiary amine use due to the potential for suboptimal response. Consider an alternative drug not metabolized by CYP2C19. TCAs without major CYP2C19 metabolism include the secondary amines nortriptyline and desipramine. If a tertiary amine is warranted, utilize therapeutic drug monitoring to guide dose adjustments.

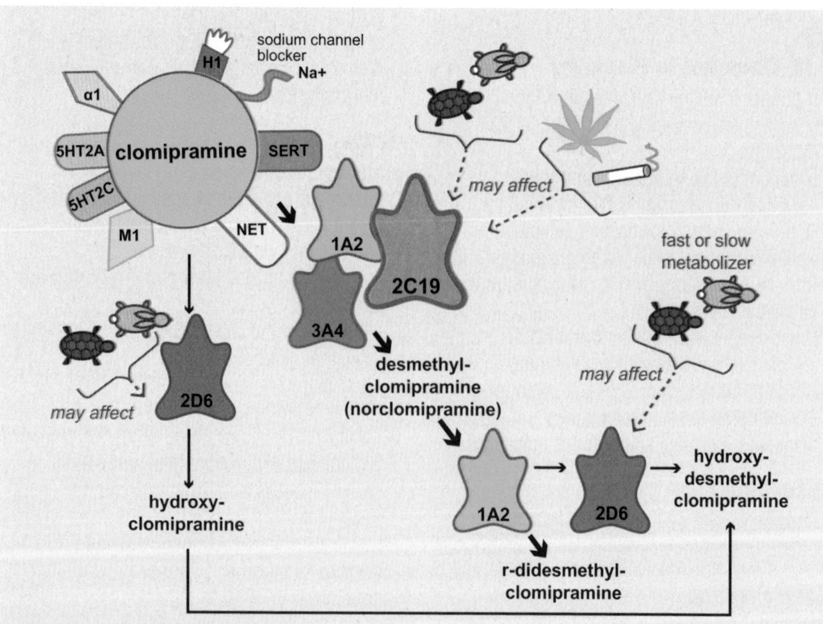

Figure 1 Clomipramine metabolism.

- **CYP2C19 poor metabolizers (optional):** Avoid tertiary amine use due to the potential for suboptimal response. Consider an alternative drug not metabolized by CYP2C19. TCAs without major CYP2C19 metabolism include secondary amines, nortriptyline, and desipramine. For tertiary amines, consider a 50% reduction of the recommended starting dose. Utilize therapeutic drug monitoring to guide dose adjustments.

Drug Interactions

- Tramadol reported to increase the risk of seizures in patients taking an antidepressant
- Can cause a fatal "serotonin syndrome" when combined with MAO inhibitors, so do not use with MAO inhibitors or for at least 14 days after MAOIs are stopped
- Do not start an MAO inhibitor for at least 5 weeks after discontinuing clomipramine
- Use of TCAs with anticholinergic drugs may result in paralytic ileus or hyperthermia
- Fluoxetine, paroxetine, bupropion, duloxetine, and other CYP2D6 inhibitors may increase TCA concentrations
- Fluvoxamine, a CYP1A2 inhibitor, decreases the conversion of clomipramine to desmethylclomipramine, and increases clomipramine plasma concentrations. Adding fluvoxamine to clomipramine has been used by experts to shift the ratio of clomipramine to its major metabolite desmethylclomipramine (norclomipramine) (see Pearls).
- Cimetidine may increase plasma concentrations of TCAs and cause anticholinergic symptoms
- Phenothiazines or haloperidol may raise TCA blood concentrations
- May alter effects of antihypertensive drugs
- Use of TCAs with sympathomimetic agents may increase sympathetic activity
- TCAs may inhibit hypotensive effects of clonidine

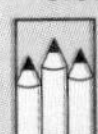

Dosing Tips

- Plasma levels are higher in lower-weight children; therefore, starting and target doses may be lower and longer intervals between dose increases may be needed (see How to Dose)
- Doses over 250 mg/day can increase risk for seizures
- Adolescents often need and receive adult doses
- Be aware that metabolism changes during puberty and entry into adolescence and becomes more like adults (i.e., slower than in children)
- If a child on a stable dose begins to have more side effects upon entering adolescence, this may signal the need for a dose reduction due to changing metabolism
- The long half-lives of clomipramine and its active metabolite mean that dose changes will not be fully reflected in plasma for 2–3 weeks, lengthening titration to final dose and extending withdrawal from treatment
- If given in a single dose, should generally be administered at bedtime because of its sedative properties
- If given in split doses, largest dose should generally be given at bedtime because of its sedative properties
- If patients experience nightmares, split dose and do not give large dose at bedtime
- Patients treated for chronic pain may require lower doses
- Patients treated for OCD may often require doses at the high end of the range (e.g., 200–250 mg/day)

How to Switch

- From another antidepressant to clomipramine:
    - When tapering a prior antidepressant, see its entry in this manual for how to stop and how to taper off that specific drug
    - In situations when there are antidepressant-related side effects, try to stop the first agent before starting clomipramine so that new side effects of clomipramine can be distinguished from withdrawal effects of the first agent
    - If urgent, cross taper
- Off clomipramine to another antidepressant:
    - Generally, try to stop clomipramine before starting another antidepressant
    - Taper to avoid withdrawal effects (dizziness, nausea, stomach cramps, sweating, tingling, dysesthesias)
    - Can reduce clomipramine dose by 50% every 3 days, or slower if this rate still causes withdrawal symptoms
    - If necessary, can cross taper off clomipramine this way while dosing up on another antidepressant simultaneously in urgent situations, being aware of all specific drug interactions to avoid

How to Stop

- Taper to avoid withdrawal effects (dizziness, nausea, sweating, tingling, dysesthesias) (Strawn et al., 2023)
- Even with gradual dose reduction some withdrawal symptoms may appear within the first 2 weeks
- Many patients tolerate 50% dose reduction for 3 days, then another 50% reduction for 3 days, then discontinuation
- If withdrawal symptoms emerge during discontinuation, raise dose to stop symptoms and then restart withdrawal much more slowly

WHAT TO EXPECT

Onset of Action

- Some patients may experience increased energy or activation early after initiation of treatment
- Full onset of therapeutic actions in depression is usually delayed by 2–4 weeks
- Onset of therapeutic action in pediatric OCD can be delayed 6–12 weeks, although meta-analyses in children and adolescents with OCD suggest that the bulk of improvement from clomipramine occurs early in treatment (Varigonda et al. 2016)
- If it is not working for OCD within 8 weeks at a therapeutic level, it may not work at all

Duration of Action

- Effects are consistent over a 24-hour period
- May continue to work for many years to prevent relapse of symptoms

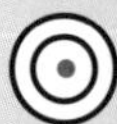

Primary Target Symptoms

- Obsessions, compulsions
- Anxiety (fear and worry are often target symptoms, but clomipramine can occasionally and transiently increase these symptoms short term before improving them)
- Prior to initiation of treatment, it is helpful to develop a list of target symptoms of OCD and anxiety to monitor during treatment to better assess treatment response

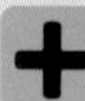

What Is Considered a Positive Result?

- The goal of treatment of OCD is complete remission of current symptoms as well as prevention of future relapses
- In practice, many patients have only a partial response where some symptoms are improved but others persist (especially insomnia, fatigue, and problems concentrating in depression), in which case higher doses of clomipramine, adding a second agent, or switching to an agent with a different mechanism of action can be considered
- If treatment works, it most often reduces or even eliminates symptoms, but is not a cure since symptoms can recur after medicine is stopped
- The goal of treatment of chronic neuropathic pain is to reduce symptoms as much as possible, especially in combination with other treatments

How Long to Treat

- After symptoms are sufficiently reduced/eliminated, continue treating for 12 months for the first episode of depression. For patients with anxiety disorders, 9 months may be advisable (Hathaway et al., 2018).
- For second and subsequent episodes of depression, treatment may need to be longer. In general, in youth, relapse is most likely in the first 1–3 months after discontinuing an antidepressant (Emslie et al., 2004).
- For OCD and anxiety disorders, treatment may need to be indefinite
- Use in other anxiety disorders and chronic pain may also need to be indefinite, but long-term treatment is not well studied in these conditions

What If It Stops Working?

- Some patients who have an initial response may relapse even though they continue treatment, sometimes called "poop-out"
- Some patients may experience apparent lack of consistent efficacy due to activation syndrome or latent or underlying or newly evolved bipolar disorder, or major depressive episodes with mixed features, and require antidepressant discontinuation and a switch to a second generation antipsychotic

What If It Doesn't Work?

- Consider evaluation for another diagnosis (especially bipolar illness or depression with mixed features) or for a comorbid condition (e.g., medical illness, substance abuse)
- Be mindful of family conflict contributing to the presentation; sometimes treating parental depression can improve psychiatric and social function without any treatment of youth. Also, accommodation is common in families of youth with anxiety disorders and may need to be addressed specifically, as it can perpetuate symptoms
- Consider factors associated with poor response to SSRIs in treatment-resistant depression or anxiety disorders, such as severe symptoms, long-lasting symptoms, poor treatment adherence, prior nonresponse to other treatments, and the presence of comorbid disorders
- Consider other important potential factors such as ongoing conflicts, family psychopathology, and an adverse environment (e.g., poverty, chaos, violence, prior and ongoing psychological trauma, abuse, neglect). Additionally, when symptoms are prominent at school, consider the presence of a learning disorder.
- Institute trauma-informed care for appropriate children and adolescents
- A 2007 meta-analysis of published and unpublished trials in pediatric patients found that antidepressants had a number needed to treat (NNT) of 10 for depression, 6 for OCD, and 3 for anxiety disorders; thus, clomipramine may not work in all children, so consider switching to another antidepressant (Bridge et al., 2007)
- Consider a dose adjustment
- Consider augmenting options:
  - Experts may consider augmentation with fluvoxamine (see below)
  - Cognitive behavioral therapy (CBT), interpersonal psychotherapy for adolescents (IPT-A), light therapy, family therapy, and exercise especially in adolescents. For youth with OCD, it is important to ensure that CBT involves exposure as these appear to be the vehicle for improvement.
  - For insomnia: sleep hygiene, CBT for insomnia, melatonin. It's probably best to avoid alpha 2 agonists in TCA-treated patients
  - For anxiety: antihistamines or perhaps buspirone (although pediatric data are mixed)
  - Add lithium or atypical antipsychotics for bipolar depression, psychotic depression, treatment-resistant depression, or treatment-resistant anxiety disorders
  - TMS (transcranial magnetic stimulation) may have a role although pediatric trials of TMS have been hampered by high sham response rates (Croarkin et al., 2021).

TALKING TO PATIENTS AND CAREGIVERS

What to Tell Parents About Efficacy

- Doesn't work right away; full therapeutic benefits may take 2–8 weeks, yet parents and teachers might see improvement before the patient does
- While the medicine helps by reducing symptoms and improving function, it is not a cure, and it is therefore necessary to keep taking the medication to sustain its therapeutic effects
- Since every treatment consideration depends on a risk/benefit analysis, parents should fully understand short- and long-term risks as well as benefits
- One of the antidepressants specifically approved for children and adolescents with OCD (obsessive-compulsive disorder)
- After successful treatment, continuation of clomipramine may be necessary to prevent relapse, especially in those who have had more than one episode or a very severe episode
- Often a good idea to tell parents whether the medication chosen is specifically approved for the disorder being treated, or whether it is being given for "unapproved" or "off-label" reasons based on good clinical practice, expert consensus, and/or prudent extrapolation of controlled data from adults

What to Tell Children and Adolescents About Efficacy

- We are trying to make you feel better
- It may be a good idea to give the medication a try; if it's not working very well, we can stop the medication and try something else

- A good try takes 2 to 3 months or even longer
- If it does make you feel better, you cannot stop it right away or you may get sick again
- Medications don't change who you are as a person; they give you the opportunity to be the best person you can be

What to Tell Parents About Side Effects

- Explain that side effects are expected in many when starting and are most common in the first 2–3 weeks of starting or increasing the dose
- Tell parents many side effects go away and do so about the same time that therapeutic effects start
- Predict side effects in advance (you will look clever and competent to the parents, unless you scare them with too much information and cause nocebo effects, in which case you won't look so clever when the patient develops lots of side effects and stops medication; use your judgment here); a balanced but honest presentation is an art rather than a science
- Ask them to help monitor for increased suicidality and if present, report any such symptoms immediately
- Ask parents to support the patient while side effects are occurring
- Parents should fully understand short- and long-term risks as well as benefits
- Explaining to the parents what to expect from medication treatment, and especially potential side effects, can help prevent early termination of medication

What to Tell Children and Adolescents About Side Effects

- Even if you get side effects, most of them get better or go away in a few days to a few weeks
- Consider having a conversation about sexual side effects in some adolescents who can find these side effects confusing and especially burdensome
- Explaining to child/adolescent what to expect from medication treatment, and especially potential side effects, can help prevent early termination of medication
- Tell adolescents and children capable of understanding that some young patients, especially those who are depressed, may develop thoughts of hurting themselves, and if this happens, not to be alarmed but to tell their parents right away

What to Tell Teachers About the Medication (If Parents Consent)

- Clomipramine can make children/adolescents jittery or restless
- If the patient is sleepy, ask whether the medication is keeping them up at night
- It is not abusable
- Encourage dialogue with parents/guardians about any behavior or mood changes

SPECIAL POPULATIONS

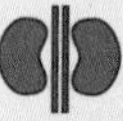

Renal Impairment

- Use with caution

Hepatic Impairment

- Use with caution

Cardiac Impairment

- ECG is recommended at baseline and after dose titrations
- TCAs have been reported to cause arrhythmias, prolongation of conduction time, orthostatic hypotension, sinus tachycardia
- TCAs produce QTc prolongation, which may be enhanced by the existence of bradycardia, hypokalemia, congenital or acquired long QTc interval, which should be evaluated prior to administering clomipramine
- Use with caution if treating concomitantly with a medication likely to produce prolonged bradycardia, hypokalemia, slowing of intracardiac conduction, or prolongation of the QTc interval
- Avoid TCAs in patients with a known history of QTc prolongation
- Risk/benefit ratio may not justify use of TCAs in cardiac impairment

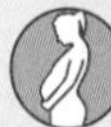

Pregnancy

- Controlled studies have not been conducted in pregnant women
- Clomipramine crosses the placenta
- Adverse effects have been reported in infants whose mothers took a TCA (lethargy, withdrawal symptoms, fetal malformations)

- Must weigh the risk of treatment (first trimester fetal development, third trimester newborn delivery) to the child against the risk of no treatment (recurrence of depression, worsening of OCD, maternal health, infant bonding) to the mother and child
- For many patients this may mean continuing treatment during pregnancy

Breast Feeding

- Some drug is found in breast milk
- Recommended either to discontinue drug or formula feed
- Immediate postpartum period is a high-risk time for depression and worsening of OCD, especially in women who have had prior depressive episodes or OCD symptoms, so drug may need to be reinstituted late in the third trimester or shortly after childbirth to prevent a recurrence or exacerbation during the postpartum period
- Must weigh benefits of breast feeding with risks and benefits of antidepressant treatment versus nontreatment to both the infant and the mother
- For many patients this may mean continuing treatment during breast feeding

THE ART OF PSYCHOPHARMACOLOGY

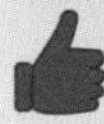

Potential Advantages

- In children:
  - One of four agents specifically approved for OCD in children (also fluvoxamine, fluoxetine, and paroxetine)
- In adolescents:
  - One of four agents specifically approved for OCD in adolescents (also fluvoxamine, fluoxetine, and paroxetine)
- All ages:
  - Patients with insomnia
  - Severe or treatment-resistant depression
  - Patients with comorbid OCD and depression
  - Patients with cataplexy

Potential Disadvantages

- In children:
  - Those who are already psychomotor agitated, angry, or irritable, and who do not have a psychiatric diagnosis
  - Those who may possibly have a mood disorder with mixed or bipolar features, especially those with these features and a family history of bipolar disorder
  - All randomized trials in youth with depression fail to show efficacy of TCAs
  - Approval for OCD is based on a single 8-week study
  - Patients with seizure disorders
- In adolescents:
  - Those who may possibly have a mood disorder with mixed or bipolar features, especially those with these features and a family history of bipolar disorder
  - All randomized trials in youth with depression fail to show efficacy of TCAs
  - Approval for OCD is based on a single 8-week study
  - Patients with seizure disorders
- All ages:
  - Cardiac patients
  - Patients with seizure disorders

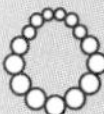

Pearls

- Only TCA with proven efficacy in OCD
- In a meta-analysis of more than 800 youth with OCD, clomipramine produced greater benefits than SSRIs and most of the improvement emerged early in the course of treatment (Varigonda et al., 2016)
- Normally, clomipramine, a potent serotonin reuptake blocker, at steady state is metabolized extensively to its active metabolite desmethylclomipramine, a potent noradrenaline reuptake blocker, by CYP1A2
- Thus, at steady state, plasma drug activity is generally more noradrenergic (with higher desmethylclomipramine levels) than serotonergic (with lower clomipramine levels)
- For experts, the addition of the SSRI and CYP1A2 inhibitor fluvoxamine blocks this conversion and results in higher clomipramine levels than desmethylclomipramine levels. This benefit has recently been demonstrated (Fung et al., 2021). Adding fluvoxamine to clomipramine inhibits the metabolism of clomipramine to desmethylclomipramine and enhances the serotonergic potency of clomipramine – it shifts the typical ratio of clomipramine < desmethylclomipramine to clomipramine > desmethylclomipramine by inhibiting CYP1A2. However, this approach

requires close monitoring. Experienced clinicians may consider starting with clomipramine and adding fluvoxamine for patients with refractory OCD.

- Unique among TCAs, clomipramine has a potentially fatal interaction with MAOIs in addition to the danger of hypertension characteristic of all MAOI–TCA combinations
- A potentially fatal serotonin syndrome with high fever, seizures, and coma, analogous to that caused by SSRIs and MAOIs, can occur with clomipramine and SSRIs, presumably due to clomipramine's potent serotonin reuptake blocking properties
- Alcohol should be avoided because of additive CNS effects
- Underweight patients may be more susceptible to adverse cardiovascular effects
- Children, patients with inadequate hydration, and patients with cardiac disease may be more susceptible to TCA-induced cardiotoxicity than healthy adults
- Patients on TCAs should be aware that they may experience symptoms such as photosensitivity or blue-green urine
- Patients who are poor CYP2D6 metabolizers may experience side effects at low or normal doses; in such cases consider switching to another antidepressant not metabolized by CYP2D6

SUGGESTED READING

Bridge JA, Iyengar S, Salary CB et al. Clinical response and risk for reported suicidal ideation and suicide attempts in pediatric antidepressant treatment: a meta-analysis of randomized controlled trials. JAMA 2007;297(15):1683–96.

Cipriani A, Zhou X, Del Giovane C et al. Comparative efficacy and tolerability of antidepressants for major depressive disorder in children and adolescents: a network meta-analysis. Lancet 2016;388:881–90.

Croarkin PE, Elmaadawi AZ, Aaronson ST et al. Left prefrontal transcranial magnetic stimulation for treatment-resistant depression in adolescents: a double-blind, randomized, sham-controlled trial. Neuropsychopharmacology 2021;46(2):462–9.

Emslie GJ, Heiligenstein JH, Hoog SL et al. Fluoxetine treatment for prevention of relapse of depression in children and adolescents: a double-blind, placebo-controlled study. J Am Acad Child Adolesc Psychiatry 2004;43(11):1397–405.

Fung R, Elbe D, Stewart SE. Retrospective review of fluvoxamine-clomipramine combination therapy in obsessive-compulsive disorder in children and adolescents. J Can Acad Child Adolesc Psychiatry 2021;30(3):150–5.

Hathaway EE, Walkup JT, Strawn JR. Antidepressant treatment duration in pediatric depressive and anxiety disorders: how long is long enough? Curr Probl Pediatr Adolesc Health Care 2018;48(2):31–9.

Hazell P, Mirzaie M. Tricyclic drugs for depression in children and adolescents. Cochrane Database Syst Rev 2013;2013(6):CD002317. doi: 10.1002/14651858.CD002317.pub2.

Hebert AA, Glaser DA, Green L et al. Long-term efficacy and safety of topical glycopyrronium tosylate for the treatment of primary axillary hyperhidrosis: post hoc pediatric subgroup analysis from a 44-week open-label extension study. Pediatr Dermatol 2020;37(3):490–7.

Hicks JK, Sangkuhl K, Swen JJ et al. Clinical Pharmacogenetics Implementation Consortium guideline (CPIC) for CYP2D6 and CYP2C19 genotypes and dosing of tricyclic antidepressants: 2016 update. Clin Pharmacol Ther 2017;102(1):37–44.

Remington C, Ruth J, Hebert AA. Primary hyperhidrosis in children: a review of therapeutics. Pediatr Dermatol 2021;38(3):561–7.

Strawn JR, Poweleit EA, Uppugunduri CRS, Ramsey LB. Pediatric therapeutic drug monitoring for selective serotonin reuptake inhibitors. Front Pharmacol 2021;12:749692.

Strawn JR, Mills JA, Poweleit EA, Ramsey LB, Croarkin PE. Adverse effects of antidepressant medications and their management in children and adolescents. Pharmacotherapy 2023;43(7):675–90.

Varigonda AL, Jakubovski E, Bloch MH. Systematic review and meta-analysis: early treatment responses of selective serotonin reuptake inhibitors and clomipramine in pediatric obsessive-compulsive disorder. J Am Acad Child Adolesc Psychiatry 2016;55(10):851–9.

THERAPEUTICS

Brands
- Klonopin

Generic
Yes

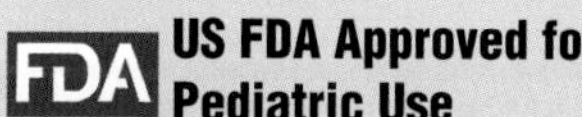

US FDA Approved for Pediatric Use
- None

Off-Label for Pediatric Use
- Approved in adults
  - Panic disorder, with or without agoraphobia
  - Lennox–Gastaut syndrome (petit mal variant)
  - Akinetic seizure
  - Myoclonic seizure
  - Absence seizure (petit mal)
- Other off-label uses
  - Atonic seizures
  - Other seizure disorders
  - Other anxiety disorders
  - Acute mania (adjunctive)
  - Acute psychosis (adjunctive)
  - Insomnia
  - Catatonia

Class and Mechanism of Action
- Neuroscience-based Nomenclature: GABA positive allosteric modulator (GABA-PAM)
- Benzodiazepine (anxiolytic, anticonvulsant)
- As positive allosteric modulators of GABA-A receptors, benzodiazepines (in the presence of GABA) increase the frequency of opening of the inhibitory chloride channels (although it does not increase the conductance of chloride across the individual channels or the time that the channel is open). This enhances the inhibitory effects of GABA.
- Inhibits neuronal activity presumably in amygdala-centered fear circuits to provide therapeutic benefits in anxiety disorders
- Inhibitory actions in the cerebral cortex may provide therapeutic benefits in seizure disorders

SAFETY AND TOLERABILITY

Notable Side Effects
- Sedation, fatigue, depression
- Dizziness, ataxia, slurred speech, weakness
- Forgetfulness, confusion
- Agitation and irritability
- Sialorrhea, dry mouth
- Rare hallucinations, mania
- Rare hypotension

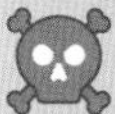

Life-Threatening or Dangerous Side Effects
- Respiratory depression, especially when taken with CNS depressants in overdose
- Rare hepatic dysfunction, renal dysfunction, blood dyscrasias

Growth and Maturation
- Not studied

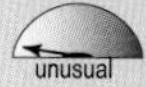

Weight Gain
- Reported but not expected

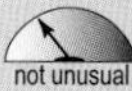

Sedation
- Occurs in significant minority
- Especially at initiation of treatment or when dose increases
- Tolerance often develops over time

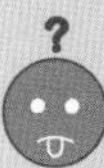

What to Do About Side Effects
- Wait
- Wait
- Wait
- Lower the dose
- Take largest dose at bedtime to avoid sedative effects during the day
- Switch to another agent
- Administer flumazenil if side effects are severe or life threatening

How Drug Causes Side Effects
- Same mechanism for side effects as for therapeutic effects – namely due to excessive actions at benzodiazepine receptors
- Long-term adaptations in benzodiazepine receptors may explain the development of dependence, tolerance, and withdrawal
- Side effects are generally immediate, but immediate side effects often disappear in time

Warnings and Precautions

- Boxed warning regarding the increased risk of CNS depressant effects when benzodiazepines and opioid medications are used together, including specifically the risk of slowed or difficulty breathing and death
- If alternatives to the combined use of benzodiazepines and opioids are not available, clinicians should limit the dosage and duration of each drug to the minimum possible while still achieving therapeutic efficacy
- Patients and their caregivers should be warned to seek medical attention if unusual dizziness, lightheadedness, sedation, slowed or difficulty breathing, or unresponsiveness occur
- Dosage changes should be made in collaboration with prescriber
- Use with caution in patients with pulmonary disease; rare reports of death after initiation of benzodiazepines in patients with severe pulmonary impairment
- History of drug or alcohol abuse often creates greater risk for dependency
- Clonazepam may induce grand mal seizures in patients with multiple seizure disorders
- Use only with extreme caution if patient has obstructive sleep apnea
- Some depressed patients may experience a worsening of suicidal ideation
- Some patients may exhibit abnormal thinking or behavioral changes similar to those caused by other CNS depressants (i.e., either depressant actions or disinhibiting actions)

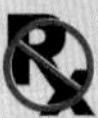

When Not to Prescribe

- If patient has angle-closure glaucoma
- If patient has severe liver disease
- If there is a proven allergy to clonazepam or any benzodiazepine

Long-Term Use

- May lose efficacy for seizures; dose increase may restore efficacy
- Risk of dependence, particularly for treatment periods longer than 12 weeks and especially in patients with past or current polysubstance abuse

Habit Forming

- Clonazepam is a Schedule IV drug
- Patients may develop dependence and/or tolerance with long-term use

Overdose

- Rarely fatal in monotherapy; sedation, confusion, coma, diminished reflexes

DOSING AND USE

Usual Dosage Range

- Panic/anxiety: 0.5–2 mg/day either as divided doses or once at bedtime

Dosage Forms

- Tablet 0.5 mg scored, 1 mg, 2 mg
- Disintegrating (wafer) 0.125 mg, 0.25 mg, 0.5 mg, 1 mg, 2 mg
- Suspension 0.1 mg/mL can be compounded by some pharmacies (requires refrigeration)

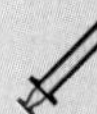

How to Dose

- Panic/anxiety: 1 mg/day; start at 0.25 mg divided into 2 doses, raise to 1 mg/day after 4–5 days; dose either twice daily or once at bedtime; maximum dose generally 2–3 mg/day in children and adolescents

Options for Administration

- Available as an oral disintegrating wafer

Tests

- In patients with seizure disorders, concomitant medical illness, and/or those with multiple concomitant long-term medications, periodic liver tests and blood counts may be prudent

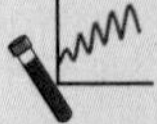

Pharmacokinetics

- After oral administration, clonazepam is rapidly absorbed from the gastrointestinal tract. The absorption rate may vary among individuals, but it generally takes about 1 to 2 hours for peak plasma concentrations to be reached.
- The presence of food in the stomach can delay the absorption of clonazepam
- Clonazepam is extensively distributed throughout the body, including the central nervous system. It readily crosses the blood–brain barrier, resulting in its sedative and anticonvulsant effects.

- The drug is highly protein-bound, primarily to albumin. The degree of protein binding can be lower in children compared to adults, potentially leading to higher free drug concentrations.
- Clonazepam undergoes extensive hepatic metabolism, primarily via CYP3A4 (Figure 1), and is metabolized into its major active metabolite, 7-aminoclonazepam, which also exhibits pharmacological activity
- The elimination half-life of clonazepam in children and adolescents can range from approximately 18 to 50 hours, with an average of around 30 hours. The prolonged half-life in children is primarily due to their lower clearance rates compared to adults.
- Long half-life compared to other benzodiazepine anxiolytics

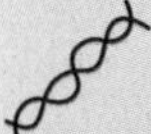

Pharmacogenetics

- No recommendations

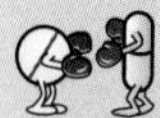

Drug Interactions

- Increased depressive effects when taken with other CNS depressants
- Inhibitors of CYP3A4 may affect the clearance of clonazepam
- Flumazenil (used to reverse the effects of benzodiazepines) may precipitate seizures and should not be used in patients treated for seizure disorders with clonazepam
- Use of clonazepam with valproate may cause absence status

Dosing Tips

- For anxiety disorders, use lowest possible effective dose for the shortest possible period of time (a benzodiazepine-sparing strategy). In adolescents, these medications may be administered prior to some anxiety-producing situations and can help to facilitate returning to school in patients with school refusal.
- Assess need for continuous treatment regularly
- Risk of dependence may increase with dose and duration of treatment and with more lipophilic benzodiazepines (e.g., alprazolam)
- For interdose symptoms of anxiety, can either increase dose or maintain same daily dose but divide into more frequent doses
- Because seizure disorder can require doses much higher than 2 mg/day, the risk of dependence may be greater in these patients
- Frequency of dosing in practice is often different than predicted from half-life, as duration for benzodiazepines is often related to redistribution (Stimpfl et al., 2023)
- Clonazepam is generally dosed half the dosage of alprazolam
- Escalation of dose may be necessary if tolerance develops in seizure disorders
- Escalation of dose usually not necessary in anxiety disorders, as tolerance to clonazepam does not generally develop in the treatment of anxiety disorders

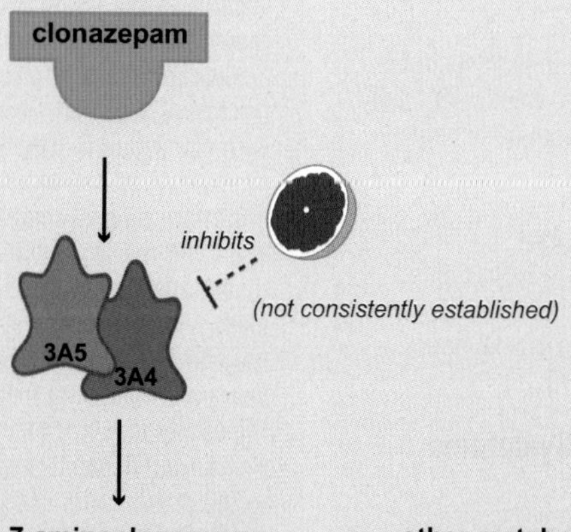

Figure 1 Clonazepam metabolism.

How to Switch

- Use the accompanying equivalence table to convert from the clonazepam dose to the dose of the new benzodiazepine

Approximate equivalent dosage (mg)	
Alprazolam (Xanax)	0.5
Chlordiazepoxide (Librium)	25
Clonazepam (Klonopin)	0.25–0.5
Diazepam (Valium)	5
Lorazepam (Ativan)	1

How to Stop

- Patients with history of seizures may seize upon withdrawal, especially if withdrawal is abrupt
- Taper by 0.25 mg every 3 days to reduce chances of withdrawal effects
- For difficult to taper cases, consider reducing dose much more slowly after reaching 1.5 mg/day, perhaps by as little as 0.125 mg per week or less
- Be sure to differentiate the reemergence of symptoms requiring reinstitution of treatment from withdrawal symptoms
- Benzodiazepine-dependent anxiety patients and insulin-dependent diabetics are not addicted to their medications. When benzodiazepine-dependent patients stop their medication, disease symptoms can reemerge, disease symptoms can worsen (rebound), and/or withdrawal symptoms can emerge.

WHAT TO EXPECT

Onset of Action

- Some immediate relief with first dosing is common; can take several weeks with daily dosing for maximal therapeutic benefit

Duration of Action

- Duration of action varies for benzodiazepines, including clonazepam, in pediatric patients, but is generally considered to be between 10–12 hours

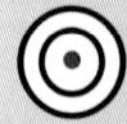

Primary Target Symptoms

- Panic attacks
- Anxiety
- Frequency and duration of seizures
- Spike and wave discharges in absence seizures (petit mal)

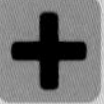

What Is Considered a Positive Result?

- The goal of treatment for anxiety is complete remission of current symptoms as well as prevention of future relapses
- If treatment works, it most often reduces or even eliminates symptoms, but is not a cure since symptoms can recur after medicine is stopped

How Long to Treat

- For short-term symptoms of anxiety: after a few weeks, discontinue use or use on an "as-needed" basis
- For long-term symptoms of anxiety, consider switching to an SSRI or SNRI for long-term maintenance
- If long-term maintenance with a benzodiazepine is necessary, continue treatment for 6 months after symptoms resolve, and then taper dose slowly
- For long-term treatment of seizure disorders, development of tolerance dose escalation and loss of efficacy necessitating adding or switching to other anticonvulsants is not uncommon

What If It Stops Working?

- If anxiety symptoms reemerge, consider an SSRI, and re-trying psychotherapeutic approaches

What If It Doesn't Work?

- Consider a trial of an SSRI
- When treating youth with anxiety disorders, many patients will have had significant anxiety for years prior to beginning treatment. As such, when anxiety is treated with clonazepam, their symptoms may be improved, but the patient has likely missed important developmental milestones (e.g., spending the night with friends, being able to ask questions in class). Developing these skills will take time. Beyond this, the family may have lived with the anxious child for years and following treatment of the child, the family may need to readjust.
- Be mindful of family conflict contributing to the presentation; sometimes treating parental depression or anxiety disorders improves psychiatric and social function

without any treatment of youth. Also, accommodation is common in families of youth with anxiety disorders and may need to be addressed specifically, as it can perpetuate symptoms.

TALKING TO PATIENTS AND CAREGIVERS

What to Tell Parents About Efficacy

- While the medicine helps by reducing symptoms and improving function, it is not a cure, and it is therefore necessary to keep taking the medication to sustain its therapeutic effects
- Since every treatment consideration depends on a risk/benefit analysis, parents should fully understand short- and long-term risks as well as benefits
- Often a good idea to tell parents whether the medication chosen is specifically approved for the disorder being treated, or whether it is being given for "unapproved" or "off-label" reasons based on good clinical practice, expert consensus, and/or prudent extrapolation of controlled data from adults

What to Tell Children and Adolescents About Efficacy

- We are trying to make you feel better
- It may be a good idea to give the medication a try; if it's not working very well, we can stop the medication and try something else
- Medications don't change who you are as a person; they give you the opportunity to be the best person you can be

What to Tell Parents About Side Effects

- Explain that mild side effects are expected at initiation or when increasing the dose and are usually transitory
- Predict side effects in advance (you will look clever and competent to the parents, unless you scare them with too much information and cause nocebo effects, in which case you won't look so clever when the patient develops lots of side effects and stops medication; use your judgment here); a balanced but honest presentation is an art rather than a science
- Ask parents to support the patient while side effects are occurring
- Parents should fully understand short- and long-term risks as well as benefits
- Explaining to the parents what to expect from medication treatment, and especially potential side effects, can help prevent early termination of medication

What to Tell Children and Adolescents About Side Effects

- Even if you get side effects, most of them get better or go away in a few days to a few weeks; however, we will likely not use this medication for a long time
- Explaining to child/adolescent what to expect from medication treatment, and especially potential side effects, can help prevent early termination of medication

What to Tell Teachers About the Medication (If Parents Consent)

- Clonazepam can make children/adolescents sleepy and make it difficult for children or adolescents to pay attention. In these situations, it is important to notify the clinician so that the dose can be decreased.
- Clonazepam may interfere with children's ability to engage in some activities at recess and in physical education class
- Encourage dialogue with parents/guardians about any behavior or mood changes

SPECIAL POPULATIONS

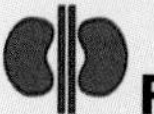

Renal Impairment

- Dose should be reduced

Hepatic Impairment

- Dose should be reduced

Cardiac Impairment

- No data available

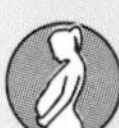

Pregnancy

- Possible increased risk of birth defects when benzodiazepines taken during pregnancy
- Because of the potential risks, clonazepam is not generally recommended as treatment for anxiety during pregnancy, especially during the first trimester

- Drug should be tapered if discontinued
- Infants whose mothers received a benzodiazepine late in pregnancy may experience withdrawal effects
- Neonatal flaccidity has been reported in infants whose mothers took a benzodiazepine during pregnancy
- Seizures, even mild seizures, may cause harm to the embryo/fetus

Breast Feeding

- Some drug is found in breast milk
- Recommended either to discontinue drug or formula feed
- Effects on infant have been observed and include feeding difficulties, sedation, and weight loss

THE ART OF PSYCHOPHARMACOLOGY

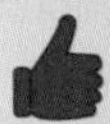

Potential Advantages

- Rapid onset of action
- Less sedation than some other benzodiazepines
- Longer duration of action than some other benzodiazepines
- Availability of oral disintegrating wafer or suspension (if compounded)

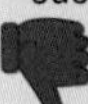

Potential Disadvantages

- Development of tolerance may require dose increases, especially in seizure disorders
- Abuse especially risky in past or present substance users

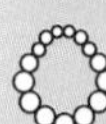

Pearls

- Despite trials of benzodiazepines in adults with anxiety disorders consistently demonstrating benefit, trials of benzodiazepines in pediatric patients have produced mixed results:
  - Small double-blind placebo-controlled trials and meta-analyses do not reveal differences between benzodiazepines and placebo for the management of anxiety disorders. However, these studies were small and included very young children and high doses of short-acting benzodiazepines (e.g., alprazolam).
  - By contrast, for acute anxiety in children and adolescents, a meta-analysis of nearly 1,500 patients suggested that benzodiazepines are more effective than placebo in treating acute anxiety; in this meta-analysis, there was no significant difference in the risk of developing irritability or behavioral changes between benzodiazepine and control groups (Kuang et al., 2017)
- One double-blind placebo-controlled trial evaluated the efficacy of clonazepam in children and young adolescents (ages 7 to 13 years). This was a short trial (4 weeks) and placebo response rates were very high (Graae et al., 1994).
- In the pediatric benzodiazepine trials, the poor tolerability – particularly in younger patients – may relate to age-related pharmacodynamic factors (Strawn and Stahl, 2023)
- The pharmacodynamics of the GABA receptor in children and adolescents differ from adults, with adult expression/function not being achieved until ages 14–17½ years for subcortical regions and 18–22 years for cortical regions, although girls reach adult expression of GABA receptors slightly earlier than boys (Chugani et al. 2001)
- In adults with anxiety disorders, benzodiazepines may be a very useful adjunct to SSRIs and SNRIs in the treatment of numerous anxiety disorders; however, the evidence for this is limited in children and adolescents
- Easier to taper than some other benzodiazepines because of long half-life
- Grapefruit significantly affects the pharmacokinetics of most benzodiazepines (and other medications that are metabolized by CYP3A4) (Figure 1). In fact, grapefruit increases peak benzodiazepine blood levels (Cmax) by almost 60%, increases the time to maximum concentration (Tmax) by 80%, and boosts absorption by up to 50%.
- May have less abuse potential than some other benzodiazepines
- May cause less depression, euphoria, or dependence than some other benzodiazepines
- Clonazepam is often considered a "longer-acting alprazolam-like anxiolytic" with improved tolerability features in terms of less euphoria, abuse, dependence, and withdrawal problems, but this has not been proven
- When using to treat insomnia, remember that insomnia may be a symptom of some other primary disorder itself, and thus

warrant evaluation for comorbid psychiatric and/or medical conditions
- Though not systematically studied, benzodiazepines have been used effectively to treat catatonia and are the initial recommended treatment

SUGGESTED READING

Allen LV Jr, Erickson MA III. Stability of acetazolamide, allopurinol, azathioprine, clonazepam, and flucytosine in extemporaneously compounded oral liquids. Am J Health-Syst Pharm 1996;53: 1944–9.

Chugani DC, Muzik O, Juhász C et al. Postnatal maturation of human GABAA receptors measured with positron emission tomography. Ann Neurol 2001;49(5):618–26.

Graae F, Milner J, Rizzotto L, Klein RG. Clonazepam in childhood anxiety disorders. J Am Acad Child Adolesc Psychiatry 1994;33(3):372–6.

Kuang H, Johnson JA, Mulqueen JM, Bloch MH. The efficacy of benzodiazepines as acute anxiolytics in children: a meta-analysis. Depress Anxiety 2017;34(10):888–96.

Lin AE, Peller AJ, Westgate MN et al. Clonazepam use in pregnancy and the risk of malformations. Birth Defects Res A Clin Mol Teratol 2004;70(8):534–6.

Nicotra CM, Strawn JS. Advances in pharmacotherapy for pediatric anxiety disorders. Child Adolesc Psychiatr Clin N Am 2023;32(3):573–87.

Sidorchuk A, Isomura K, Molero Y et al. Benzodiazepine prescribing for children, adolescents, and young adults from 2006 through 2013: a total population register-linkage study. PLoS Med 2018;15(8):e1002635.

Stimpfl JN, Mills JA, Strawn JR. Pharmacologic predictors of benzodiazepine response trajectory in anxiety disorders: a Bayesian hierarchical modeling meta-analysis. CNS Spectr 2023;28(1):53–60.

Strawn JR, Lu L, Peris TS, Levine A, Walkup JT. Research review: pediatric anxiety disorders – what have we learnt in the last 10 years? J Child Psychol Psychiatry 2021;62(2):114–39.

Strawn JR, Stahl SM. Case Studies: Stahl's Essential Psychopharmacology: Volume 4: Children and Adolescents. New York: Cambridge University Press, 2023.

THERAPEUTICS

Brands

- Kapvay, others for hypotension

Generic

Yes

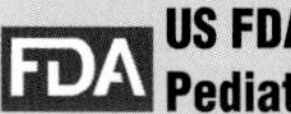

US FDA Approved for Pediatric Use

- Attention deficit hyperactivity disorder (Kapvay, ages 6 to 17, adjunct and monotherapy)

Off-Label for Pediatric Use

- Approved in adults
  - Hypertension (Jenloga, Catapres, Duraclon, others)
- Other off-label uses
  - Motor tics
  - Tourette syndrome
  - Oppositional defiant disorder
  - Conduct disorder
  - Pervasive developmental disorders
  - Substance withdrawal, including opiates and alcohol
  - Anxiety disorders, including posttraumatic stress disorder (PTSD) and social anxiety disorder
  - Clozapine-induced sialorrhea
  - Menopausal flushing
  - Severe pain in cancer patients that is not adequately relieved by opioid analgesics alone (combination with opiates)

Class and Mechanism of Action

- Neuroscience-based Nomenclature: norepinephrine receptor agonist (N-RA)
- Centrally acting alpha 2A agonist; antihypertensive; nonstimulant for ADHD
- For ADHD, theoretically has central actions on postsynaptic alpha 2A receptors in the prefrontal cortex
- The prefrontal cortex is thought to be responsible for modulation of working memory, attention, impulse control, and planning
- For hypertension, stimulates alpha 2A adrenergic receptors in the brainstem, reducing sympathetic outflow from the CNS and decreasing peripheral resistance, renal vascular resistance, heart rate, and blood pressure
- An imidazoline, so also interacts at imidazoline receptors

SAFETY AND TOLERABILITY

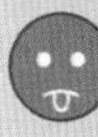

Notable Side Effects

- Dry mouth, constipation
- Dizziness, sedation
- Weakness, fatigue
- Hypotension
- Impotence, loss of libido
- Insomnia, headache, depression
- Dermatological reactions (especially with transdermal clonidine)
- Tachycardia, occasional syncope
- Nervousness, agitation
- Nausea, vomiting

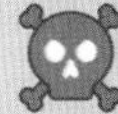

Life-Threatening or Dangerous Side Effects

- Sinus bradycardia, atrioventricular block
- During withdrawal, hypertensive encephalopathy, cerebrovascular accidents, and death (rare)

Growth and Maturation

- Clonidine is not expected to have an adverse effect on growth
- Clonidine stimulates growth hormone secretion (no chronic effects have been observed); growth hormone response to clonidine may be reduced during menses; alcohol may reduce the effects of clonidine on growth hormone

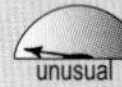

Weight Gain

- Reported but not expected

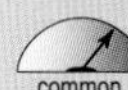

Sedation

- Many experience and/or can be significant in amount
- Some patients may not tolerate it
- Can abate with time

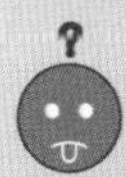

What to Do About Side Effects

- Wait, wait, wait: mild side effects are common, happen early, and usually improve with time, but treatment benefits can be delayed and often begin just as the side effects wear off
- Take larger dose at bedtime to avoid daytime sedation

- Often best to try another monotherapy prior to resorting to augmentation strategies to treat side effects
- Monitor side effects closely, especially when initiating treatment
- For withdrawal and discontinuation reactions, may need to reinstate clonidine and taper very slowly when stabilized

How Drug Causes Side Effects

- Excessive actions on alpha 2 receptors and/or on imidazoline receptors

Warnings and Precautions

- In children and adolescents:
  - Safety and efficacy not established in children under age 6
  - Use in young children should be reserved for the expert
  - Consider distributing brochures provided by the FDA and the drug companies
- All ages:
  - Carefully weigh the risks and benefits of pharmacological treatment against the risks and benefits of nonpharmacological treatment and it is a good idea to document this in the patient's chart
  - There have been cases of hypertensive encephalopathy, cerebrovascular accidents, and death after abrupt discontinuation
  - If used with a beta blocker, the beta blocker should generally be stopped several days before tapering clonidine
  - Excessive heat may exacerbate some of the side effects, such as dizziness and drowsiness
  - Use with caution in patients at risk for hypotension, heart block, and bradycardia
  - Be aware that forgetting to take clonidine or running out of medication can lead to abrupt discontinuation and associated withdrawal reactions and complications
  - In patients who have developed localized contact sensitization to transdermal clonidine, continuing transdermal dosing on other skin areas or substituting with oral clonidine may be associated with the development of a generalized skin rash, urticaria, or angioedema
  - Certain transdermal patches containing even small traces of aluminum or other metals in the adhesive backing can cause skin burns if worn during MRI, so warn patients taking the transdermal formulation about this possibility and advise them to disclose this information if they need an MRI

When Not to Prescribe

- If there is a proven allergy to clonidine

Long-Term Use

- Long-term use for ADHD has not been studied in controlled trials
- Shown to be safe and effective for treatment of hypertension; patients may develop tolerance to the antihypertensive effects

Habit Forming

- Reports of some abuse by nonopioid-dependent patients

Overdose

- Hypotension, hypertension, miosis, respiratory depression, seizures, bradycardia, hypothermia, coma, sedation, decreased reflexes, weakness, irritability, dysrhythmia

DOSING AND USE

Usual Dosage Range

- Extended-release for ADHD: 0.1–0.4 mg/day in divided doses
- Immediate-release for hypertension or off-label for ADHD: 0.2–0.6 mg/day in divided doses
- Opioid withdrawal: 0.1 mg 3 times daily (can be higher in inpatient setting)

Dosage Forms

- Extended-release tablet 0.1 mg, 0.2 mg
- Immediate-release tablet 0.1 mg scored, 0.2 mg scored, 0.3 mg scored
- Topical (7-day administration) 0.1 mg/24 hours, 0.2 mg/24 hours, 0.3 mg/24 hours
- Injection 0.1 mg/mL, 0.5 mg/mL

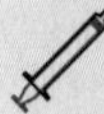

How to Dose

- Oral, extended-release (for ADHD): initial 0.1 mg at bedtime; can increase by 0.1 mg/day each week with dosing divided and larger dose at bedtime; maximum dose generally 0.4 mg/day in divided doses
- For opioid withdrawal: 0.1 mg 3 times daily; next dose should be withheld if

blood pressure falls below 90/60 mmHg; outpatients should not be given more than a 3-day supply, detoxification can usually be achieved in 4–6 days for short-acting opioids
- Oral, immediate-release (for hypertension): initial 0.1 mg in 2 divided doses, morning and night; can increase by 0.1 mg/day each week; maximum dose generally 2.4 mg/day
- Topical (for hypertension): apply once every 7 days in hairless area; change location with each application
- Injection (for hypertension): initial 30 mcg/hr; maximum 40 mcg/hr; 500 mcg/mL must be diluted
- For PTSD symptoms in youth: typically start at 0.05 to 0.1 mg at night, increase by 0.05 to 0.1 mg every 3 nights to a maximum dose of 0.2 to 0.5 mg/day (Strawn et al., 2023)

Options for Administration

- Multiple formulation options, although only oral extended-release is approved for ADHD

Tests

- Blood pressure (sitting and standing) and pulse should be measured at baseline and monitored following dose increases and periodically during treatment

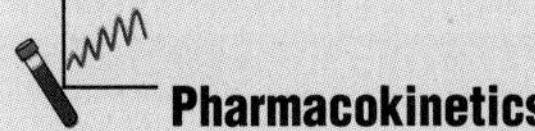

Pharmacokinetics

- Well absorbed from the gastrointestinal tract. The rate and extent of absorption may vary among individuals. After oral administration, clonidine reaches peak plasma concentration (Cmax) within 1 to 3 hours.
- Highly protein-bound, primarily to albumin, and the extent of protein binding remains relatively constant across different age groups
- Half-life of immediate-release formulation is 12–16 hours in adults; similar elimination half-lives were observed with extended-release formulation in adults
- Plasma clonidine concentrations in children and adolescents with ADHD are greater than those in adults with hypertension, with children and adolescents receiving higher doses on a mg/kg basis
- Clonidine undergoes extensive hepatic metabolism, primarily through CYP2D6 and to a lesser extent CYP3A4, as well as CYP1A2. The major metabolite formed is 4-hydroxyclonidine, which possesses approximately half the alpha 2 adrenergic agonist activity of the parent compound, but is not lipophilic (Figure 1).
- Clonidine is excreted renally

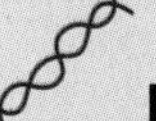

Pharmacogenetics

- No recommendations; however, CYP2D6 significantly impacts clonidine metabolism and clinicians may consider a patient's CYP2D6 phenotype when dosing clonidine

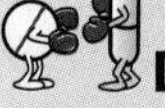

Drug Interactions

- The likelihood of severe discontinuation reactions with CNS and cardiovascular

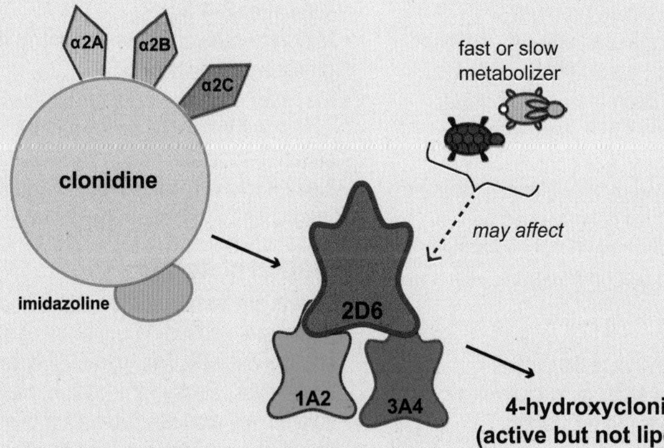

Figure 1 Clonidine metabolism.

symptoms may be greater when clonidine is combined with beta blocker treatment
- Increased depressive and sedative effects when taken with other CNS depressants
- Tricyclic antidepressants may reduce the hypotensive effects of clonidine
- Using clonidine in combination with another antihypertensive agent may attenuate the development of tolerance to clonidine's antihypertensive effects
- Use of clonidine with agents that affect sinus node function or AV nodal function (e.g., digitalis, calcium channel blockers, beta blockers) may result in bradycardia or AV block

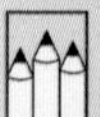

Dosing Tips

- Plasma levels are higher in lower-weight children; therefore, starting and target doses may be lower and longer intervals between dose increases may be needed (see How to Dose)
- Plasma clonidine concentrations in children and adolescents with ADHD are greater than those in adults with hypertension with children and adolescents receiving higher doses on a mg/kg basis
- Many children require tid dosing for immediate-release forms for best results
- Do not substitute different clonidine products for each other on a mg-per-mg basis, because they have different pharmacokinetic profiles
- Adverse effects are dose related and usually transient
- Extended-release tablets should not be crushed, chewed, or broken, as this could alter controlled-release properties
- If clonidine is terminated abruptly, rebound hypertension may occur within 2–4 days, so taper dose in decrements of no more than 0.1 mg every 3 to 7 days when discontinuing
- If administered with a beta blocker, stop the beta blocker first for several days before the gradual discontinuation of clonidine in cases of planned discontinuation

How to Switch

- Clonidine is always tapered when discontinuing, whether or not another medication is going to be started
- Taper in decrements of no more than 0.1 mg every 3 to 7 days to minimize the risk of an increase in blood pressure upon discontinuation
- Discontinue one formulation of clonidine by taper over several days before beginning another formulation of clonidine
- Discontinue guanfacine before beginning clonidine
- Be aware of drug interactions with other agents if cross tapering/combining with other agents

How to Stop

- Discontinuation reactions are common and sometimes severe
- Sudden discontinuation can result in nervousness, agitation, headache, and tremor, with rapid rise in blood pressure
- Rare instances of hypertensive encephalopathy, cerebrovascular accident, and death have been reported after clonidine withdrawal
- Taper in decrements of no more than 0.1 mg every 3 to 7 days to minimize the risk of an increase in blood pressure upon discontinuation
- If administered with a beta blocker, stop the beta blocker first for several days before the gradual discontinuation of clonidine in cases of planned discontinuation

WHAT TO EXPECT

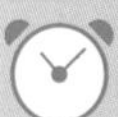

Onset of Action

- For ADHD, can take a few weeks to see maximum therapeutic benefits
- Blood pressure may be lowered 30–60 minutes after first dose; greatest reduction seen after 2–4 hours
- May take several weeks to control blood pressure adequately
- May take several weeks for dizziness and syncope from blood pressure effects, or sedation to abate, and in some cases, these side effects will not disappear and another medication will have to be given

Duration of Action

- Effects are consistent for 2 to 4 hours minimum; depending upon the patient and the patient's age, particularly for the immediate-release formulation, multiple daily doses may need to be administered to obtain consistent clinical results over a 24-hour period

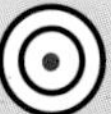

Primary Target Symptoms

- Concentration, attention span, distractibility
- Motor hyperactivity
- Oppositional and impulsive behavior
- High blood pressure
- Tics

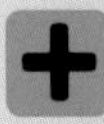

What Is Considered a Positive Result?

- The goal of treatment of ADHD is reduction of symptoms of inattentiveness, motor hyperactivity, and/or impulsiveness and tics that disrupt social, school, and/or occupational functioning
- The goal of treatment is complete remission of symptoms
- If treatment works, it most often reduces or even eliminates symptoms, but is not a cure since symptoms often recur after medicine is stopped

How Long to Treat

- ADHD is typically a lifelong illness; if any symptoms improve, hyperactivity is more likely to improve than inattention
- Can tell parents there is some chance that their child can grow out of this in adulthood, but many adults continue to have symptoms of ADHD throughout adolescence and adulthood
- Tics are typically a lifelong symptom
- However, oppositional and impulsive behaviors may diminish with neurodevelopment from childhood to adolescence to adulthood
- Continue treatment until all symptoms are under control or improvement is stable and then continue treatment as long as improvement persists
- Reevaluate the need for treatment periodically; some clinicians advise to periodically taper ADHD medication in patients who are not severely symptomatic to observe how the patient responds, but not routinely done by most clinicians
- Treatment for ADHD begun in childhood may need to be continued into adolescence and adulthood if continued benefit is documented

What If It Stops Working?

- Some patients may experience apparent lack of consistent efficacy due to activation of latent or underlying or newly evolved bipolar disorder, major depressive episodes with mixed features of mania, new onset of major depression or an anxiety disorder (GAD, OCD, PD), and require medication discontinuation and a switch to the clinically appropriate medication(s)

What If It Doesn't Work?

- In practice, many patients have only a partial response where some symptoms are improved but others persist, in which case higher doses or more frequent doses of clonidine or augmenting with a stimulant can be considered
- Consider evaluation for another diagnosis or for a comorbid condition (e.g., medical illness, substance abuse). Also, when treating ADHD, consider the possibility of a learning disorder or learning weakness and consider school-based interventions.
- Consider the presence of nonadherence and counsel patient and parents
- Some ADHD patients may experience lack of consistent efficacy due to activation of latent or underlying bipolar disorder, and require either augmenting with a mood stabilizer or switching to a mood stabilizer
- Augmenting options:
  - Organizational skills training/executive function coaching
  - Exercise
  - Parent Management Training (PMT)
  - Coordinating with school for appropriate support
  - Augmentation with a stimulant is commonly used for treatment-resistant ADHD, particularly oppositional/aggressive/impulsive behaviors inadequately responding to stimulants alone
- Consider factors associated with poor response to any psychotropic medication in children and adolescents, such as severe symptoms, long-lasting symptoms, poor treatment adherence, prior nonresponse to other treatments, and the presence of comorbid psychiatric disorders or learning disorders
- Consider other important potential factors such as ongoing conflicts, family psychopathology, and an adverse environment (e.g., poverty, chaos, violence, prior and ongoing psychological trauma,

abuse, bullying, less than ideal school placement, neglect)
- Institute trauma-informed care for appropriate children and adolescents

TALKING TO PATIENTS AND CAREGIVERS

What to Tell Parents About Efficacy

- It is a good idea to explain why this medication was chosen instead of a stimulant, or to use in combination with a stimulant, and if there are specific target symptoms for this medication compared to those for a stimulant
- Often works within several days once the dose is correct, although full therapeutic benefits may take a few weeks
- While the medicine helps ADHD by reducing symptoms and improving function, there are no cures for ADHD and it is therefore necessary to keep taking the medication to sustain its therapeutic effects
- Since every treatment consideration depends on a risk/benefit analysis, parents should fully understand short- and long-term risks as well as benefits compared to nontreatment of ADHD
- Often a good idea to tell parents whether the medication chosen is specifically approved for the disorder being treated, or whether it is being given for "unapproved" or "off-label" reasons based on good clinical practice, expert consensus, and/or prudent extrapolation of controlled data from adults
- The American Academy of Child & Adolescent Psychiatry (AACAP) has helpful handouts for parents

What to Tell Children and Adolescents About Efficacy

- Be specific about the symptoms being targeted: we are trying to help you remember things better, do your best at school, follow the rules, get into less trouble (as applicable)
- It may be a good idea to give the medication a try; if it's not working very well, we can stop the medication and try something else
- You can be part of a special plan to help us figure out if the medicine is helpful for you. Would you like to do that? (for the parents and prescriber, can consider here a trial both on and then off medication, and then on again to see if the effects are clear and thus worth continuing the medication)
- The medication often doesn't work right away, so a good try can take a few months to find the right dose and see if it works for you
- Even if it does make you feel better, it will wear off and no longer work shortly after you stop it
- The medication can help you decide what you want to do, like making good choices versus bad choices; the medicine does not make you do something you don't want to do
- Medications don't change who you are as a person; they give you the opportunity to be the best person you can be

What to Tell Parents About Side Effects

- Explain that side effects are expected in many when starting
- Tell parents many side effects often go away in a few days to weeks, but if they don't we will change the treatment
- Predict side effects in advance (you will look clever and competent to the parents, unless you scare them with too much information and cause nocebo effects, in which case you won't look so clever when the patient develops lots of side effects and stops medication; use your judgment here); a balanced but honest presentation is an art rather than a science
- Ask parents to support the patient while side effects are occurring
- Parents should fully understand short- and long-term risks as well as benefits
- Explaining to the parents what to expect from medication treatment, and especially what potential side effects to expect, can help prevent early termination
- Tell parents this medication – unlike stimulants – should be tapered rather than abruptly withdrawn when discontinuing it to avoid withdrawal side effects, some of which can be rarely dangerous; don't purposely skip a dose or stop over the weekend, for example, like you can do with stimulants

What to Tell Children and Adolescents About Side Effects

- When a medicine starts to work, your body can first experience this by giving you unpleasant sensations – just like if you take a cough medicine it may taste bad. So, just like with a cough medicine, the bad taste will often go away before the medicine begins to stop the cough – many medicines work like that. It's important for you to pay attention to what your body is telling you, and we'll go over some of the ways that can happen.

- Even if you get a side effect, it's not permanent (it won't last forever)
- Explaining to child/adolescent what to expect from medication treatment, and especially potential side effects, can help prevent early termination
- Make sure you tell your parents or your doctor if you decide to stop your medication, because stopping it all at once can cause you side effects, some of which can be dangerous

What to Tell Teachers About the Medication (If Parents Consent)

- Clonidine can be helpful in improving the symptoms of ADHD: namely, inattention, impulsivity, and hyperactivity
- Some students will experience side effects from the medications that you may notice in or outside the classroom; many of these side effects can be modified
- Clonidine can make children/adolescents sleepy (often) or can make them dizzy or faint (not common)

SPECIAL POPULATIONS

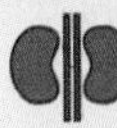

Renal Impairment

- Use with caution and possibly reduce dose

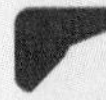

Hepatic Impairment

- Use with caution

Cardiac Impairment

- Use with caution in patients with conduction disturbances

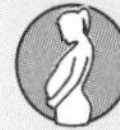

Pregnancy

- Controlled studies have not been conducted in pregnant women
- Some animal studies have shown adverse effects
- Use in women of childbearing potential requires weighing potential benefits to the mother against potential risks to the fetus
- For ADHD patients, clonidine should generally be discontinued before anticipated pregnancies

Breast Feeding

- Some drug is found in breast milk
- No adverse effects have been reported in nursing infants
- If irritability or sedation develop in nursing infant, may need to discontinue drug or formula feed

THE ART OF PSYCHOPHARMACOLOGY

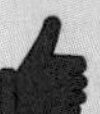

Potential Advantages

- In children:
  - For patients whose parents do not want them to take a stimulant or who cannot tolerate or do not respond to stimulants
  - For patients with oppositional and impulsive symptoms inadequately responsive to stimulants
- In adolescents:
  - For patients who have a history of diverting or abusing stimulants
  - Can improve school performance and grades, especially if ADHD has been unrecognized and untreated prior to adolescence
  - Can improve performance in high school and college students whose ADHD is compromising academic performance due to the increased demands of higher levels of study
- All ages:
  - No known abuse potential; not a controlled substance

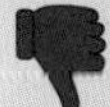

Potential Disadvantages

- All ages:
  - Withdrawal reactions
  - Nonadherent patients
  - Patients on concomitant CNS medications

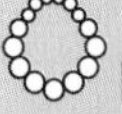

Pearls

- In children:
  - For children with comorbid ADHD and Tourette syndrome, and whose tics worsen with stimulant treatment,

clonidine may improve both ADHD symptoms and tics
  - Effects may be delayed and less robust on ADHD symptoms than stimulants; however, may add to the efficacy of stimulants when used in combination
  - May be particularly helpful in targeting aggressive, impulsive, and oppositional behaviors associated with ADHD
- In adolescents:
  - For adolescents with comorbid ADHD and Tourette syndrome, and whose tics are worse with stimulant treatment, clonidine may improve both ADHD symptoms and tics
  - Unlike stimulants, clonidine is not abusable and has little or no value to friends of adolescent patients who may otherwise divert stimulant medications, especially when responsible for self-administration of medications in college settings
- All ages:
  - Clonidine extended-release is approved for ADHD in children ages 6–17
  - Unlike stimulants approved for ADHD, clonidine does not have abuse potential and is not a scheduled substance
  - As monotherapy or in combination with methylphenidate for ADHD with conduct disorder or oppositional defiant disorder, may improve aggression, oppositional, and conduct disorder symptoms
  - Clonidine is sometimes used in combination with stimulants to reduce side effects and enhance therapeutic effects on motor hyperactivity
  - Doses of 0.1 mg in 3 divided doses have been reported to reduce stimulant-induced insomnia as well as impulsivity
  - Clonidine may also be effective for treatment of tic disorders, including Tourette syndrome
  - May suppress tics especially in severe Tourette syndrome, and may be even better at reducing explosive violent behaviors in Tourette syndrome
  - Sedation is often unacceptable in various patients despite improvement in CNS symptoms and leads to discontinuation of treatment, especially for ADHD and Tourette syndrome
  - Considered an investigational treatment for most other CNS applications
  - May block the autonomic symptoms in anxiety and panic disorders (e.g., palpitations, sweating) and improve subjective anxiety as well, although this has not been evaluated in children or adolescents
  - May be useful in decreasing the autonomic arousal of PTSD, and there are open-label reports of clonidine in young children with PTSD
  - May block autonomic symptoms of opioid withdrawal (e.g., palpitations, sweating) especially in inpatients, but muscle aches, irritability, and insomnia may not be well suppressed by clonidine
  - Often prescribed with naltrexone to suppress symptoms of opioid withdrawal; this requires monitoring of the patient for 8 hours on the first day due to the potential severity of naltrexone-induced withdrawal and the potential blood pressure effects of clonidine
  - May be useful in decreasing the hypertension, tachycardia, and tremulousness associated with alcohol withdrawal, but not the seizures or delirium tremens in complicated alcohol withdrawal
  - Guanfacine ER is a related, centrally active alpha 2 agonist also approved for ADHD, and may work better or be tolerated better than clonidine in some children/adolescents, although no head-to-head studies
  - Although both guanfacine and clonidine are alpha 2 adrenergic agonists, guanfacine is relatively more selective for alpha 2A receptors, whereas clonidine binds not only alpha 2A, 2B, and 2C receptors, but also imidazoline receptors, hypothetically causing more sedation, hypotension, and side effects than guanfacine in some patients

SUGGESTED READING

Catalá-López F, Hutton B, Nuñez-Beltrán A et al. The pharmacological and non-pharmacological treatment of attention deficit hyperactivity disorder in children and adolescents: a systematic review with network meta-analyses of randomised trials. PLoS One 2017;12(7):e0180355.

Croxtall JD. Clonidine extended-release: in attention-deficit hyperactivity disorder. Paediatr Drugs 2011;13(5):329–36.

Kemper AR, Maslow GR, Hill S et al. Attention Deficit Hyperactivity Disorder: Diagnosis And Treatment In Children And Adolescents. Comparative Effectiveness Review No. 203. AHRQ Publication No. 18-EHC005-EF. Rockville, MD: Agency for Healthcare Research and Quality; January 2018.

Kollins SH, Jain R, Brams M et al. Clonidine extended-release tablets as add-on therapy to psychostimulants in children and adolescents with ADHD. Pediatrics 2011;127(6):e1406-13.

Pliszka S ; AACAP Work Group on Quality Issues. Practice parameter for the assessment and treatment of children and adolescents with attention-deficit/hyperactivity disorder. J Am Acad Child Adolesc Psychiatry 2007;46(7):894–921.

Strawn JR, Keeshin BR, Cohen JA. Posttraumatic stress disorder in children and adolescents: treatment and overview. UpToDate 2023. Last updated Sept. 6, 2023.

THERAPEUTICS

Brands
- Clozaril
- FazaClo ODT (oral disintegrating tablet)
- Leponex
- Versacloz (oral suspension)

Generic
Yes

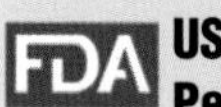

US FDA Approved for Pediatric Use
- None

Off-Label for Pediatric Use
- Approved in adults
  - Treatment-resistant schizophrenia
  - Reduction in risk of recurrent suicidal behavior in patients with schizophrenia or schizoaffective disorder
- Other off-label uses
  - Other psychotic disorder
  - Treatment-resistant bipolar disorder
  - Violent aggressive patients with psychosis and other severe neurodevelopmental disorders not responsive to other treatments

Class and Mechanism of Action
- Neuroscience-based Nomenclature: dopamine, serotonin, norepinephrine receptor antagonist (DSN-RAn)
- Atypical antipsychotic (serotonin-dopamine antagonist; second generation antipsychotic; also a mood stabilizer)
- Blocks dopamine 2 receptors, reducing positive symptoms of psychosis and stabilizing affective symptoms
- Blockade of serotonin type 2A receptors may also contribute at clinical doses to the enhancement of dopamine release in certain brain regions, thus theoretically reducing motor side effects
- Interactions at a myriad of other neurotransmitter receptors may contribute to clozapine's efficacy
- Specifically, interactions at 5HT2C and 5HT1A receptors may contribute to efficacy for cognitive and affective symptoms in some patients
- Mechanism of efficacy for psychotic patients who do not respond to other antipsychotics is unknown but is presumed to be a mechanism other than D2 antagonism

SAFETY AND TOLERABILITY

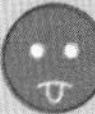

Notable Side Effects
- In children:
  - Limited data
- In adults:
  - Orthostasis
  - Sialorrhea
  - Constipation
  - Sedation
  - Tachycardia
  - Weight gain
  - Dyslipidemia and hyperglycemia
  - Benign fever (~20%)
- Risk of tardive dyskinesia may be higher in children than it is in adults, although overall risk of tardive dyskinesia for adults may be very low and clozapine may even improve tardive dyskinesia in some patients

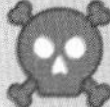

Life-Threatening or Dangerous Side Effects
- Severe neutropenia
- Myocarditis (first 6 weeks of treatment)
- Paralytic ileus
- Seizures (risk increases with dose)
- Hyperglycemia, in some cases extreme and associated with ketoacidosis or hyperosmolar coma or death, has been reported in patients taking atypical antipsychotics
- Pulmonary embolism (may include deep vein thrombosis or respiratory symptoms)
- Dilated cardiomyopathy
- Rare neuroleptic malignant syndrome (NMS) may cause hyperpyrexia, muscle rigidity, delirium, and autonomic instability with elevated creatine phosphokinase, myoglobinuria (rhabdomyolysis), and acute renal failure (much reduced risk compared to conventional antipsychotics; may be more likely when clozapine is used with another agent)

Growth and Maturation
- Long-term effects are unknown

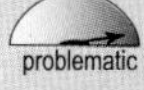

Weight Gain
- Frequent and can be significant in amount
- May be more risk of weight gain and metabolic effects in children than in adults
- May increase risk for aspiration events
- Should be managed aggressively

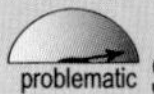

Sedation

- Frequent and can be significant in amount
- May be more likely to be sedating in children than in adults
- Can reemerge as dose increases and then wear off again over time

What to Do About Side Effects

- The ability to manage side effects is the secret to success with clozapine
- Wait, wait, wait: mild side effects are common, happen early, and usually improve with time, but treatment benefits can be delayed
- Monitor side effects closely, especially when initiating treatment
- Reduce the dose, or split into two or three daily doses
- Orthostasis and sedation:
  - Slow titration
  - Minimize use of other alpha 1 antagonists
  - Take largest dose at bedtime to help reduce daytime sedation
- Sialorrhea:
  - Atropine 1% drops sublingually at bedtime; can use up to 3 times per day if needed and if tolerated
  - Ipratropium bromide 0.06% spray, intra-orally at bedtime; can use up to 3 times per day if needed and if tolerated
  - Avoid use of systemic anticholinergic agents, which increases risk of ileus (benztropine, glycopyrrolate, etc.)
- Constipation:
  - Avoid psyllium, as it may worsen symptoms
  - All patients should receive docusate when starting clozapine
  - If needed, add polyethylene glycol (Miralax)
  - If docusate + polyethylene glycol (Miralax) are ineffective, add either bisacodyl or sennosides
  - If constipation still remains a problem, anecdotal evidence in adults suggests a possible role for lubiprostone
  - Advise patient to contact a healthcare professional right away if they have difficulty having a bowel movement, do not have a bowel movement at least 3 times a week or less than their normal frequency, or are unable to pass gas
- Weight gain and metabolic effects:
  - All patients should be referred for lifestyle management and exercise
  - Consider prophylactic metformin with a goal of 2 g/day in adolescents
  - Omega-3 fatty acids may be helpful in reducing second generation antipsychotic-induced hypertriglyceridemia
- Chest pain during the first 6 weeks:
  - Obtain workup for myocarditis
- Fever:
  - In the absence of elevated troponin and myocarditis symptoms, fever is usually self-limited and there is no need to stop
- Seizures:
  - Avoid phenytoin and carbamazepine because of pharmacokinetic interactions

How Drug Causes Side Effects

- Mechanism of agranulocytosis unknown
- Blocking alpha 1 adrenergic receptors can cause dizziness, hypotension, and syncope
- Blocking muscarinic cholinergic receptors can cause dry mouth, blurred vision, urinary retention, constipation, and paralytic ileus
- By blocking histamine 1 receptors in the brain, it can cause sedation and possibly weight gain
- Mechanism of any possible weight gain is unknown but may relate to effects at 5HT2C receptors
- Mechanism of any possible increased incidence of diabetes or dyslipidemia is unknown, but insulin regulation may be impaired by blocking pancreatic M3 muscarinic receptors
- By blocking dopamine 2 receptors in the striatum, it can cause motor side effects (very rare)

Warnings and Precautions

- Consider distributing brochures provided by the FDA and the drug companies or have the pharmacy do this for the parents
- Carefully weigh the risks and benefits of pharmacological treatment against the risks and benefits of treating with clozapine against treatment with another antipsychotic and it is a good idea to document this in the patient's chart

- Use with caution if at all in patients on other anticholinergic agents (benztropine, trihexyphenidyl, olanzapine, quetiapine, chlorpromazine, oxybutynin, and other antimuscarinics)
- Constipation caused by clozapine can uncommonly lead to serious bowel complications, so advise patients of the risk and the need to stay hydrated, question patients about their bowel movements throughout treatment, and advise them to contact a healthcare professional right away if they have difficulty having a bowel movement, do not have a bowel movement at least 3 times a week or less than their normal frequency, or are unable to pass gas
- Should not be used in conjunction with agents that are known to cause neutropenia
- Myocarditis is rare and occurs in the first 6 weeks of treatment
- Cardiomyopathy is a late complication (consider annual echocardiogram)
- Use with caution in patients with glaucoma
- Atypical antipsychotics have the potential for cognitive and motor impairment, especially related to sedation
- Atypical antipsychotics can cause body temperature dysregulation; use caution in patients who may experience conditions that increase body temperature (e.g., strenuous exercise, saunas, extreme heat, dehydration, or concomitant anticholinergic medication)
- As with any antipsychotic, use with caution in patients with history of seizures

When Not to Prescribe

- In patients with myeloproliferative disorder
- In patients with uncontrolled epilepsy
- In patients with paralytic ileus
- In patients with CNS depression
- If there is a proven allergy to clozapine

Long-Term Use

- Medication of choice for treatment-refractory schizophrenia in adults

Habit Forming

- No

Overdose

- Sometimes lethal; changes in heart rhythm, excess salivation, respiratory depression, altered state of consciousness

DOSING AND USE

Usual Dosage Range

- Depends on plasma clozapine levels more than upon oral dose; threshold for response is trough plasma level of 350 ng/mL

Dosage Forms

- Tablet 12.5 mg, 25 mg scored, 50 mg, 100 mg scored, 200 mg
- Orally disintegrating tablet 12.5 mg, 25 mg, 100 mg, 150 mg, 200 mg
- Oral suspension 50 mg/mL

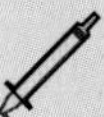

How to Dose

- Initial dose 12.5 mg at night; increase by 12.5–25 mg/day every 2–3 days as tolerated; typically administered in 2–3 divided doses. Titrate more slowly in outpatients (dose increases every 5–7 days).
- Threshold for response is 350 ng/mL
- Levels greater than 700 ng/mL are often not well tolerated
- No evidence to support dosing that results in plasma levels greater than 1,000 ng/mL
- Doses greater than 500 mg per day may require a split dose

Options for Administration

- Oral solution and orally disintegrating tablet provide alternatives for patients who have difficulty swallowing pills

Tests

- Before starting clozapine:
- Evaluate bowel function before starting a patient on clozapine
- Liver function testing, electrocardiogram, general physical exam, and assessment of baseline cardiac status
- Lower ANC threshold for starting clozapine:
  - General population: ≥1,500/μL
  - Benign ethnic neutropenia (BEN): ≥1,000/μL
- Plan to monitor weight and metabolic parameters more closely than in adults since children and adolescents may be more prone to metabolic side effects than adults
- Weigh all patients and monitor weight gain against that expected for normal growth, using the pediatric height/weight chart to monitor. In particular, monitor BMI percentiles.

- Get baseline personal and family history of diabetes, obesity, dyslipidemia, hypertension, and cardiovascular disease
- Obtain blood pressure, fasting plasma glucose (or hemoglobin A1C), and a lipid profile
- Tests for myocarditis:
  - Myocarditis is rare and almost only occurs in the first 6 weeks of treatment
- Consider baseline: check troponin I/T, CRP
  - Weekly troponin I/T and CRP for the first month
  - Fever is usually benign and self-limited; suspicion of myocarditis should only be raised based on elevated troponin and other features of myocarditis
  - Clozapine should be stopped if troponin ≥ 2 × ULN or CRP >100 mg/L, although in pediatric patients, consultation with a pediatric cardiologist should be considered if myocarditis is suspected
  - Cardiomyopathy is a late complication; consider annual echocardiogram in adults (pediatric recommendations are limited)
- After starting clozapine:
  - BMI percentile monthly for 3 months, then quarterly
  - Consider monitoring fasting triglycerides monthly in patients at high risk for metabolic complications
  - Blood pressure, fasting plasma glucose (or hemoglobin A1C), lipid profile within 3 months and then annually
  - Treat or refer for treatment and consider switching to another atypical antipsychotic for patients who become overweight, obese, have impaired glucose metabolism, or are dyslipidemic while receiving an atypical antipsychotic
  - Even in patients without known diabetes, be vigilant for the rare but life-threatening onset of diabetic ketoacidosis, which always requires immediate treatment, by monitoring for the rapid onset of polyuria, polydipsia, weight loss, nausea, vomiting, dehydration, rapid respiration, weakness, and clouding of sensorium, even coma
  - Liver tests may be necessary in patients who develop nausea, vomiting, or anorexia
  - Patients should be monitored periodically for the development of abnormal movements using neurological exam and the Abnormal Involuntary Movement Scale (AIMS)

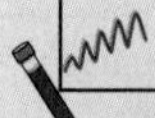

Pharmacokinetics

- Clozapine is well absorbed after oral administration. It undergoes extensive first-pass metabolism in the liver, resulting in a relatively low bioavailability of approximately 27% to 50%. The time to peak plasma concentration (Tmax) ranges from 1 to 4 hours.
- Clozapine has a large volume of distribution, indicating that it distributes extensively into tissues throughout the body. It readily crosses the blood–brain barrier, contributing to its central nervous system effects. Clozapine is highly protein-bound, primarily to albumin.
- Half-life in adults is 5–16-hours
- Inhibits CYP2D6
- Metabolized primarily by CYP1A2 and to a lesser extent by CYP2D6 and 3A4 (Figure 1)
- Plasma level to dose ratios significantly vary by age (Figure 2)

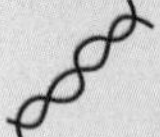

Pharmacogenetics

- No recommendations

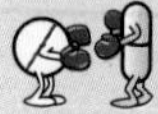

Drug Interactions

- Use clozapine plasma levels to guide treatment due to the propensity for drug interactions
- In presence of a strong CYP1A2 inhibitor (e.g., fluvoxamine, ciprofloxacin): use 1/3 the dose of clozapine
- In the presence of a strong CYP1A2 inducer (e.g., cigarette smoke), clozapine plasma levels are decreased
- May need to decrease clozapine dose by up to 50% during periods of extended smoking cessation (>1 week)
- Strong CYP2D6 inhibitors (e.g., bupropion, duloxetine, paroxetine, fluoxetine) can raise clozapine levels; dose adjustment may be necessary
- Strong CYP3A4 inhibitors (e.g., ketoconazole) can raise clozapine levels; dose adjustment may be necessary
- May increase effect of antihypertensive agents

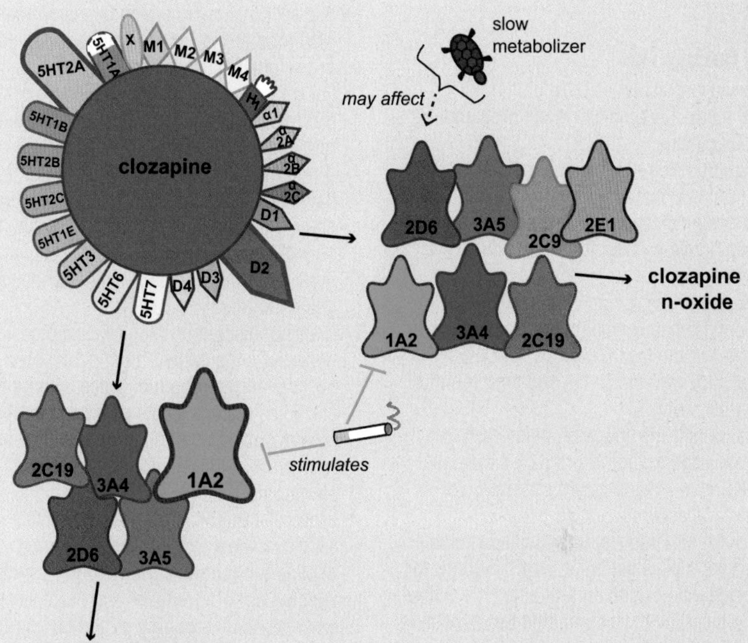

Figure 1 Clozapine metabolism. Clozapine is extensively metabolized in the liver with the main routes being demethylation to n-desmethylclozapine and oxidation to clozapine n-oxide. Variation in clozapine blood levels is related to dose, gender, age, and smoking, and these factors account for approximately 50% of variability in serum clozapine. The remaining 50% is likely related to genetic variation in drug metabolizing enzymes and to concomitant medications.

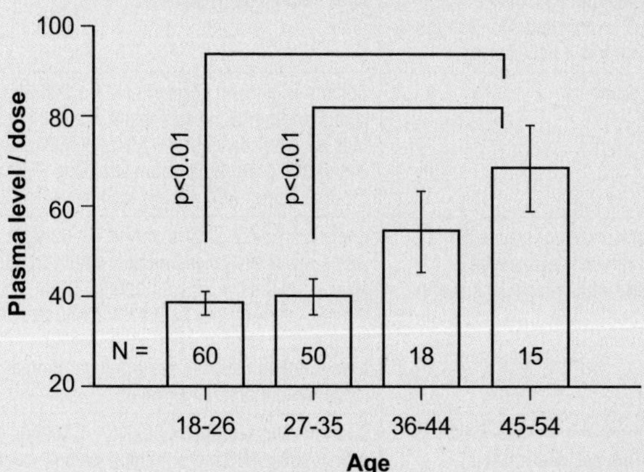

Figure 2 Clozapine concentrations relative to dose vary considerably and are influenced by age. Reproduced from Haring et al., 1989.

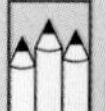

Dosing Tips

- Start low, go slow as clozapine not well studied, especially in children and adolescents
- Be guided more by plasma drug levels than by total oral dose
- Get trough clozapine levels simultaneously when blood is taken for blood count monitoring
- Because of the monitoring schedule, prescriptions are generally given 1 week at a time for the first 6 months, then every 2 weeks for months 6–12, and then monthly after 12 months
- Plasma half-life suggests twice-daily administration, but in practice it may be given once a day at night especially for older adolescents
- Prior to initiating treatment with clozapine, a baseline ANC must be at least 1,500/μL for the general population and at least 1,000/μL for patients with documented benign ethnic neutropenia (BEN)
- See accompanying tables for recommended ANC monitoring for the general population or for individuals with BEN
- For treatment resistance, consider obtaining plasma drug levels to guide dosing above recommended levels
- If treatment is discontinued for more than 2 days, reinitiate with 12.5 mg once or twice daily; if that dose is tolerated, the dose may be increased to the previously therapeutic dose more quickly than recommended for initial treatment
- If abrupt discontinuation of clozapine is necessary, the patient must be covered for cholinergic rebound; those with higher clozapine plasma levels may need extremely high doses of anticholinergic medications to prevent delirium and other rebound symptoms
- Slow off-titration is strongly preferred for clozapine if at all possible to avoid cholinergic rebound and rebound psychosis which are more frequent and more severe when abruptly stopping clozapine compared to other antipsychotics

Recommended ANC monitoring for the general population		
ANC level	Recommendation	ANC monitoring
Normal range (at least 1,500 μL)	Initiate treatment If treatment is interrupted for <30 days, continue monitoring as before If treatment is interrupted for 30 days or more, monitor as if new patient	First 6 months: weekly Second 6 months: every 2 weeks After 1 year: every month
Mild neutropenia (1,000–1,499 μL)	Continue treatment	Confirm all initial reports of ANC < 1,500/μL with a repeat ANC measurement within 24 hours Monitor 3 times/week until ANC ≥ 1,500/μL Once ANC ≥ 1,500/μL, return to patient's last "normal range" ANC monitoring interval
Moderate neutropenia (500–999 μL)	Interrupt treatment for suspected clozapine-induced neutropenia Recommend hematology consultation	Confirm all initial reports of ANC < 1,500/μL with a repeat ANC measurement within 24 hours Monitor ANC daily until ≥ 1,000/μL THEN Monitor 3 times/week until ANC ≥ 1,500/μL Once ANC ≥ 1,500/μL, check ANC weekly for 4 weeks, then return to patient's last "normal range" ANC monitoring interval
Severe neutropenia (<500 μL)	Interrupt treatment for suspected clozapine-induced neutropenia Recommend hematology consultation Do not rechallenge unless prescriber determines benefits outweigh risks	Confirm all initial reports of ANC < 1,500/μL with a repeat ANC measurement within 24 hours Monitor ANC daily until ≥ 1,000/μL THEN Monitor 3 times/week until ANC ≥ 1,500/μL If patient is rechallenged, resume treatment as a new patient under "normal range" monitoring once ANC ≥ 1,500/μL

Abbreviation: ANC: absolute neutrophil count

Recommended ANC monitoring for BEN patients		
ANC level	Recommendation	ANC monitoring
Normal BEN range (established ANC bsaseline ≥ 1,000 μL)	Obtain at least 2 baseline ANC levels before initiating treatment If treatment is interrupted for <30 days, continue monitoring as before If treatment is interrupted for 30 days or more, monitor as if new patient	First 6 months: weekly Second 6 months: every 2 weeks After 1 year: every month
BEN neutropenia (500–999 μL)	Continue treatment Recommend hematology consultation	Confirm all initial reports of ANC < 1,500/μL with a repeat ANC measurement within 24 hours Monitor 3 times/week until ANC ≥ 1,000/μL or ≥ patient's known baseline Once ANC ≥ 1,000/μL or above patient's known baseline, check ANC weekly for 4 weeks, then return to patient's last "normal BEN range" ANC monitoring interval
BEN severe neutropenia (<500 μL)	Interrupt treatment for suspected clozapine-induced neutropenia Recommend hematology consultation Do not rechallenge unless prescriber determines benefits outweigh risks	Confirm all initial reports of ANC < 1,500/μL with a repeat ANC measurement within 24 hours Monitor ANC daily until ≥ 500/μL THEN Monitor 3 times/week until ANC ≥ patient's baseline If patient is rechallenged, resume treatment as a new patient under "normal BEN range" monitoring once ANC ≥ 1,000/μL or at patient's known baseline

Abbreviations: ANC: absolute neutrophil count; BEN: benign ethnic neutropenia

How to Switch

- From another antipsychotic to clozapine:
  - When tapering a prior antipsychotic, see its entry in this manual for how to stop and how to taper off that specific drug
  - Generally, try to stop the first agent before starting clozapine so that new side effects of clozapine can be distinguished from withdrawal effects of the first agent
  - If urgent, cross taper off the other antipsychotic while clozapine is started at a low dose, with dose adjustments down of the other antipsychotic, and up for clozapine every 3 to 7 days
  - Be especially cautious and alert to worsening anticholinergic side effects during cross taper from other antipsychotics with strong anticholinergic side effects
- Off clozapine to another antipsychotic:
  - Generally, try to stop clozapine before starting the new antipsychotic so that new side effects of the next drug can be distinguished from any withdrawal effects from clozapine
  - In nonurgent situations, clozapine is the antipsychotic generally recommended to be the slowest in tapering off, since rapid taper faster than 4 weeks is often associated with rebound psychosis
  - If urgent, such as in a medical emergency, abruptly stop clozapine and be prepared for rebound psychosis while starting a new antipsychotic and consider hospitalization

How to Stop

- Whenever possible, discontinue by slow down-titration over at least 4 weeks
- See tables under Dosing Tips for guidance on stopping due to neutropenia
- Rapid oral discontinuation may lead to withdrawal dyskinesias, which are generally reversible in the pediatric population. Of note, withdrawal dyskinesias are more common in pediatric patients than in adults.
- Make down-titration even slower if any signs of rebound psychosis or of anticholinergic rebound such as tachycardia, tremor, gastrointestinal symptoms

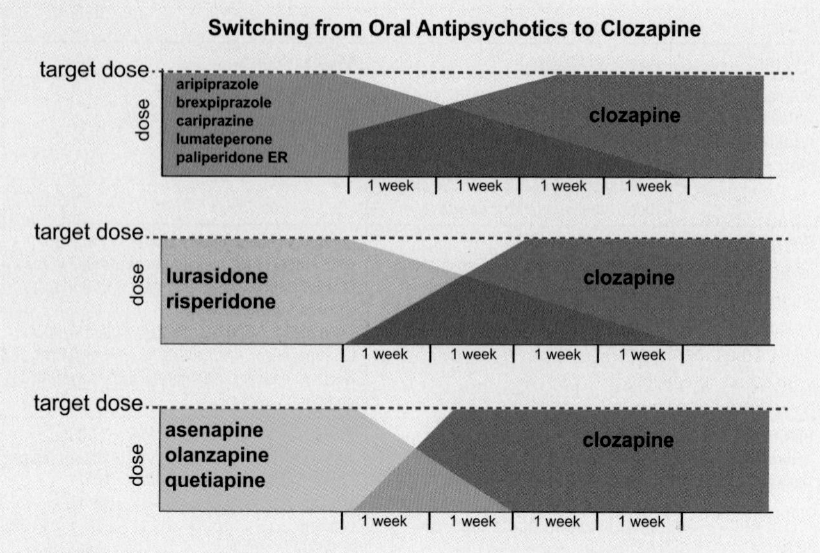

WHAT TO EXPECT

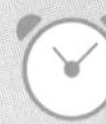

Onset of Action

- Likelihood of response depends on achieving trough plasma levels of at least 350 ng/mL
- Median time to response after achieving therapeutic plasma levels (350 ng/mL) is approximately 3 weeks
- If there is no response after 3 weeks of therapeutic plasma levels, recheck plasma levels and continue titration
- Onset of action can be several weeks, and full therapeutic effects can slowly emerge over many months

Duration of Action

- Effects are consistent over a 24-hour period
- May continue to work for many years to prevent relapse of symptoms

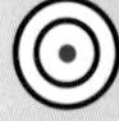

Primary Target Symptoms

- Treatment-resistant positive symptoms of psychosis
- Negative symptoms of psychosis
- Cognitive symptoms
- Affective symptoms
- Suicidal behavior
- Treatment-resistant psychotic violence and aggression

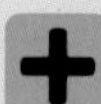

What Is Considered a Positive Result?

- In schizophrenia:
  - In strictly defined refractory schizophrenia, 50–60% of adult patients will respond to clozapine
  - The response rate to other atypical antipsychotics in the refractory patient population ranges from 0–9%
  - Can improve negative symptoms, as well as aggressive, cognitive, and affective symptoms but less so than for positive symptoms although more so than for other antipsychotics
  - In children or adolescents with a first episode of psychosis, initial response may be greater than for recurrent episodes of psychosis in adults
- In other disorders:
  - Many patients with bipolar disorder and other disorders with psychotic, aggressive, violent, impulsive, and other types of behavioral disturbances may respond to clozapine when other agents have failed

How Long to Treat

- Continue treatment until reaching a plateau of improvement
- After reaching a satisfactory plateau, continue treatment for at least a year after

first episode of psychosis; treatment may need to be indefinite

What If It Stops Working?

- Check for nonadherence, possibly by checking plasma drug level, and consider switching to another antipsychotic with fewer side effects
- Growth/developmental changes may contribute to apparent loss of efficacy as well as to new onset of side effects as metabolism slows and drug levels rise in transition from childhood to adolescence; dose adjustment (increase or decrease) should be considered
- Also consider new onset cigarette smoking or increased smoking since this can lower plasma clozapine levels
- Screen for the development of a new comorbid disorder, especially substance use
- Screen for adverse changes in the home or school environment

What If It Doesn't Work?

- Consider evaluation for another diagnosis (especially bipolar illness or depression with mixed features) or for a comorbid condition (e.g., medical illness, substance use)
- Consider other important potential factors such as ongoing conflicts, family psychopathology, and an adverse environment (e.g., poverty, chaos, violence, prior and ongoing psychological trauma, abuse, neglect)
- Institute trauma-informed care for appropriate children and adolescents
- Obtain clozapine plasma levels and continue titration
- Levels greater than 700 ng/mL are often not well tolerated; no evidence to support dosing that results in plasma levels greater than 1,000 ng/mL
- Consider augmentation with valproate, lithium, or lamotrigine, but use caution with valproate as it can also cause bone marrow suppression and be sedating
- Rather than high dosing of clozapine, consider adding another antipsychotic with caution and by an expert
- Consider initiating psychotherapy. In adolescents with bipolar disorder (and those with affective symptoms who are at risk of developing bipolar disorder), family-focused psychotherapy can be particularly helpful (Miklowitz et al., 2020).
- Consider presence of concomitant drug abuse

TALKING TO PATIENTS AND CAREGIVERS

What to Tell Parents About Efficacy

- Clozapine is a special medication being given off-label because your child has failed to respond adequately to other antipsychotics
- Explain which use clozapine is being chosen for, how to tell if the drug is working by targeting specific symptoms, and why this is being done
- Clozapine can work when other antipsychotics fail to work
- Clozapine can cause problems with your child's blood count and for that reason your child must have blood counts monitored while taking clozapine
- You must inform your pediatrician of any serious infection or fever while taking clozapine
- While the medicine helps by reducing symptoms and improving function, it is not a cure, and it therefore may be necessary to keep taking the medication long term to sustain its therapeutic effects
- Since every treatment consideration depends on a risk/benefit analysis, parents should fully understand short- and long-term risks as well as benefits

What to Tell Children and Adolescents About Efficacy

- Be specific about the symptoms being targeted: we are trying to help you …
- Give the medication a try; if it's not working very well, we can stop the medication and try something else
- A good try often takes several weeks
- If it does make you feel better, you cannot stop it right away or you may get sick again
- Medications don't change who you are as a person; they give you the opportunity to be the best person you can be
- You will need to have blood counts measured while taking this medication

What to Tell Parents About Side Effects

- Explain that side effects are expected with clozapine and that clozapine has more side effects than other antipsychotics but it also may have more efficacy
- Explain sialorrhea, sedation, constipation, and weight gain and other side effects as deemed appropriate
- Tell parents some side effects may go away with time but that many will not
- This medication will require regular blood counts because of a specific side effect that rarely can reduce blood cells and be very dangerous
- Ask parents to support the patient while side effects are occurring
- Parents should fully understand short- and long-term risks as well as benefits
- Explaining to the parents what to expect from medication treatment, and especially what potential side effects to expect, can help prevent early termination of medication
- Keep in closer touch with your mental health professional and your pediatrician if any unexplained problems arise

What to Tell Children and Adolescents About Side Effects

- This medication may make you tired, constipated, gain weight, have too much saliva
- Let your parents know if you are experiencing abdominal pain or constipation
- Drink lots of fluids
- If you have side effects that are bothering you, tell your parents and your parents should tell me
- Explaining to child/adolescent what to expect from medication treatment, and especially potential side effects, can help prevent early termination of medication

What to Tell Teachers About the Medication (If Parents Consent)

- Clozapine can make children/adolescents sedated and have excessive salivation
- If student complains of fever, the student should be sent to the school nurse's office to have their temperature checked
- Consider bathroom passes, as students may need to use the bathroom more frequently as a result of bowel regimens
- Encourage students to have frequent access to water
- It is not abusable
- Encourage dialogue with parents/guardians about any behavior or mood changes
- Notify the clinician of increased restlessness or akathisia symptoms, which may be apparent in the school setting

SPECIAL POPULATIONS

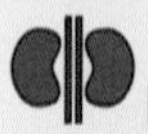

Renal Impairment

- Should be used with caution

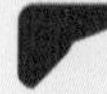

Hepatic Impairment

- Should be used with caution

Cardiac Impairment

- Use in patients with cardiac impairment has not been studied; however, the risk of orthostatic hypotension in pediatric patients is less than in adults, as children rely less on peripheral vasoconstriction to regulate blood pressure
- Use with caution if patient is taking concomitant antihypertensive or alpha 1 antagonist

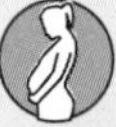

Pregnancy

- Controlled studies have not been conducted in pregnant women
- There is a risk of abnormal muscle movements and withdrawal symptoms in newborns whose mothers took an antipsychotic during the third trimester; symptoms may include agitation, abnormally increased or decreased muscle tone, tremor, sleepiness, severe difficulty breathing, and difficulty feeding
- Animal studies have not shown adverse effects
- Psychotic symptoms may worsen during pregnancy, and some form of treatment may be necessary
- Clozapine should be used only when the potential benefits outweigh potential risks to the fetus
- National Pregnancy Registry for Atypical Antipsychotics: 1-866-961-2388 or http://womensmentalhealth.org/clinical-and-research-programs/pregnancyregistry/

Breast Feeding

- Unknown if clozapine is secreted in human breast milk, but all psychotropics assumed to be secreted in breast milk
- Recommended either to discontinue drug or formula feed
- Infants of women who choose to breast feed while on clozapine should be monitored for possible adverse effects; sedation, failure to thrive, jitteriness, tremor, and abnormal muscle movements have been reported

THE ART OF PSYCHOPHARMACOLOGY

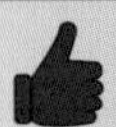

Potential Advantages

- In children and adolescents:
  - When all other options have failed
- All ages:
  - Treatment-resistant schizophrenia
  - Violent, aggressive patients
  - Patients with tardive dyskinesia
  - Patients with suicidal behavior
  - Superior efficacy for psychotic symptoms
  - Low/no drug-induced parkinsonism/ akathisia
  - Low/no hyperprolactinemia
  - Low/no tardive dyskinesia; can even improve tardive dyskinesia
  - Use in Lewy body dementia (adults)
  - Use in Parkinson's psychosis (adults)

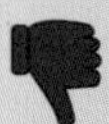

Potential Disadvantages

- In children and adolescents:
  - May be more susceptible to side effects, including sedation and weight gain
  - Those who have unacceptable weight gain
- All ages:
  - Patients with diabetes, obesity, and/or dyslipidemia
  - Sialorrhea, sedation, and orthostasis may be intolerable for some
- Barriers to adopting clozapine:
  - Wishing to avoid side effects
  - Wishing to avoid blood monitoring
  - Not knowing how to manage side effects if they arise
  - Not knowing when termination of clozapine treatment is warranted or how it can be avoided
  - Not knowing when to rechallenge after adverse effects

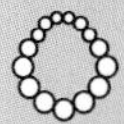

Pearls

- The secret to successful use of clozapine is knowing how to manage side effects
- The secret to managing side effects of clozapine is anticipating them, detecting them early, and aggressively treating them early
- The secret as to how to do this may be experience with clozapine or close collaboration with someone who has experience with clozapine
- Therefore, removing the barriers to adopting clozapine means learning how to avoid or manage key side effects including when to continue, discontinue, or rechallenge with clozapine
- Specific side effects of clozapine to become expert in managing:
  - Ileus/constipation
  - Blood monitoring/agranulocytosis/ neutropenia/eosinophilia
  - Myocarditis/QTc prolongation/tachycardia
  - Neuroleptic malignant syndrome
  - Sialorrhea
- Clozapine is the gold-standard treatment for refractory schizophrenia in adults
- Clozapine is not used first line due to side effects and monitoring burden
- Reduces suicide in schizophrenia
- Some studies in adults have shown that clozapine was associated with the lowest risk of mortality among the antipsychotics, due largely to reducing suicide, causing some to question if its use should continue to be restricted to resistant adult cases
- However, there is no argument against restricting off-label clozapine use in children and adolescents to treatment-resistant cases
- May reduce violence and aggression in difficult cases, including forensic cases
- May reduce substance abuse
- May improve tardive dyskinesia
- Cigarette smoke can decrease clozapine levels (Figure 1), and patients may be at risk for relapse if they begin or increase smoking
- Patients can have much better responses to clozapine than to any other agent, but not always

- To treat constipation and reduce risk of paralytic ileus and bowel obstruction, taper off other anticholinergic agents and start all patients routinely on docusate
- The FDA has changed the requirements for monitoring, prescribing, dispensing, and receiving clozapine in order to address concerns related to neutropenia; in addition to updating the prescribing information for clozapine, the FDA has approved a new, shared risk evaluation and mitigation strategy (REMS)
- The Clozapine REMS program replaces the six existing clozapine registries, which are maintained by individual clozapine manufacturers. Prescribers, pharmacies, and patients will now be required to enroll in a single centralized program; patients already treated with clozapine will be automatically transferred. In order to prescribe and dispense clozapine, prescribers and pharmacies will be required to be certified in the Clozapine REMS Program. Visit the Clozapine REMS Program homepage at www.newclozapinerems.com/home# for more information.
- Antipsychotic-related weight gain significantly affects adherence and survey data suggest that many young patients would start pharmacological treatment to mitigate antipsychotic-related weight gain at treatment initiation, while parents and clinicians are more hesitant (Klein et al., 2020)

SUGGESTED READING

Correll CU, Agid O, Crespo-Facorro B et al. A guideline and checklist for initiating and managing clozapine treatment in patients with treatment-resistant schizophrenia. CNS Drugs 2022;36(7):659–79.

Gogtay N, Rapoport J. Clozapine use in children and adolescents. Expert Opin Pharmacother 2008;9(3):459–65.

Haring C, Meise Y, Humpel C et al. Dose-related plasma levels of clozapine: influence of smoking behaviour, sex and age. Psychopharmacology (Berl) 1989:99 Suppl:S38–40.

Klein CC, Topalian AG, Starr B et al. The importance of second-generation antipsychotic-related weight gain and adherence barriers in youth with bipolar disorders: patient, parent, and provider perspectives. J Child Adolesc Psychopharmacol 2020;30(6):376–80.

Kumra S, Frazier JA, Jacobsen LK et al. Childhood-onset schizophrenia. A double-blind clozapine-haloperidol comparison. Arch Gen Psychiatry 1996;53(12):1090–7.

Masuda T, Misawa F, Takase M, Kane JM, Correll CU. Association with hospitalization and all-cause discontinuation among patients with schizophrenia on clozapine vs other oral second-generation antipsychotics: a systematic review and meta-analysis of cohort studies. JAMA Psychiatry 2019;76(10):1052–62.

Meyer JM, Stahl SM. Stahl's Handbooks: The Clozapine Handbook. New York: Cambridge University Press, 2019.

Miklowitz DJ, Schneck CD, Walshaw PD et al. Effects of family-focused therapy vs enhanced usual care for symptomatic youths at high risk for bipolar disorder: a randomized clinical trial. JAMA Psychiatry 2020 1;77(5):455–63.

Pillay J, Boylan K, Carrey N et al. First- and Second-Generation Antipsychotics in Children and Young Adults: Systematic Review Update [Internet]. Rockville, MD: Agency for Healthcare Research and Quality (US); 2017 Mar. Report No.: 17-EHC001-EF. AHRQ Comparative Effectiveness Reviews.

Strawn JR, Stahl SM. Case Studies: Stahl's Essential Psychopharmacology: Volume 4: Children and Adolescents. New York: Cambridge University Press, 2023

THERAPEUTICS

Brands
- Periactin

Generic
Yes

US FDA Approved for Pediatric Use
- Allergy symptoms (ages 2 and older)

Off-Label for Pediatric Use
- Approved in adults
  - None
- Other off-label uses
  - Insomnia
  - Anxiety
  - Migraine prophylaxis
  - Appetite stimulation
  - Serotonin syndrome

Class and Mechanism of Action
- Antihistamine (anxiolytic, hypnotic, antiemetic)
- Antagonism at serotonin receptors
- At higher concentrations, cyproheptadine has anticholinergic, antiserotonergic, and antidopaminergic activities
  - Of the serotonin receptors, it is an especially potent antagonist of the 5HT2 receptors; in adults, it blocks 85% of 5HT2 receptors at 12 mg/day and 95% of 5HT2 receptors at 18 mg/day (Kapur et al., 1997)
  - Antagonism at muscarinic 1 receptors occurs at high doses

SAFETY AND TOLERABILITY

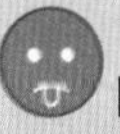

Notable Side Effects
- Sedation, dizziness
- Constipation, nausea
- Dry mouth, blurred vision

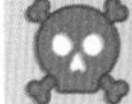

Life-Threatening or Dangerous Side Effects
- Rare convulsions
- Urinary retention
- Tachycardia, cardiac arrhythmias
- Confusion
- Rare hepatotoxicity

Growth and Maturation
- Not studied

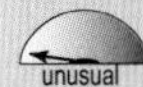

Weight Gain
- Cyproheptadine is used off-label for appetite stimulation and weight gain

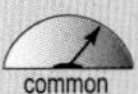

Sedation
- Many experience and/or can be significant in amount

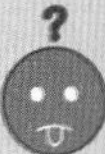

What to Do About Side Effects
- Wait
- For dry mouth, interventions include lozenges, sprays, mouth rinses, gels, oils, and chewing gum, which broadly fall into two categories: saliva stimulants and saliva substitutes
- If side effects persist or are intolerable, switch to another agent

How Drug Causes Side Effects
- Blocking histamine 1 receptors can cause sedation
- Preventing the action of acetylcholine on muscarinic receptors can cause anticholinergic effects such as dry mouth, blurred vision, constipation

Warnings and Precautions
- Cyproheptadine may potentiate the effects of CNS depressants, including alcohol
- Antihistamines such as cyproheptadine may reduce mental alertness
- Cyproheptadine has an atropine-like effect and should be used with caution in patients with history of bronchial asthma, increased intraocular pressure, hyperthyroidism, cardiovascular disease, and hypertension
- May have additive effects if taken with anticholinergic agents
- In younger children, antihistamines such as cyproheptadine may cause disinhibition

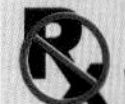

When Not to Prescribe
- If patient is breast feeding
- In children under the age of 2
- If patient is taking an MAOI
- If patient has acute angle glaucoma, stenosing peptic ulcer, bladder obstruction, or pyloroduodenal obstruction

- If there is a proven allergy to cyproheptadine

Long-Term Use
- Not studied

Habit Forming
- No

Overdose
- Hallucinations, central nervous system depression, seizure
- Respiratory and cardiac arrest, death

DOSING AND USE

Usual Dosage Range
- Total daily dosage may be calculated on the basis of body weight or body area using approximately 0.25 mg/kg/day or 8 mg per square meter of body surface
- Ages 2–6: maximum daily dose 12 mg/day
- Ages 7–14: maximum daily dose 16 mg/day
- Ages 15 and older: 12–16 mg/day; maximum daily dose should not exceed 0.5 mg/kg/day or 32 mg/day, whichever is less

Dosage Forms
- Oral syrup 2 mg/5 mL
- Tablet 4 mg

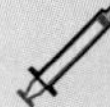

How to Dose
- Appetite stimulation and anxiety in children: consider 2 mg bid for 3–4 days and then 2 mg tid. In older children, increase to 4 mg tid.
- Appetite stimulation and anxiety in adolescents: consider beginning at 4 mg bid and increasing to 4 mg tid in 3 to 4 days. Depending on the improvement seen within the first week of treatment, may consider increasing to 8 mg tid.
- Insomnia in children: consider 2–4 mg qHS
- Insomnia in adolescents: consider 4–8 mg qHS

Options for Administration
- Available as an oral solution and as a tablet; tablet can be divided in half

Tests
- None for healthy individuals

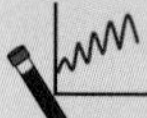

Pharmacokinetics
- Extensively metabolized in the liver via CYP3A4 and CYP2D6. Several metabolites are formed, including the active metabolite norcyproheptadine, which contributes to its prolonged duration of action.
- The elimination half-life of cyproheptadine in pediatric patients ranges from 12 to 21 hours, depending on age
- Cyproheptadine is well absorbed after oral administration, with peak plasma concentrations reached within 1 to 3 hours. Food intake may slightly delay absorption but does not significantly affect the overall bioavailability.

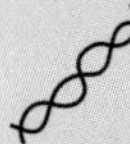

Pharmacogenetics
- No recommendations

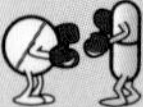

Drug Interactions
- May potentiate the effects of other CNS depressants
- If anticholinergic agents are used with cyproheptadine, the anticholinergic effects may be enhanced

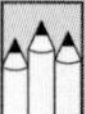

Dosing Tips
- Can be taken with or without food, but when used for appetite stimulation and anxiety is generally given tid
- When used for insomnia, is generally given qHS

How to Switch
- Tapering generally not necessary

How to Stop
- Tapering generally not necessary

WHAT TO EXPECT

Onset of Action
- When used for appetite stimulation, effects will generally emerge in 1–2 days
- When used for anxiety, effects generally emerge within the first day of treatment

Duration of Action
- Approximately 8 hours

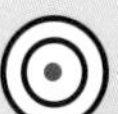

Primary Target Symptoms

- Insomnia
- Anxiety
- Decreased appetite

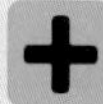

What Is Considered a Positive Result?

- The goal of treatment of insomnia is to improve the quality of sleep, including effects on total wake time and number of nighttime awakenings
- The goal of treatment for anxiety is complete remission of current symptoms as well as prevention of future relapses
- The goal of treatment in patients with appetite suppression is a restoration of normal growth trajectory

How Long to Treat

- For insomnia and short-term symptoms of anxiety: not intended for use beyond two weeks
- For long-term symptoms of anxiety, consider switching to an SSRI or SNRI for long-term maintenance
- For appetite stimulation, longer-term treatment may be needed

What If It Stops Working?

- If anxiety symptoms reemerge, consider an SSRI, and re-trying psychotherapeutic approaches
- If the primary target symptom is insomnia, consider an alternative medication or melatonin and re-trying CBT for insomnia (CBT-I)
- If the primary symptom is appetite suppression, consider an alternative strategy, referral to nutritionist, lowering the dose of the stimulant medication, or switching to a stimulant medication that is less likely to produce appetite suppression (e.g., isomeric form)

What If It Doesn't Work?

- For anxiety, consider switching to an SSRI or SNRI
- If insomnia does not improve, it may be a manifestation of a primary psychiatric or physical illness, which requires independent evaluation. Also, re-trying other interventions for insomnia may be helpful.
- For appetite stimulation, consider an alternative strategy, referral to nutritionist, lowering the dose of the stimulant medication, or switching to a stimulant medication that is less likely to produce appetite suppression (e.g., isomeric form)

TALKING TO PATIENTS AND CAREGIVERS

What to Tell Parents About Efficacy

- While the medicine helps by reducing symptoms and improving function, it is not a cure, and it is therefore necessary to keep taking the medication to sustain its therapeutic effects
- Since every treatment consideration depends on a risk/benefit analysis, parents should fully understand short- and long-term risks as well as benefits
- Often a good idea to tell parents whether the medication chosen is specifically approved for the disorder being treated, or whether it is being given for "unapproved" or "off-label" reasons based on good clinical practice, expert consensus, and/or prudent extrapolation of controlled data from adults

What to Tell Children and Adolescents About Efficacy

- We are trying to make you feel better
- It may be a good idea to give the medication a try; if it's not working very well, we can stop the medication and try something else
- Medications don't change who you are as a person; they give you the opportunity to be the best person you can be

What to Tell Parents About Side Effects

- Explain that mild side effects are expected at initiation or when increasing the dose
- Predict side effects in advance (you will look clever and competent to the parents, unless you scare them with too much information and cause nocebo effects, in which case you won't look so clever when the patient develops lots of side effects and stops medication; use your judgment here); a balanced but honest presentation is an art rather than a science
- Ask parents to support the patient while side effects are occurring

- Parents should fully understand short- and long-term risks as well as benefits
- Explaining to the parents what to expect from medication treatment, and especially potential side effects, can help prevent early termination of medication

What to Tell Children and Adolescents About Side Effects

- Even if you get side effects, most of them get better or go away in a few days to a few weeks
- Explaining to child/adolescent what to expect from medication treatment, and especially potential side effects, can help prevent early termination of medication

What to Tell Teachers About the Medication (If Parents Consent)

- Cyproheptadine can make children/ adolescents sleepy
- It is not abusable

SPECIAL POPULATIONS

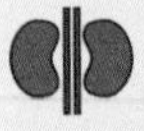

Renal Impairment

- No dose adjustment necessary

Hepatic Impairment

- Dose reduction may be necessary since cyproheptadine is extensively metabolized in the liver

Cardiac Impairment

- Not systematically evaluated in patients with cardiac impairment

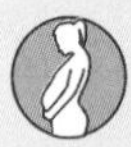

Pregnancy

- Two studies in pregnant women have not shown that cyproheptadine increases the risk of abnormalities when administered during the first, second, and third trimesters of pregnancy; no teratogenic effects were observed in any of the newborns
- Cyproheptadine is not generally recommended for use during pregnancy

Breast Feeding

- Unknown if cyproheptadine is secreted in human breast milk, but all psychotropics assumed to be secreted in breast milk
- Cyproheptadine may lower prolactin concentrations, which could interfere with breast feeding
- Recommended either to discontinue drug or formula feed

THE ART OF PSYCHOPHARMACOLOGY

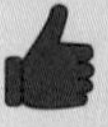

Potential Advantages

- Patients with dermatitis and itching
- No abuse liability, dependence, or withdrawal

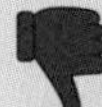

Potential Disadvantages

- Sedation
- Need to dose multiple times per day when using for appetite stimulation and anxiety

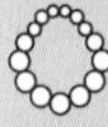

Pearls

- Cyproheptadine is commonly used to stimulate appetite in children and adolescents who are experiencing stimulant-associated appetite suppression
- In double-blind, controlled trials of children and adolescents, cyproheptadine is associated with improved weight and height velocities as well as improvements in insulin-like growth factor-I
- Cyproheptadine has been used as an adjunctive treatment for serotonin syndrome because of its ability to block 5HT2 and potentially 5HT1 receptors. Case reports suggest that it may be helpful in pediatric serotonin syndrome.
- In general, the sedating effects wane quickly with H1 antagonists as a result of tachyphylaxis; however, the effects of cyproheptadine on appetite stimulation seems to persist in youth
- Cyproheptadine has also been used to decrease nightmares in adults and pediatric patients with PTSD, although alpha-1 antagonists remain the first-line pharmacological treatment for these symptoms

SUGGESTED READING

Bertrand V, Massy N, Vegas N et al. Safety of cyproheptadine, an orexigenic drug. Analysis of the French national pharmacovigilance data-base and systematic review. Front Pediatr 2021;9:712413.

Cyproheptadine. Lexicomp. Wolters Kluwer Health, Inc. [Internet] Updated June 2021.

Gupta M, Gupta N, Madabushi J. Off-label cyproheptadine in children and adolescents: psychiatric comorbidities, interacting variables, safety, and risks of hepatotoxicity. Cureus 2023;15(1):e33745.

Harrison ME, Norris ML, Robinson A et al. Use of cyproheptadine to stimulate appetite and body weight gain: a systematic review. Appetite 2019;137:62–72.

Kapur S, Zipursky RB, Jones C et al. Cyproheptadine: a potent in vivo serotonin antagonist. Am J Psychiatry 1997;154(6):884.

Mahachoklertwattana P, Wanasuwankul S, Poomthavorn P, Choubtum L, Sriphrapradang A. Short-term cyproheptadine therapy in underweight children: effects on growth and serum insulin-like growth factor-I. J Pediatr Endocrinol Metab 2009;22(5):425–32.

Simons FE, Simons KJ. H1 Antihistamines: current status and future directions. World Allergy Organ J 2008;1(9):145–55.

THERAPEUTICS

Brands
- DDAVP
- Nocdurna

Generic
Yes

US FDA Approved for Pediatric Use
- Primary nocturnal enuresis (ages 6 and older)
- To evaluate capacity of the kidneys to concentrate urine (pediatric patients ages 3 and older)
- Central diabetes insipidus

Off-Label for Pediatric Use
- Approved in adults
  - Hemophilia A (injection)
  - Von Willebrand's disease (mild to moderate) (injection)

Class and Mechanism of Action
- Desmopressin acts as an agonist at the renal collecting duct by binding to vasopressin2 (V_2) receptor. These receptors trigger the translocation of aquaporin channels to the apical membrane of the collecting duct, and these channels increase water reabsorption from the urine.
- Arginine vasopressin (AVP), which is also known as antidiuretic hormone (ADH), stimulates kidneys to retain water, but not sodium. In effect, urine is concentrated, and urine volume is reduced.

SAFETY AND TOLERABILITY

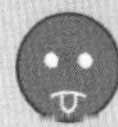

Notable Side Effects
- Headache, facial flushing, tachycardia

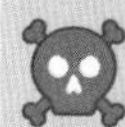

Life-Threatening or Dangerous Side Effects
- Hyponatremia (risk is higher with intranasal formulation)

Growth and Maturation
- Not studied

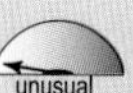

Weight Gain
- Not expected
- Rapid weight gain due to fluid retention may occur with overdose

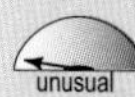

Sedation
- No

What to Do About Side Effects
- If hyponatremia occurs, desmopressin may need to be temporarily or permanently discontinued

How Drug Causes Side Effects
- Agonist action at V_2 receptors leads to water reabsorption from the urine, which may decrease serum sodium concentration; this can cause headaches, fluid retention, and hyponatremia

Warnings and Precautions
- Desmopressin can cause hyponatremia and should not be used in patients at increased risk of severe hyponatremia, such as those with excessive fluid intake or illnesses that can cause fluid or electrolyte imbalances, or in patients using loop diuretics or glucocorticoids
- Limit fluid intake to a minimum from 1 hour before until 8 hours after administration; treatment without concomitant reduction of fluid intake may lead to fluid retention and hyponatremia
- Desmopressin is not recommended for patients at risk of increased intracranial pressure or history of urinary retention

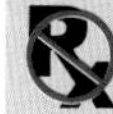

When Not to Prescribe
- In patients with hyponatremia or history of hyponatremia
- In patients with polydipsia
- In patients taking loop diuretics or systemic or inhaled glucocorticoids
- In patients with renal impairment
- In patients with syndrome of inappropriate antidiuretic hormone secretion (SIADH)
- During illnesses that can cause fluid or electrolyte imbalance
- In patients with heart failure
- If there is a proven allergy to desmopressin

Long-Term Use
- Continually reevaluate need for treatment; in most cases nocturnal enuresis resolves spontaneously, and cases continuing into adolescence are rare

Habit Forming
- No

Overdose
- Confusion, drowsiness, continuing headache, problems passing urine, rapid weight gain due to fluid retention

DOSING AND USE

Usual Dosage Range
- 0.2–0.4 mg at bedtime

Dosage Forms
- Tablet 0.1 mg, 0.2 mg
- Sublingual formulation 0.0277 mg, 0.0553 mg (not available in the United States)
- Nasal spray 0.01 mg/spray (not recommended)
- Injection 0.004 mg/mL

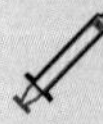

How to Dose
- Patients should limit fluid intake to a minimum from 1 hour before administration until the next morning or at least 8 hours after administration
- Oral tablet: initial dose is 0.2 mg orally at bedtime; maximum dose is 0.6 mg orally at bedtime

Options for Administration
- Nasal spray should not be used in pediatric patients

Tests
- Consider measuring serum sodium within 1 week and approximately 1 month after starting, as well as periodically during treatment

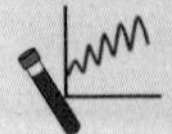

Pharmacokinetics
- Desmopressin produces peak concentrations quickly (within 1 hour, Figure 1 top), and its effects on diuresis can also be seen quickly
- Additionally, the duration of action for sublingual is approximately 8 hours compared to 6 hours with the tablet formulation (Figure 1 bottom) (Michelet et al., 2020)
- DDAVP tablet has a low protein binding of approximately 20%. It distributes rapidly throughout the body, including the central nervous system. The drug has a relatively small volume of distribution, indicating limited tissue distribution.
- Metabolism of desmopressin is minimal, and it is mainly eliminated unchanged. Therefore, there are no significant metabolic pathways or active metabolites.
- Relatively short elimination half-life of 1–3 hours
- Undergoes glomerular filtration in the kidneys and is excreted unchanged in the urine

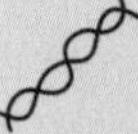

Pharmacogenetics
- No recommendations

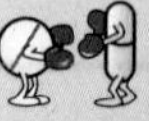

Drug Interactions
- Concomitant use with medications that increase risk of hyponatremia requires more frequent monitoring of serum sodium
- Concomitant use with vasoconstrictors may increase blood pressure and require lower desmopressin dose

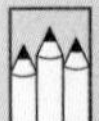

Dosing Tips
- Taking desmopressin sublingually in the fasted state increases concentrations over time by 50% and similarly increases the effect on diuresis by about 50%. However, in the United States, most desmopressin is administered orally.

How to Switch
- Taper not necessary

How to Stop
- Taper not necessary

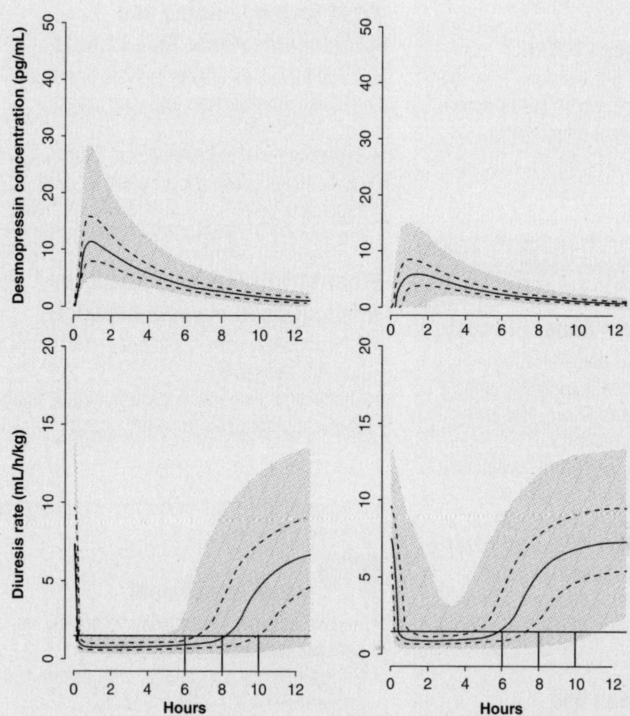

Figure 1 Simulation results after desmopressin sublingual formulation (left) or tablet (right). On top, the plasma concentration–time profiles are shown, whereas the pharmacodynamic (clinical) response, depicted as the diuresis rate per kilogram body weight, is shown in the bottom portion. The horizontal line marks the target of 1.5 mL/h/kg, and the solid line marks the median response, with the shaded area representing the 90% prediction interval and the dashed lines representing the 25th–75th percentiles. Vertical lines mark the targets of 6 h effect, 8 h effect, and no more than 10 h effect. Adapted from Michelet et al., 2020.

WHAT TO EXPECT

Onset of Action

- Once the target dose is reached, it may resolve nocturnal enuresis or significantly decrease bedwetting within the first several doses

Duration of Action

- Approximately 8 hours for sublingual compared to 6 hours with the tablet formulation (Michelet et al., 2020)

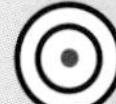

Primary Target Symptoms

- Nocturnal enuresis

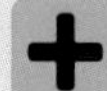

What Is Considered a Positive Result?

- Reduction or elimination of nocturnal enuresis

How Long to Treat

- Continually reevaluate need for treatment; in most cases nocturnal enuresis resolves spontaneously, and cases continuing into adolescence are rare

What If It Stops Working?

- Consider behavioral interventions (e.g., bell and pad conditioning), which are effective and may have persistent effects after discontinuation, unlike pharmacological interventions wherein enuresis will typically recur when the medication is stopped

What If It Doesn't Work?

- Consider behavioral interventions (e.g., bell and pad conditioning), which are effective and may have persistent effects after discontinuation

TALKING TO PATIENTS AND CAREGIVERS

What to Tell Parents About Efficacy

- Since every treatment consideration depends on a risk/benefit analysis, parents should fully understand short- and long-term risks as well as benefits
- Often a good idea to tell parents whether the medication chosen is specifically approved for the disorder being treated, or whether it is being given for "unapproved" or "off-label" reasons based on good clinical practice, expert consensus, and/or prudent extrapolation of controlled data from adults

What to Tell Children and Adolescents About Efficacy

- Be specific about the symptoms being targeted: we are trying to help you ...
- Give the medication a try; if it's not working very well, we can stop the medication and try something else

What to Tell Parents About Side Effects

- Explain the importance of fluid intake restriction to prevent hyponatremia with water intoxication
- Explain that treatment should be suspended during acute illness characterized by fluid and/or electrolyte imbalance or under conditions of extremely hot weather, vigorous exercise, or other conditions associated with increased water intake
- Parents should fully understand short- and long-term risks as well as benefits
- Explaining to the parents what to expect from medication treatment, and especially what potential side effects to expect, can help prevent early termination of medication

What to Tell Children and Adolescents About Side Effects

- If you have side effects that are bothering you, tell your parents and your parents should tell me
- Explaining to child/adolescent what to expect from medication treatment, and especially potential side effects, can help prevent early termination of medication

What to Tell Teachers About the Medication (If Parents Consent)

- Desmopressin can cause headache
- It is not abusable
- Encourage dialogue with parents/guardians about any behavior or mood changes

SPECIAL POPULATIONS

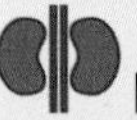

Renal Impairment

- Risk of adverse events may be greater in patients with renal impairment
- Contraindicated in patients with severe renal impairment (ClCr < 50 mL/min)

Hepatic Impairment

- Dose adjustment not necessary

Cardiac Impairment

- No data available

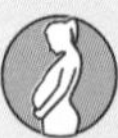

Pregnancy

- Controlled studies have not been conducted in pregnant women
- Published data and case reports have not shown an increased risk of major birth defects, miscarriage, or adverse maternal or fetal outcomes
- In vitro studies with human placenta show poor placental transfer of desmopressin
- In animal studies, administration of desmopressin to pregnant rats and rabbits during organogenesis did not lead to adverse developmental outcomes at doses approximately < 1 and 38 times the maximum recommended human dose

Breast Feeding

- Some drug is found in breast milk

THE ART OF PSYCHOPHARMACOLOGY

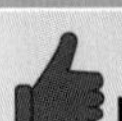

Potential Advantages

- Effective at reducing nocturnal enuresis

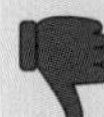

Potential Disadvantages

- Requires careful monitoring of fluid intake

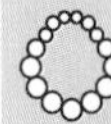

Pearls

- DDAVP is the first-line pharmacological intervention for youth with nocturnal enuresis; however, the FDA alert has called attention to the potential risk of hyponatremia and seizures as well as some deaths related to intranasal desmopressin. The intranasal formulation should no longer be used in pediatric patients.
- Care should be taken not to use desmopressin in patients who are predisposed to electrolyte imbalances, and if a patient is ill with a condition that acutely may case electrolyte imbalances, desmopressin should be withheld
- Nocturnal enuresis has a high rate of spontaneous remission, typically remitting in most patients between ages 5 and 7. Cases of nocturnal enuresis persisting into adolescence are generally rare.
- When evaluating a child with enuresis, obtain a thorough history with particular attention to developmental milestones and behavioral interventions. This evaluation should also focus on anxiety. For example, in some children, fear of the dark may produce nocturnal enuresis, given that the child is afraid to get up from bed to go to the bathroom.
- In evaluating nocturnal enuresis, many clinicians use a calendar tracking method to record the frequency of these events; this is also helpful in establishing a baseline before beginning treatment
- Behavioral interventions (e.g., bell and pad conditioning) is effective and may have persistent effects after discontinuation, unlike pharmacological interventions wherein enuresis will typically recur when the medication is stopped

SUGGESTED READING

Dossche L, Michelet R, de Bruyne P et al. Desmopressin oral lyophilisate in young children: new insights in pharmacokinetics and pharmacodynamics. Arch Dis Childhood 2021;106(6):597–602.

Glazener CMA, Evans JHC. Desmopressin for nocturnal enuresis in children. Cochrane Database Syst Rev 2002;(3):CD002112. Doi:10.1002/14651858.CD002112.

Keten T, Aslan Y, Balci M et al. Comparison of the efficacy of desmopressin fast-melting formulation and enuretic alarm in the treatment of monosymptomatic nocturnal enuresis. J Pediatr Urol 2020;16(5):645.e1–645e7.

Michelet R, Dossche L, van Herzeele et al. An integrated paediatric population PK/PD analysis of dDAVP: how do PK differences translate to clinical outcomes? Clin Pharmacokinet 2020;59(1):81–96.

Strawn JR, Stahl SM. Case Studies in Psychopharmacology: Children & Adolescents. New York: Cambridge University Press, 2023.

THERAPEUTICS

Brands

- Pristiq

Generic

Yes

US FDA Approved for Pediatric Use

- None

Off-Label for Pediatric Use

- Approved in adults
  - Major depressive disorder
- Other off-label uses
  - Generalized anxiety disorder (GAD)
  - Social anxiety disorder
  - Panic disorder
  - Separation anxiety disorder
  - Premenstrual dysphoric disorder (PMDD)
  - Posttraumatic stress disorder (PTSD)

Class and Mechanism of Action

- Neuroscience-based Nomenclature: serotonin norepinephrine reuptake inhibitor (SN-RI)
- SNRI (dual serotonin and norepinephrine reuptake inhibitor); often classified as a drug for depression (i.e., antidepressant), but it is not just an antidepressant
- Desvenlafaxine presumably increases serotonergic neurotransmission by blocking the serotonin reuptake pump (transporter, SERT), which results in the desensitization of serotonin receptors, especially serotonin 1A receptors
- Desvenlafaxine presumably increases noradrenergic neurotransmission by blocking the norepinephrine reuptake pump (transporter, NET), which results in the desensitization of beta adrenergic receptors
- Since dopamine is inactivated by norepinephrine reuptake in the frontal cortex, which largely lacks dopamine transporters, desvenlafaxine can increase dopamine neurotransmission in this part of the brain
- Desvenlafaxine weakly blocks the dopamine reuptake pump (dopamine transporter) and may increase dopamine neurotransmission

SAFETY AND TOLERABILITY

Notable Side Effects

- Most side effects increase with higher doses, at least transiently
- Mostly central nervous system side effects (insomnia but also sedation, especially if not sleeping at night; agitation, tremors, headache, dizziness)
- Note: patients with diagnosed or undiagnosed bipolar or psychotic disorders may be more vulnerable to CNS-activating actions of antidepressants like desvenlafaxine; pay particular attention to signs of activation in children with developmental disorders or autism spectrum disorders
- Treatment-emergent activation syndrome (TEAS) includes agitation, anxiety, panic attacks, irritability, aggression, impulsivity, and insomnia; however, in pediatric patients, this is less with SNRIs compared to SSRIs (Mills and Strawn, 2020)
- TEAS can represent side effects but should not be confused with bipolar mania or the onset of suicidality and should be monitored and investigated with consideration of discontinuing or decreasing the dose of desvenlafaxine or addition of another agent or switching to another agent to reduce these symptoms
- Gastrointestinal (decreased appetite, nausea, diarrhea, constipation, dry mouth)
- Sexual dysfunction (boys: delayed ejaculation, erectile dysfunction; boys and girls: decreased sexual desire, anorgasmia)
- Autonomic (sweating)
- Syndrome of inappropriate antidiuretic hormone secretion (SIADH)

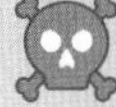

Life-Threatening or Dangerous Side Effects

- Rare seizures
- Rare hyponatremia
- Rare induction of mania
- Rare suicidal ideation and behavior (suicidality) (short-term regulatory studies did not show any actual suicides in any age group and also did not show an increase in the risk of suicidality with antidepressants compared to placebo beyond age 24)

Growth and Maturation

- Limited data suggest less than expected weight gain and less than expected height increases in children and adolescents taking desvenlafaxine; the differences between observed and expected growth rates were greater for children than for adolescents

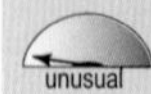

Weight Gain

- Limited data suggest weight loss in children and adolescents taking desvenlafaxine

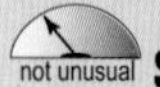

Sedation

- Occurs in significant minority

What to Do About Side Effects

- Wait, wait, wait: mild side effects are common, happen early, and usually improve with time, but treatment benefits can be delayed and often begin just as the side effects wear off
- Monitor side effects closely, especially when initiating treatment
- For activation (jitteriness, anxiety, insomnia):
  - Administer dose in the morning
  - Consider a temporary dose reduction or a more gradual up-titration
  - Consider switching to another antidepressant
  - Optimize psychotherapeutic interventions
  - Activation and agitation may represent the induction of a bipolar state, especially a mixed dysphoric bipolar II condition sometimes associated with suicidal ideation, and may require the addition of lithium or an atypical antipsychotic and/or discontinuation of desvenlafaxine
- Often best to try another monotherapy prior to resorting to augmentation strategies to treat side effects
- For insomnia: consider adding melatonin
- For GI upset: try giving medication with a meal
- For sexual dysfunction:
  - Probably best to reduce dose or discontinue and try another agent
  - Consider adding daytime exercise, bupropion, or buspirone
- For emotional flattening, apathy: consider adding bupropion (with caution, as little experience in children)

How Drug Causes Side Effects

- Theoretically due to increases in serotonin and norepinephrine concentrations at receptors in parts of the brain and body other than those that cause therapeutic actions (e.g., unwanted actions of serotonin in sleep centers causing insomnia, unwanted actions of norepinephrine on acetylcholine release causing constipation and dry mouth)

Warnings and Precautions

- Consider distributing the brochures provided by the FDA and the drug companies as well as the medication guides from the American Academy of Child & Adolescent Psychiatry (AACAP)
- Carefully consider monitoring patients regularly and within the practical limits, particularly during the first several weeks of treatment
- Warn patients and their caregivers when possible about the possibility of activating side effects and advise them to report such symptoms immediately
- Carefully weigh the risks and benefits of pharmacological treatment against the risks and benefits of nontreatment with antidepressants and it is a good idea to document this in the patient's chart
- Use with caution in patients with heart disease
- As with any antidepressant, use with caution in patients with history of seizure
- As with any antidepressant, use with caution in patients with bipolar disorder unless treated with concomitant mood-stabilizing agent
- Monitor patients for activation and suicidal ideation and involve parents/guardians

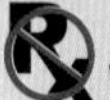

When Not to Prescribe

- If patient is taking an MAO inhibitor
- If patient has uncontrolled angle-closure glaucoma
- If there is a proven allergy to venlafaxine or desvenlafaxine

Long-Term Use

- Growth should be monitored; long-term effects are unknown
- Regularly monitor blood pressure

Habit Forming

- No

Overdose

- No fatalities have been reported as monotherapy; headache, vomiting, agitation, dizziness, nausea, constipation, diarrhea, dry mouth, paresthesia, tachycardia
- Desvenlafaxine is the active metabolite of venlafaxine; fatal toxicity index data from the UK suggest a higher rate of deaths from overdose with venlafaxine than with SSRIs; it is unknown whether this is related to differences in patients who receive venlafaxine or to potential cardiovascular toxicity of venlafaxine

DOSING AND USE

Usual Dosage Range

In adults: the usual dose is 50 mg once daily for depression

Dosage Forms

- Tablet (extended-release) 25 mg, 50 mg, 100 mg

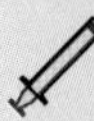

How to Dose

- In children: initial dose 25 mg once daily; maximum recommended dose generally 100 mg once daily
- In adolescents: initial dose 50 mg once daily; maximum recommended dose generally 100 mg once daily
- In adults: initial dose 50 mg once daily; maximum recommended dose generally 100 mg once daily; doses up to 400 mg once daily have been shown to be effective but higher doses are associated with increased side effects

Options for Administration

- Do not cut or crush extended-release capsules

Tests

- Check blood pressure before initiating treatment and regularly during treatment
- Monitor weight and height against that expected for normal growth

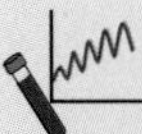

Pharmacokinetics

- Compared to other antidepressants, desvenlafaxine has low protein binding (30%)
- Desvenlafaxine absorption from the gastrointestinal tract is lower in children and adolescents than in adults
- The time to maximum concentration is approximately 5 hours in children ages 7–11 years and 8–9 hours in adolescents ages 12–17 years (Figure 1)
- The half-life of venlafaxine is approximately 8–12 hours in both children and adolescents

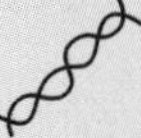

Pharmacogenetics

- No recommendations

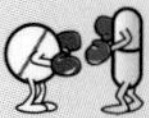

Drug Interactions

- Tramadol reported to increase the risk of seizures in adults taking an antidepressant
- Can cause a fatal "serotonin syndrome" when combined with MAO inhibitors, so do not use with MAO inhibitors or for at least 14 days after MAOIs are stopped
- Do not start an MAO inhibitor for at least 5 half-lives (5 to 7 days for most drugs) after discontinuing desvenlafaxine
- Few known adverse drug interactions
- False-positive urine immunoassay screening tests for phencyclidine (PCP) and amphetamine have been reported in patients taking desvenlafaxine, due to a lack of specificity of the screening tests. False-positive test results may be expected for several days following discontinuation of desvenlafaxine

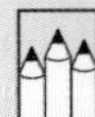

Dosing Tips

- Desvenlafaxine is the active metabolite (O-desmethylvenlafaxine) of venlafaxine, and is formed as the result of CYP2D6
- Has greater inhibition of NET relative to SERT compared to venlafaxine
- Do not break or chew desvenlafaxine XR tablets, as this will alter controlled-release properties
- The more anxious and agitated the patient, the lower the starting dose, the slower the titration

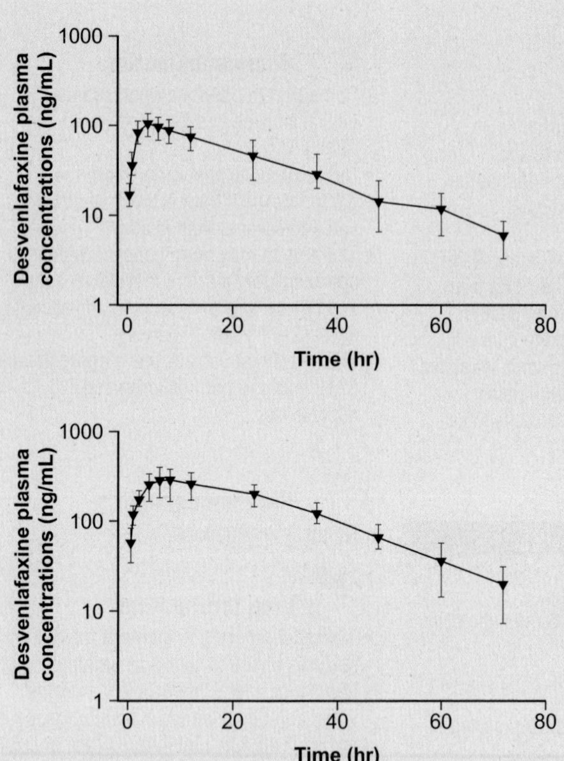

Figure 1 Concentration–time curves for desvenlafaxine (50 mg) in children (top) and adolescents (bottom).
Source: Desvenlafaxine Clinical Study Report (4206315), www.fda.gov

- If intolerable anxiety, insomnia, agitation, akathisia, or activation occurs either upon dosing initiation or discontinuation, consider the possibility of activated bipolar disorder and switch to an atypical antipsychotic or a mood stabilizer
- These symptoms may also indicate the need to evaluate for a mixed features episode and thus discontinuing desvenlafaxine and considering an atypical antipsychotic or a mood stabilizer or lithium

How to Switch

- From another antidepressant to desvenlafaxine:
  - When tapering a prior antidepressant, see its entry in this manual for how to stop and how to taper off that specific drug
  - In situations when there are antidepressant-related side effects, try to stop the first agent before starting desvenlafaxine so that new side effects of desvenlafaxine can be distinguished from withdrawal effects of the first agent

- If urgent, cross taper
- Off desvenlafaxine to another antidepressant:
  - Generally, try to stop desvenlafaxine before starting another antidepressant
  - Taper to avoid withdrawal effects (dizziness, nausea, stomach cramps, sweating, tingling, dysesthesias)
  - Many patients tolerate 50% dose reduction for 5–7 days, then another 50% reduction for 5–7 days, then discontinuation
  - If necessary, can cross taper off desvenlafaxine this way while dosing up on another antidepressant simultaneously in urgent situations, being aware of all specific drug interactions to avoid

How to Stop

- Withdrawal effects can be more common or more severe with desvenlafaxine than with some other antidepressants
- Taper to avoid withdrawal effects (dizziness, nausea, stomach cramps, sweating, tingling, dysesthesias)
- Many patients tolerate 50% dose reduction for 5–7 days, then another 50% reduction for 5–7 days, then discontinuation
- If withdrawal symptoms emerge during discontinuation, raise dose to stop symptoms and then restart withdrawal much more slowly
- For some patients with severe problems discontinuing desvenlafaxine, it may be useful to add an SSRI with a long half-life, especially fluoxetine, prior to taper of desvenlafaxine; while maintaining fluoxetine dosing, first slowly taper desvenlafaxine and then taper fluoxetine
- Be sure to differentiate between reemergence of symptoms requiring reinstitution of treatment and withdrawal symptoms

WHAT TO EXPECT

Onset of Action

- Some patients may experience increased energy or activation early after initiation of treatment
- Full onset of therapeutic actions is usually delayed by 2–4 weeks
- If it is not working within 6–8 weeks, it may require a dosage increase or it may not work at all

Duration of Action

- Effects are consistent over a 24-hour period
- May continue to work for many years to prevent relapse of symptoms

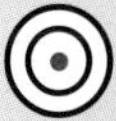

Primary Target Symptoms

- Depressed and/or irritable mood
- Energy, motivation, and interest
- Sleep disturbance
- Anxiety (fear and worry are often target symptoms, but desvenlafaxine can occasionally and transiently increase these symptoms short term before improving them)
- Prior to initiation of treatment, it is helpful to develop a list of target symptoms of depression and/or anxiety to monitor during treatment to better assess treatment response

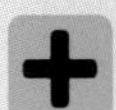

What Is Considered a Positive Result?

- The goal of treatment is complete remission of current symptoms as well as prevention of future relapses
- In practice, many patients have only a partial response where some symptoms are improved but others persist (especially insomnia, fatigue, and problems concentrating in depression), in which case higher doses of desvenlafaxine, adding a second agent, or switching to an agent with a different mechanism of action can be considered
- If treatment works, it most often reduces or even eliminates symptoms, but is not a cure since symptoms can recur after medicine is stopped

How Long to Treat

- For adolescents with depression, generally, 9–12 months of antidepressant treatment is recommended (Hathaway et al., 2018)
- For anxiety disorders, 6–9 months of antidepressant treatment may be sufficient, though many clinicians extend treatment to 12 months based on extrapolation of data from adults with anxiety disorders (Hathaway et al., 2018; Strawn et al., 2021)

- Extended treatment periods may decrease the risk of long-term morbidity and recurrence; however, the goal of treatment is ultimately remission rather than duration of antidepressant pharmacotherapy (Hathaway et al., 2018)
- In terms of the length of antidepressant treatment, evidence-based guidelines represent a starting point; appropriate treatment duration varies, and patient-specific response, psychological factors, and timing of discontinuation must be considered for individual pediatric patients (Hathaway et al., 2018)

What If It Stops Working?

- Some patients who have an initial response may relapse even though they continue treatment, sometimes called "poop-out"
- Some patients may experience apparent lack of consistent efficacy due to activation syndrome or latent or underlying or newly evolved bipolar disorder, or major depressive episodes with mixed features of mania, and require antidepressant discontinuation and a switch to a second generation antipsychotic

What If It Doesn't Work?

- Consider evaluation for another diagnosis (especially bipolar illness or depression with mixed features) or for a comorbid condition (e.g., medical illness, substance abuse)
- Be mindful of family conflict contributing to the presentation; sometimes treating parental depression or anxiety disorders improves psychiatric and social function without any treatment of youth. Also, accommodation is common in families of youth with anxiety disorders and may need to be addressed specifically, as it can perpetuate symptoms.
- Consider factors associated with poor response to antidepressants in treatment-resistant depression (Dwyer et al., 2020) or anxiety disorders (Strawn et al., 2023), such as severe symptoms, long-lasting symptoms, poor treatment adherence, prior nonresponse to other treatments, and the presence of comorbid disorders
- Consider other important potential factors such as ongoing conflicts, family psychopathology, and an adverse environment (e.g., poverty, chaos, violence, prior and ongoing psychological trauma, abuse, neglect). Additionally, when symptoms are prominent at school, consider the presence of a learning disorder.
- Institute trauma-informed care for appropriate children and adolescents
- A 2007 meta-analysis of published and unpublished trials in pediatric patients found that antidepressants had a number needed to treat (NNT) of 10 for depression, 6 for OCD, and 3 for anxiety disorders; thus, desvenlafaxine may not work in all children, so consider switching to another antidepressant (Bridge et al., 2007)
- Consider a dose adjustment
- Consider augmenting options:
  - Cognitive behavioral therapy (CBT), interpersonal psychotherapy for adolescents (IPT-A), light therapy, family therapy, and exercise, especially in adolescents
  - For partial response (depression): use caution when adding medications to desvenlafaxine, especially in children since there are not sufficient studies of augmentation in children or adolescents; however, for the expert, consider bupropion, aripiprazole, or other atypical antipsychotics such as quetiapine; use combinations of antidepressants with caution, as this may activate bipolar disorder and suicidal ideation
  - For insomnia: sleep hygiene, CBT for insomnia, melatonin, or alpha 2 agonists
  - For anxiety: buspirone, antihistamines
  - Add lithium or atypical antipsychotics for bipolar depression, psychotic depression, treatment-resistant depression, or treatment-resistant anxiety disorders
  - TMS (transcranial magnetic stimulation) may have a role, although pediatric trials of TMS have been hampered by high sham response rates (Croarkin et al., 2021)
  - ECT (case studies show effectiveness; cognitive side effects are similar to those in adults; reserve for treatment-resistant cases)

TALKING TO PATIENTS AND CAREGIVERS

What to Tell Parents About Efficacy

- Doesn't work right away; full therapeutic benefits may take up to 8 weeks, yet parents and teachers might see improvement before the patient does
- While the medicine helps by reducing symptoms and improving function, it is not a cure, and it is therefore necessary to keep taking the medication to sustain its therapeutic effects
- Since every treatment consideration depends on a risk/benefit analysis, parents should fully understand short- and long-term risks as well as benefits
- After successful treatment, continuation of desvenlafaxine may be necessary to prevent relapse, especially in those who have had more than one episode or a very severe episode. In general, when treating depression in children and adolescents, medications are continued for 12 months after symptoms have resolved, while for anxiety disorders, clinicians have generally treated for 6–9 months (Hathaway et al., 2018).
- Often a good idea to tell parents whether the medication chosen is specifically approved for the disorder being treated, or whether it is being given for "unapproved" or "off-label" reasons based on good clinical practice, expert consensus, and/or prudent extrapolation of controlled data from adults

What to Tell Children and Adolescents About Efficacy

- We are trying to make you feel better
- It may be a good idea to give the medication a try; if it's not working very well, we can stop the medication and try something else
- A good try takes 2 to 3 months or even longer
- If it does make you feel better, you cannot stop it right away or you may feel sad or worried again
- Medications don't change who you are as a person; they give you the opportunity to be the best person you can be

What to Tell Parents About Side Effects

- Explain that side effects are expected in many when starting and are most common in the first 2–3 weeks of starting or increasing the dose
- Tell parents many side effects go away and do so about the same time that therapeutic effects start
- Predict side effects in advance (you will look clever and competent to the parents, unless you scare them with too much information and cause nocebo effects, in which case you won't look so clever when the patient develops lots of side effects and stops medication; use your judgment here); a balanced but honest presentation is an art rather than a science
- Ask them to help monitor for increased suicidality and if present, report any such symptoms immediately
- Ask parents to support the patient while side effects are occurring
- Parents should fully understand short- and long-term risks as well as benefits
- Explaining to the parents what to expect from medication treatment, and especially potential side effects, can help prevent early termination of medication

What to Tell Children and Adolescents About Side Effects

- Even if you get side effects, most of them get better or go away in a few days to a few weeks
- Consider having a conversation about sexual side effects in some adolescents who can find these side effects confusing and especially burdensome
- Explaining to child/adolescent what to expect from medication treatment, and especially potential side effects, can help prevent early termination of medication
- Tell adolescents and children capable of understanding that some young patients, especially those who are depressed, may develop thoughts of hurting themselves, and if this happens, not to be alarmed but to tell their parents right away

What to Tell Teachers About the Medication (If Parents Consent)

- Desvenlafaxine can make children/adolescents jittery or restless

- If the patient is sleepy, ask whether the medication is keeping them up at night
- It is not abusable
- Encourage dialogue with parents/guardians about any behavior or mood changes

SPECIAL POPULATIONS

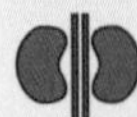

Renal Impairment

- For moderate impairment, recommended dose in adults is 50 mg/day
- For severe impairment, recommended dose in adults is 50 mg every other day
- Patients on dialysis should not receive subsequent dose until dialysis is completed

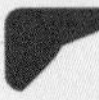

Hepatic Impairment

- In adults, doses greater than 100 mg/day not recommended

Cardiac Impairment

- Drug should be used with caution
- Hypertension should be controlled prior to initiation of desvenlafaxine and should be monitored regularly during treatment. In children and adolescents, desvenlafaxine is associated with increases in heart rate, although increases in blood pressure were not consistently observed in these studies.
- Desvenlafaxine is the active metabolite of venlafaxine, which is contraindicated in patients with heart disease in the UK
- Venlafaxine can block cardiac ion channels in vitro

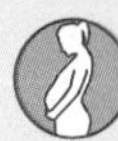

Pregnancy

- Controlled studies have not been conducted in pregnant women
- Not generally recommended for use during pregnancy, especially during first trimester
- Nonetheless, continuous treatment during pregnancy may be necessary and has not been proven to be harmful to the fetus
- Must weigh the risk of treatment (first trimester fetal development, third trimester newborn delivery) to the child against the risk of no treatment (recurrence of depression, maternal health, infant bonding) to the mother and child
- For many patients this may mean continuing treatment during pregnancy
- Neonates exposed to SSRIs or SNRIs late in the third trimester have developed complications requiring prolonged hospitalization, respiratory support, and tube feeding; reported symptoms are consistent with either a direct toxic effect of SSRIs and SNRIs or, possibly, a drug discontinuation syndrome, and include respiratory distress, cyanosis, apnea, seizures, temperature instability, feeding difficulty, vomiting, hypoglycemia, hypotonia, hypertonia, hyperreflexia, tremor, jitteriness, irritability, and constant crying

Breast Feeding

- Some drug is found in breast milk
- Trace amounts may be present in nursing children whose mothers are on desvenlafaxine
- If child becomes irritable or sedated, breast feeding or drug may need to be discontinued
- Immediate postpartum period is a high-risk time for depression, especially in women who have had prior depressive episodes, so drug may need to be reinstituted late in the third trimester or shortly after childbirth to prevent a recurrence during the postpartum period
- Must weigh benefits of breast feeding with risks and benefits of antidepressant treatment versus nontreatment to both the infant and the mother
- For many patients, this may mean continuing treatment during breast feeding

THE ART OF PSYCHOPHARMACOLOGY

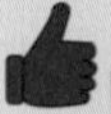

Potential Advantages

- In children and adolescents:
  - May be helpful in treatment-resistant depression or anxiety disorders; however, it should be used cautiously in patients who have higher suicidality prior to treatment, as these patients are at greater risk for suicide attempts when treated with venlafaxine (the parent drug of desvenlafaxine) (Brent et al., 2009)
- All ages:
  - Patients with atypical depression (hypersomnia, increased appetite)

- Depressed patients with somatic symptoms, fatigue, and pain
- Patients who do not respond or remit on treatment with SSRIs; however, data from the Treatment of SSRI-Resistant Depression in Adolescents (TORDIA) Study (Brent et al., 2008) suggest that patients who have not responded to an initial SSRI should receive a trial of a second SSRI before pursuing a trial of an SNRI (Suresh et al., 2020)

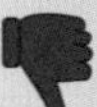

Potential Disadvantages

- In children:
  - Those who are already psychomotor agitated, angry, or irritable, and who do not have a psychiatric diagnosis
  - Randomized controlled trials of children with MDD have failed to show benefit of desvenlafaxine compared to placebo
- In adolescents:
  - Those who may possibly have a mood disorder with mixed or bipolar features, especially those with these features and a family history of bipolar disorder
  - Randomized controlled trials of children with MDD have failed to show benefit of desvenlafaxine compared to placebo
  - In meta-analyses of adolescents with anxiety disorders (Strawn et al., 2018) and SSRI-resistant depression (Suresh et al., 2020), SSRIs produce larger and faster improvement compared to SNRIs
- All ages:
  - Patients who may already have weight loss related to their depression
  - Patients with cardiac disease

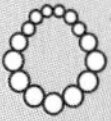

Pearls

- SNRIs appear less effective than SSRIs in reducing depressive and anxiety symptoms in youth (Strawn et al., 2018; Suresh et al., 2020)
- Many SSRIs and SNRIs have an even smaller effect and sometimes no effect in controlled clinical trials of child and adolescent depression
- Venlafaxine (the parent drug of desvenlafaxine) has been associated with more treatment-emergent suicidality in adolescents compared to other SNRIs or SSRIs in multiple studies and meta-analyses (Brent et al., 2009; Dobson et al., 2019)
- Because desvenlafaxine is only minimally metabolized by CYP3A4 and is not metabolized at all by CYP2D6, as venlafaxine is, it may have more consistent plasma levels than venlafaxine
- In addition, although desvenlafaxine, like venlafaxine, is more potent at the serotonin transporter (SERT) than the norepinephrine transporter (NET), it has relatively greater actions on NET versus SERT than venlafaxine does at comparable doses
- Blood pressure increases and heart rate increases have been observed with venlafaxine in pediatric populations and may be more common in patients treated with higher doses
- More withdrawal reactions reported upon discontinuation than for some other antidepressants

SUGGESTED READING

Atkinson S, Lubaczewski S, Ramaker S et al. Desvenlafaxine versus placebo in the treatment of children and adolescents with major depressive disorder. J Child Adolesc Psychopharmacol 2018;28(1):55–65.

Bousman CA, Stevenson JM, Ramsey LB et al. Clinical Pharmacogenetics Implementation Consortium (CPIC) guideline for CYP2D6, CYP2C19, CYP2B6, SLC6A4, and HTR2A genotypes and serotonin reuptake inhibitor antidepressants. Clin Pharmacol Ther 2023;114(1):51–68.

Brent D, Emslie G, Clarke G et al. Switching to another SSRI or to venlafaxine with or without cognitive behavioral therapy for adolescents with SSRI-resistant depression: the TORDIA randomized controlled trial. JAMA 2008;299(8):901–13.

Brent DA, Emslie GJ, Clarke GN et al. Predictors of spontaneous and systematically assessed suicidal adverse events in the Treatment of SSRI-Resistant Depression in Adolescents (TORDIA) study. Am J Psychiatry 2009;166(4):418–26.

Bridge JA, Iyengar S, Salary CB et al. Clinical response and risk for reported suicidal ideation and suicide attempts in pediatric antidepressant treatment: a meta-analysis of randomized controlled trials. JAMA 2007;297(15):1683–96.

Croarkin PE, Elmaadawi AZ, Aaronson ST et al. Left prefrontal transcranial magnetic stimulation for treatment-resistant depression in adolescents: a double-blind, randomized, sham-controlled trial. Neuropsychopharmacology 2021;46(2):462–9.

Dobson ET, Bloch MH, Strawn JR. Efficacy and tolerability of pharmacotherapy for pediatric anxiety disorders: a network meta-analysis. J Clin Psychiatry 2019;80(1):17r12064.

Doroudgar S, Perry PJ, Lackey GD et al. An 11-year retrospective review of venlafaxine ingestion in children from the California Poison Control System. Hum Exp Toxicol 2016;35(7):767–74.

Dwyer JB, Stringaris A, Brent DA, Bloch MH. Annual Research Review: Defining and treating pediatric treatment-resistant depression. J Child Psychol Psychiatry 2020;61(3):312–32.

Emslie GJ, Findling RL, Yeung PP, Kunz NR, Li Y. Venlafaxine ER for the treatment of pediatric subjects with depression: results of two placebo-controlled trials. J Am Acad Child Adolesc Psychiatry 2007;46(4):479–88.

Findling RL, Groark J, Chiles D et al. Safety and tolerability of desvenlafaxine in children and adolescents with major depressive disorder. J Child Adolesc Psychopharmacol 2014;24(4):201–9.

Findling RL, Groark J, Tourian KA et al. Pharmacokinetics and tolerability of single-ascending doses of desvenlafaxine administered to children and adolescents with major depressive disorder. J Child Adolesc Psychopharmacol 2016;26(10):909–21.

Hathaway EE, Walkup JT, Strawn JR. Antidepressant treatment duration in pediatric depressive and anxiety disorders: how long is long enough? Curr Probl Pediatr Adolesc Health Care 2018;48(2):31–9.

Mills JA, Strawn JR. Antidepressant tolerability in pediatric anxiety and obsessive-compulsive disorders: a Bayesian hierarchical modeling meta-analysis. J Am Acad Child Adolesc Psychiatry 2020;59(11):1240–51.

Rynn MA, Riddle MA, Yeung PP, Kunz NR. Efficacy and safety of extended-release venlafaxine in the treatment of generalized anxiety disorder in children and adolescents: two placebo-controlled trials. Am J Psychiatry 2007;164(2):290–300.

Sangkuhl K, Stingl JC, Turpeinen M, Altman RB, Klein TE. PharmGKB summary: venlafaxine pathway. Pharmacogenet Genomics 2014;24(1):62–72.

Strawn JR, Lu L, Peris TS, Levine A, Walkup JT. Research review: pediatric anxiety disorders – what have we learnt in the last 10 years? J Child Psychol Psychiatry 2021 Feb;62(2):114–39.

Strawn JR, Mills JA, Sauley BA, Welge JA. The impact of antidepressant dose and class on treatment response in pediatric anxiety disorders: a meta-analysis. J Am Acad Child Adolesc Psychiatry 2018;57(4):235–44.e2

Strawn JR, Mills JA, Poweleit EA, Ramsey LB, Croarkin PE. Adverse effects of antidepressant medications and their management in children and adolescents. Pharmacotherapy 2023;43(7):675–90.

Suresh V, Mills JA, Croarkin PE, Strawn JR. What next? A Bayesian hierarchical modeling re-examination of treatments for adolescents with selective serotonin reuptake inhibitor-resistant depression. Depress Anxiety 2020;37(9):926–34.

Weihs KL, Murphy W, Abbas R, et al. Desvenlafaxine versus placebo in a fluoxetine-referenced study of children and adolescents with major depressive disorder. J Child Adolesc Psychopharmacol 2018;28(1):36–46.

THERAPEUTICS

Brands
- Diastat
- Valium

Generic
Yes

US FDA Approved for Pediatric Use
- Status epilepticus (injection; age 30 days and older)

Off-Label for Pediatric Use
- Approved in adults
  - Anxiety disorder
  - Symptoms of anxiety (short term)
  - Acute agitation, tremor, impending or acute delirium tremens and hallucinosis in acute alcohol withdrawal
  - Skeletal muscle spasm due to reflex spasm to local pathology
  - Spasticity caused by upper motor neuron disorder
  - Athetosis
  - Stiffman syndrome
  - Convulsive disorder (adjunctive)
  - Anxiety during endoscopic procedures (adjunctive) (injection only)
  - Preoperative anxiety (injection only)
  - Anxiety relief prior to cardioversion (intravenous)
- Other off-label uses
  - Insomnia
  - Catatonia

Class and Mechanism of Action
- Neuroscience-based Nomenclature: GABA positive allosteric modulator (GABA-PAM)
- Benzodiazepine (anxiolytic, muscle relaxant, anticonvulsant)
- As positive allosteric modulators of GABA A receptors, benzodiazepines (in the presence of GABA) increase the frequency of opening of the inhibitory chloride channels (although it does not increase the conductance of chloride across the individual channels or the time that the channel is open). This enhances the inhibitory effects of GABA.
- Inhibits neuronal activity presumably in amygdala-centered fear circuits to provide therapeutic benefits in anxiety disorders
- Inhibiting actions in the cerebral cortex may provide therapeutic benefits in seizure disorders
- Inhibitory actions in spinal cord may provide therapeutic benefits for muscle spasms

SAFETY AND TOLERABILITY

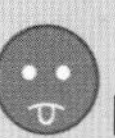

Notable Side Effects
- Sedation, fatigue, depression
- Dizziness, ataxia, slurred speech, weakness
- Forgetfulness, confusion
- Agitation and irritability
- Sialorrhea, dry mouth
- Rare hallucinations, mania
- Rare hypotension
- Pain at injection site

Life-Threatening or Dangerous Side Effects
- Respiratory depression, especially when taken with CNS depressants in overdose
- Rare hepatic dysfunction, renal dysfunction, blood dyscrasias

Growth and Maturation
- Not studied

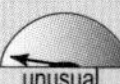

Weight Gain
- Reported but not expected

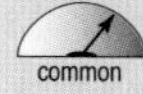

Sedation
- Many experience and/or can be significant in amount
- Especially at initiation of treatment or when dose increases
- Tolerance often develops over time

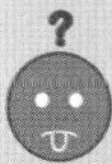

What to Do About Side Effects
- Wait
- Wait
- Wait
- Lower the dose
- Take largest dose at bedtime to avoid sedative effects during the day
- Switch to another agent
- Administer flumazenil if side effects are severe or life threatening

How Drug Causes Side Effects

- Same mechanism for side effects as for therapeutic effects – namely due to excessive actions at benzodiazepine receptors
- Long-term adaptations in benzodiazepine receptors may explain the development of dependence, tolerance, and withdrawal
- Side effects are generally immediate, but immediate side effects often disappear in time

Warnings and Precautions

- Boxed warning regarding the increased risk of CNS depressant effects when benzodiazepines and opioid medications are used together, including specifically the risk of slowed or difficulty breathing and death
- If alternatives to the combined use of benzodiazepines and opioids are not available, clinicians should limit the dosage and duration of each drug to the minimum possible while still achieving therapeutic efficacy
- Patients and their caregivers should be warned to seek medical attention if unusual dizziness, lightheadedness, sedation, slowed or difficulty breathing, or unresponsiveness occurs
- Dosage changes should be made in collaboration with prescriber
- Use with caution in patients with pulmonary disease; rare reports of death after initiation of benzodiazepines in patients with severe pulmonary impairment
- History of drug or alcohol abuse often creates greater risk for dependency
- Some depressed patients may experience a worsening of suicidal ideation
- Some patients may exhibit abnormal thinking or behavioral changes similar to those caused by other CNS depressants (i.e., either depressant actions or disinhibiting actions)

When Not to Prescribe

- In patients under 6 months of age (rectal gel formulation is not intended for use in children under age 2)
- If patient has myasthenia gravis, severe respiratory insufficiency, severe hepatic insufficiency, or sleep apnea syndrome
- If patient has angle-closure glaucoma
- If there is a proven allergy to diazepam or any benzodiazepine

Long-Term Use

- Evidence of efficacy up to 16 weeks
- Risk of dependence, particularly for treatment periods longer than 12 weeks and especially in patients with past or current polysubstance abuse
- Not recommended for long-term treatment of seizure disorders

Habit Forming

- Diazepam is a Schedule IV drug
- Patients may develop dependence and/or tolerance with long-term use

Overdose

- Fatalities can occur; hypotension, tiredness, ataxia, confusion, coma

DOSING AND USE

Usual Dosage Range

- Oral: initial 1–2.5 mg, 3–4 times/day; increase gradually as needed
- Intravenous: 0.25 mg/kg every 3 minutes

Dosage Forms

- Tablet 2 mg, 5 mg, 10 mg
- Nasal 5 mg/spray, 7.5 mg/spray, 10 mg/spray
- Concentrate 5 mg/mL
- Solution 5 mg/5 mL
- Injection 10 mg/2 mL, 50 mg/10 mL
- Rectal gel 2.5 mg/0.5 mL, 10 mg/2 mL, 20 mg/4 mL

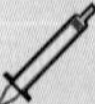

How to Dose

- Oral (anxiety, muscle spasm, seizure): initial 1–2.5 mg, 3–4 times/day; increase gradually as needed
- Liquid formulation should be mixed with water or fruit juice, applesauce, or pudding
- Because of risk of respiratory depression, rectal diazepam treatment should not be given more than once in 5 days or more than twice during a treatment course. Recently, intranasal diazepam has been preferred for acute repetitive seizures, as it has less pharmacokinetic variability and reliable bioavailability compared with the diazepam rectal gel.

Options for Administration

- Available in a liquid formulation and as a nasal spray

Tests

- In patients with seizure disorders, concomitant medical illness, and/or those with multiple concomitant long-term medications, periodic liver tests and blood counts may be prudent

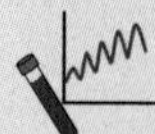

Pharmacokinetics

- Diazepam is well absorbed after oral administration, although the rate and extent of absorption can vary among individuals. For oral use, bioavailability is high but varies by other routes of administration.
- Following oral ingestion, peak plasma concentrations are typically reached within 30–90 min, but this varies by route of administration (see accompanying table)

Route	Peak plasma levels (min)	Bioavailability
Oral	30–90	94%
Intramuscular	30–60	60–90%
Rectal	10–45	80–90%
Intranasal	>60	97%

- Food intake may delay the absorption of diazepam
- Diazepam is extensively distributed throughout the body, including the CNS, is highly lipophilic and has a large volume of distribution
- Diazepam is extensively bound to plasma proteins, primarily albumin
- In children ages 3–8, the mean half-life is 18 hours
- Diazepam is *N*-demethylated by CYP3A4 and CYP2C19 to the active metabolite *N*-desmethyldiazepam (also known as nordiazepine), and is hydroxylated by CYP3A4 to the active metabolite temazepam (Figure 1)

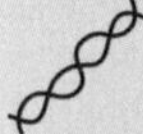

Pharmacogenetics

- No recommendations. However; the FDA notes that variation in CYP2C19 may affect diazepam exposure, and PharmGKB notes that patients with decreased CYP2C19 metabolism have decreased metabolism of diazepam as compared to patients carrying two normal function alleles.

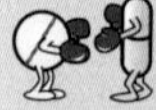

Drug Interactions

- Increased depressive effects when taken with other CNS depressants
- Cimetidine, ketoconazole, fluvoxamine, fluoxetine, omeprazole, and grapefruit

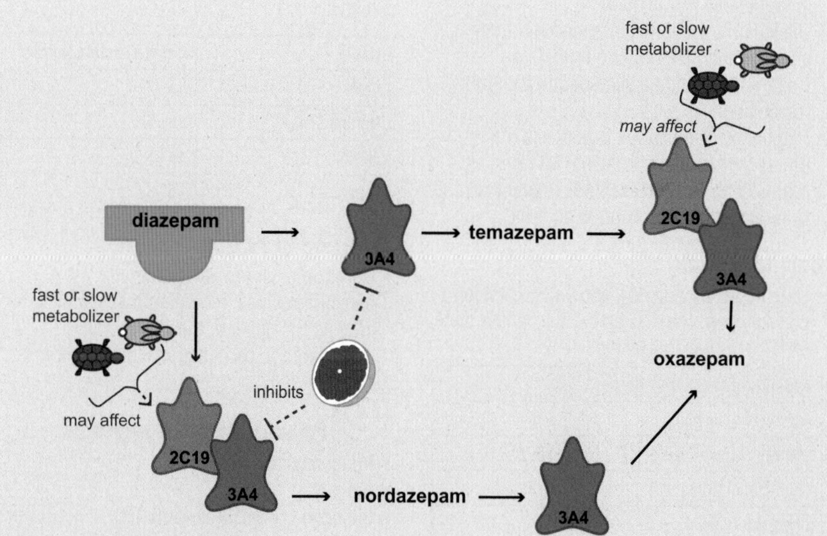

Figure 1 Diazepam metabolism.

juice may reduce the clearance and raise the levels of diazepam, which may lead to increased sedation
- The FDA notes that "inducers of CYP2C19 and CYP3A4 could increase the rate of elimination of diazepam"
- Flumazenil (used to reverse the effects of benzodiazepines) may precipitate seizures and should not be used in patients treated for seizure disorders with diazepam

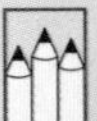

Dosing Tips

- For anxiety disorders, use lowest possible effective dose for the shortest possible period of time (a benzodiazepine-sparing strategy). In adolescents, these medications may be administered prior to some anxiety-producing situations and can help to facilitate returning to school in patients with school refusal.
- Assess need for continuous treatment regularly
- Risk of dependence may increase with dose and duration of treatment and with more lipophilic benzodiazepines (e.g., alprazolam)
- For interdose symptoms of anxiety, can either increase dose or maintain same daily dose but divide into more frequent doses
- Only benzodiazepine with a formulation specifically for rectal administration
- One of the few benzodiazepines available in an oral liquid formulation
- One of the few benzodiazepines available in an injectable formulation
- Diazepam injection is intended for acute use; patients who require long-term treatment should be switched to the oral formulation
- Frequency of dosing in practice is often different than predicted from half-life, as duration for benzodiazepines is often related to redistribution (Stimpfl et al., 2023)

How to Switch

- Use the accompanying equivalence table to convert from the diazepam dose to the dose of the new benzodiazepine

Approximate equivalent dosage (mg)	
Alprazolam (Xanax)	0.5
Chlordiazepoxide (Librium)	25
Clonazepam (Klonopin)	0.25–0.5
Diazepam (Valium)	5
Lorazepam (Ativan)	1

How to Stop

- Patients with history of seizure may seize upon withdrawal, especially if withdrawal is abrupt
- Taper by 2 mg every 5–7 days to reduce chances of withdrawal effects
- For difficult to taper cases, consider reducing dose much more slowly after reaching 20 mg/day, perhaps by as little as 0.5–1 mg every week or less
- Be sure to differentiate the reemergence of symptoms requiring reinstitution of treatment from withdrawal symptoms
- Benzodiazepine-dependent anxiety patients and insulin-dependent diabetics are not addicted to their medications. When benzodiazepine-dependent patients stop their medication, disease symptoms can reemerge, disease symptoms can worsen (rebound), and/or withdrawal symptoms can emerge.

WHAT TO EXPECT

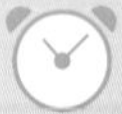

Onset of Action

- Some immediate relief with first dosing is common; however, onset of action varies by route of administration; it can take several weeks with daily dosing for maximal therapeutic benefit (see accompanying table)

Route	Onset of action (min)
Oral	15–60
Intramuscular	15–30
Rectal	5–10
Intranasal	<5

Duration of Action

- Duration of action varies for benzodiazepines, including diazepam, in pediatric patients but is generally considered to be between 8 and 10 hours

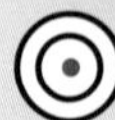

Primary Target Symptoms

- Panic attacks
- Anxiety
- Incidence of seizures (adjunct)
- Muscle spasms

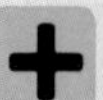

What Is Considered a Positive Result?

- The goal of treatment for anxiety is complete remission of current symptoms as well as prevention of future relapses
- If treatment works, it most often reduces or even eliminates symptoms, but is not a cure since symptoms can recur after medicine is stopped

How Long to Treat

- For short-term symptoms of anxiety or muscle spasms – after a few weeks, discontinue use or use on an "as-needed" basis
- For long-term symptoms of anxiety, consider switching to an SSRI or SNRI for long-term maintenance
- If long-term maintenance with a benzodiazepine is necessary, continue treatment for 6 months after symptoms resolve, and then taper dose slowly
- Chronic muscle spasms may require chronic diazepam treatment

What If It Stops Working?

- If anxiety symptoms reemerge, consider an SSRI, and re-trying psychotherapeutic approaches

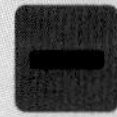

What If It Doesn't Work?

- Consider a trial of an SSRI
- When treating youth with anxiety disorders, many patients will have had significant anxiety for years prior to beginning treatment. As such, when anxiety is treated with diazepam, their symptoms may be improved, but the patient has likely missed important developmental milestones (e.g., spending the night with friends, being able to ask questions in class). Developing these skills will take time. Beyond this, the family may have lived with the anxious child for years and following treatment of the child, the family may need to readjust.
- Be mindful of family conflict contributing to the presentation; sometimes treating parental depression or anxiety disorders improves psychiatric and social function without any treatment of youth. Also, accommodation is common in families of youth with anxiety disorders and may need to be addressed specifically, as it can perpetuate symptoms.

TALKING TO PATIENTS AND CAREGIVERS

What to Tell Parents About Efficacy

- While the medicine helps by reducing symptoms and improving function, it is not a cure, and it is therefore necessary to keep taking the medication to sustain its therapeutic effects
- Since every treatment consideration depends on a risk/benefit analysis, parents should fully understand short- and long-term risks as well as benefits
- Often a good idea to tell parents whether the medication chosen is specifically approved for the disorder being treated, or whether it is being given for "unapproved" or "off-label" reasons based on good clinical practice, expert consensus, and/or prudent extrapolation of controlled data from adults

What to Tell Children and Adolescents About Efficacy

- We are trying to make you feel better
- It may be a good idea to give the medication a try; if it's not working very well, we can stop the medication and try something else
- Medications don't change who you are as a person; they give you the opportunity to be the best person you can be

What to Tell Parents About Side Effects

- Explain that mild side effects are expected at initiation or when increasing the dose and are usually transitory
- Predict side effects in advance (you will look clever and competent to the parents, unless you scare them with too much information and cause nocebo effects, in which case you won't look so clever when the patient develops lots of side effects and stops medication; use your judgment here); a balanced but honest presentation is an art rather than a science
- Ask parents to support the patient while side effects are occurring
- Parents should fully understand short- and long-term risks as well as benefits
- Explaining to the parents what to expect from medication treatment, and especially potential side effects, can help prevent early termination of medication

What to Tell Children and Adolescents About Side Effects

- Even if you get side effects, most of them get better or go away in a few days to a few weeks; however, we will likely not use this medication for a long time
- Explaining to child/adolescent what to expect from medication treatment, and especially potential side effects, can help prevent early termination of medication

What to Tell Teachers About the Medication (If Parents Consent)

- Diazepam can make children/adolescents sleepy and make it difficult for children or adolescents to pay attention. In these situations, it is important to notify the clinician so that the dose can be decreased.
- Diazepam may interfere with children's ability to engage in some activities at recess and in physical education class
- Encourage dialogue with parents/guardians about any behavior or mood changes

SPECIAL POPULATIONS

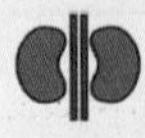

Renal Impairment

- Initial 2–2.5 mg, 1–2 times/day; increase gradually as needed

Hepatic Impairment

- Initial 2–2.5 mg, 1–2 times/day; increase gradually as needed

Cardiac Impairment

- No data available

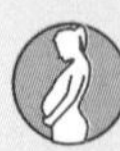

Pregnancy

- Possible increased risk of birth defects when benzodiazepines taken during pregnancy
- Because of the potential risks, diazepam is not generally recommended as treatment for anxiety during pregnancy, especially during the first trimester
- Drug should be tapered if discontinued
- Infants whose mothers received a benzodiazepine late in pregnancy may experience withdrawal effects
- Neonatal flaccidity has been reported in infants whose mothers took a benzodiazepine during pregnancy
- Seizures, even mild seizures, may cause harm to the embryo/fetus

Breast Feeding

- Some drug is found in breast milk
- Recommended either to discontinue drug or formula feed
- Effects on infant have been observed and include feeding difficulties, sedation, and weight loss

THE ART OF PSYCHOPHARMACOLOGY

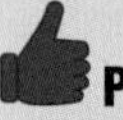

Potential Advantages

- Rapid onset of action
- Availability of oral liquid, rectal, intranasal, and injectable dosage formulations

Potential Disadvantages

- Abuse especially risky in past or present substance users
- Can be sedating at doses necessary to treat moderately severe anxiety disorders

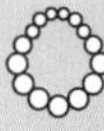

Pearls

- Despite trials of benzodiazepines in adults with anxiety disorders consistently demonstrating benefit, trials of benzodiazepines in pediatric patients have produced mixed results:
  - Small double-blind placebo-controlled trials and meta-analyses do not reveal differences between benzodiazepines and placebo for the management of anxiety disorders. However, these studies were small and included very young children and high doses of short-acting benzodiazepines (e.g., alprazolam).
  - By contrast, for acute anxiety in children and adolescents, a meta-analysis of nearly 1,500 patients suggests that benzodiazepines are more effective than placebo in treating acute anxiety; in this meta-analysis, there was no significant difference in the risk of developing irritability or behavioral changes between benzodiazepine and control groups (Kuang et al., 2017)

- In the pediatric benzodiazepine trials, the poor tolerability – particularly in younger patients – may relate to age-related pharmacodynamic factors (Strawn and Stahl, 2023)
- The pharmacodynamics of the GABA receptor in children and adolescents differ from adults, with adult expression/function not being achieved until ages 14–17½ years for subcortical regions and 18–22 years for cortical regions, although girls reach adult expression of GABA receptors slightly earlier than boys (Chugani et al., 2001)
- In adults with anxiety disorders, benzodiazepines may be a very useful adjunct to SSRIs and SNRIs in the treatment of numerous anxiety disorders; however, the evidence for this is limited in children and adolescents, and even in adults diazepam is not used as frequently as other benzodiazepines for this purpose
- Grapefruit significantly affects the pharmacokinetics of most benzodiazepines (and other medications that are metabolized by CYP3A4). In fact, grapefruit increases peak benzodiazepine blood levels (Cmax) by almost 60%, increases the time to maximum concentration (Tmax) by 80%, and boosts absorption by up to 50%.
- Diazepam is often the first-choice benzodiazepine to treat status epilepticus and is administered intranasally, intravenously, or rectally. However, intranasal diazepam has been preferred for acute repetitive seizures, as it has less pharmacokinetic variability and reliable bioavailability compared with the diazepam rectal gel.
- Diazepam suppresses stage 4 sleep
- Multiple dosage formulations (oral tablet, oral liquid, rectal gel, injectable, intranasal) allow more flexibility of administration compared to most other benzodiazepines
- When using to treat insomnia, remember that insomnia may be a symptom of some other primary disorder itself, and thus warrant evaluation for comorbid psychiatric and/or medical conditions
- Though not systematically studied, benzodiazepines have been used effectively to treat catatonia and are the initial recommended treatment

SUGGESTED READING

Boddu SHS, Kumari S. A short review on the intranasal delivery of diazepam for treating acute repetitive seizures. Pharmaceutics 2020;12(12):1167.

Chugani DC, Muzik O, Juhász C et al. Postnatal maturation of human GABAA receptors measured with positron emission tomography. Ann Neurol 2001;49(5):618–26.

Kuang H, Johnson JA, Mulqueen JM, Bloch MH. The efficacy of benzodiazepines as acute anxiolytics in children: a meta-analysis. Depress Anxiety 2017;34(10):888–96.

Nicotra CM, Strawn JS. Advances in pharmacotherapy for pediatric anxiety disorders. Child Adolesc Psychiatr Clin N Am 2023;32(3):573–87.

Sidorchuk A, Isomura K, Molero Y et al. Benzodiazepine prescribing for children, adolescents, and young adults from 2006 through 2013: a total population register-linkage study. PloS Med 2018;15(8):e1002635.

Stimpfl JN, Mills JA, Strawn JR. Pharmacologic predictors of benzodiazepine response trajectory in anxiety disorders: a Bayesian hierarchical modeling meta-analysis. CNS Spectr 2023;28(1):53–60.

Strawn JR, Lu L, Peris TS, Levine A, Walkup JT. Research review: pediatric anxiety disorders – what have we learnt in the last 10 years? J Child Psychol Psychiatry 2021;62(2):114–39.

Strawn JR, Stahl SM. Case Studies: Stahl's Essential Psychopharmacology: Volume 1: Children and Adolescents. New York: Cambridge University Press, 2023.

THERAPEUTICS

Brands
- Benadryl
- Sominex, other

Generic
Yes

US FDA Approved for Pediatric Use
- Insomnia (ages 12 and older)
- Allergy symptoms (ages 6 and older)
- Motion sickness (ages 6 and older)
- Drug-induced extrapyramidal symptoms

Off-Label for Pediatric Use
- Approved in adults
  - Antiparkinsonism
  - Itchy skin
- Other off-label uses
  - Anxiety

Class and Mechanism of Action
- Antihistamine (anxiolytic, hypnotic, antiemetic); anticholinergic agent

SAFETY AND TOLERABILITY

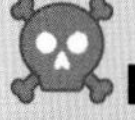

Notable Side Effects
- Sedation, dizziness
- Constipation, nausea
- Dry mouth, blurred vision

Life-Threatening or Dangerous Side Effects
- Rare convulsions (at high doses)
- Urinary retention
- Tachycardia, cardiac arrhythmias
- Confusion
- Paralytic ileus/bowel obstruction

Growth and Maturation
- Not studied

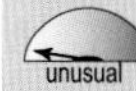

Weight Gain
- Although histamine 1 antagonism may be associated with increased appetite/weight gain, this is not a common side effect with short-term use of diphenhydramine

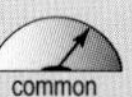

Sedation
- Many experience and/or can be significant in amount

What to Do About Side Effects
- Wait; side effects are usually mild
- For sedation, lower the dose and/or take the entire dose at night
- For dry mouth, chew gum or drink water
- If side effects persist or are intolerable, switch to another agent

How Drug Causes Side Effects
- Blocking histamine 1 receptors can cause sedation
- Preventing the action of acetylcholine on muscarinic receptors can cause anticholinergic effects such as dry mouth, blurred vision, constipation

Warnings and Precautions
- Use with caution in patients with a history of bronchial asthma, lower respiratory disease, increased intraocular pressure, hyperthyroidism, cardiovascular disease, or hypertension
- Diphenhydramine may potentiate the effects of CNS depressants, including alcohol
- May have additive effects if taken with anticholinergic agents
- Antihistamines such as diphenhydramine may reduce mental alertness
- In younger children, antihistamines such as diphenhydramine may cause hyperactivation or excitation

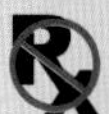

When Not to Prescribe
- If patient is breast feeding
- In children under the age of 2
- In patients with glaucoma, particularly narrow angle glaucoma
- In patients with pyloric or duodenal obstruction, stenosing peptic ulcers, or bladder obstructions
- If patient is taking an MAOI
- If there is a proven allergy to diphenhydramine

Long-Term Use
- Not intended for long-term/chronic use in children or adolescents

Habit Forming

- No

Overdose

- CNS depression, CNS stimulation (more likely in pediatric patients), dry mouth, dilated pupils, flushing, gastrointestinal symptoms, hallucinations, heart problems, seizures, coma, death

DOSING AND USE

Usual Dosage Range

Weight range, lb (kg)	Age (years)	Dose (mg)
24–35 (11–16)	2–3	6.25
36–47 (16–21)	4–5	12.5
48–59 (22–27)	6–8	18.75
60–71 (27–32)	9–10	25
72–95 (33–43)	11	32.25
n/a	12–17	50

Dosage Forms

- Prescription:
  - Elixir 12.5 mg/5 mL
  - Injectable 50 mg/mL
- Over-the-Counter:
  - Liquid 12.5 mg/5 mL
  - Chewable tablet 12.5 mg
- Also available in formulations in combination with other medications

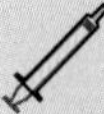

How to Dose

- Ages 2–6: recommended oral dose is 1 to 1.25 mg/kg per dose; this can be administered every 6 to 8 hours as needed, but should not exceed 37.5 mg per dose
- Ages 6–12: recommended oral dose is 1 to 2 mg/kg per dose; this can be administered every 6 to 8 hours as needed, but should not exceed 50 mg per dose
- Maximum doses are indication specific

Options for Administration

- Oral solution and chewable tablets are available as options

Tests

- None for healthy individuals

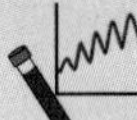

Pharmacokinetics

- Diphenhydramine is well absorbed after oral administration, with peak plasma concentrations typically reached within 2 hours. The presence of food may slightly delay the absorption but does not significantly affect overall bioavailability. Additionally, time to maximum concentration is similar in children ages 2–5 compared to those ages 6–11 compared to those ages 12–17, although half-life is slightly lower in younger patients compared to adolescents (Figure 1).
- Diphenhydramine has a moderate volume of distribution and readily crosses the blood–brain barrier, leading to its central nervous system effects. It is extensively bound to plasma proteins, primarily albumin.
- The metabolism of diphenhydramine primarily occurs in the liver through CYP2D6 and minor demethylation by CYP1A2, CYP2C9, and CYP2C19 (Figure 2). Several metabolites are formed, including the active metabolite, nordiphenhydramine, which contributes to the drug's effects.
- Elimination half-life is shorter in children (approximately 5 hours, range 4–7 hours) than in adults (approximately 9 hours, range 7–12 hours)
- Bioavailability is 40–60%

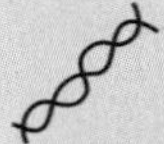

Pharmacogenetics

- No recommendations

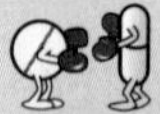

Drug Interactions

- May potentiate the effects of other CNS depressants
- If anticholinergic agents are used with diphenhydramine, the anticholinergic effects may be enhanced

Dosing Tips

- Can be taken with or without food

How to Switch

- Tapering generally not necessary

How to Stop

- Tapering generally not necessary

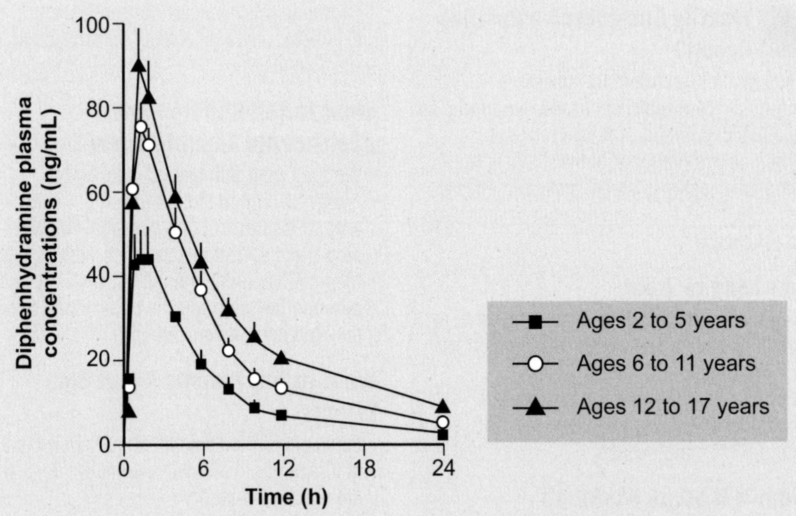

Figure 1 Diphenhydramine concentration time profiles. Individuals aged 2–5 received 10.2 mg, those aged 6–11 years received 24.2 mg, and those aged 12–17 received a 50 mg dose. Adapted from Gelotte et al., Clinical Pharmacology in Drug Development, 2018.

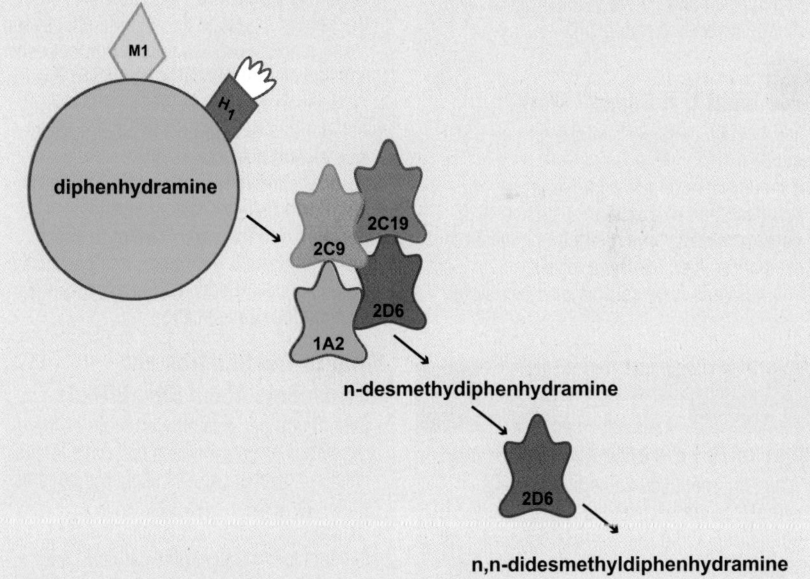

Figure 2 Diphenhydramine metabolism.

WHAT TO EXPECT

Onset of Action

- Onset of action typically occurs within 1 hour

Duration of Action

- Duration of action is generally 4–6 hours

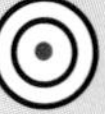

Primary Target Symptoms

- Anxiety
- Insomnia

What Is Considered a Positive Result?

- The goal of treatment for anxiety is complete remission of current symptoms as well as prevention of future relapses
- The goal of treatment of insomnia is to improve quality of sleep, including effects on total wake time and number of nighttime awakenings

How Long to Treat

- For insomnia and short-term symptoms of anxiety: after a few weeks, discontinue use or use on an "as-needed" basis
- For long-term symptoms of anxiety, consider switching to an SSRI or SNRI for long-term maintenance

What If It Stops Working?

- If anxiety symptoms reemerge, consider an SSRI, and re-trying psychotherapeutic approaches
- If the primary target symptom is insomnia, consider an alternative medication or melatonin and re-trying CBT-I

What If It Doesn't Work?

- For anxiety, consider switching to an SSRI or SNRI
- If insomnia does not improve, it may be a manifestation of a primary psychiatric or physical illness, which requires independent evaluation. Also, re-trying other interventions for insomnia may be helpful.

TALKING TO PATIENTS AND CAREGIVERS

What to Tell Parents About Efficacy

- While the medicine helps by reducing symptoms and improving function, it is not a cure, and it is therefore necessary to keep taking the medication to sustain its therapeutic effects
- Since every treatment consideration depends on a risk/benefit analysis, parents should fully understand short- and long-term risks as well as benefits
- Often a good idea to tell parents whether the medication chosen is specifically approved for the disorder being treated, or whether it is being given for "unapproved" or "off-label" reasons based on good clinical practice, expert consensus, and/or prudent extrapolation of controlled data from adults

What to Tell Children and Adolescents About Efficacy

- We are trying to make you feel better
- It may be a good idea to give the medication a try; if it's not working very well, we can stop the medication and try something else
- Medications don't change who you are as a person; they give you the opportunity to be the best person you can be

What to Tell Parents About Side Effects

- Explain that mild side effects are expected at initiation or when increasing the dose and are usually transitory
- Predict side effects in advance (you will look clever and competent to the parents, unless you scare them with too much information and cause nocebo effects, in which case you won't look so clever when the patient develops lots of side effects and stops medication; use your judgment here); a balanced but honest presentation is an art rather than a science
- Ask parents to support the patient while side effects are occurring
- Parents should fully understand short- and long-term risks as well as benefits
- Explaining to the parents what to expect from medication treatment, and especially potential side effects, can help prevent early termination of medication

What to Tell Children and Adolescents About Side Effects

- Even if you get side effects, most of them get better or go away in a few days to a few weeks; however, we will likely not use this medication for a long time
- Explaining to child/adolescent what to expect from medication treatment, and especially potential side effects, can help prevent early termination of medication

What to Tell Teachers About the Medication (If Parents Consent)

- Diphenhydramine can make children/adolescents sleepy
- It is not abusable
- Encourage dialogue with parents/guardians about any behavior or mood changes

SPECIAL POPULATIONS

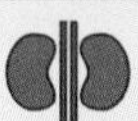

Renal Impairment

- No dose adjustment necessary

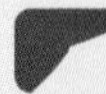

Hepatic Impairment

- Dose reduction may be necessary since diphenhydramine is extensively metabolized in the liver

Cardiac Impairment

- Not systematically evaluated in patients with cardiac impairment

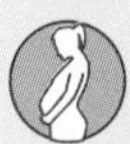

Pregnancy

- Controlled studies have not been conducted in pregnant women
- Animal studies have not shown adverse effects

Breast Feeding

- Contraindicated

THE ART OF PSYCHOPHARMACOLOGY

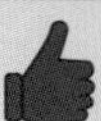

Potential Advantages

- Patients with dermatitis and itching
- No abuse liability, dependence, or withdrawal

Potential Disadvantages

- Can be too sedating for some patients
- Can cause cognitive side effects with chronic use

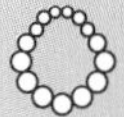

Pearls

- Disinhibition has been described with all antihistamines in pediatric patients; however, while this may be more common in younger children, it is uncommon in older children and adolescents. Also, some patients who have experienced disinhibition at a younger age may not experience it when they are older.

SUGGESTED READING

Blyden GT, Greenblatt DJ, Scavone JM, et al. Pharmacokinetics of diphenhydramine and a demethylated metabolite following intravenous and oral administration. J Clin Pharmacol 1986;26(7):529–33.

Brost BC, Scardo JA, Newman RB. Diphenhydramine overdose during pregnancy: lessons from the past. Am J Obstet Gynecol 1996;175(5):1376–7.

Gelotte CK, Zimmerman BA, Thompson GA. Single-dose pharmacokinetic study of diphenhydramine hcl in children and adolescents. Clin Pharmacol Drug Dev 2018;7(4):400–7.

Ito S, Blajchman A, Stephenson M et al. Prospective follow-up of adverse reactions in breast-fed infants exposed to maternal medication. Am J Obstet Gynecol 1993;168(5):1393–9.

Lessard E, Yessine MA, Hamelin BA et al. Diphenhydramine alters the disposition of venlafaxine through inhibition of CYP2D6 activity in humans. J Clin Psychopharmacol 2001;21:175–84.

Messinis IE, Souvatzoglou A, Fais N et al. Histamine H1 receptor participation in the control of prolactin secretion in postpartum. J Endocrinol Invest 1985;8(2):143–6.

Simons KJ, Watson WT, Martin TJ, Chen XY, Simons FE. Diphenhydramine: pharmacokinetics and pharmacodynamics in elderly adults, young adults, and children. J Clin Pharmacol 1990;30:665–71.

THERAPEUTICS

Brands

- Unisom

Generic

Yes

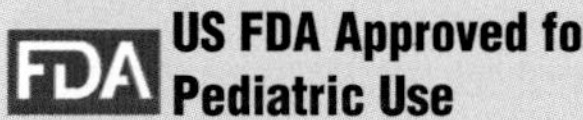

US FDA Approved for Pediatric Use

- Insomnia (ages 12 and older)
- Allergy symptoms (ages 6 and older)

Off-Label for Pediatric Use

- Approved in adults
  - None
- Other off-label uses
  - Anxiety

Class and Mechanism of Action

- Antihistamine (anxiolytic, hypnotic, antiemetic); anticholinergic agent

SAFETY AND TOLERABILITY

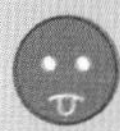

Notable Side Effects

- Sedation, dizziness
- Constipation, nausea
- Dry mouth, blurred vision

Life-Threatening or Dangerous Side Effects

- Rare convulsions
- Urinary retention
- Bradycardia, tachycardia, cardiac arrhythmias
- Confusion

Growth and Maturation

- Not studied

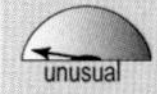

Weight Gain

- Although histamine 1 antagonism may be associated with increased appetite/weight gain, this is not a common side effect with short-term use of doxylamine

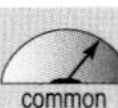

Sedation

- Many experience and/or can be significant in amount

What to Do About Side Effects

- Wait
- For dry mouth, chew gum or drink water
- If side effects persist or are intolerable, switch to another agent

How Drug Causes Side Effects

- Blocking histamine 1 receptors can cause sedation
- Preventing the action of acetylcholine on muscarinic receptors can cause anticholinergic effects such as dry mouth, blurred vision, constipation

Warnings and Precautions

- Doxylamine may potentiate the effects of CNS depressants, including alcohol
- Antihistamines such as doxylamine may reduce mental alertness
- Doxylamine has anticholinergic properties and should be used with caution in patients with conditions such as GI or bladder obstruction, closed-angle glaucoma, or increased intraocular pressure
- May have additive effects if taken with anticholinergic agents
- In younger children, antihistamines such as doxylamine may cause hyperactivation or excitation

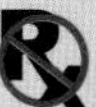

When Not to Prescribe

- If patient is breast feeding
- In children under the age of 2
- If there is a proven allergy to doxylamine

Long-Term Use

- Not intended for long-term use

Habit Forming

- No

Overdose

- Dry mouth, dilated pupils, sedation, mental confusion, tachycardia, seizures, rhabdomyolysis, acute renal failure, death

DOSING AND USE

Usual Dosage Range

- Insomnia (ages 12 and older): 25 mg 30 minutes before bedtime as needed

Dosage Forms

- Over-the-Counter
  - Tablet 25 mg

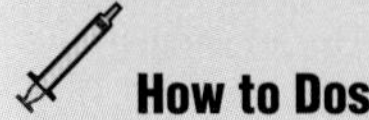

How to Dose

- For insomnia, dose should be administered 30 minutes prior to bedtime
- Nonprescription use of doxylamine for insomnia should be limited to 2 weeks
- Not recommended for insomnia in children under 12 years of age

Options for Administration

- Only available as a tablet

Tests

- None for healthy individuals

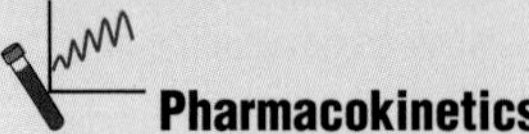

Pharmacokinetics

- Doxylamine is rapidly and well absorbed following oral administration (Figure 1). The onset of action typically occurs within 30 minutes.
- Bioavailability is high when administered orally
- Doxylamine undergoes extensive hepatic metabolism. The main metabolic pathway involves *N*-demethylation by CYP2D6 and CYP2C19.
- Primary metabolic route is *N*-dealkylation and *N*-acetyl conjugation in the liver
- Elimination half-life is approximately 16 hours in children ages 2–17

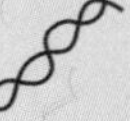

Pharmacogenetics

- No recommendations

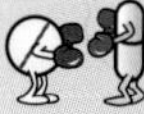

Drug Interactions

- May potentiate the effects of other CNS depressants
- If anticholinergic agents are used with doxylamine, the anticholinergic effects may be enhanced; concomitant use with opioids should be avoided due to the increased risk of anticholinergic side effects

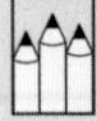

Dosing Tips

- Can be taken with or without food

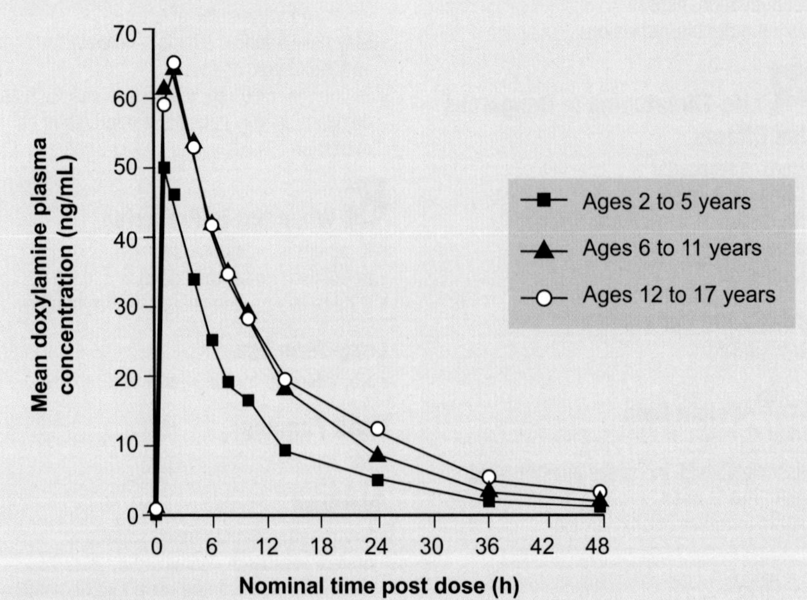

Figure 1 Doxylamine plasma concentration–time profiles by age group following single oral dose. Adapted from Balan et al, Journal of Clinical Pharmacology, 2013.

- In children and adolescents, tachyphylaxis is common with repeated use, which results in decreased efficacy over time. Therefore, for antihistamines, prn use may be preferred.

How to Switch

- Tapering generally not necessary

How to Stop

- Tapering generally not necessary

WHAT TO EXPECT

Onset of Action

- Clinical effects can occur within 30–45 minutes

Duration of Action

- Effects on anxiety and sleep are consistent over 6 hours

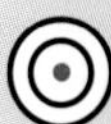

Primary Target Symptoms

- Insomnia
- Anxiety

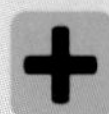

What Is Considered a Positive Result?

- The goal of treatment of insomnia is to improve quality of sleep, including effects on total wake time and number of nighttime awakenings
- The goal of treatment for anxiety is complete remission of current symptoms as well as prevention of future relapses

How Long to Treat

- For insomnia and short-term symptoms of anxiety: not intended for use beyond 2 weeks
- For long-term symptoms of anxiety, consider switching to an SSRI or SNRI for long-term maintenance

What If It Stops Working?

- If being used to treat anxiety and anxiety symptoms reemerge, consider treatment with an SSRI or SNRI
- If the primary target symptom is insomnia, consider an alternative medication or melatonin and re-trying CBT-I

What If It Doesn't Work?

- For anxiety, consider switching to an SSRI or SNRI
- If insomnia does not improve, it may be a manifestation of a primary psychiatric or physical illness, which requires independent evaluation. Also, re-trying other interventions for insomnia may be helpful.

TALKING TO PATIENTS AND CAREGIVERS

What to Tell Parents About Efficacy

- While the medicine helps by reducing symptoms and improving function, it is not a cure, and it is therefore necessary to keep taking the medication to sustain its therapeutic effects
- Since every treatment consideration depends on a risk/benefit analysis, parents should fully understand short- and long-term risks as well as benefits
- Often a good idea to tell parents whether the medication chosen is specifically approved for the disorder being treated, or whether it is being given for "unapproved" or "off-label" reasons based on good clinical practice, expert consensus, and/or prudent extrapolation of controlled data from adults

What to Tell Children and Adolescents About Efficacy

- We are trying to make you feel better
- It may be a good idea to give the medication a try; if it's not working very well, we can stop the medication and try something else
- Medications don't change who you are as a person; they give you the opportunity to be the best person you can be

What to Tell Parents About Side Effects

- Explain that mild side effects are expected at initiation or when increasing the dose and are usually transitory
- Predict side effects in advance (you will look clever and competent to the parents, unless you scare them with too much information and cause nocebo effects, in which case you won't look so clever when the patient develops lots of side effects and

stops medication; use your judgment here); a balanced but honest presentation is an art rather than a science
- Ask parents to support the patient while side effects are occurring
- Parents should fully understand short- and long-term risks as well as benefits
- Explaining to the parents what to expect from medication treatment, and especially potential side effects, can help prevent early termination of medication

What to Tell Children and Adolescents About Side Effects

- Even if you get side effects, most of them get better or go away in a few days to a few weeks
- Explaining to child/adolescent what to expect from medication treatment, and especially potential side effects, can help prevent early termination of medication

What to Tell Teachers About the Medication (If Parents Consent)

- Doxylamine can make children/adolescents sleepy
- It is not abusable
- Encourage dialogue with parents/guardians about any behavior or mood changes

SPECIAL POPULATIONS

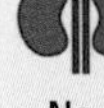

Renal Impairment

- No dose adjustment necessary

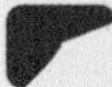

Hepatic Impairment

- Dose reduction may be necessary since doxylamine is extensively metabolized in the liver

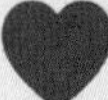

Cardiac Impairment

- Not systematically evaluated in patients with cardiac impairment

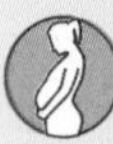

Pregnancy

- Controlled studies have not been conducted in pregnant women
- Meta-analysis of epidemiological studies did not show increased risk for malformations from first trimester exposure
- Doxylamine is not recommended for use during pregnancy

Breast Feeding

- Unknown if doxylamine is secreted in human breast milk, but all psychotropics assumed to be secreted in breast milk
- Recommended either to discontinue drug or formula feed

THE ART OF PSYCHOPHARMACOLOGY

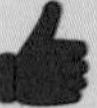

Potential Advantages

- Patients with dermatitis and itching
- No abuse liability, dependence, or withdrawal

Potential Disadvantages

- Morning sedation
- Anticholinergic side effects

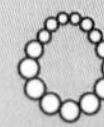

Pearls

- Doxylamine in combination with pyridoxine is approved for the treatment of nausea/vomiting of pregnancy in women who do not respond to conservative treatment

SUGGESTED READING

Balan G, Thompson GA, Gibb R et al. Doxylamine pharmacokinetics following single dose oral administration in children ages 2–17 years. J Clin Pharmacol 2013;53(11):1177–85.

Derinöz-Güleryüz O. Doxylamine succinate overdose: slurred speech and visual hallucination. Turk J Pediatr 2018;60(4):439–42.

THERAPEUTICS

Brands
- Cymbalta
- Drizalma

Generic
Yes

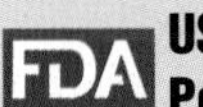

US FDA Approved for Pediatric Use
- Generalized anxiety disorder (ages 7 and older)

Off-Label for Pediatric Use
- Approved in adults
  - Major depressive disorder
  - Diabetic peripheral neuropathic pain (DPNP)
  - Fibromyalgia
  - Chronic musculoskeletal pain
- Other off-label uses
  - Stress urinary incontinence
  - Neuropathic pain/chronic pain
  - Other anxiety disorders

Class and Mechanism of Action
- Neuroscience-based Nomenclature: serotonin norepinephrine reuptake inhibitor (SN-RI)
- SNRI (dual serotonin and norepinephrine reuptake inhibitor); often classified as a drug for depression (i.e., antidepressant), but it is not just an antidepressant
- Duloxetine presumably increases serotonergic neurotransmission by blocking the serotonin reuptake pump (transporter, SERT), which results in the desensitization of serotonin receptors, especially serotonin 1A receptors
- Duloxetine presumably increases noradrenergic neurotransmission by blocking the norepinephrine reuptake pump (transporter, NET), which results in the desensitization of beta adrenergic receptors
- Since dopamine is inactivated by norepinephrine reuptake in the frontal cortex, which largely lacks dopamine transporters, duloxetine can increase dopamine neurotransmission in this part of the brain
- Duloxetine weakly blocks the dopamine reuptake pump (dopamine transporter), and may increase dopamine neurotransmission

SAFETY AND TOLERABILITY

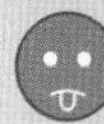

Notable Side Effects
- Unlike for some antidepressants, side effects for duloxetine do not appear to be related to dose
- Mostly central nervous system side effects (insomnia but also sedation, especially if not sleeping at night; agitation, tremors, headache, dizziness)
- Note: patients with diagnosed or undiagnosed bipolar or psychotic disorders may be more vulnerable to CNS-activating actions of antidepressants like duloxetine; pay particular attention to signs of activation in children with developmental disorders or autism spectrum disorders
- Treatment-emergent activation syndrome (TEAS) includes agitation, anxiety, panic attacks, irritability, aggression, impulsivity, and insomnia
- TEAS can represent side effects but should not be confused with bipolar mania or the onset of suicidality and should be monitored and investigated with consideration of discontinuing or decreasing the dose of duloxetine or addition of another agent or switching to another agent to reduce these symptoms
- Gastrointestinal (decreased appetite, nausea, diarrhea constipation, dry mouth)
- Sexual dysfunction (boys: delayed ejaculation, erectile dysfunction; boys and girls: decreased sexual desire, anorgasmia)
- In pediatric trials, duloxetine increases resting heart rate and diastolic blood pressure, and these effects are not dose-related syndrome of inappropriate antidiuretic hormone secretion (SIADH)

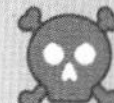

Life-Threatening or Dangerous Side Effects
- Rare seizures
- Rare induction of mania
- Rare suicidal ideation and behavior (suicidality) (short-term regulatory studies did not show any actual suicides in any age group and also did not show an increase in the risk of suicidality with antidepressants compared to placebo beyond age 24)

Growth and Maturation

- Limited data suggest weight loss, at least in the short term. This was added to the pediatric labeling for duloxetine following several large trials of youth with generalized anxiety disorder and MDD.

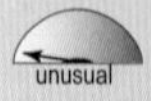

Weight Gain

- Unlikely
- Pediatric patients may experience decreased weight/less than expected weight gain

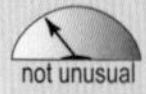

Sedation

- Occurs in significant minority

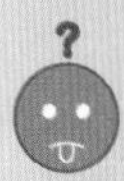

What to Do About Side Effects

- Wait, wait, wait: mild side effects are common, happen early, and usually improve with time, but treatment benefits can be delayed and often begin just as the side effects wear off
- Monitor side effects closely, especially when initiating treatment
- May wish to try dosing every other day to deal with side effects, or wash out for a week and try again at half dose or every other day
- May wish to give some drugs at night if not tolerated during the day, particularly if the medication is associated with sedation
- For activation (jitteriness, anxiety, insomnia):
  - Administer dose in the morning
  - Consider a temporary dose reduction or a more gradual up-titration
  - Consider switching to another antidepressant
  - Optimize psychotherapeutic interventions
  - Activation and agitation may represent the induction of a bipolar state, especially a mixed dysphoric bipolar II condition sometimes associated with suicidal ideation, and may require the addition of lithium or an atypical antipsychotic, and/or discontinuation of duloxetine
- Often best to try another monotherapy prior to resorting to augmentation strategies to treat side effects
- For insomnia: consider adding melatonin
- For GI upset: try giving medication with a meal
- For sexual dysfunction:
  - Probably best to reduce dose or discontinue and try another agent
  - Consider adding daytime exercise, bupropion, or buspirone
- For emotional flattening, apathy: consider adding bupropion (with caution as little experience in children)

How Drug Causes Side Effects

- Theoretically due to increases in serotonin and norepinephrine concentrations at receptors in parts of the brain and body other than those that cause therapeutic actions (e.g., unwanted actions of serotonin in sleep centers causing insomnia, unwanted actions of norepinephrine on acetylcholine release causing decreased appetite, increased blood pressure, urinary retention)

Warnings and Precautions

- Consider distributing the brochures provided by the FDA and the drug companies as well as the medication guides from the American Academy of Child & Adolescent Psychiatry (AACAP)
- Carefully consider monitoring patients regularly and within the practical limits, particularly during the first several weeks of treatment
- Warn patients and their caregivers when possible about the possibility of activating side effects and advise them to report such symptoms immediately
- Carefully weigh the risks and benefits of pharmacological treatment against the risks and benefits of nontreatment with antidepressants and it is a good idea to document this in the patient's chart
- Rare reports of hepatotoxicity; although causality has not been established, duloxetine should be discontinued in patients who develop jaundice or other evidence of significant liver dysfunction
- Duloxetine may increase blood pressure, so blood pressure should be monitored during treatment
- As with any antidepressant, use with caution in patients with history of seizure
- As with any antidepressant, use with caution in patients with bipolar disorder unless treated with concomitant mood-stabilizing agent
- Monitor patients for activation and suicidal ideation and involve parents/guardians

When Not to Prescribe

- If patient is taking an MAO inhibitor
- If patient has uncontrolled angle-closure glaucoma
- If patient has substantial alcohol use
- If patient is taking thioridazine
- Not generally recommended in patients taking tricyclic antidepressants (see Drug Interactions)
- If there is a proven allergy to duloxetine

Long-Term Use

- Growth should be monitored; long-term effects are unknown
- See doctor regularly to monitor blood pressure

Habit Forming

- No

Overdose

- Rare fatalities have been reported; serotonin syndrome, sedation, vomiting, seizures, coma, change in blood pressure

DOSING AND USE

Usual Dosage Range

- Children (for GAD): 30–60 mg once daily (studied up to 120 mg/day)
- Adolescents (for GAD): 30–60 mg once daily (studied up to 120 mg/day)

Dosage Forms

- Capsule 20 mg, 30 mg, 40 mg, 60 mg
- Capsule (sprinkles) 20 mg, 40 mg

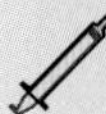

How to Dose

- Children (for GAD): initial dose 30 mg/day; can increase to 60 mg/day after 2 weeks if necessary; can increase in increments of 30 mg once daily up to a maximum dose of 120 mg/day if necessary
- Adolescents (for GAD): initial dose 30 mg/day; can increase to 60 mg/day after 2 weeks if necessary; can increase in increments of 30 mg once daily up to a maximum dose of 120 mg/day if necessary

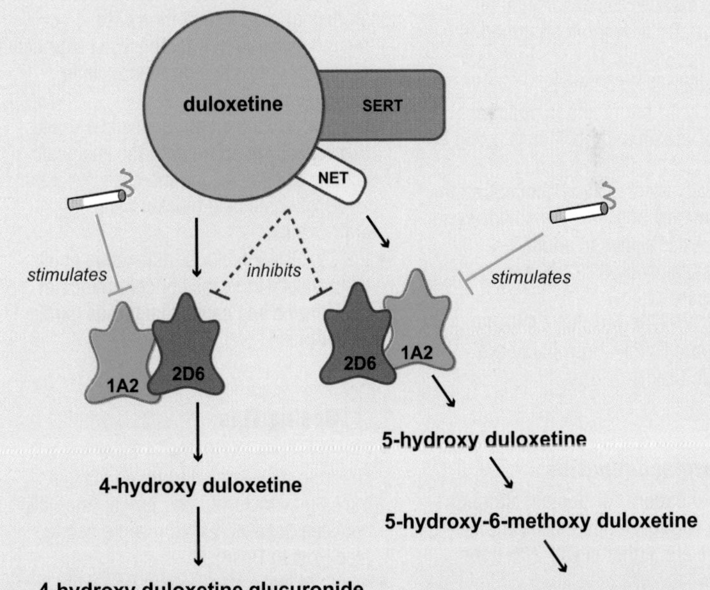

Figure 1 Duloxetine metabolism. Duloxetine is extensively metabolized in the liver and its major circulating metabolites 4-hydroxy duloxetine glucuronide and 5-hydroxy-6-methoxy duloxetine sulfate are inactive at serotonin and norepinephrine transporters. Duloxetine concentrations are higher in non-smokers compared to smokers, and strong CYP1A2 inhibitors should be avoided.

Options for Administration

- Capsule should not be cut or crushed; however, capsules containing duloxetine sprinkles may be opened

Tests

- Check blood pressure and heart rate before initiating treatment and regularly during treatment
- Monitor weight and height against that expected for normal growth, using the pediatric height/weight chart to monitor

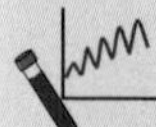

Pharmacokinetics

- Duloxetine is well absorbed, and peak concentrations occur approximately 5 hours after administration of duloxetine delayed-release capsules
- Interestingly, administering in the evening delays absorption by approximately 3 hours compared to morning administration
- Food has minimal effects on absorption of duloxetine and has not been specifically evaluated in youth, although in adults, administering duloxetine with a high-fat, high-calorie meal delays absorption by about 2 hours (total amount absorbed is unaffected)
- Elimination half-life in adults is approximately 12 hours and in pediatric patients is approximately 10 hours (Lobo et al., 2014)
- Average steady-state plasma concentrations are approximately 30% lower in children and adolescents relative to adults
- Metabolized mainly by CYP2D6 and CYP1A2 (Figure 1)
- Inhibitor of CYP2D6 (possibly clinically significant) and CYP1A2 (probably not clinically significant)

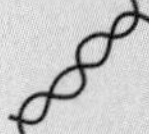

Pharmacogenetics

- No recommendations for dosing, although limited data suggest that concentrations of duloxetine are higher in CYP2D6 poor metabolizers

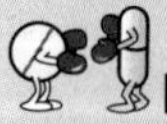

Drug Interactions

- Tramadol reported to increase the risk of seizures in adults taking an antidepressant
- Can increase tricyclic antidepressant (TCA) levels; use with caution with tricyclic antidepressants or when switching from a TCA to duloxetine
- Can cause a fatal "serotonin syndrome" when combined with MAO inhibitors, so do not use with MAO inhibitors or for at least 14 days after MAOIs are stopped
- Do not start an MAO inhibitor for at least 5 half-lives (5 to 7 days for most drugs) after discontinuing duloxetine
- Possible increased risk of bleeding
- Inhibitors of CYP1A2, such as fluvoxamine, increase plasma levels of duloxetine and may require a dosage reduction of duloxetine
- Cigarette smoking induces CYP1A2 and may reduce plasma levels of duloxetine, but dosage modifications are not recommended for smokers
- Inhibitors of CYP2D6, such as paroxetine, fluoxetine, and quinidine, may increase plasma levels of duloxetine and require a dosage reduction of duloxetine
- Via CYP1A2 inhibition, duloxetine could theoretically reduce clearance of theophylline and clozapine; however, studies of coadministration with theophylline did not demonstrate significant effects of duloxetine on theophylline pharmacokinetics
- Via CYP2D6 inhibition, duloxetine could theoretically interfere with the analgesic actions of codeine and increase the plasma levels of some beta blockers and of atomoxetine
- Via CYP2D6 inhibition, duloxetine could theoretically increase concentrations of thioridazine and cause dangerous cardiac arrhythmias

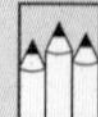

Dosing Tips

- Plasma levels are higher in lower-weight children; therefore, starting and target doses may be lower, and longer intervals between dose increases may be needed (see How to Dose)
- If a child loses efficacy between daily doses, it may indicate rapid metabolism and the need to increase the dose
- Adolescents often need and receive adult doses

- Studies have not demonstrated increased efficacy beyond 60 mg/day, although the trial that gave rise to the FDA indication for duloxetine in children and adolescents with GAD examined doses up to 120 mg/day. In these studies, because of the flexible titration, duloxetine was not titrated aggressively in many patients. Some patients may require up to 120 mg/day.
- In relapse prevention studies in depression (adults), a significant percentage of patients who relapsed on 60 mg/day responded and remitted when the dose was increased to 120 mg/day
- In adults with neuropathic pain and fibromyalgia, doses above 60 mg/day are associated with increased side effects without an increase in efficacy
- Some studies suggest that both serotonin and norepinephrine reuptake blockade are present at 40–60 mg/day
- If intolerable anxiety, insomnia, agitation, akathisia, or activation occurs either upon dosing initiation or discontinuation, consider the possibility of activated bipolar disorder and switch to an atypical antipsychotic or a mood stabilizer
- These symptoms may also indicate the need to evaluate for a mixed features episode and thus discontinuing duloxetine and considering an atypical antipsychotic or a mood stabilizer or lithium

How to Switch

- From another antidepressant to duloxetine:
  - When tapering a prior antidepressant, see its entry in this manual for how to stop and how to taper off that specific drug
  - In situations when there are antidepressant-related side effects, try to stop the first agent before starting duloxetine so that new side effects of duloxetine can be distinguished from withdrawal effects of the first agent
  - If urgent, cross taper
- Off duloxetine to another antidepressant:
  - Generally, try to stop duloxetine before starting another antidepressant
  - Taper to avoid withdrawal effects (dizziness, nausea, stomach cramps, sweating, tingling, dysesthesias)
  - Many patients tolerate 50% dose reduction for 3 days, then another 50% reduction for 3 days, then discontinuation
  - If necessary, can cross taper off duloxetine this way while dosing up on another antidepressant simultaneously in urgent situations, being aware of all specific drug interactions to avoid

How to Stop

- Taper to avoid withdrawal effects (dizziness, nausea, stomach cramps, sweating, tingling, dysesthesias)
- Many patients tolerate 50% dose reduction for 7–10 days, then another 50% reduction for 7–10 days, then discontinuation. However, clinical experience discontinuing duloxetine in youth suggests that this may need to be done over a longer interval.
- If withdrawal symptoms emerge during discontinuation, raise dose to stop symptoms and then restart withdrawal much more slowly

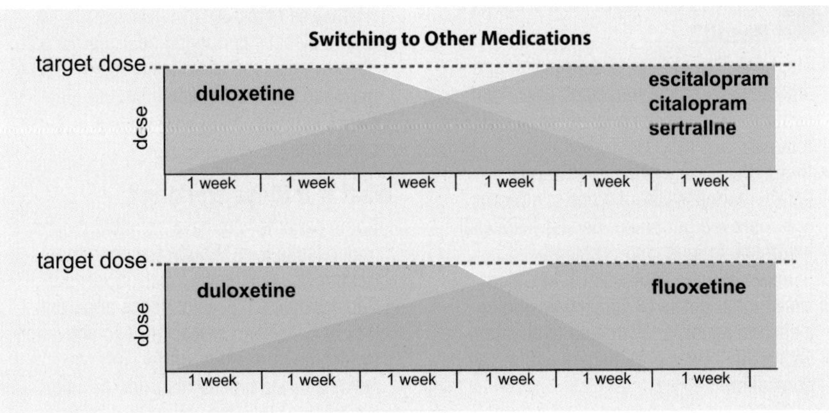

WHAT TO EXPECT

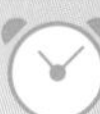

Onset of Action

- Some patients may experience increased energy or activation early after initiation of treatment
- Full onset of therapeutic actions is usually delayed by 2–4 weeks, although in the trial of duloxetine in children and adolescents with GAD, separation from placebo occurred at week 2
- If it is not working within 6–8 weeks for depression or anxiety, it may require a dosage increase or it may not work at all
- Can reduce neuropathic pain within a week, but onset can take longer

Duration of Action

- Effects are consistent over a 24-hour period
- May continue to work for many years to prevent relapse of symptoms

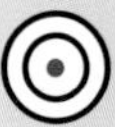

Primary Target Symptoms

- Depressed and/or irritable mood
- Energy, motivation, and interest
- Sleep disturbance
- Anxiety (fear and worry are often target symptoms, but duloxetine can occasionally and transiently increase these symptoms short term before improving them)
- Physical symptoms, pain
- Prior to initiation of treatment, it is helpful to develop a list of target symptoms of depression and/or anxiety to monitor during treatment to better assess treatment response

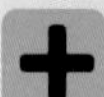

What Is Considered a Positive Result?

- The goal of treatment of depression and anxiety is complete remission of current symptoms as well as prevention of future relapses
- In practice, many patients have only a partial response where some symptoms are improved but others persist (especially insomnia, fatigue, and problems concentrating in depression), in which case higher doses of duloxetine, adding a second agent, or switching to an agent with a different mechanism of action can be considered
- If treatment works, it most often reduces or even eliminates symptoms, but is not a cure since symptoms can recur after medicine is stopped
- The goal of treatment of diabetic peripheral neuropathic pain and fibromyalgia and chronic neuropathic pain is to reduce symptoms as much as possible, especially in combination with other treatments
- Treatment of diabetic peripheral neuropathic pain, fibromyalgia, and chronic neuropathic pain may reduce symptoms, but rarely eliminates them completely, and is not a cure since symptoms can recur after medicine is stopped

How Long to Treat

- For adolescents with depression, generally, 9–12 months of antidepressant treatment is recommended (Hathaway et al., 2018)
- For anxiety disorders, 6–9 months of antidepressant treatment may be sufficient, though many clinicians extend treatment to 12 months based on extrapolation of data from adults with anxiety disorders (Hathaway et al., 2018; Strawn et al., 2023)
- Extended treatment periods may decrease the risk of long-term morbidity and recurrence; however, the goal of treatment is ultimately remission, rather than duration of antidepressant pharmacotherapy (Hathaway et al., 2018)
- In terms of the length of antidepressant treatment, evidence-based guidelines represent a starting point; appropriate treatment duration varies, and patient-specific response, psychological factors, and timing of discontinuation must be considered for individual pediatric patients (Hathaway et al., 2018)
- Use in diabetic peripheral neuropathic pain, fibromyalgia, and chronic neuropathic pain may also need to be indefinite, but long-term treatment is not well studied in these conditions

What If It Stops Working?

- Some patients who have an initial response may relapse even though they continue treatment, sometimes called "poop-out"
- Some patients may experience apparent lack of consistent efficacy due to activation syndrome or latent or underlying or newly evolved bipolar disorder, or major depressive episodes with mixed features,

and require antidepressant discontinuation and a switch to a second generation antipsychotic

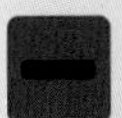

What If It Doesn't Work?

- Consider evaluation for another diagnosis (especially bipolar illness or depression with mixed features) or for a comorbid condition (e.g., medical illness, substance abuse)
- Be mindful of family conflict contributing to the presentation; sometimes treating parental depression or anxiety disorders improves psychiatric and social function without any treatment of youth. Also, accommodation is common in families of youth with anxiety disorders and may need to be addressed specifically, as it can perpetuate symptoms.
- Consider factors associated with poor response to SSRIs in treatment-resistant depression or anxiety disorders, such as severe symptoms, long-lasting symptoms, poor treatment adherence, prior nonresponse to other treatments, and the presence of comorbid disorders
- Consider other important potential factors such as ongoing conflicts, family psychopathology, and an adverse environment (e.g., poverty, chaos, violence, prior and ongoing psychological trauma, abuse, neglect). Additionally, when symptoms are prominent at school, consider the presence of a learning disorder.
- Institute trauma-informed care for appropriate children and adolescents
- A 2007 meta-analysis of published and unpublished trials in pediatric patients found that antidepressants had a number needed to treat (NNT) of 10 for depression, 6 for OCD, and 3 for anxiety disorders; thus, duloxetine may not work in all children, so consider switching to another antidepressant (Bridge et al., 2007)
- Consider a dose adjustment
- Consider augmenting options:
    - Cognitive behavioral therapy (CBT), interpersonal psychotherapy for adolescents (IPT-A), light therapy, family therapy, and exercise especially in adolescents
    - For partial response (depression): use caution when adding medications to duloxetine, especially in children since there are not sufficient studies of augmentation in children or adolescents; however, for the expert, consider bupropion, aripiprazole, or other atypical antipsychotics such as quetiapine; use combinations of antidepressants with caution as this may activate bipolar disorder and suicidal ideation
    - For insomnia: sleep hygiene, CBT for insomnia, melatonin, or alpha 2 agonists
    - For anxiety: buspirone, antihistamines
    - Add mood stabilizers or atypical antipsychotics for bipolar depression, psychotic depression, treatment-resistant depression, or treatment-resistant anxiety disorders
    - TMS (transcranial magnetic stimulation) may have a role although pediatric trials of TMS have been hampered by high sham response rates (Croarkin et al., 2021)
    - ECT (case studies show effectiveness; cognitive side effects are similar to those in adults; reserve for treatment-resistant cases)
    - For pain, consider biofeedback or hypnosis

TALKING TO PATIENTS AND CAREGIVERS

What to Tell Parents About Efficacy

- Doesn't work right away; full therapeutic benefits may take up to 8 weeks, yet parents and teachers might see improvement before the patient does
- While the medicine helps by reducing symptoms and improving function, it is not a cure, and it is therefore necessary to keep taking the medication to sustain its therapeutic effects
- Since every treatment consideration depends on a risk/benefit analysis, parents should fully understand short- and long-term risks as well as benefits
- After successful treatment, continuation of duloxetine may be necessary to prevent relapse, especially in those who have had more than one episode or a very severe episode. In general, when treating depression in children and adolescents, medications are continued for 12 months after symptoms have resolved, while for anxiety disorders, clinicians have generally

treated for 6–9 months (Hathaway et al., 2018).
- Often a good idea to tell parents whether the medication chosen is specifically approved for the disorder being treated, or whether it is being given for "unapproved" or "off-label" reasons based on good clinical practice, expert consensus, and/or prudent extrapolation of controlled data from adults

What to Tell Children and Adolescents About Efficacy

- We are trying to make you feel better
- It may be a good idea to give the medication a try; if it's not working very well, we can stop the medication and try something else
- A good try takes 2 to 3 months or even longer
- If it does make you feel better, you cannot stop it right away or you may feel sad or worried again
- Medications don't change who you are as a person; they give you the opportunity to be the best person you can be

What to Tell Parents About Side Effects

- Explain that side effects are expected in many when starting and are most common in the first 2–3 weeks of starting or increasing the dose
- Tell parents many side effects go away and do so about the same time that therapeutic effects start
- Predict side effects in advance (you will look clever and competent to the parents, unless you scare them with too much information and cause nocebo effects, in which case you won't look so clever when the patient develops lots of side effects and stops medication; use your judgment here); a balanced but honest presentation is an art rather than a science
- Ask them to help monitor for increased suicidality and if present, report any such symptoms immediately
- Ask parents to support the patient while side effects are occurring
- Parents should fully understand short- and long-term risks as well as benefits
- Explaining to the parents what to expect from medication treatment, and especially potential side effects, can help prevent early termination of medication

What to Tell Children and Adolescents About Side Effects

- Even if you get side effects, most of them get better or go away in a few days to a few weeks
- Consider having a conversation about sexual side effects in some adolescents who can find these side effects confusing and especially burdensome
- Explaining to child/adolescent what to expect from medication treatment, and especially potential side effects, can help prevent early termination of medication
- Tell adolescents and children capable of understanding that some young patients, especially those who are depressed, may develop thoughts of hurting themselves, and if this happens, not to be alarmed but to tell their parents right away

What to Tell Teachers About the Medication (If Parents Consent)

- Duloxetine can make children/adolescents jittery or restless
- If the patient is sleepy, ask whether the medication is keeping them up at night
- It is not abusable
- Encourage dialogue with parents/guardians about any behavior or mood changes

SPECIAL POPULATIONS

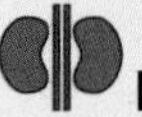

Renal Impairment

- Dose adjustment generally not necessary for mild to moderate impairment
- Not recommended for use in patients with end-stage renal disease (requiring dialysis) or severe renal impairment

Hepatic Impairment

- Not to be administered to patients with any hepatic insufficiency
- Not recommended for use in patients with substantial alcohol use
- Increased risk of elevation of serum transaminase levels

Cardiac Impairment

- Drug should be used with caution
- Duloxetine may raise heart rate (by 2 BPM on average) in pediatric and may increase

blood pressure in youth by, on average, 2 mmHg (Strawn et al., 2015)

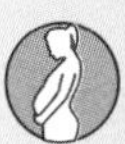

Pregnancy

- Controlled studies have not been conducted in pregnant women
- Not generally recommended for use during pregnancy, especially during first trimester
- Nonetheless, continuous treatment during pregnancy may be necessary and has not been proven to be harmful to the fetus
- Must weigh the risk of treatment (first trimester fetal development, third trimester newborn delivery) to the child against the risk of no treatment (recurrence of depression, maternal health, infant bonding) to the mother and child
- For many patients this may mean continuing treatment during pregnancy
- Neonates exposed to SSRIs or SNRIs late in the third trimester have developed complications requiring prolonged hospitalization, respiratory support, and tube feeding; reported symptoms are consistent with either a direct toxic effect of SSRIs and SNRIs or, possibly, a drug discontinuation syndrome, and include respiratory distress, cyanosis, apnea, seizures, temperature instability, feeding difficulty, vomiting, hypoglycemia, hypotonia, hypertonia, hyperreflexia, tremor, jitteriness, irritability, and constant crying

Breast Feeding

- Some drug is found in breast milk
- If child becomes irritable or sedated, breast feeding or drug may need to be discontinued
- Immediate postpartum period is a high-risk time for depression, especially in women who have had prior depressive episodes, so drug may need to be reinstituted late in the third trimester or shortly after childbirth to prevent a recurrence during the postpartum period
- Must weigh benefits of breast feeding with risks and benefits of antidepressant treatment versus nontreatment to both the infant and the mother
- For many patients, this may mean continuing treatment during breast feeding

THE ART OF PSYCHOPHARMACOLOGY

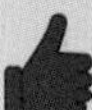

Potential Advantages

- In children:
  - Specifically approved by the US FDA for generalized anxiety disorder in children
- In adolescents:
  - Specifically approved by the US FDA for generalized anxiety disorder in adolescents
- All ages:
  - Patients with atypical depression (hypersomnia, increased appetite)
  - Patients with comorbid anxiety
  - Patients with depression may have higher remission rates on SNRIs than on SSRIs
  - Depressed patients with somatic symptoms, fatigue, and pain
  - Patients who do not respond or remit on treatment with SSRIs

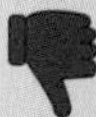

Potential Disadvantages

- In children and adolescents:
  - Those who are already psychomotor agitated, angry, or irritable, and who do not have a psychiatric diagnosis
  - Those who may possibly have a mood disorder with mixed or bipolar features, especially those with these features and a family history of bipolar disorder
- All ages:
  - Patients sensitive to nausea

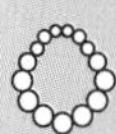

Pearls

- SSRIs and SNRIs show a small to medium effect in reducing childhood and adolescent anxiety in controlled clinical trials but may have more robust effects in clinical practice
- Many SSRIs and SNRIs have an even smaller effect and sometimes no effect in controlled clinical trials of child and adolescent depression yet can show robust efficacy in clinical practice
- Overall, adolescents respond better than children to SSRIs/SNRIs
- Duloxetine has well-documented efficacy for the painful physical symptoms of depression
- Duloxetine has only somewhat greater potency for serotonin reuptake blockade than for norepinephrine reuptake blockade, but this is of unclear clinical significance as a differentiator from other SNRIs

- No head-to-head studies, but may have less hypertension than venlafaxine XR
- Powerful pro-noradrenergic actions may occur at doses greater than 60 mg/day
- Not well studied in ADHD, but may be effective
- Approved in many countries for stress urinary incontinence
- Patients may have higher remission rate for depression on SNRIs than on SSRIs

- Add or switch to or from pro-noradrenergic agents (e.g., atomoxetine, reboxetine, other SNRIs, mirtazapine, maprotiline, nortriptyline, desipramine, bupropion) with caution
- Add or switch to or from CYP2D6 substrates with caution (e.g., atomoxetine, maprotiline, nortriptyline, desipramine)
- Mechanism of action as SNRI suggests it may be effective in some patients who fail to respond to SSRIs

SUGGESTED READING

Bridge JA, Iyengar S, Salary CB et al. Clinical response and risk for reported suicidal ideation and suicide attempts in pediatric antidepressant treatment: a meta-analysis of randomized controlled trials. JAMA 2007;297(15):1683–96.

Croarkin PE, Elmaadawi AZ, Aaronson ST et al. Left prefrontal transcranial magnetic stimulation for treatment-resistant depression in adolescents: a double-blind, randomized, sham-controlled trial. Neuropsychopharmacology 2021;46(2):462–9.

Emslie GJ, Wells TG, Prakash A et al. Acute and longer-term safety results from a pooled analysis of duloxetine studies for the treatment of children and adolescents with major depressive disorder. J Child Adolesc Psychopharmacol 2015;25(4):293–305.

Hathaway EE, Walkup JT, Strawn JR. Antidepressant treatment duration in pediatric depressive and anxiety disorders: how long is long enough? Curr Probl Pediatr Adolesc Health Care 2018;48(2):31–9.

Lobo ED, Quinlan T, Prakash A. Pharmacokinetics of orally administered duloxetine in children and adolescents with major depressive disorder. Clin Pharmacokinet 2014;53(8):731–40.

Strawn JR, Prakash A, Zhang Q et al. A randomized, placebo-controlled study of duloxetine for the treatment of children and adolescents with generalized anxiety disorder. J Am Acad Child Adolesc Psychiatry 2015;54(4):283–93.

Strawn JR, Mills JA, Poweleit EA, Ramsey LB, Croarkin PE. Adverse effects of antidepressant medications and their management in children and adolescents. Pharmacotherapy 2023;43(7):675–90.

ESCITALOPRAM

THERAPEUTICS

Brands

- Chemmart
- Cipralex
- Lexapro

Generic

Yes

US FDA Approved for Pediatric Use

- Major depressive disorder (ages 12 and older)
- Generalized anxiety disorder (ages 7 and older)

Off-Label for Pediatric Use

- Approved in adults
  - None
- Other off-label uses
  - Separation anxiety disorder
  - Obsessive-compulsive disorder (OCD)
  - Social anxiety disorder
  - Panic disorder
  - Premenstrual dysphoric disorder
  - Posttraumatic stress disorder (PTSD)

Class and Mechanism of Action

- Neuroscience-based Nomenclature: serotonin reuptake inhibitor (S-RI)
- SSRI (selective serotonin reuptake inhibitor); often classified as a drug for depression (i.e., antidepressant), but it is not just an antidepressant
- Escitalopram presumably increases serotonergic neurotransmission by blocking the serotonin reuptake pump (transporter, SERT), which results in the desensitization of serotonin receptors, especially serotonin 1A receptors. Escitalopram also binds allosterically at the SERT which increases its binding at the active site.
- In adolescents with anxiety disorders, escitalopram (but not placebo) increases the connections between the amygdala and regions of the brain that dampen the activity of the amygdala (i.e., prefrontal cortex) (Lu et al., 2022). These changes in brain circuits in adolescents who are treated with escitalopram predict more clinical improvement (Lu et al., 2022).

SAFETY AND TOLERABILITY

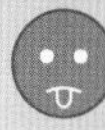

Notable Side Effects

- Several central nervous system side effects (insomnia but also sedation, especially if not sleeping at night, agitation, headache, dizziness)
- Note: patients with diagnosed or undiagnosed bipolar or psychotic disorders may be more vulnerable to CNS-activating actions of SSRIs like escitalopram; pay particular attention to signs of activation in children with developmental disorders or autism spectrum disorders
- Treatment-emergent activation syndrome (TEAS) includes agitation, anxiety, panic attacks, irritability, aggression, impulsivity, and insomnia. For citalopram/escitalopram in pediatric patients, the risk of activation is greater in slower CYP2C19 metabolizers and has been associated with greater blood levels of citalopram/escitalopram.
- TEAS can represent side effects but should not be confused with bipolar mania or the onset of suicidality and should be monitored and investigated with consideration of discontinuing or decreasing the dose of escitalopram or addition of another agent or switching to another agent to reduce these symptoms
- Gastrointestinal (nausea, diarrhea, constipation, dry mouth)
- Sexual dysfunction (boys: delayed ejaculation, erectile dysfunction; boys and girls: decreased sexual desire, anorgasmia)
- Autonomic (sweating)
- Bruising and rare bleeding
- Syndrome of inappropriate antidiuretic hormone secretion (SIADH)

Life-Threatening or Dangerous Side Effects

- Rare seizures
- Rare induction of mania
- Rare suicidal ideation and behavior (suicidality) (short-term regulatory studies did not show any actual suicides in any age group and also did not show an increase in the risk of suicidality with antidepressants compared to placebo beyond age 24)

Growth and Maturation

- In adolescents, escitalopram may increase visceral fat mass and have unclear effects on bone mineralization

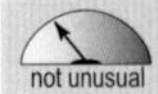

Weight Gain

- Weight gain is dose related and more common in adolescents who are slower CYP2C19 metabolizers

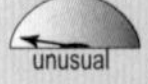

Sedation

- Reported but not common

What to Do About Side Effects

- Wait, wait, wait: mild side effects are common, happen early, and usually improve with time, but treatment benefits can be delayed and often begin just as the side effects wear off. However, some side effects may emerge later such as weight gain.
- Monitor side effects closely, especially when initiating treatment
- May wish to give in the evening or at bedtime, particularly if the medication is associated with sedation
- For activation (jitteriness, anxiety, insomnia):
    - Activation with escitalopram is dose related and more likely in slower CYP2C19 metabolizers. Consider a temporary dose reduction or a more gradual up-titration.
    - Administer dose in the morning
    - Consider switching to another SSRI or potentially an SNRI (other than venlafaxine)
    - Optimize psychotherapeutic interventions
    - Activation and agitation may represent the induction of a bipolar state, especially a mixed dysphoric bipolar II condition sometimes associated with suicidal ideation, and may require the addition of lithium, or an atypical antipsychotic, and/or discontinuation of escitalopram
- Often best to try another monotherapy prior to resorting to augmentation strategies to treat side effects
- For insomnia: consider adding melatonin
- For GI upset: try giving medication with a meal
- For sexual dysfunction:
    - Probably best to reduce dose or discontinue and try another agent
    - Consider adding daytime exercise, bupropion, or buspirone
- For emotional flattening, apathy: consider adding bupropion (with caution as little experience in children)

How Drug Causes Side Effects

- Theoretically due to increases in serotonin concentrations at serotonin receptors in parts of the brain and body other than those that cause therapeutic actions (e.g., unwanted actions of serotonin in sleep centers causing insomnia, unwanted actions of serotonin in the gut causing diarrhea)
- Increasing serotonin can cause diminished dopamine release and might contribute to emotional flattening, cognitive slowing, and apathy in some patients
- As escitalopram has no known important secondary pharmacological properties, its side effects are presumably all mediated by its serotonin reuptake blockade

Warnings and Precautions

- Consider distributing the brochures provided by the FDA and the drug companies as well as the medication guides from the American Academy of Child & Adolescent Psychiatry (AACAP)
- Carefully consider monitoring patients regularly and within the practical limits, particularly during the first several weeks of treatment
- Warn patients and their caregivers when possible about the possibility of activating side effects and advise them to report such symptoms
- Carefully weigh the risks and benefits of pharmacological treatment against the risks and benefits of nontreatment with antidepressants and make sure to document this in the patient's chart
- As with any antidepressant, use with caution in patients with history of seizure
- As with any antidepressant, use with caution in patients with bipolar disorder unless treated with concomitant mood-stabilizing agent
- Monitor patients for activation and suicidal ideation and involve parents/guardians

When Not to Prescribe

- If patient is taking an MAO inhibitor
- If patient is taking pimozide
- If there is a proven allergy to escitalopram

Long-Term Use

- Weight gain has been observed in citalopram-treated youth, so growth should be monitored; long-term effects are unknown

Habit Forming

- No

Overdose

- Rare fatalities have been reported; symptoms include convulsions, coma, dizziness, hypotension, insomnia, nausea, vomiting, sinus tachycardia, somnolence, and ECG changes

DOSING AND USE

Usual Dosage Range

- In children: 5–20 mg/day
- In adolescents: 10–20 mg/day

Dosage Forms

- Tablet 5 mg, 10 mg (scored), 20 mg (scored)
- Oral solution 5 mg/5 mL

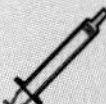

How to Dose

- In children (depression and anxiety disorders): initial dose 5 mg/day; after 1–2 weeks can increase to 10 mg/day, and after another 2 weeks can increase to 20 mg/day
- In adolescents (depression): initial dose 10 mg/day; after 2 weeks can increase to 20 mg/day. However, in anxious youth may consider starting at 5 mg/day for 2 days and then increasing to 10 mg/day.
- Because escitalopram concentrations vary significantly in adolescents based on their CYP2C19 activity, clinicians could consider adjusting the dose based on CYP2C19 activity (Figure 1).

Options for Administration

- Liquid formulation can be beneficial for patients requiring very slow titration and in those who cannot swallow tablets

Tests

- None for healthy individuals

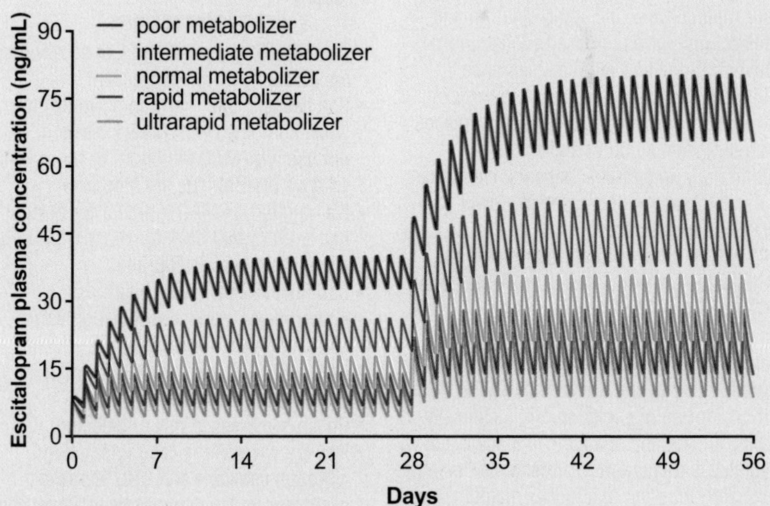

Figure 1 Escitalopram plasma concentrations in adolescents with different CYP2C19 phenotypes. Treatment was initiated at 10 mg daily and increased to 20 mg daily at week 4. There is considerable variation in blood concentrations of escitalopram among the CYP2C19 phenotypes, as demonstrated in this series of adolescent patients. Adapted from Strawn et al., 2019.

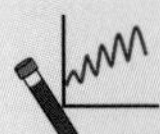

Pharmacokinetics

- Mean terminal half-life is 27–32 hours in adults. In children and adolescents, its half-life is related to CYP2C19 metabolism. Children and adolescents who are normal metabolizers have a half-life of 20.9 hours, while poor metabolizers have a half-life of 61 hours, and ultrarapid metabolizers have a half-life of 16 hours (Poweleit et al., 2023).
- Steady-state plasma concentrations achieved within 1 week
- Substrate for CYP2C19 and 3A4 as well as CYP2D6 (Figure 2)
- Escitalopram has low protein binding (56%) and is not likely to cause interactions with highly protein-bound drugs
- No significant actions on CYP450 enzymes
- Peak blood levels (Cmax) occur at about 5 hours after dosing and food does not alter escitalopram absorption

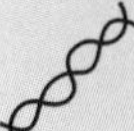

Pharmacogenetics

- Because citalopram, escitalopram, and sertraline are extensively metabolized by CYP2C19, variants impacting CYP2C19 activity may alter drug exposure. CYP2C19 poor metabolizers, including children and adolescents, have increased escitalopram concentrations and reduced clearance (Figure 3), which may increase the risk of adverse drug reactions, including increased drug discontinuation or switching. Additionally, in pediatric patients, clearance of escitalopram is decreased in slower CYP2C19 metabolizers.
  - **CYP2C19 ultrarapid metabolizers:** The Clinical Pharmacogenetics Implementation Consortium (CPIC) recommends clinicians consider a clinically appropriate alternative antidepressant not predominantly metabolized by CYP2C19. If citalopram or escitalopram is clinically appropriate, and adequate efficacy is not achieved at standard maintenance dosing, consider titrating to a higher maintenance dose.
  - **CYP2C19 normal metabolizers:** CPIC recommends that clinicians initiate therapy with recommended starting dose. If patient does not adequately respond to recommended maintenance dosing, consider titrating to a higher maintenance dose or switching to a clinically appropriate alternative antidepressant not predominantly metabolized by CYP2C19.
  - **CYP2C19 intermediate metabolizers:** CPIC recommends (moderate) that clinicians initiate the standard starting dose but consider a slower titration and lower maintenance dose than normal metabolizers.
  - **CYP2C19 poor metabolizers:** CPIC recommends that clinicians consider an antidepressant not predominantly metabolized by CYP2C19. If citalopram or escitalopram is clinically appropriate, consider a lower starting dose, slower titration, and 50% reduction of the standard maintenance dose as compared to normal metabolizers.
  - Additionally, per the FDA warning, citalopram 20 mg/day is the maximum recommended dose in CYP2C19 poor metabolizers due to the risk of QTc prolongation. FDA product labeling additionally cautions that citalopram dose should be limited to 20 mg/day in patients with hepatic impairment and in those taking a CYP2C19 inhibitor.

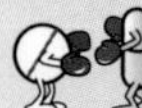

Drug Interactions

- Tramadol increases the risk of seizures in adults taking an antidepressant
- Can cause a fatal "serotonin syndrome" when combined with MAO inhibitors, so do not use with MAO inhibitors or for at least 14 days after MAOIs are stopped
- Do not start an MAO inhibitor for at least 5 half-lives (5 to 7 days for most drugs) after discontinuing escitalopram
- Can theoretically cause weakness, hyperreflexia, and incoordination when combined with sumatriptan, or possibly with other triptans, requiring careful monitoring of patient
- Possible increased risk of bleeding
- Few known adverse drug interactions, although cannabis and CBD increase escitalopram concentrations in adolescents (Vaughn et al., 2021). Also, proton pump inhibitors (e.g., omeprazole) will increase the concentrations of escitalopram by approximately 50%.

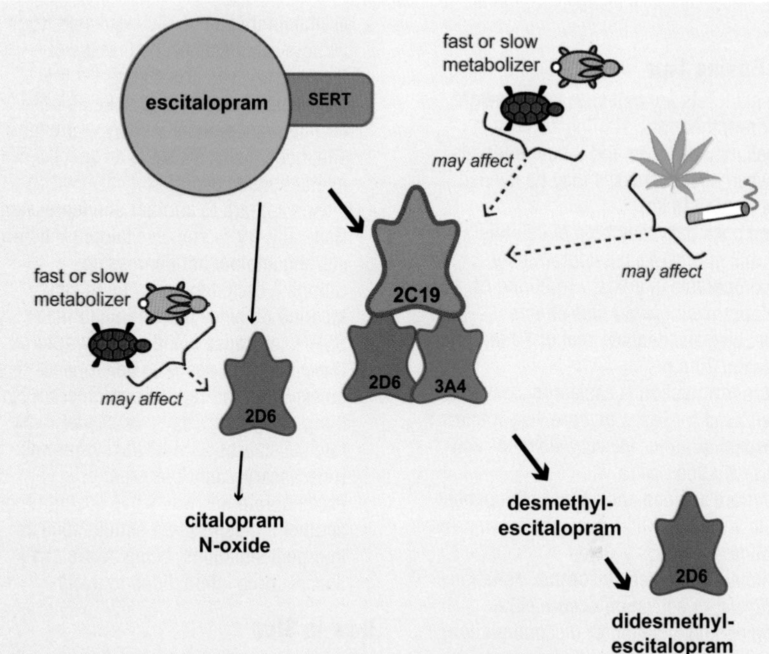

Figure 2 Escitalopram metabolism. Escitalopram is metabolized primarily through CYP2C19 and variation in CYP2C19 activity produces differences in escitalopram exposure (i.e., blood levels over time) in children and adolescents.

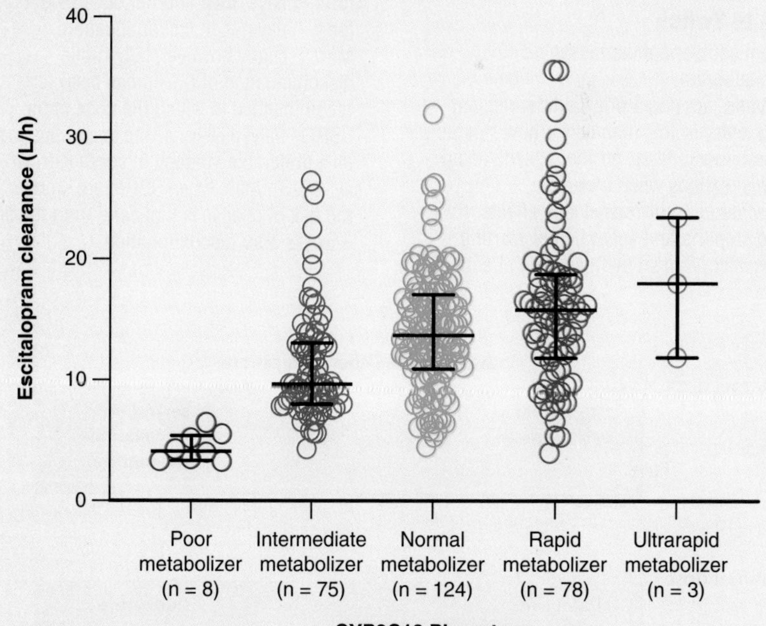

Figure 3 CYP2C19 phenotype effect on escitalopram clearance in children and adolescents. Adapted from Poweleit et al., Clinical Pharmacokinetics, 2023.

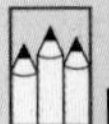

Dosing Tips

- Plasma levels are higher in lower-weight children; therefore, starting and target doses may be lower and longer intervals between dose increases may be needed (see How to Dose)
- Given once daily, any time of day tolerated
- Ten milligrams of escitalopram may be comparable in efficacy to 20 mg of citalopram with fewer side effects
- Thus, give an adequate trial of 10 mg prior to giving 20 mg
- Liquid formulation is easiest for low doses when used for cases that are very intolerant to escitalopram or for very slow up- and down-titration needs
- The more anxious and agitated the patient, the lower the starting dose, the slower the titration
- If intolerable anxiety, insomnia, agitation, akathisia, or activation occurs either upon dosing initiation or discontinuation, consider an alternative SSRI. Importantly, the risk of activation with one SSRI does not predict the likelihood of activation with another SSRI.

How to Switch

- From another antidepressant to escitalopram:
  - When tapering a prior antidepressant, see its entry in this manual for how to stop and how to taper off that specific drug
  - In situations when there are antidepressant-related side effects, try to stop the first agent before starting escitalopram so that new side effects of escitalopram can be distinguished from withdrawal effects of the first agent
  - If necessary, can cross taper off the prior antidepressant and dose up on escitalopram simultaneously in urgent situations, being aware of all specific drug interactions to avoid
- Off escitalopram to another antidepressant:
  - Generally, try to stop escitalopram before starting another antidepressant
  - Stopping escitalopram often means tapering off since discontinuing many SSRIs can cause withdrawal symptoms
  - If escitalopram needs to be stopped quickly, one can reduce escitalopram by 5 mg every 3 to 7 days, or slower if this rate still causes withdrawal symptoms
  - If necessary, can cross taper off escitalopram this way while dosing up on another antidepressant simultaneously in urgent situations, being aware of all specific drug interactions to avoid

How to Stop

- Taper may not be necessary; however, tapering to avoid potential withdrawal reactions is generally prudent
- Many patients tolerate 50% dose reduction for 4–6 days, then another 50% reduction for 4–6 days, then discontinuation. More recently however, hyperbolic discontinuation of SSRIs has been recommended in which the dose of the SSRI is halved every 4 weeks and this may be a preferable strategy in youth (Strawn et al., 2023). Also, when SSRIs are stopped, the risk of relapse is highest during the first 8 weeks after discontinuation.

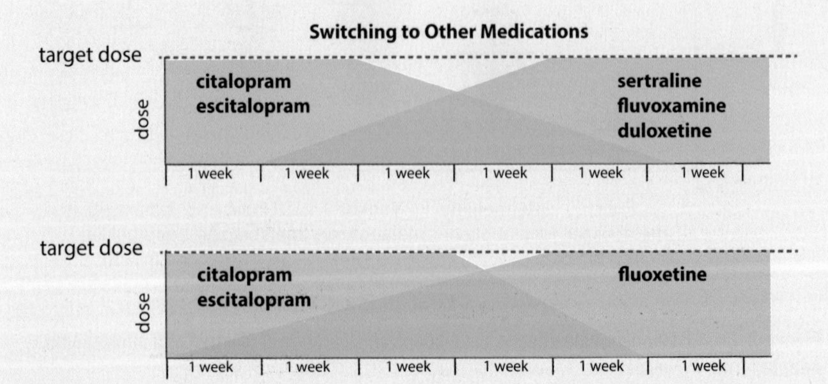

- If withdrawal symptoms emerge during discontinuation, raise dose to stop symptoms and then restart withdrawal much more slowly such as reducing escitalopram by 5 mg every 10 days

WHAT TO EXPECT

Onset of Action

- Some patients may experience increased energy or activation early after initiation of treatment
- Full onset of therapeutic actions is usually delayed by 2–4 weeks. However, two double-blind, placebo-controlled trials in adolescents suggest that benefit may occur within the first 2 weeks (Strawn et al., 2020, 2023)
- If it is not working within 6–8 weeks, it may require a dosage increase or it may not work at all

Duration of Action

- Effects are consistent over a 24-hour period
- May continue to work for many years to prevent relapse of symptoms

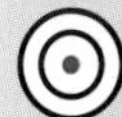

Primary Target Symptoms

- Depressed and/or irritable mood
- Anxiety (fear and worry are often target symptoms, but escitalopram can occasionally and transiently increase these symptoms short term before improving them)
- Sleep disturbance, both hypersomnia and insomnia (eventually, but can actually cause insomnia, especially short term)
- Prior to initiation of treatment, it is helpful to develop a list of target symptoms of depression and/or anxiety to monitor during treatment to better assess treatment response

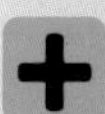

What Is Considered a Positive Result?

- The goal of treatment is complete remission of current symptoms as well as prevention of future relapses
- In practice, many patients have only a partial response where some symptoms are improved but others persist (especially insomnia, fatigue, and problems concentrating in depression), in which case higher doses of escitalopram, adding a second agent, or switching to an agent with a different mechanism of action can be considered
- If treatment works, it most often reduces or even eliminates symptoms, but is not a cure since symptoms can recur after medicine is stopped

How Long to Treat

- For adolescents with depression, generally, 9–12 months of antidepressant treatment is recommended (Hathaway et al., 2018)
- For anxiety disorders, 6–9 months of antidepressant treatment may be sufficient, though many clinicians extend treatment to 12 months based on extrapolation of data from adults with anxiety disorders (Hathaway et al., 2018; Strawn et al., 2020)
- Extended treatment periods may decrease the risk of long-term morbidity and recurrence; however, the goal of treatment is ultimately remission, rather than duration of antidepressant pharmacotherapy (Hathaway et al., 2018)
- In terms of the length of antidepressant treatment, evidence-based guidelines represent a starting point; appropriate treatment duration varies, and patient-specific response, psychological factors, and timing of discontinuation must be considered for individual pediatric patients (Hathaway et al., 2018)

What If It Stops Working?

- Some patients who have an initial response may relapse even though they continue treatment, sometimes called "poop-out"
- Some patients may experience apparent lack of consistent efficacy due to activation syndrome or latent or underlying or newly evolved bipolar disorder, or major depressive episodes with mixed features, and require antidepressant discontinuation and a switch to a second generation antipsychotic

What If It Doesn't Work?

- Consider evaluation for another diagnosis (especially bipolar illness or depression with mixed features) or for a comorbid condition (e.g., medical illness, substance abuse)

- When treating youth with anxiety disorders, many patients will have had significant anxiety for years prior to beginning treatment. As such, when anxiety is treated with an SSRI, their symptoms may be improved, but the patient has likely missed important developmental milestones (e.g., spending the night with friends, being able to ask questions in class). Developing these skills will take time. Beyond this, the family may have lived with the anxious child for years and following treatment of the child, the family may need to readjust.
- Be mindful of family conflict contributing to the presentation; sometimes treating parental depression or anxiety disorders improves psychiatric and social function without any treatment of youth. Also, accommodation is common in families of youth with anxiety disorders and may need to be addressed specifically, as it can perpetuate symptoms.
- Consider factors associated with poor response to SSRIs in treatment-resistant depression or anxiety disorders, such as severe symptoms, long-lasting symptoms, poor treatment adherence, prior nonresponse to other treatments, and the presence of comorbid disorders
- Consider other important potential factors such as ongoing conflicts, family psychopathology, and an adverse environment (e.g., poverty, chaos, violence, prior and ongoing psychological trauma, abuse, neglect). Additionally, when symptoms are prominent at school, consider the presence of a learning disorder.
- Institute trauma-informed care for appropriate children and adolescents
- A 2007 meta-analysis of published and unpublished trials in pediatric patients found that antidepressants had a number needed to treat (NNT) of 10 for depression, 6 for OCD, and 3 for anxiety disorders; thus, escitalopram may not work in all children, so consider switching to another antidepressant (Bridge et al., 2007)
- Consider a dose adjustment in escitalopram-treated patients, particularly if the patient is a CYP2C19 ultrarapid metabolizer
- Consider augmenting options:
    - Cognitive behavioral therapy (CBT), interpersonal psychotherapy for adolescents (IPT-A), light therapy, family therapy, and exercise especially in adolescents
    - For partial response (depression): use caution when adding medications to escitalopram, especially in children, since there are not sufficient studies of augmentation in children or adolescents; however, for the expert, consider bupropion, aripiprazole, or other atypical antipsychotics such as quetiapine; use combinations of antidepressants with caution as this may activate bipolar disorder and suicidal ideation
    - For insomnia: sleep hygiene, CBT for insomnia, melatonin, or alpha 2 agonists
    - For anxiety: buspirone, antihistamines
    - Add lithium or atypical antipsychotics for bipolar depression, psychotic depression, treatment-resistant depression, or treatment-resistant anxiety disorders
    - TMS (transcranial magnetic stimulation) may have a role although pediatric trials of TMS have been hampered by high sham response rates (Croarkin et al., 2021)
    - ECT (case studies show effectiveness; cognitive side effects are similar to those in adults; reserve for treatment-resistant cases)

TALKING TO PATIENTS AND CAREGIVERS

What to Tell Parents About Efficacy

- Doesn't work right away; full therapeutic benefits may take up to 8 weeks, yet parents and teachers might see improvement before the patient does
- While the medicine helps by reducing symptoms and improving function, it is not a cure, and it is therefore necessary to keep taking the medication to sustain its therapeutic effects
- Since every treatment consideration depends on a risk/benefit analysis, parents should fully understand short- and long-term risks as well as benefits
- One of the SSRIs specifically approved for adolescents with depression and has been studied extensively in children and adolescents with anxiety disorders

- After successful treatment, continuation of escitalopram may be necessary to prevent relapse, especially in those who have had more than one episode or a very severe episode. In general, when treating depression in children and adolescents, medications are continued for 12 months after symptoms have resolved, while for anxiety disorders, clinicians have generally treated for 6–9 months (Hathaway et al., 2018).
- Often a good idea to tell parents whether the medication chosen is specifically approved for the disorder being treated, or if it is "unapproved" or "off-label" but nevertheless good clinical practice and based upon prudent extrapolation of controlled data from adults and from experience in children and adolescents instead of formal FDA approval

What to Tell Children and Adolescents About Efficacy

- We are trying to make you feel better
- It may be a good idea to give the medication a try; if it's not working very well, we can stop the medication and try something else
- A good try takes 2 to 3 months or even longer
- If it does make you feel better, you cannot stop it right away or you may feel sad or worried again
- Medications don't change who you are as a person; they give you the opportunity to be the best person you can be

What to Tell Parents About Side Effects

- Explain that side effects are expected in many when starting and are most common in the first 2–3 weeks of starting or increasing the dose
- Some SSRI side effects emerge early and resolve quickly (e.g., activation, gastrointestinal symptoms). In contrast, other side effects are late-emerging (e.g., weight gain) or persistent (e.g., sexual dysfunction). Discussing the temporal course of the side effects and distinguishing between persistent and transient side effects is critical. Ensuring that patients are aware not only of side effects but the tendency of some side effects to be transient is important and should be part of discussions with patients and their families. For many, knowing that a side effect is likely transient, as opposed to persistent, may significantly influence the patient and family's anxiety or fears related to medication (Strawn et al., 2023).
- Tell parents many side effects go away and do so about the same time that therapeutic effects start
- Predict side effects in advance (you will look clever and competent to the parents, unless you scare them with too much information and cause nocebo effects, in which case you won't look so clever when the patient develops lots of side effects and stops medication; use your judgment here); a balanced but honest presentation is an art rather than a science
- Ask them to help monitor for increased suicidality and if present, report any such symptoms immediately
- Ask parents to support the patient while side effects are occurring
- Parents should fully understand short- and long-term risks as well as benefits
- Explaining to the parents what to expect from medication treatment, and especially potential side effects, can help prevent early termination of medication

What to Tell Children and Adolescents About Side Effects

- Even if you get side effects, most of them get better or go away in a few days to a few weeks
- Consider having a conversation about sexual side effects in some adolescents who can find these side effects confusing and especially burdensome
- Explaining to child/adolescent what to expect from medication treatment, and especially potential side effects, can help prevent early termination of medication
- Tell adolescents and children capable of understanding that some young patients, especially those who are depressed, may develop thoughts of hurting themselves, and if this happens, not to be alarmed but to tell their parents right away

What to Tell Teachers About the Medication (If Parents Consent)

- It is not abusable
- Encourage dialogue with parents/guardians about any behavior or mood changes

SPECIAL POPULATIONS

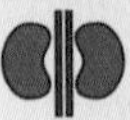

Renal Impairment

- No dose adjustment for mild to moderate impairment
- Use cautiously in patients with severe impairment

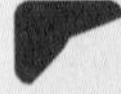

Hepatic Impairment

- Recommended dose 10 mg/day

Cardiac Impairment

- Not systematically evaluated in patients with cardiac impairment
- In a study using US claims data, the crude incident rate of adverse cardiac events in pediatric patients taking escitalopram was 19.5/10,000 person-years (Czaja et al., 2013)
- None of the randomized controlled trials of escitalopram in pediatric patients suggests increased QTc in escitalopram-treated youth

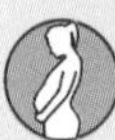

Pregnancy

- Controlled studies have not been conducted in pregnant women
- Not generally recommended for use during pregnancy, especially during first trimester
- Nonetheless, continuous treatment during pregnancy may be necessary and has not been proven to be harmful to the fetus
- At delivery there may be more bleeding in the mother and transient irritability or sedation in the newborn
- Must weigh the risk of treatment (first trimester fetal development, third trimester newborn delivery) to the child against the risk of no treatment (recurrence of depression, maternal health, infant bonding) to the mother and child
- For many patients, this may mean continuing treatment during pregnancy
- Exposure to SSRIs early in pregnancy may be associated with increased risk of septal heart defects (absolute risk is small)
- SSRI use beyond the 20th week of pregnancy may be associated with increased risk of pulmonary hypertension in newborns, although this is not proven
- Exposure to SSRIs late in pregnancy may be associated with increased risk of gestational hypertension and preeclampsia
- Neonates exposed to SSRIs or SNRIs late in the third trimester have developed complications requiring prolonged hospitalization, respiratory support, and tube feeding; reported symptoms are consistent with either a direct toxic effect of SSRIs and SNRIs or, possibly, a drug discontinuation syndrome, and include respiratory distress, cyanosis, apnea, seizures, temperature instability, feeding difficulty, vomiting, hypoglycemia, hypotonia, hypertonia, hyperreflexia, tremor, jitteriness, irritability, and constant crying

Breast Feeding

- Some drug is found in breast milk
- Trace amounts may be present in nursing children whose mothers are on escitalopram
- If child becomes irritable or sedated, breast feeding or drug may need to be discontinued
- Immediate postpartum period is a high-risk time for depression, especially in women who have had prior depressive episodes, so drug may need to be reinstituted late in the third trimester or shortly after childbirth to prevent a recurrence during the postpartum period
- Must weigh benefits of breast feeding with risks and benefits of antidepressant treatment versus nontreatment to both the infant and the mother
- For many patients, this may mean continuing treatment during breast feeding

THE ART OF PSYCHOPHARMACOLOGY

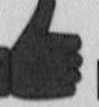

Potential Advantages

- In adolescents:
  - One of only two agents approved for depression in adolescents (also fluoxetine)
  - One of only two agents approved for generalized anxiety disorder in children and adolescents (also duloxetine)
- All ages:
  - Patients taking concomitant medications (few drug interactions and fewer even than with citalopram)
  - Patients requiring faster onset of action
  - In general, escitalopram may be better tolerated than some other SSRIs, with

fewer drug interactions and without the warning for high dose QTc prolongation given to citalopram

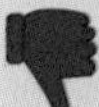

Potential Disadvantages

- Those who are already psychomotor agitated, angry, or irritable, and who do not have a psychiatric diagnosis
- Those who may possibly have a mood disorder with mixed or bipolar features, especially those with these features and a family history of bipolar disorder
- Approval of escitalopram for depression in adolescents is based on a single randomized controlled trial

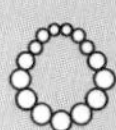

Pearls

- SSRIs show greater efficacy in pediatric anxiety disorders compared to depression
- In anxious youth, SSRIs produce faster and greater improvement compared to SNRIs (Strawn et al., 2018)
- In adolescents with anxiety disorders, escitalopram produces statistically significant improvement in emotional processing within two weeks and enhances the connection between the prefrontal cortex and the amygdala
- Can cause cognitive and affective "flattening"
- Escitalopram metabolism in children and adolescents is related to CYP2C19 metabolism. Poor metabolizers have nearly a threefold increase in half-life compared to normal metabolizers. Adjusting dosing can address this (see Pharmacogenetics).
- R-citalopram may interfere with the binding of S-citalopram at the serotonin transporter
- For this reason, S-citalopram may be more than twice as potent as R,S-citalopram (i.e., citalopram)
- Thus, 10 mg starting dose of S-citalopram may have the therapeutic efficacy of 20–40 mg of R,S-citalopram
- Thus, escitalopram may have faster onset and better efficacy with reduced side effects compared to R,S-citalopram
- Cannabis and cannabidiol (CBD) may increase escitalopram concentrations in adolescents through their effects at CYP2C19 (Vaughn et al., 2021)
- Escitalopram is commonly used with augmenting agents, as it is the SSRI with the least interaction at either CYP2D6 or CYP3A4, therefore causing fewer pharmacokinetically mediated drug interactions with augmenting agents than other SSRIs
- Some side effects of escitalopram, including weight gain and activation, are related to blood levels or CYP2C19 metabolism. Slower CYP2C19 metabolizers experience more side effects, but have faster improvement.

SUGGESTED READING

Aldrich SL, Poweleit EA, Prows CA et al. Influence of CYP2C19 metabolizer status on escitalopram/citalopram tolerability and response in youth with anxiety and depressive disorders. Front Pharmacol 2019;10:99.

Bridge JA, Iyengar S, Salary CB et al. Clinical response and risk for reported suicidal ideation and suicide attempts in pediatric antidepressant treatment: a meta-analysis of randomized controlled trials. JAMA 2007;297(15):1683–96.

Croarkin PE, Elmaadawi AZ, Aaronson ST et al. Left prefrontal transcranial magnetic stimulation for treatment-resistant depression in adolescents: a double-blind, randomized, sham-controlled trial. Neuropsychopharmacology 2021;46(2):462–9.

Czaja AS, Valuck RJ, Anderson HD. Comparative safety of selective serotonin reuptake inhibitors among pediatric users with respect to adverse cardiac events. Pharmacoepidemiol Drug Saf 2013;22(6):607–14.

Emslie GJ, Ventura D, Korotzer A, Tourkodimitris S. Escitalopram in the treatment of adolescent depression: a randomized placebo-controlled multisite trial. J Am Acad Child Adolesc Psychiatry 2009;48(7):721–9.

Hathaway EE, Walkup JT, Strawn JR. Antidepressant treatment duration in pediatric depressive and anxiety disorders: how long is long enough? Curr Probl Pediatr Adolesc Health Care 2018;48(2):31–9.

Lu L, Li H, Baumel WT et al. Acute neurofunctional effects of escitalopram during emotional processing in pediatric anxiety: a double-blind, placebo-controlled trial. Neuropsychopharmacology 2022;47(5):1081–7.

Poweleit EA, Taylor ZL, Mizuno T et al. Escitalopram and sertraline population pharmacokinetic analysis in pediatric patients. Clin Pharmacokinet 2023;62(11):1621–37.

Strawn JR, Mills JA, Sauley BA, Welge JA. The impact of antidepressant dose and class on treatment response in pediatric anxiety disorders: a meta-analysis. J Am Acad Child Adolesc Psychiatry 2018;57(4):235–244.e2.

Strawn JR, Poweleit EA, Ramsey LB. CYP2C19-guided escitalopram and sertraline dosing in pediatric patients: a pharmacokinetic modeling study. J Child Adolesc Psychopharmacol 2019;29(5):340–7.

Strawn JR, Mills JA, Schroeder H et al. Escitalopram in adolescents with generalized anxiety disorder: a double-blind, randomized, placebo-controlled study. J Clin Psychiatry 2020;81(5):20m13396.

Strawn JR, Lu L, Peris TS, Levine A, Walkup JT. Research review: pediatric anxiety disorders – what have we learnt in the last 10 years? J Child Psychol Psychiatry 2021;62(2):114–39.

Strawn JR, Mills JA, Poweleit EA, Ramsey LB, Croarkin PE. Adverse effects of antidepressant medications and their management in children and adolescents. Pharmacotherapy 2023;43(7):675–90.

Vaughn SE, Strawn JR, Poweleit EA, Sarangdhar M, Ramsey LB. The impact of marijuana on antidepressant treatment in adolescents: clinical and pharmacologic considerations. J Pers Med 2021;11(7):615.

Wagner KD, Jonas J, Findling RL, Ventura D, Saikali K. A double-blind, randomized, placebo-controlled trial of escitalopram in the treatment of pediatric depression. J Am Acad Child Adolesc Psychiatry 2006;45(3):280–8.

THERAPEUTICS

Brands

- Spravato

Generic

No

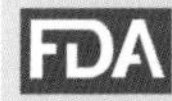

US FDA Approved for Pediatric Use

- None

Off-Label for Pediatric Use

- Approved in adults
  - Treatment-resistant depression in adults (adjunct)
  - Depressive symptoms in adults with major depressive disorder (MDD) with acute suicidal ideation or behavior (adjunct)

Class and Mechanism of Action

- Esketamine is a nonselective, noncompetitive open channel inhibitor of the NMDA receptor; specifically, it binds to the phencyclidine site of the NMDA receptor
- This leads to downstream glutamate release and consequent stimulation of other glutamate receptors, including AMPA receptors
- Theoretically, esketamine may have antidepressant effects because activation of AMPA receptors leads to activation of signal transduction cascades, including mTORC1, and an increase in growth factors such as BDNF, that cause the expression of synaptic proteins and an increase in the density of dendritic spines

SAFETY AND TOLERABILITY

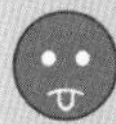

Notable Side Effects

- In pediatric patients with depression, the most common side effects are dizziness, nausea, dissociation, headache, dysgeusia, and somnolence
- In adolescents with depression, dissociative symptoms, measured by the Clinician Administered Dissociative States Scale total score, peak at 40 minutes and generally resolved by 1.5 hour post-dose
- In adults, numbness, hypoesthesia, blood pressure increase, and euphoric mood have been described. Of note, no changes in euphoria were seen in adolescent trials.
- Lower urinary tract symptoms, including increased frequency of urination (pollakiuria), have been described in adults

Life-Threatening or Dangerous Side Effects

- Dissociation, sedation (in the United States as part of the Risk Evaluation and Mitigation Strategy [REMS] there is a required monitoring for at least 2 hours at each treatment session)
- Increased blood pressure (peaks at approximately 40 minutes post-administration and lasts approximately 4 hours)
- Short-term cognitive impairment (generally resolves by 2 hours post-dose)

Growth and Maturation

- Not studied

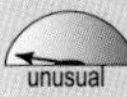

Weight Gain

- Reported but not expected

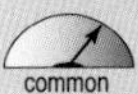

Sedation

- Many experience and/or can be significant in amount

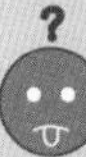

What to Do About Side Effects

- Use lower dose (56 mg rather than 84 mg)
- For CNS side effects, if clinically appropriate, discontinuation of nonessential centrally acting medications may help
- If blood pressure remains high, promptly seek consultation
- Refer patients experiencing symptoms of a hypertensive crisis (e.g., chest pain, shortness of breath) or hypertensive encephalopathy (e.g., sudden severe headache, visual disturbances, seizures, diminished consciousness or focal neurological deficits) immediately for emergency care

How Drug Causes Side Effects

- Direct effect on NMDA receptors

Warnings and Precautions

- Because of the risks of sedation and dissociation and of abuse and misuse, in the United States esketamine is only available through a restricted program under a REMS; healthcare settings and pharmacies must be certified in the REMS program, and pharmacies must only dispense esketamine to healthcare settings that are certified in the program
- Esketamine can raise blood pressure; patients with cardiovascular and cerebrovascular conditions and risk factors may be at an increased risk of associated adverse effects
- Blood pressure should be monitored post-administration of esketamine, and prompt medical care should be sought if blood pressure remains high; refer patients experiencing symptoms of a hypertensive crisis or hypertensive encephalopathy for immediate emergency care; in the United States, at least 2 hours' monitoring is required
- In patients with a history of hypertensive encephalopathy, more intensive monitoring, including more frequent blood pressure and symptom assessment, is warranted because these patients are at higher risk for developing encephalopathy with even small increases in blood pressure
- Because of the risks of delayed or prolonged sedation and dissociation, patients must be monitored at each treatment session, followed by an assessment to determine when the patient is clinically stable and ready to leave the healthcare facility; in the United States, at least 2 hours' monitoring is required
- Because of the risk of dissociation, carefully assess patients with psychosis before administering esketamine and only initiate treatment if the potential benefits outweigh the risks
- Esketamine may impair attention, judgment, thinking, reaction speed, and motor skills
- Esketamine may impair ability to drive and operate machinery; patients should not drive or operate machinery until the next day after a restful sleep
- Warn patients and their caregivers if possible about the possibility of activating side effects and advise them to report such symptoms immediately
- Monitor patients for activation of suicidal ideation, especially children and adolescents

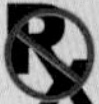

When Not to Prescribe

- If patient has aneurysmal vascular disease (including thoracic and abdominal aorta, intracranial and peripheral arterial vessels) or arteriovenous malformation
- If patient has a history of intracerebral hemorrhage
- If patient has had a recent (within 6 weeks) cardiovascular event, including myocardial infarction (MI)
- If there is a proven allergy to esketamine or ketamine

Long-Term Use

- Long-term cognitive effects of esketamine have not been evaluated beyond 1 year
- Long-term cognitive and memory impairment has been reported with repeated ketamine misuse or abuse

Habit Forming

- Esketamine is a Schedule III drug and in the United States is available only through a restricted program under a REMS

Overdose

- With racemic ketamine, symptoms of overdose include restlessness, psychosis, hallucinations, stupor, respiratory depression

DOSING AND USE

Usual Dosage Range (Treatment-Resistant Depression)

- Administer in conjunction with an oral antidepressant
- In adults, during the induction phase (weeks 1–4), administer twice per week; day 1 starting dose 56 mg; subsequent doses 56 mg or 84 mg. During the maintenance phase (weeks 5–8): administer once weekly; 56 mg or 84 mg. Finally, in weeks 9 and after, administer every 2 weeks or once weekly (use least-frequent dosing to maintain remission/response); 56 mg or 84 mg

Usual Dosage Range (MDD with Acute Suicidality)

- Administer in conjunction with an oral antidepressant
- In adolescents (clinical trial dosing), patients received intranasal esketamine 28, 56, or 84 mg twice per week for 4 weeks
- In adults, during the first 4 weeks of treatment, patients received 84 mg twice per week; dosage may be reduced to 56 mg twice per week based on tolerability
- After 4 weeks of treatment, evidence of therapeutic benefit should be evaluated to determine need for continued treatment

Dosage Forms

- 56 mg dose (two 28 mg nasal spray devices)
- 84 mg dose (three 28 mg nasal spray devices)
- In EU: 28 mg dose (for patients > 65 years old or adults of Japanese ancestry)

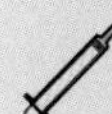

How to Dose

- Given in conjunction with an oral antidepressant
- Administered intranasally under the supervision of a healthcare clinician
- Each nasal spray device delivers two sprays containing a total of 28 mg of esketamine
- To prevent loss of medication, do not prime the device before use
- Patient should recline head at about 45 degrees during administration to keep medication inside the nose
- Patient should blow nose before first administration
- After patient self-administers both sprays (one in each nostril), check that the indicator shows no green dots; if there is a green dot, have patient spray again into the second nostril
- Use two devices (for a 56 mg dose) or three devices (for an 84 mg dose) with a 5-minute rest period between each device
- Blood pressure must be assessed before administration; if blood pressure is elevated, weigh the risks versus benefits of esketamine administration
- After dosing with esketamine, blood pressure should be reassessed at approximately 40 minutes and subsequently as clinically warranted
- Because of the possibility of sedation, dissociation, and elevated blood pressure, patients must be monitored by a healthcare professional until the patient is considered clinically stable and ready to leave the healthcare setting
- In the United States as part of the REMS, patients must be monitored for at least 2 hours at each treatment session; if blood pressure is decreasing and patient is clinically stable for at least 2 hours, the patient may be discharged; if not, continue to monitor
- Advise the patient not to engage in potentially hazardous activities, such as driving or operating machinery, until the next day after a restful sleep; patients will need to arrange transportation home

Options for Administration

- Available as a nasal spray

Tests

- Assess blood pressure prior to dosing: if baseline blood pressure is elevated (e.g., >140 mmHg systolic, >90 mmHg diastolic), consider the risks of short-term increases in blood pressure and benefit of esketamine treatment, and do not administer esketamine if an increase in blood pressure or intracranial pressure poses a serious risk
- Given its potential to induce dissociative effects, carefully assess patients with psychosis before administering esketamine

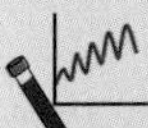

Pharmacokinetics

- When administered intranasally, it is rapidly absorbed through the nasal mucosa and enters the systemic circulation. In adults, time to maximum plasma concentration (Cmax) is approximately 20 to 40 minutes after the last administered nasal spray.
- Bioavailability of intranasal esketamine is variable, with approximately 48% to 55% of the dose absorbed
- Relatively large volume of distribution, indicating that it distributes extensively into tissues beyond the bloodstream. It is known to cross the blood–brain barrier, which is important for its antidepressant effects.
- Binds strongly to plasma proteins (approximately 94%), mainly to albumin
- Extensive hepatic metabolism, primarily through the cytochrome P450 system,

with CYP3A4 playing a significant role and CYP2B6, CYP2C9, and CYP2A6 playing minor roles (Figure 1)
- Metabolized into various metabolites, including noresketamine, which also has pharmacological activity (Figure 1)
- Elimination half-life of esketamine is relatively short, typically around 2 to 3 hours
- After intranasal administration, esketamine and its metabolites are mainly excreted in the urine (approximately 51% of the dose), with a smaller portion being excreted in the feces

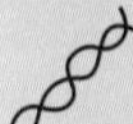

Pharmacogenetics

- No recommendations

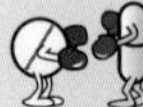

Drug Interactions

- Little potential to affect metabolism of drugs cleared by CYP enzymes
- Use with caution with other drugs that are NMDA antagonists (amantadine, memantine, dextromethorphan)
- Esketamine may increase the effects of other sedatives, including benzodiazepines, barbiturates, opioids, anesthetics, and alcohol
- Concomitant use with stimulants or monoamine oxidase inhibitors may increase blood pressure

Dosing Tips

- Nausea and vomiting are potential side effects, so advise patients to avoid food for at least 2 hours before administration and liquids for at least 30 minutes before administration
- Nasal corticosteroid or nasal decongestant should not be used within an hour prior to administration of esketamine
- If a patient misses treatment sessions and there is a worsening of symptoms, consider returning to the previous dosing schedule (i.e., every 2 weeks to once weekly, weekly to twice weekly)
- For treatment-resistant depression, evidence of therapeutic benefit should be evaluated at the end of the induction phase to determine the need for continued treatment
- For MDD with acute suicidality (FDA approval only), evidence of therapeutic benefit should be evaluated after 4 weeks to determine the need for continued treatment; use beyond 4 weeks has not been systematically evaluated

How to Switch

- Esketamine is used as an adjunct to an oral antidepressant

How to Stop

- Taper not necessary

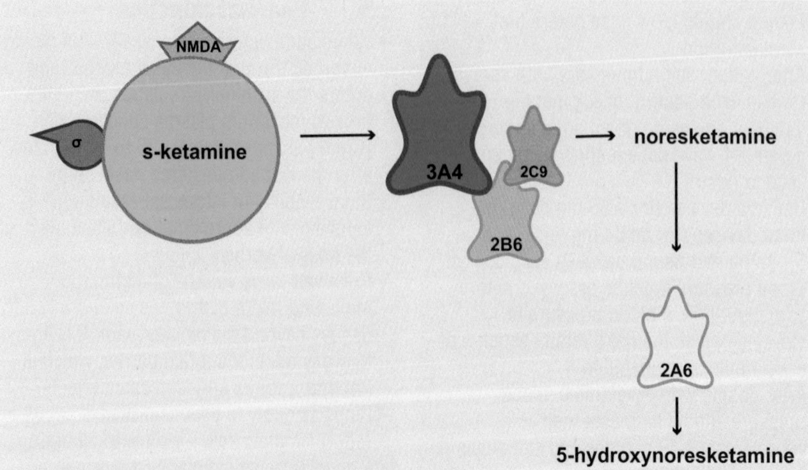

Figure 1 Metabolism of esketamine.

WHAT TO EXPECT

Onset of Action

- Antidepressant effects can occur within 24 hours

Duration of Action

- May continue to work for many years to prevent relapse of symptoms

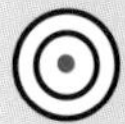

Primary Target Symptoms

- Treatment-resistant depression

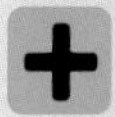

What Is Considered a Positive Result?

- Can immediately alleviate depressed mood and suicidal ideation
- Use of esketamine does not preclude the need for hospitalization if clinically warranted, even if patients experience improvement after an initial dose of esketamine

How Long to Treat

- Continue treatment until all symptoms are gone or until improvement is stable and then continue treating indefinitely as long as improvement persists

What If It Stops Working?

- Consider any prior antidepressant approaches that have not been exhausted and optimize psychosocial treatment
- Consider neuromodulation-based treatments
- Screen for the development of a new comorbid disorder, especially substance abuse
- Screen for adverse changes in the home or school environment

What If It Doesn't Work?

- Consider any prior antidepressant approaches that have not been exhausted and optimize psychosocial treatment
- Consider neuromodulation-based treatments
- Consider evaluation for another diagnosis or for a comorbid condition (e.g., medical illness, substance abuse)
- Consider other important potential factors such as ongoing conflicts, family psychopathology, and an adverse environment (e.g., poverty, chaos, violence, prior and ongoing psychological trauma, abuse, neglect)
- Institute trauma-informed care for appropriate children and adolescents

TALKING TO PATIENTS AND CAREGIVERS

What to Tell Parents About Efficacy

- For acute symptoms, it can work right away
- Explain which use esketamine is being chosen for, how to tell if the drug is working by targeting specific symptoms, and why this is being done
- Since every treatment consideration depends on a risk/benefit analysis, parents should fully understand short- and long-term risks as well as benefits
- Often a good idea to tell parents whether the medication chosen is specifically approved for the disorder being treated, or whether it is being given for "unapproved" or "off-label" reasons based on good clinical practice, expert consensus, and/or prudent extrapolation of controlled data from adults

What to Tell Children and Adolescents About Efficacy

- Be specific about the symptoms being targeted: we are trying to help you ...
- Give the medication a try; if it's not working very well, we can stop the medication and try something else
- If it does make you feel better, you cannot stop it right away or you may get sick again
- Medications don't change who you are as a person; they give you the opportunity to be the best person you can be

What to Tell Parents About Side Effects

- Explain that side effects are expected in many when starting
- Tell parents many side effects go away and do so about the same time that therapeutic effects start
- Predict side effects in advance (you will look clever and competent to the parents, unless you scare them with too much information and cause nocebo effects, in which case you won't look so clever when the patient develops lots of side effects and stops medication; use your judgment here);

a balanced but honest presentation is an art rather than a science
- Ask parents to support the patient while side effects are occurring
- Parents should fully understand short- and long-term risks as well as benefits
- Explaining to the parents what to expect from medication treatment, and especially what potential side effects to expect, can help prevent early termination of medication

What to Tell Children and Adolescents About Side Effects
- Even if you get a side effect, we can usually reduce it over time
- If you have side effects that are bothering you, tell your parents and your parents should tell me
- Explaining to child/adolescent what to expect from medication treatment, and especially potential side effects, can help prevent early termination of medication

What to Tell Teachers About the Medication (If Parents Consent)
- Esketamine can make children/adolescents sedated
- Encourage dialogue with parents/guardians about any behavior or mood changes

SPECIAL POPULATIONS

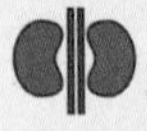

Renal Impairment
- No dose adjustment necessary

Hepatic Impairment
- Patients with moderate impairment may need to be monitored for adverse reactions for a longer period of time
- Not recommended for use in patients with severe impairment

Cardiac Impairment
- Contraindicated in patients with aneurysmal vascular disease (including thoracic and abdominal aorta, intracranial and peripheral arterial vessels) or arteriovenous malformation
- Patients with cardiovascular and cerebrovascular conditions and risk factors may be at an increased risk of associated adverse effects

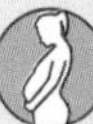

Pregnancy
- Controlled studies have not been conducted in pregnant women
- Not recommended for use during pregnancy; if a woman becomes pregnant while being treated with esketamine, treatment with esketamine should be discontinued and the patient should be counseled about the potential risk to the fetus
- In pregnant primates, use of NMDA receptor antagonists during the period of peak brain development increased neuronal apoptosis in the developing brain of the fetuses
- In rabbits, skeletal malformations were observed when ketamine was administered intranasally at estimated esketamine exposures of 0.3 times the maximum recommended human dose
- In rats, delay in sensorimotor development in pups was observed when esketamine was administered intranasally at exposures similar to the maximum recommended human dose
- Because of the risk for fetal harm, consider pregnancy planning and prevention in females of reproductive potential
- National Pregnancy Registry for Antidepressants: 1-844-405-6185

Breast Feeding
- Some drug is found in breast milk
- Animal studies have shown neurotoxicity in juvenile animals when NMDA antagonists were administered during a window of vulnerability that correlates with exposures in the third trimester through the first several months of life, but this window may extend out to approximately 3 years of age in humans
- Recommended either to discontinue drug or formula feed

THE ART OF PSYCHOPHARMACOLOGY

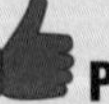

Potential Advantages
- Moderate to severe treatment-resistant depression
- Suicidal ideation

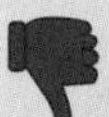

Potential Disadvantages

- In the United States, only available through a restricted program under a REMS
- Must be administered in presence of a healthcare professional
- Requires post-administration monitoring until patient is clinically stable and ready to leave the healthcare setting (in the United States, requires monitoring for at least 2 hours)

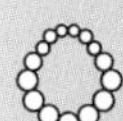

Pearls

- Esketamine is the "s" enantiomer of ketamine
- Esketamine has been evaluated in two controlled trials of adolescents with treatment-resistant depression (Zhou et al., 2023; DelBello et al, 2023):
  - In the first study, 54 adolescents (ages 13–18 years) with MDD and suicidal ideation received either three infusions of esketamine (0.25 mg/kg) or midazolam (0.045 mg/kg) over 5 days. Esketamine produced greater improvement in suicidal ideation and change in Montgomery–Asberg Depression Rating Scale (MADRS) scores and greater antidepressant response at 4 weeks posttreatment (Zhou et al., 2023).
  - In the second study, which used intranasal esketamine (three fixed doses: 28 mg, 56 mg, and 84 mg) compared with midazolam in youth ages 12–17 years who were at imminent risk for suicide, adolescents also received comprehensive standard of care, including initial hospitalization, oral antidepressant, and psychotherapy. In this study (N = 82), esketamine doses (56 mg, 84 mg) were superior to midazolam in reducing depressive symptoms at 24 hours (p = 0.037) and the severity of suicidality improved in all groups, including midazolam (DelBello et al., 2023).
- For ketamine, there has been considerable focus on the role of dissociation and its relationship to response; however, current data do not show a relationship between acute dissociative effects and antidepressant response to ketamine in pediatric treatment-resistant depression (Lineham et al., 2023)
- In clinical trials, treatment-resistant depression was defined as a DSM-5 diagnosis for MDD in adults who have not responded adequately to at least two different antidepressants of adequate dose and duration in the current depressive episode
- A randomized, active-placebo-controlled trial of 3-dose intravenous esketamine in adolescents with major depressive disorder offered preliminary findings that it may be efficacious and well-tolerated

SUGGESTED READING

DelBello M. Efficacy and safety of intranasal esketamine for the rapid reduction of depressive symptoms in adolescents with MDD at imminent risk for suicide: results of a double-blind, randomized, psychoactive controlled study. Presented at the annual meeting of the American Academy of Child & Adolescent Psychiatry. October 25, 2023.

Dwyer JB, Stringaris A, Brent DA, Bloch MH. Annual research review: defining and treating pediatric treatment-resistant depression. J Child Psychol Psychiatry 2020;61(3):312–32.

Dwyer JB, Landeros-Weisenberger A, Johnson JA et al. Efficacy of intravenous ketamine in adolescent treatment-resistant depression: a randomized midazolam-controlled trial. Am J Psychiatry 2021;178(4):352–62.

Fu DJ, Ionescu DF, Li X, et al. Esketamine nasal spray for rapid reduction of major depressive disorder symptoms in patients who have active suicidal ideation with intent: double-blind randomized study (ASPIRE I). J Clin Psychiatry 2020;81(3):19m13191.

Ionescu DF, Fu DJ, Qiu X, et al. Esketamine nasal spray for rapid reduction of depressive symptoms in patients with major depressive disorder who have active suicidal ideation with intent: results of a phase 3, double-blind, randomized study (ASPIRE II). Int J Neuropsychopharmacol 2021;24(1):22–31.

Lineham A, Avila-Quintero VJ, Bloch MH, Dwyer J. The relationship between acute dissociative effects induced by ketamine and treatment response in adolescent patients with treatment-resistant depression. J Child Adolesc Psychopharmacol 2023;33(1):20–6.

Zhou Y, Lan X, Wang C et al. Effect of repeated intravenous esketamine on adolescents with major depressive disorder and suicidal ideation: a randomized active-placebo-controlled trial. J Am Acad Child Adolesc Psychiatry 2023;S0890-8567(23):00373–8.

THERAPEUTICS

Brands

- Prozac (fluoxetine)
- Prozac weekly (fluoxetine weekly)
- Sarafem
- Symbyax (in combination with olanzapine)

Generic

Yes

US FDA Approved for Pediatric Use

- Major depressive disorder (fluoxetine, ages 8 and older)
- Obsessive-compulsive disorder (fluoxetine, ages 7 and older)
- Bipolar depression [in combination with olanzapine (Symbyax), ages 10 and older]

Off-Label for Pediatric Use

- Approved in adults
    - Panic disorder (fluoxetine, fluoxetine weekly)
    - Premenstrual dysphoric disorder (Sarafem)
    - Bulimia nervosa (fluoxetine, fluoxetine weekly)
    - Treatment-resistant depression [in combination with olanzapine (Symbyax)]
- Other off-label uses
    - Separation anxiety disorder
    - Social anxiety disorder
    - Generalized anxiety disorder

Class and Mechanism of Action

- Neuroscience-based Nomenclature: serotonin reuptake inhibitor (S-RI)
- SSRI (selective serotonin reuptake inhibitor); often classified as a drug for depression (i.e., antidepressant), but it is not just an antidepressant
- Fluoxetine presumably increases serotonergic neurotransmission by blocking the serotonin reuptake pump (transporter, SERT), which results in the desensitization of serotonin receptors, especially serotonin 1A receptors
- Fluoxetine also has antagonist properties at serotonin 2C receptors, which could increase norepinephrine and dopamine neurotransmission

SAFETY AND TOLERABILITY

Notable Side Effects

- Mostly central nervous system side effects (insomnia but also sedation especially if not sleeping at night; agitation, tremors, headache, dizziness)
- Note: patients with diagnosed or undiagnosed bipolar or psychotic disorders may be more vulnerable to CNS-activating actions of SSRIs; pay particular attention to signs of activation in children with developmental disorders or autism spectrum disorders
- Treatment-emergent activation syndrome (TEAS) includes agitation, anxiety, panic attacks, irritability, aggression, impulsivity, and insomnia
- TEAS can represent side effects but should not be confused with bipolar mania or the onset of suicidality and should be monitored and investigated with consideration of discontinuing or decreasing the dose of fluoxetine or addition of another agent or switching to another agent to reduce these symptoms
- Gastrointestinal (decreased appetite, nausea, diarrhea, constipation, dry mouth)
- Sexual dysfunction (boys: delayed ejaculation, erectile dysfunction; boys and girls: decreased sexual desire, anorgasmia)
- Autonomic (sweating)
- Bruising and rare bleeding
- Syndrome of inappropriate antidiuretic hormone secretion (SIADH)

Life-Threatening or Dangerous Side Effects

- Rare seizures
- Rare induction of mania
- Rare suicidal ideation and behavior (suicidality) (short-term regulatory studies did not show any actual suicides in any age group and also did not show an increase in the risk of suicidality with antidepressants compared to placebo beyond age 24)

Growth and Maturation

- Children taking fluoxetine may have slower growth; long-term effects are unknown

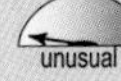

Weight Gain

- Reported but not expected

- Weight loss has been observed in children and adolescents

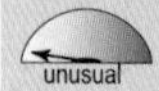

Sedation

- Reported but not expected

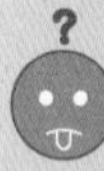

What to Do About Side Effects

- Wait, wait, wait: mild side effects are common, happen early, and usually improve with time, but treatment benefits can be delayed and often begin just as the side effects wear off
- Monitor side effects closely, especially when initiating treatment
- May wish to try dosing every other day to deal with side effects, or wash out for a week and try again at half dose or every other day
- May wish to give some drugs at night if not tolerated during the day, although this may not be useful for fluoxetine
- Fluoxetine may be one of the most activating agents in its class
- For activation (jitteriness, anxiety, insomnia):
  - Consider a temporary dose reduction or a more gradual up-titration
  - Consider switching to another SSRI or potentially an SNRI (other than venlafaxine)
  - Optimize psychotherapeutic interventions
  - Activation and agitation may represent the induction of a bipolar state, especially a mixed dysphoric bipolar II condition sometimes associated with suicidal ideation, and may require the addition of lithium, or an atypical antipsychotic, and/or discontinuation of fluoxetine
- Often best to try another monotherapy prior to resorting to augmentation strategies to treat side effects (Suresh et al., 2020)
- For insomnia: consider adding melatonin. Use caution with adding trazodone to fluoxetine as this has been associated with worse outcomes in depressed youth.
- For GI upset: try giving medication with a meal. Giving antidepressants with food will, in general, decrease peak plasma concentrations and increase the time required for absorption (Strawn et al., 2021, 2023).
- For sexual dysfunction:
  - Probably best to reduce dose or discontinue and try another agent
  - Consider adding daytime exercise, bupropion, or buspirone
- For emotional flattening, apathy: consider adding bupropion (with caution as little experience in children)

How Drug Causes Side Effects

- Theoretically due to increases in serotonin concentrations at serotonin receptors in parts of the brain and body other than those that cause therapeutic actions (e.g., unwanted actions of serotonin in sleep centers causing insomnia, unwanted actions of serotonin in the gut causing diarrhea)
- Increasing serotonin can cause diminished dopamine release and might contribute to emotional flattening, cognitive slowing, and apathy in some patients
- Fluoxetine's 5HT2C antagonist properties could contribute to agitation, anxiety, and undesirable activation, especially early in dosing

Warnings and Precautions

- Consider distributing brochures provided by the FDA and the drug companies as well as the medication guides from the American Academy of Child & Adolescent Psychiatry (AACAP)
- Carefully consider monitoring patients regularly within the practical limits, particularly during the first several weeks of treatment
- Warn patients and their caregivers when possible about the possibility of activating side effects and advise them to report such symptoms
- Carefully weigh the risks and benefits of pharmacological treatment against the risks and benefits of nontreatment with antidepressants and it is a good idea to document this in the patient's chart
- Add or initiate other antidepressants with caution for up to 5 weeks after discontinuing fluoxetine (fluoxetine has a long half-life and takes a long time to wash out)
- As with any antidepressant, use with caution in patients with history of seizure
- As with any antidepressant, use with caution in patients with bipolar disorder

unless treated with concomitant mood-stabilizing agent
- Monitor patients for activation and suicidal ideation and involve parents/guardians

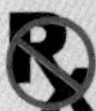

When Not to Prescribe
- If patient is taking an MAO inhibitor
- If patient is taking thioridazine
- If patient is taking pimozide
- If patient is taking tamoxifen
- Not generally recommended in patients taking tricyclic antidepressants (see Drug Interactions)
- If there is a proven allergy to fluoxetine

Long-Term Use
- Children taking fluoxetine may have slower growth; long-term effects are unknown

Habit Forming
- No

Overdose
- Rarely lethal in monotherapy overdose; symptoms can include respiratory depression (especially with alcohol), ataxia, sedation, and possible seizures, especially in overdoses mixed with other psychotropic medications

DOSING AND USE

Usual Dosage Range
- In children:
  - Depression: 10–40 mg/day; can go up to 60 mg/day if medically indicated and no side effects
  - OCD: 10–40 mg/day; can go up to 60 mg/day if medically indicated and no side effects
  - Bipolar depression: fluoxetine/olanzapine as 3 mg/25 mg–12 mg/50 mg once daily in the evening
- In adolescents:
  - Depression: 20–60 mg/day; can go up to 80 mg/day if medically indicated and no side effects
  - OCD: 20–60 mg/day; can go up to 80 mg/day if medically indicated and no side effects
  - Bipolar depression: fluoxetine/olanzapine as 3 mg/25 mg–12 mg/50 mg once daily in the evening

Dosage Forms
- Capsule 10 mg, 20 mg, 40 mg
- Tablet 10 mg, 15 mg, 20 mg, 60 mg
- Liquid 20 mg/5 mL–120 mL
- Weekly capsule 90 mg
- Olanzapine–fluoxetine combination capsule (mg equivalent olanzapine / mg equivalent fluoxetine) 3 mg/25 mg, 6 mg/25 mg, 6 mg/50 mg, 12 mg/25 mg, 12 mg/50 mg

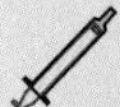

How to Dose
- In children:
  - Depression: initial dose 10 mg/day; after 2 weeks can increase to 20 mg/day; can go up to 60 mg/day if medically indicated and no side effects
  - OCD: initial dose 10 mg/day; after 2 weeks can increase to 20 mg/day (wait several weeks for lower-weight children); consider additional dose increases up to 60 mg/day after several more weeks if there is insufficient response
  - Bipolar depression: initial 2.5 mg olanzapine/20 mg fluoxetine once daily in the evening; adjust based on tolerability/efficacy; usual dose 3 mg/25 mg–12 mg/50 mg once daily in the evening
- In adolescents:
  - Depression: initial dose 10 mg/day; after 1 week can increase to 20 mg/day; can go up to 80 mg/day if medically indicated and no side effects
  - In general, for doses higher than 20 mg/day fluoxetine may be best administered in divided doses twice daily (in the morning and at noon)
  - OCD: initial dose 10 mg/day; after 2 weeks can increase to 20 mg/day; consider additional dose increases after several more weeks if there is insufficient response; usual dose range is 20–60 mg/day
  - Bipolar depression: initial 2.5 mg olanzapine/20 mg fluoxetine once daily in the evening; adjust based on tolerability/efficacy; usual dose 3 mg/25 mg–12 mg/50 mg once daily in the evening

Options for Administration
- Liquid formulation can be beneficial for patients requiring very slow titration and in those who cannot swallow tablets or capsules

Tests

- None for healthy individuals

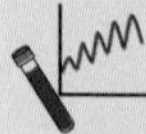

Pharmacokinetics

- Active metabolite (norfluoxetine) has a 2-week half-life (based on adult studies)
- Parent drug has 2–3-day half-life (based on adult studies)
- Inhibits CYP2D6
- Inhibits CYP3A4
- Inhibits CYP2C19
- Fluoxetine serum concentrations in children (ages 6–12) may be higher than in adolescents (ages 13–17) and concentrations of the metabolite norfluoxetine are almost twice as high in children compared to adolescents. These differences are largely related to differences in weight (Wilens et al., 2002).

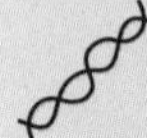

Pharmacogenetics

- The Clinical Pharmacogenetics Implementation Consortium does not provide dosing recommendations for fluoxetine in youth, although in CYP2D6 poor metabolizers, it may be advisable to consider an alternative medication

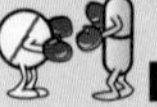

Drug Interactions

- Tramadol reported to increase the risk of seizures in adults taking an antidepressant
- Can increase tricyclic antidepressant (TCA) levels; use with caution with tricyclic antidepressants or when switching from a TCA to fluoxetine
- Can cause a fatal "serotonin syndrome" when combined with MAO inhibitors, so do not use with MAO inhibitors or for at least 14 days after MAOIs are stopped
- Do not start an MAO inhibitor for at least 5 weeks after discontinuing fluoxetine
- May displace highly protein-bound drugs (e.g., phenytoin, valproate)
- Can theoretically cause weakness, hyperreflexia, and incoordination when combined with sumatriptan, or possibly with other triptans, requiring careful monitoring of patient
- Possible increased risk of bleeding
- Via CYP2D6 inhibition, could theoretically interfere with the analgesic actions of

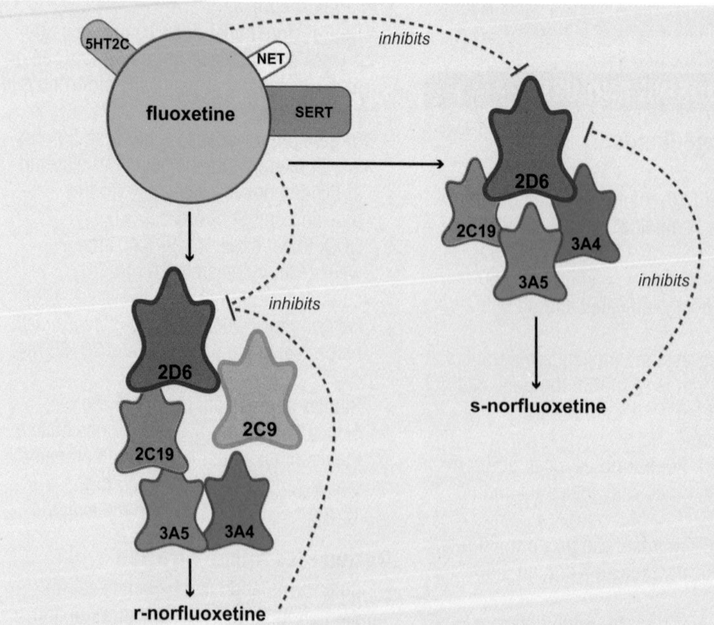

Figure 1 Fluoxetine metabolism. Fluoxetine is metabolized primarily by CYP2D6; however, fluoxetine and its metabolites (r-norfluoxetine and s-norfluoxetine) also inhibit CYP2D6.

codeine, and increase the plasma levels of some beta blockers and of atomoxetine
- Via CYP2D6 inhibition, fluoxetine could theoretically increase concentrations of thioridazine and cause dangerous cardiac arrhythmias
- Via CYP2D6 inhibition, may increase aripiprazole levels; consider up to 50% dose reduction of aripiprazole
- May reduce the clearance of diazepam or trazodone, thus increasing their levels
- Via CYP3A4 inhibition, may increase the levels of alprazolam, buspirone, and triazolam
- Via CYP3A4 inhibition, fluoxetine could theoretically increase concentrations of HMG CoA reductase inhibitors, especially simvastatin, atorvastatin, and lovastatin, but not pravastatin or fluvastatin, which would increase the risk of rhabdomyolysis; thus, coadministration of fluoxetine with certain HMG CoA reductase inhibitors should proceed with caution
- Via CYP3A4 inhibition, fluoxetine could theoretically increase the concentrations of pimozide, and cause QTc prolongation and dangerous cardiac arrhythmias
- Caution when used with drugs metabolized by CYP2D6, 3A4, and 2C19, since plasma levels of those drugs may increase in patients also taking fluoxetine

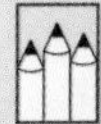

Dosing Tips

- Plasma levels are higher in lower-weight children; therefore, starting and target doses may be lower and longer intervals between dose increases may be needed (see How to Dose)
- If a child loses efficacy between daily doses, it may indicate rapid metabolism and the need to increase the dose or give twice daily even though fluoxetine has a long half-life (this is more common with other antidepressants with shorter half-lives)
- Adolescents often need and receive adult doses
- Be aware that metabolism changes during puberty and entry into adolescence and becomes more like adults (i.e., slower than in children)
- If a child on a stable dose begins to have more side effects upon entering adolescence, this may signal the need for a dose reduction due to changing metabolism
- The long half-lives of fluoxetine and its active metabolites mean that dose changes will not be fully reflected in plasma for several weeks, lengthening titration to final dose and extending withdrawal from treatment
- Liquid formulation easiest for doses below 10 mg when used for cases that are very intolerant to fluoxetine or for very slow up- and down-titration needs
- Occasionally patients are dosed above 80 mg
- The more anxious and agitated the patient, the lower the starting dose, the slower the titration
- If intolerable anxiety, insomnia, agitation, akathisia, or activation occurs either upon dosing initiation or discontinuation, consider the possibility of activated bipolar disorder and switch to an atypical antipsychotic or a mood stabilizer
- These symptoms may also indicate the need to evaluate for a mixed features episode and thus discontinuing fluoxetine and considering an atypical antipsychotic or a mood stabilizer or lithium

How to Switch

- From another antidepressant to fluoxetine:
  - When tapering a prior antidepressant, see its entry in this manual for how to stop and how to taper off that specific drug
  - In situations when there are antidepressant-related side effects, try to stop the first agent before starting fluoxetine so that new side effects of fluoxetine can be distinguished from withdrawal effects of the first agent
  - If urgent, cross taper starting fluoxetine at 10 mg/day while reducing the dose of the first agent for 2 weeks, and then increase the dose of fluoxetine to 20 mg/day while further reducing the first agent
- From fluoxetine to another antidepressant:
  - Fluoxetine tapers itself, so abrupt discontinuation leads to drug levels and active metabolite levels floating down slowly over 2–6 weeks

How to Stop

- Taper rarely necessary since fluoxetine tapers itself after immediate discontinuation, due to the long half-life of fluoxetine and its active metabolites

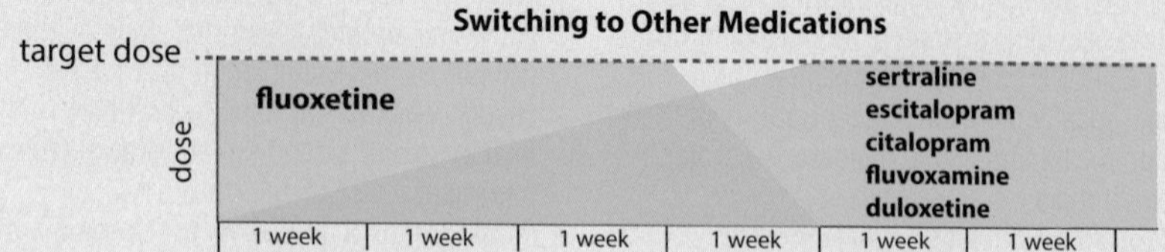

WHAT TO EXPECT

Onset of Action

- Some patients may experience increased energy or activation early after initiation of treatment
- Full onset of therapeutic actions is usually delayed by 2–4 weeks and may be faster in anxiety disorders (Strawn et al., 2018) compared to depressive disorders
- If it is not working within 6–8 weeks, it may require a dosage increase or it may not work at all. Children and adolescents who have had zero response to an antidepressant, after 8 weeks, have only a 25% chance of responding over the next 4 weeks (Strawn et al., 2017).

Duration of Action

- Effects are consistent over a 24-hour period
- May continue to work for many years to prevent relapse of symptoms

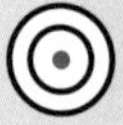

Primary Target Symptoms

- Depressed and/or irritable mood
- Energy, motivation, and interest
- Obsessions, compulsions
- Anxiety (fear and worry are often target symptoms, but fluoxetine can occasionally and transiently increase these symptoms short term before improving them)
- Prior to initiation of treatment, it is helpful to develop a list of target symptoms of depression and/or anxiety to monitor during treatment to better assess treatment response

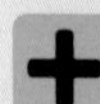

What Is Considered a Positive Result?

- The goal of treatment is complete remission of current symptoms as well as prevention of future relapses
- In practice, many patients have only a partial response where some symptoms are improved but others persist (especially insomnia, fatigue, and problems concentrating in depression), in which case higher doses of fluoxetine, adding a second agent, or switching to an agent with a different mechanism of action can be considered
- If treatment works, it most often reduces or even eliminates symptoms, but is not a cure since symptoms can recur after medicine is stopped (Emslie et al., 2004).
- Response rates in depression for psychopharmacology combined with CBT are approximately 70%

How Long to Treat

- For adolescents with depression, generally, 9–12 months of antidepressant treatment is recommended (Hathaway et al., 2018)
- For anxiety disorders, 6–9 months of antidepressant treatment may be sufficient, though many clinicians extend treatment to 12 months based on extrapolation of data from adults with anxiety disorders (Hathaway et al., 2018; Strawn et al., 2021)
- Extended treatment periods may decrease the risk of long-term morbidity and recurrence; however, the goal of treatment is ultimately remission, rather than duration of antidepressant pharmacotherapy (Hathaway et al., 2018)
- In terms of the length of antidepressant treatment, evidence-based guidelines represent a starting point; appropriate treatment duration varies, and patient-specific response, psychological factors, and timing of discontinuation must be considered for individual pediatric patients (Hathaway et al., 2018)
- For OCD and bulimia, treatment should be continued for 12 months

What If It Stops Working?

- Some patients who have an initial response may relapse even though they continue treatment, sometimes called "poop-out"
- Some patients may experience apparent lack of consistent efficacy due to activation syndrome or latent or underlying or newly evolved bipolar disorder, or major depressive episodes with mixed features, and require antidepressant discontinuation and a switch to a second generation antipsychotic

What If It Doesn't Work?

- Consider evaluation for another diagnosis (especially bipolar illness or depression with mixed features) or for a comorbid condition (e.g., medical illness, substance abuse)
- When treating youth with anxiety disorders, many patients will have had significant anxiety for years prior to beginning treatment. As such, when anxiety is treated with an SSRI, their symptoms may be improved, but the patient has likely missed important developmental milestones (e.g., spending the night with friends, being able to ask questions in class). Developing these skills will take time. Beyond this, the family may have lived with the anxious child for years and following treatment of the child, the family may need to readjust.
- Be mindful of family conflict contributing to the presentation; sometimes treating parental depression can improve psychiatric and social function without any treatment of youth. Also, accommodation is common in families of youth with anxiety disorders and may need to be addressed specifically, as it can perpetuate symptoms.
- Consider factors associated with poor response to SSRIs in treatment-resistant depression or anxiety disorders, such as severe symptoms, long-lasting symptoms, poor treatment adherence, prior nonresponse to other treatments, and the presence of comorbid disorders
- Consider other important potential factors such as ongoing conflicts, family psychopathology, and an adverse environment (e.g., poverty, chaos, violence, prior and ongoing psychological trauma, abuse, neglect). Additionally, when symptoms are prominent at school, consider the presence of a learning disorder.
- Institute trauma-informed care for appropriate children and adolescents
- A 2007 meta-analysis of published and unpublished trials in pediatric patients found that antidepressants had a number needed to treat (NNT) of 10 for depression, 6 for OCD, and 3 for anxiety disorders; thus, fluoxetine may not work in all children, so consider switching to another antidepressant (Bridge et al., 2007)
- Consider a dose adjustment
- Consider augmenting options:
  - Cognitive behavioral therapy (CBT), interpersonal psychotherapy for adolescents (IPT-A), light therapy, family therapy, and exercise especially in adolescents
  - For partial response (depression): use caution when adding medications to fluoxetine, especially in children, since there are not sufficient studies of augmentation in children or adolescents; however, for the expert, consider bupropion, aripiprazole, or other atypical antipsychotics such as quetiapine; use combinations of antidepressants with caution as this may activate bipolar disorder and suicidal ideation
  - For insomnia: sleep hygiene, CBT for insomnia, melatonin, or alpha 2 agonists. Trazodone is not recommended for use with fluoxetine given that pediatric studies have shown this combination results in poorer outcomes (Shamseddeen et al., 2012).
  - For anxiety: buspirone, antihistamines
  - Add lithium or atypical antipsychotics for bipolar depression, psychotic depression, treatment-resistant depression, or treatment-resistant anxiety disorders
  - Fluoxetine is specifically approved in combination with olanzapine for bipolar depression (ages 10 and older) and treatment-resistant unipolar depression (adults only)
  - TMS (transcranial magnetic stimulation) may have a role although pediatric trials of TMS have been hampered by high sham response rates (Croarkin et al., 2021)
  - ECT (case studies show effectiveness; cognitive side effects are similar to those in adults; reserve for treatment-resistant cases)

TALKING TO PATIENTS AND CAREGIVERS

What to Tell Parents About Efficacy

- Doesn't work right away; full therapeutic benefits may take up to 8 weeks, yet parents and teachers might see improvement before the patient does
- While the medicine helps by reducing symptoms and improving function, it is not a cure, and it is therefore necessary to keep taking the medication to sustain its therapeutic effects
- Since every treatment consideration depends on a risk/benefit analysis, parents should fully understand short- and long-term risks as well as benefits
- Only drug with regulatory approval for depression in both adolescents and children
- One of the SSRIs specifically approved for children and adolescents with OCD (obsessive-compulsive disorder)
- Only combination product (with olanzapine) approved in children and adolescents for bipolar depression
- Fluoxetine is perhaps the SSRI with the most clinical experience for use in children and adolescents
- Fluoxetine has some of the most robust clinical trial results of any agent in the class for children and adolescents
- After successful treatment, continuation of fluoxetine may be necessary to prevent relapse, especially in those who have had more than one episode or a very severe episode. In general, when treating depression in children and adolescents, medications are continued for 12 months after symptoms have resolved, while for anxiety disorders, clinicians have generally treated for 6–9 months (Hathaway et al., 2018).
- Often a good idea to tell parents whether the medication chosen is specifically approved for the disorder being treated, or whether it is being given for "unapproved" or "off-label" reasons based on good clinical practice, expert consensus, and/or prudent extrapolation of controlled data from adults

What to Tell Children and Adolescents About Efficacy

- We are trying to make you feel better
- It may be a good idea to give the medication a try; if it's not working very well, we can stop the medication and try something else
- A good try takes 2 to 3 months or even longer
- If it does make you feel better, you cannot stop it right away or you may feel sad or worried again
- Medications don't change who you are as a person; they give you the opportunity to be the best person you can be

What to Tell Parents About Side Effects

- Explain that side effects are expected in many when starting and are most common in the first 2–3 weeks of starting or increasing the dose
- Some SSRI side effects emerge early and resolve quickly (e.g., activation, gastrointestinal symptoms). In contrast, other side effects are late-emerging (e.g., weight gain) or persistent (e.g., sexual dysfunction). Discussing the temporal course of the side effects and distinguishing between persistent and transient side effects is critical. Ensuring that patients are aware not only of side effects but the tendency of some side effects to be transient is important and should be part of discussions with patients and their families. For many, knowing that a side effect is likely transient, as opposed to persistent, may significantly influence the patient and family's anxiety or fears related to medication (Strawn et al., 2023).
- Tell parents many side effects go away and do so about the same time that therapeutic effects start
- Predict side effects in advance (you will look clever and competent to the parents, unless you scare them with too much information and cause nocebo effects, in which case you won't look so clever when the patient develops lots of side effects and stops medication; use your judgment here); a balanced but honest presentation is an art rather than a science
- Ask them to help monitor for increased suicidality and if present, report any such symptoms immediately
- Ask parents to support the patient while side effects are occurring
- Parents should fully understand short- and long-term risks as well as benefits

- Explaining to the parents what to expect from medication treatment, and especially potential side effects, can help prevent early termination of medication

What to Tell Children and Adolescents About Side Effects

- Even if you get side effects, most of them get better or go away in a few days to a few weeks
- Consider having a conversation about sexual side effects in some adolescents who can find these side effects confusing and especially burdensome
- Explaining to child/adolescent what to expect from medication treatment, and especially potential side effects, can help prevent early termination of medication
- Tell adolescents and children capable of understanding that some young patients, especially those who are depressed, may develop thoughts of hurting themselves, and if this happens, not to be alarmed but to tell their parents right away

What to Tell Teachers About the Medication (If Parents Consent)

- Fluoxetine can make children/adolescents jittery or restless
- If the patient is sleepy, ask whether the medication is keeping them up at night
- It is not abusable
- Encourage dialogue with parents/guardians about any behavior or mood changes

SPECIAL POPULATIONS

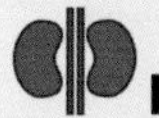

Renal Impairment

- No dose adjustment
- Not removed by hemodialysis

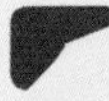

Hepatic Impairment

- Lower dose or give less frequently, perhaps by half

Cardiac Impairment

- Preliminary research suggests that fluoxetine is safe in these patients
- In a study using US claims data, the crude incident rate of adverse cardiac events in pediatric patients taking fluoxetine was 4.2/10,000 person-years (lowest of all SSRIs evaluated) (Czaja et al., 2013)

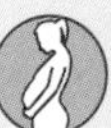

Pregnancy

- Controlled studies have not been conducted in pregnant women
- Not generally recommended for use during pregnancy, especially during first trimester
- Nonetheless, continuous treatment during pregnancy may be necessary and has not been proven to be harmful to the fetus
- Current patient registries of children whose mothers took fluoxetine during pregnancy do not show adverse consequences
- At delivery there may be more bleeding in the mother and transient irritability or sedation in the newborn
- Must weigh the risk of treatment (first trimester fetal development, third trimester newborn delivery) to the child against the risk of no treatment (recurrence of depression, maternal health, infant bonding) to the mother and child
- For many patients this may mean continuing treatment during pregnancy
- Exposure to SSRIs early in pregnancy may be associated with increased risk of septal heart defects (absolute risk is small)
- SSRI use beyond the 20th week of pregnancy may be associated with increased risk of pulmonary hypertension in newborns, although this is not proven
- Exposure to SSRIs late in pregnancy may be associated with increased risk of gestational hypertension and preeclampsia
- Neonates exposed to SSRIs or SNRIs late in the third trimester have developed complications requiring prolonged hospitalization, respiratory support, and tube feeding; reported symptoms are consistent with either a direct toxic effect of SSRIs and SNRIs or, possibly, a drug discontinuation syndrome, and include respiratory distress, cyanosis, apnea, seizures, temperature instability, feeding difficulty, vomiting, hypoglycemia, hypotonia, hypertonia, hyperreflexia, tremor, jitteriness, irritability, and constant crying
- National Pregnancy Registry for Psychiatric Medications: 1-866-961-2388 or https://womensmentalhealth.org/research/pregnancyregistry/

Breast Feeding

- Some drug is found in breast milk
- Trace amounts may be present in nursing children whose mothers are on fluoxetine
- If child becomes irritable or sedated, breast feeding or drug may need to be discontinued
- Immediate postpartum period is a high-risk time for depression, especially in women who have had prior depressive episodes, so drug may need to be reinstituted late in the third trimester or shortly after childbirth to prevent a recurrence during the postpartum period
- Must weigh benefits of breast feeding with risks and benefits of antidepressant treatment versus nontreatment to both the infant and the mother
- For many patients this may mean continuing treatment during breast feeding

THE ART OF PSYCHOPHARMACOLOGY

Potential Advantages

- In children:
  - Only agent specifically approved by the FDA for depression in children
  - One of only four agents specifically approved for OCD in children (also fluvoxamine, sertraline, and clomipramine)
- In adolescents:
  - One of only two agents approved for depression in adolescents (also escitalopram)
  - One of only four agents specifically approved for OCD in adolescents (also fluvoxamine, sertraline, and clomipramine)
- All ages:
  - Patients with atypical depression (hypersomnia, increased appetite)
  - Patients with fatigue and low energy
  - Patients with comorbid eating and affective disorders
  - Patients for whom weekly administration is desired

Potential Disadvantages

- In children and adolescents:
  - Those who are already psychomotor agitated, angry, or irritable, and who do not have a psychiatric diagnosis
  - Those who may possibly have a mood disorder with mixed or bipolar features, especially those with these features and a family history of bipolar disorder
- All ages:
  - Patients with anorexia
  - Initiating treatment in anxious, agitated patients
  - Initiating treatment in severe insomnia

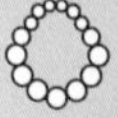

Pearls

- SSRIs show greater efficacy in pediatric anxiety disorders compared to depression
- In anxious youth, SSRIs produce faster and greater improvement compared to SNRIs (Strawn et al., 2018)
- Although fluoxetine has a more robust and consistent effect in child and adolescent depression than some other antidepressants, there are few head-to-head trials with other antidepressants
- More recent studies with antidepressants newer than fluoxetine all tend to have lower drug–placebo differences than fluoxetine, but this may be due to changes in clinical trial methodologies and not to true differences in drug efficacy
- Younger children tend to be more sensitive to adverse effects of SSRIs
- However, younger children can also have faster hepatic and renal metabolism and excretion, leading to the need to use adult-like doses in children
- For all SSRIs, and perhaps particularly for fluoxetine, children can have a two- to threefold higher incidence of behavioral activation and vomiting than adolescents, who have a somewhat higher incidence than adults
- Mood disorders can be associated with eating disorders, especially in adolescent females, and both can be treated successfully with fluoxetine
- May be a first-line choice for atypical depression (e.g., hypersomnia, hyperphagia, low energy, mood reactivity)
- Combinations of CBT (cognitive behavioral therapy) and fluoxetine may have better results than either treatment alone both for anxiety disorders and depression, especially for more severe cases
- Consider avoiding in patients with agitation and insomnia

- Can cause cognitive and affective "flattening"
- Not as well tolerated as some other SSRIs for panic disorder and other anxiety disorders, especially when dosing is initiated, unless given with co-therapies such as benzodiazepines or trazodone
- Actions at 5HT2C receptors may explain its activating properties
- Actions at 5HT2C receptors may explain in part fluoxetine's efficacy in eating disorders as a monotherapy or in combination with olanzapine for bipolar depression and treatment-resistant depression, since both agents have this property

SUGGESTED READING

Bridge JA, Iyengar S, Salary CB et al. Clinical response and risk for reported suicidal ideation and suicide attempts in pediatric antidepressant treatment: a meta-analysis of randomized controlled trials. JAMA 2007;297(15):1683–96.

Croarkin PE, Elmaadawi AZ, Aaronson ST et al. Left prefrontal transcranial magnetic stimulation for treatment-resistant depression in adolescents: a double-blind, randomized, sham-controlled trial. Neuropsychopharmacology 2021;46(2):462–9.

Czaja AS, Valuck RJ, Anderson HD. Comparative safety of selective serotonin reuptake inhibitors among pediatric users with respect to adverse cardiac events. Pharmacoepidemiol Drug Saf 2013;22(6):607–14.

Emslie GJ, Heiligenstein JH, Hoog SL et al. Fluoxetine treatment for prevention of relapse of depression in children and adolescents: a double-blind, placebo-controlled study. J Am Acad Child Adolesc Psychiatry 2004;43(11):1397–405.

Hathaway EE, Walkup JT, Strawn JR. Antidepressant treatment duration in pediatric depressive and anxiety disorders: how long is long enough? Curr Probl Pediatr Adolesc Health Care 2018;48(2):31–9.

March J, Silva S, Petrycki S et al. Fluoxetine, cognitive-behavioral therapy, and their combination for adolescents with depression: Treatment for Adolescents with Depression Study (TADS) randomized controlled trial. JAMA 2004;292:807–20.

Shamseddeen W, Clarke G, Keller MB et al. Adjunctive sleep medications and depression outcome in the treatment of serotonin-selective reuptake inhibitor resistant depression in adolescents study. J Child Adolesc Psychopharmacol 2012;22(1):29–36.

Strawn JR, Lu L, Peris TS, Levine A, Walkup JT. Research review: pediatric anxiety disorders- what have we learnt in the last 10 years? J Child Psychol Psychiatry 2021 Feb;62(2):114–39.

Strawn JR, Dobson ET, Mills JA et al. Placebo response in pediatric anxiety disorders: results from the Child/Adolescent Anxiety Multimodal Study. J Child Adolesc Psychopharmacol 2017;27(6):501–8.

Strawn JR, Mills JA, Sauley BA, Welge JA. The impact of antidepressant dose and class on treatment response in pediatric anxiety disorders: a meta-analysis. J Am Acad Child Adolesc Psychiatry 2018;57(4):235–244.e2.

Strawn JR, Poweleit EA, Uppugunduri CRS, Ramsey LB. Pediatric therapeutic drug monitoring for selective serotonin reuptake inhibitors. Front Pharmacol 2021;12:749692.

Strawn JR, Mills JA, Poweleit EA, Ramsey LB, Croarkin PE. Adverse effects of antidepressant medications and their management in children and adolescents. Pharmacotherapy 2023;43(7):675–90.

Suresh V, Mills JA, Croarkin PE, Strawn JR. What next? A Bayesian hierarchical modeling re-examination of treatments for adolescents with selective serotonin reuptake inhibitor-resistant depression. Depress Anxiety 2020;37(9):926–34.

Wilens TE, Cohen L, Biederman J et al. Fluoxetine pharmacokinetics in pediatric patients. J Clin Psychopharmacol 2002;22(6):568–75.

THERAPEUTICS

Brands
- Prolixin

Generic
Yes

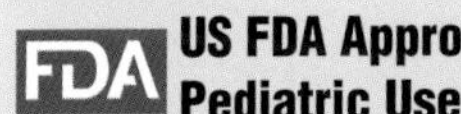

US FDA Approved for Pediatric Use
- None

Off-Label for Pediatric Use
- Approved in adults
  - Psychotic disorders
- Other off-label uses
  - Bipolar disorder

Class and Mechanism of Action
- Conventional antipsychotic (neuroleptic, phenothiazine, dopamine 2 antagonist)
- Blocks dopamine 2 receptors, reducing positive symptoms of psychosis

SAFETY AND TOLERABILITY

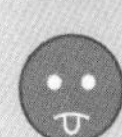

Notable Side Effects
- In adults:
  - Neuroleptic-induced deficit syndrome
  - Akathisia
  - Extrapyramidal symptoms (EPS, also called drug-induced parkinsonism)
  - Dizziness
  - Dry mouth, constipation, blurred vision
  - Decreased sweating, depression
  - Galactorrhea, amenorrhea
  - Weight gain, sedation
  - Sexual dysfunction
  - Urinary retention
  - Hypotension
  - Tardive dyskinesia, tardive dystonia (risk is higher in children than in adults)
  - Rare tachycardia, syncope

Life-Threatening or Dangerous Side Effects
- Rare neuroleptic malignant syndrome
- Rare priapism
- Rare seizures
- Rare jaundice, agranulocytosis, leukopenia

Growth and Maturation
- Long-term effects are unknown

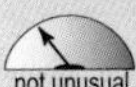

Weight Gain
- Occurs in significant minority

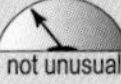

Sedation
- Occurs in significant minority

What to Do About Side Effects
- Wait, wait, wait: mild side effects are common, happen early, and usually improve with time, but treatment benefits can be delayed
- Monitor side effects closely, especially when initiating treatment
- May wish to give at night if not tolerated during the day and doesn't disrupt sleep
- Often best to try another monotherapy trial of a different antipsychotic prior to resorting to augmentation strategies to treat side effects
- Exercise and diet programs and medical management for high BMI percentiles, diabetes, dyslipidemia. Also, randomized controlled trials in youth suggest that omega-3 fatty acids can reduce SGA-related hypertriglyceridemia.
- Reduce the dose, particularly for drug-induced parkinsonism, akathisia, sedation, and tremor
- For drug-induced parkinsonism: consider reducing dose or switching to another agent. Augmenting with diphenhydramine or benztropine is less preferred in youth.
- For akathisia: reduce the dose or add a beta blocker. If these are ineffective, raising the dose of the beta blocker may be helpful.
- Using a 5HT2A antagonist such as mirtazapine or cyproheptadine to treat drug induced akathisia is less common in children and adolescents compared to adults
- Agitation due to undertreatment and inadequate dosing of the targeted disorder can be difficult to distinguish from drug-induced akathisia and activation; one approach for managing agitation/activation/akathisia when the specific side effect is difficult to distinguish is to raise the dose of fluphenazine

- If the patient improves after increasing the dose of fluphenazine, the symptoms are more likely to be due to inadequate dosing of the targeted disorder
- If the patient worsens after increasing the dose of fluphenazine, the symptoms are more likely to be drug induced and require further dose reduction, adding an agent to improve tolerability or switching to another antipsychotic

How Drug Causes Side Effects

- By blocking dopamine 2 receptors in the striatum, it can cause motor side effects, akathisia, and activation symptoms
- By blocking dopamine 2 receptors in the pituitary, it can cause elevations in prolactin
- By blocking dopamine 2 receptors excessively in the mesocortical and mesolimbic dopamine pathways, especially at high doses, it can cause worsening of negative and cognitive symptoms (neuroleptic-induced deficit syndrome)
- Anticholinergic actions may cause sedation, blurred vision, constipation, dry mouth
- Antihistaminic actions may cause sedation, weight gain
- By blocking alpha 1 adrenergic receptors, it can cause dizziness, sedation, and hypotension
- Mechanism of any possible increased incidence of diabetes or dyslipidemia is unknown

Warnings and Precautions

- Consider distributing brochures provided by the FDA and the drug companies or have the pharmacy do this for the parents
- Carefully weigh the risks and benefits of pharmacological treatment against the risks and benefits of nontreatment with an antipsychotic and it is a good idea to document this in the patient's chart
- If signs of neuroleptic malignant syndrome develop, treatment should be immediately discontinued
- Use cautiously in patients with alcohol withdrawal or convulsive disorders because of possible lowering of seizure threshold
- Avoid undue exposure to sunlight
- Use cautiously in patients with respiratory disorders
- Avoid extreme heat exposure
- Antiemetic effect can mask signs of other disorders or overdose
- Do not use epinephrine in event of overdose as interaction with some pressor agents may lower blood pressure
- As with any antipsychotic, use with caution in patients with history of seizures

When Not to Prescribe

- If patient is in a comatose state or has CNS depression
- If patient is taking cabergoline, pergolide, or metrizamide
- If there is a proven allergy to fluphenazine
- If there is a known sensitivity to any phenothiazine
- Decanoate and enanthate injectable formulations are contraindicated in children under age 12

Long-Term Use

- Some side effects may be irreversible (e.g., tardive dyskinesia)

Habit Forming

- No

Overdose

- Drug-induced parkinsonism, coma, hypotension, sedation, seizures, respiratory depression

DOSING AND USE

Usual Dosage Range

- In adults:
  - Oral: 1–20 mg/day
  - Intramuscular: generally, 1/3 to 1/2 the oral dose
  - Decanoate for intramuscular or subcutaneous administration: 12.5 mg–100 mg/2 weeks (maintenance)

Dosage Forms

- Tablet 1 mg, 2.5 mg scored, 5 mg scored, 10 mg scored
- Decanoate for long-acting intramuscular or subcutaneous administration 25 mg/mL
- Injection for acute intramuscular administration 2.5 mg/mL
- Elixir 2.5 mg/5 mL
- Concentrate 5 mg/mL

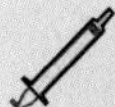

How to Dose

- In adults:
  - Oral: initial 0.5–10 mg/day in divided doses; maximum 40 mg/day
  - Intramuscular (short-acting): initial 1.25 mg; 2.5–10 mg/day can be given in divided doses every 6–8 hours; maximum dose generally 10 mg/day

Options for Administration

- Solution available for patients with difficulty swallowing pills

Tests

- Before starting fluphenazine:
  - Plan to monitor weight and metabolic parameters more closely than in adults since children and adolescents may be more prone to these side effects than adults
  - Weigh all patients and monitor weight gain against that expected for normal growth, using the pediatric height/weight chart to monitor
  - Get baseline personal and family history of diabetes, obesity, dyslipidemia, hypertension, and cardiovascular disease
  - Obtain blood pressure, fasting plasma glucose (or hemoglobin A1C), and a lipid profile
- After starting fluphenazine:
  - Monitor weight and BMI percentile
  - Consider monitoring fasting triglycerides monthly in patients at high risk for metabolic complications
  - Patients with low white blood cell count (WBC) or history of drug-induced leukopenia/neutropenia should have complete blood count (CBC) monitored frequently during the first few months and fluphenazine should be discontinued at the first sign of decline of WBC in the absence of other causative factors
  - Patients should be monitored periodically for the development of abnormal movements using neurological exam and the Abnormal Involuntary Movement Scale (AIMS)
  - Monitoring elevated prolactin levels is of dubious clinical benefit
  - Phenothiazines may cause false-positive phenylketonuria results

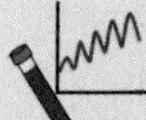

Pharmacokinetics

- Fluphenazine is well absorbed from the gastrointestinal tract, but it undergoes significant first-pass metabolism in the liver, resulting in low oral bioavailability. Intramuscular and depot formulations bypass first-pass metabolism and provide more consistent blood levels.
- Fluphenazine has a moderate to high protein binding of approximately 90–95%, primarily to albumin. It distributes widely throughout the body, including the central nervous system (CNS), due to its lipophilic nature. The drug has a relatively large volume of distribution, indicating extensive tissue distribution.
- Fluphenazine undergoes extensive hepatic metabolism, primarily via CYP2D6, and to a lesser extent CYP2C9, CYP1A2, CYP3A4, and CYP2C19 are implicated in in vitro studies. CYP3A4 is thought to account for approximately 40% of fluphenazine's *N*-dealkylation (Olesen and Linnet, 2000).
- Fluphenazine's major metabolite, norfluphenazine, also possesses antipsychotic activity but with lower potency than fluphenazine
- Fluphenazine may also inhibit CYP2D6 and 3A4
- Oral half-life approximately 12–38 hours in adults, and there are no currently available data in pediatric patients
- Decanoate half-life approximately 3 weeks

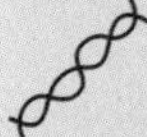

Pharmacogenetics

- No recommendations

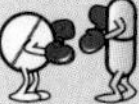

Drug Interactions

- May decrease the effects of levodopa, dopamine agonists
- May increase the effects of antihypertensive drugs except for guanethidine, whose antihypertensive actions fluphenazine may antagonize
- Additive effects may occur if used with CNS depressants
- Additive anticholinergic effects may occur if used with atropine or related compounds
- Alcohol and diuretics may increase the risk of hypotension
- Some patients taking a neuroleptic and lithium have developed an encephalopathic

syndrome similar to neuroleptic malignant syndrome
- Combined use with epinephrine may lower blood pressure

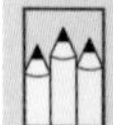

Dosing Tips

- Children should generally be dosed at the lower end of the dosage spectrum when drug is initiated
- Fluphenazine tablets 2.5 mg, 5 mg, and 10 mg contain tartrazine, which can cause allergic reactions, especially in patients sensitive to aspirin
- Oral solution should not be mixed with drinks containing caffeine, tannic acid (tea), or pectinates (apple juice)
- For treatment resistance, consider obtaining plasma drug levels to guide dosing above recommended levels
- Treatment should be suspended if absolute neutrophil count falls below 1,000/mm^3

How to Switch

- From another antipsychotic to fluphenazine:
  - When tapering a prior antipsychotic, see its entry in this manual for how to stop and how to taper off that specific drug
  - Generally, try to stop the first agent before starting fluphenazine so that new side effects of fluphenazine can be distinguished from withdrawal effects of the first agent
  - If urgent, cross taper off the other antipsychotic while fluphenazine is started at a low dose, with dose adjustments down of the other antipsychotic, and up for fluphenazine, every 3 to 7 days
- Off fluphenazine to another antipsychotic:
  - Generally, try to stop fluphenazine before starting the new antipsychotic so that new side effects of the next drug can be distinguished from any withdrawal effects from fluphenazine
  - If urgent, cross taper off fluphenazine by cutting the dose in half as the new antipsychotic is also started with dose adjustments down of fluphenazine and up for the new antipsychotic while monitoring for anticholinergic rebound symptoms from the withdrawal of fluphenazine

How to Stop

- Slow down-titration of oral formulation (over 6–8 weeks), especially when simultaneously beginning a new antipsychotic while switching (i.e., cross-titration)
- Rapid oral discontinuation may lead to rebound psychosis and worsening of symptoms
- Rapid oral discontinuation may lead to withdrawal dyskinesias, sometimes reversible, as well as anticholinergic rebound symptoms, especially in children following long-term daily use
- If antiparkinsonian agents are being used, they should be continued for a few weeks after fluphenazine is discontinued

WHAT TO EXPECT

Onset of Action

- Psychotic and manic symptoms can improve within 1 week of oral dosing, but it may take several weeks for full effect on behavior as well as on cognition and affective stabilization
- If it is not working within 6–8 weeks, it may require a dosage increase or it may not work at all
- Acute intramuscular dosing for agitation can have onset within minutes to an hour, but not well studied or specifically approved for children/adolescents

Duration of Action

- Effects of oral medication are consistent over a 24-hour period

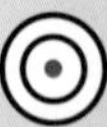

Primary Target Symptoms

- Positive symptoms of psychosis
- Motor and autonomic hyperactivity
- Violent or aggressive behavior

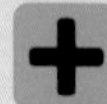

What Is Considered a Positive Result?

- Most often reduces positive symptoms but does not eliminate them
- In children or adolescents with a first episode of psychosis, initial response may be greater than for recurrent episodes of psychosis in adults

How Long to Treat

- Continue treatment until reaching a plateau of improvement
- After reaching a satisfactory plateau, continue treatment for at least a year after first episode of psychosis
- For second and subsequent episodes of psychosis, treatment may need to be indefinite

What If It Stops Working?

- Check for nonadherence, possibly by checking plasma drug level, and consider switching to another antipsychotic with fewer side effects
- Some patients who have an initial response may relapse even though they continue treatment, sometimes called "poop-out"
- Growth/developmental changes may contribute to apparent loss of efficacy as well as to new onset of side effects as metabolism slows and drug levels rise in transition from childhood to adolescence; dose adjustment (increase or decrease) should be considered
- Screen for the development of a new comorbid disorder, especially substance use
- Screen for adverse changes in the home or school environment

What If It Doesn't Work?

- Consider evaluation for another diagnosis (especially bipolar illness or depression with mixed features) or for a comorbid condition (e.g., medical illness, substance use)
- Consider other important potential factors such as ongoing conflicts, family psychopathology, and an adverse environment (e.g., poverty, chaos, violence, prior and ongoing psychological trauma, abuse, neglect)
- Institute trauma-informed care for appropriate children and adolescents
- Try one of the atypical antipsychotics
- If no first-line atypical antipsychotic is effective, can consider augmentation with valproate, lithium, or lamotrigine, although this has not been systematically studied
- Consider initiating psychotherapy. In adolescents with bipolar disorder (and those with affective symptoms who are at risk of developing bipolar disorder), family-focused psychotherapy can be particularly helpful (Miklowitz et al., 2020)
- Consider presence of concomitant drug abuse

TALKING TO PATIENTS AND CAREGIVERS

What to Tell Parents About Efficacy

- For acute symptoms, it can work right away
- This medication is being given because other antipsychotics have not worked
- Intramuscular fluphenazine can be given by a healthcare professional on an as needed basis for some symptoms like agitation associated with your child's psychotic illness; oral fluphenazine can be given by a parent under supervision by a healthcare professional off-label on an as needed basis as well
- Oral fluphenazine is usually given every day
- Explain which use fluphenazine is being chosen for, how to tell if the drug is working by targeting specific symptoms, and why this is being done
- Once the child/adolescent calms down, at some point after one dose or after several days of dosing or after long-term dosing, we should all assess whether the medication should be continued
- While the medicine helps by reducing symptoms and improving function, it is not a cure, and it therefore may be necessary to keep taking the medication long term to sustain its therapeutic effects
- Since every treatment consideration depends on a risk/benefit analysis, parents should fully understand short- and long-term risks as well as benefits
- Often a good idea to tell parents whether the medication chosen is specifically approved for the disorder being treated, or whether it is being given for "unapproved" or "off-label" reasons based on good clinical practice, expert consensus, and/or prudent extrapolation of controlled data from adults

What to Tell Children and Adolescents About Efficacy

- Be specific about the symptoms being targeted: we are trying to help you …
- Give the medication a try; if it's not working very well, we can stop the medication and try something else

- A good try often takes several weeks
- If it does make you feel better, you cannot stop it right away or you may get sick again
- Medications don't change who you are as a person; they give you the opportunity to be the best person you can be

What to Tell Parents About Side Effects

- Explain that side effects are expected in many when starting
- Tell parents many side effects go away and do so about the same time that therapeutic effects start
- Predict side effects in advance (you will look clever and competent to the parents, unless you scare them with too much information and cause nocebo effects, in which case you won't look so clever when the patient develops lots of side effects and stops medication; use your judgment here); a balanced but honest presentation is an art rather than a science
- Ask parents to support the patient while side effects are occurring
- Parents should fully understand short- and long-term risks as well as benefits
- Explaining to the parents what to expect from medication treatment, and especially what potential side effects to expect, can help prevent early termination of medication

What to Tell Children and Adolescents About Side Effects

- Even if you get side effects, most of them get better or go away in a few weeks
- If you have side effects that are bothering you, tell your parents and your parents should tell me
- Consider having a conversation about sexual side effects in some adolescents who can find these side effects confusing and especially burdensome
- Explaining to child/adolescent what to expect from medication treatment, and especially potential side effects, can help prevent early termination of medication

What to Tell Teachers About the Medication (If Parents Consent)

- Fluphenazine can make children/adolescents restless and cause tremor
- Fluphenazine can make children/adolescents sedated and cause tremor
- It is not abusable
- Encourage dialogue with parents/guardians about any behavior or mood changes
- Notify the clinician of increased restlessness or akathisia symptoms, which may be apparent in the school setting

SPECIAL POPULATIONS

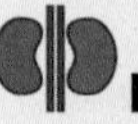

Renal Impairment

- Use with caution; titration should be slower

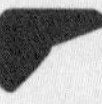

Hepatic Impairment

- Use with caution; titration should be slower

Cardiac Impairment

- Cardiovascular toxicity can occur, especially orthostatic hypotension

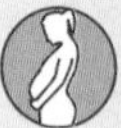

Pregnancy

- Controlled studies have not been conducted in pregnant women
- There is a risk of abnormal muscle movements and withdrawal symptoms in newborns whose mothers took an antipsychotic during the third trimester; symptoms may include agitation, abnormally increased or decreased muscle tone, tremor, sleepiness, severe difficulty breathing, and difficulty feeding
- Reports of extrapyramidal symptoms, jaundice, hyperreflexia, hyporeflexia in infants whose mothers took a phenothiazine during pregnancy
- Fluphenazine should only be used during pregnancy if clearly indicated
- Psychotic symptoms may worsen during pregnancy, and some form of treatment may be necessary
- Atypical antipsychotics may be preferable to conventional antipsychotics or is required during pregnancy

Breast Feeding

- Some drug is found in breast milk
- Effects on infant have been observed (dystonia, tardive dyskinesia, sedation)
- Recommended either to discontinue drug or formula feed

THE ART OF PSYCHOPHARMACOLOGY

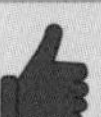

Potential Advantages

- Intramuscular formulation for emergency use

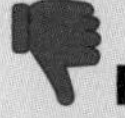

Potential Disadvantages

- In children and adolescents:
  - May be more susceptible to side effects
- All ages:
  - Patients with notable cognitive or mood symptoms

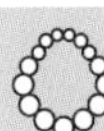

Pearls

- Fluphenazine is a high-potency phenothiazine
- Less risk of sedation and orthostatic hypotension but greater risk of extrapyramidal symptoms than with low-potency phenothiazines

SUGGESTED READING

Lytle S, McVoy M, Sajatovic M. Long-acting injectable antipsychotics in children and adolescents. J Child Adolesc Psychopharmacol 2017;27(1):2–9.

Matar HE, Almerie MQ, Sampson S. Fluphenazine (oral) versus placebo for schizophrenia. Cochrane Database Syst Rev 2013;(7):CD006352.

Miklowitz DJ, Schneck CD, Walshaw PD et al. Effects of family-focused therapy vs enhanced usual care for symptomatic youths at high risk for bipolar disorder: a randomized clinical trial. JAMA Psychiatry 2020 1;77(5):455–63.

Olesen OV, Linnet K. Identification of the human cytochrome P450 isoforms mediating in vitro N-dealkylation of perphenazine. Br J Clin Pharmacol 2000;50(6):563–71.

Sampford JR, Sampson S, Li BG et al. Fluphenazine (oral) versus atypical antipsychotics for schizophrenia. Cochrane Database Syst Rev 2016;7:CD010832.

THERAPEUTICS

Brands

- Luvox
- Luvox CR

Generic

Yes

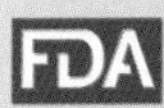

US FDA Approved for Pediatric Use

- Obsessive-compulsive disorder (OCD) (fluvoxamine, fluvoxamine CR) (ages 8 and older)

Off-Label for Pediatric Use

- Approved in adults
  - Social anxiety disorder (fluvoxamine CR)
- Other off-label uses
  - Major depressive disorder
  - Separation anxiety disorder
  - Panic disorder
  - Posttraumatic stress disorder (PTSD)
  - Generalized anxiety disorder (GAD)
  - Premenstrual dysphoric disorder (PMDD)

Class and Mechanism of Action

- Neuroscience-based Nomenclature: serotonin reuptake inhibitor (S-RI)
- SSRI (selective serotonin reuptake inhibitor); often classified as a drug for depression (i.e., antidepressant), but it is not just an antidepressant
- Fluvoxamine presumably increases serotonergic neurotransmission by blocking the serotonin reuptake pump (transporter, SERT), which results in the desensitization of serotonin receptors, especially serotonin 1A receptors
- Fluvoxamine also binds at sigma 1 receptors

SAFETY AND TOLERABILITY

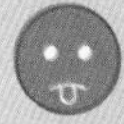

Notable Side Effects

- Mostly central nervous system side effects (insomnia but more so sedation, especially if not sleeping at night; agitation, tremors, headache, dizziness)
- Note: patients with diagnosed or undiagnosed bipolar or psychotic disorders may be more vulnerable to CNS-activating actions of SSRIs like fluvoxamine; pay particular attention to signs of activation in children with developmental disorders or autism spectrum disorders
- Treatment-emergent activation syndrome (TEAS) includes agitation, anxiety, panic attacks, irritability, aggression, impulsivity, and insomnia
- TEAS can represent side effects but should not be confused with bipolar mania or the onset of suicidality and should be monitored and investigated with consideration of discontinuing or decreasing the dose of escitalopram or addition of another agent or switching to another agent to reduce these symptoms
- Gastrointestinal (decreased appetite, nausea, diarrhea, constipation, dry mouth)
- Sexual dysfunction (boys: delayed ejaculation, erectile dysfunction; boys and girls: decreased sexual desire, anorgasmia)
- Autonomic (sweating)
- Bruising and rare bleeding
- Syndrome of inappropriate antidiuretic hormone secretion (SIADH)

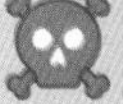

Life-Threatening or Dangerous Side Effects

- Rare seizures
- Rare hyponatremia
- Rare induction of mania
- Rare suicidal ideation and behavior (suicidality) (short-term regulatory studies did not show any actual suicides in any age group and also did not show an increase in the risk of suicidality with antidepressants compared to placebo beyond age 24)

Growth and Maturation

- Decreased appetite and weight loss have been observed in patients taking SSRIs, so growth should be monitored

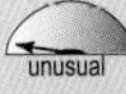

Weight Gain

- Reported but not expected
- Patients may actually experience weight loss

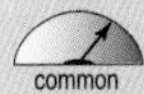

Sedation

- Many experience and/or can be significant in amount

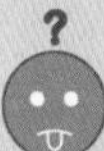

What to Do About Side Effects

- Wait, wait, wait: mild side effects are common, happen early, and usually improve with time, but treatment benefits can be delayed and often begin just as the side effects wear off
- Monitor side effects closely, especially when initiating treatment
- May wish to try dosing every other day to deal with side effects, or wash out for a week and try again at half dose or every other day
- May wish to give some drugs at night if not tolerated during the day, particularly if the medication is associated with sedation
- For activation (jitteriness, anxiety, insomnia):
  - Administer dose in the morning
  - Consider a temporary dose reduction or a more gradual up-titration
  - Consider switching to another SSRI or potentially an SNRI (other than venlafaxine)
  - Optimize psychotherapeutic interventions
  - Activation and agitation may represent the induction of a bipolar state, especially a mixed dysphoric bipolar II condition sometimes associated with suicidal ideation, and may require the addition of lithium, a mood stabilizer or an atypical antipsychotic, and/or discontinuation of fluvoxamine
- Often best to try another monotherapy prior to resorting to augmentation strategies to treat side effects
- For insomnia: consider adding melatonin
- For GI upset: try giving medication with a meal
- For sexual dysfunction:
  - Probably best to reduce dose or discontinue and try another agent
  - Consider adding daytime exercise, bupropion, or buspirone
- For emotional flattening, apathy: consider adding bupropion (with caution as little experience in children)

How Drug Causes Side Effects

- Theoretically due to increases in serotonin concentrations at serotonin receptors in parts of the brain and body other than those that cause therapeutic actions (e.g., unwanted actions of serotonin in sleep centers causing insomnia, unwanted actions of serotonin in the gut causing diarrhea)
- Increasing serotonin can cause diminished dopamine release and might contribute to emotional flattening, cognitive slowing, and apathy in some patients
- Fluvoxamine's sigma 1 antagonist properties may contribute to sedation and fatigue in some patients

Warnings and Precautions

- Consider distributing the brochures provided by the FDA and the drug companies as well as the medication guides from the American Academy of Child & Adolescent Psychiatry (AACAP)
- Carefully consider monitoring patients regularly and within the practical limits, particularly during the first several weeks of treatment
- Warn patients and their caregivers when possible about the possibility of activating side effects and advise them to report such symptoms immediately
- Carefully weigh the risks and benefits of pharmacological treatment against the risks and benefits of nontreatment with antidepressants and it is a good idea to document this in the patient's chart
- Add or initiate other antidepressants with caution for up to 2 weeks after discontinuing fluvoxamine
- As with any antidepressant, use with caution in patients with history of seizure
- As with any antidepressant, use with caution in patients with bipolar disorder unless treated with concomitant mood-stabilizing agent
- Monitor patients for activation and suicidal ideation and involve parents/guardians
- May cause photosensitivity

When Not to Prescribe

- If patient is taking an MAO inhibitor
- If patient is taking thioridazine, pimozide, tizanidine, alosetron, or ramelteon
- Not generally recommended in patients taking tricyclic antidepressants (see Drug Interactions)
- If there is a proven allergy to fluvoxamine

Long-Term Use

- Decreased appetite and weight loss have been observed in patients taking SSRIs, so growth should be monitored; long-term effects are unknown

Habit Forming

- No

Overdose

- Rare fatalities have been reported, both in combination with other drugs and alone; sedation, dizziness, vomiting, diarrhea, irregular heartbeat, seizures, coma, breathing difficulty

DOSING AND USE

Usual Dosage Range

- In children: 50–200 mg/day
- In adolescents: 50–300 mg/day

Dosage Forms

- Tablet 25 mg, 50 mg scored, 100 mg scored
- Controlled-release capsule 100 mg, 150 mg

How to Dose

- In children (immediate-release): initial dose 25 mg at bedtime; can increase by 25 mg every 4–7 days; maximum dose 200 mg/day; daily doses over 50 mg should be divided
- In adolescents (immediate-release): initial dose 25 mg at bedtime; can increase by 25 mg every 4–7 days; maximum dose 300 mg/day; daily doses over 50 mg should be divided

Options for Administration

- Controlled-release capsules should not be cut or crushed
- The lowest available controlled-release dose (100 mg) may not be appropriate for pediatric patients naïve to fluvoxamine

Tests

- None for healthy individuals

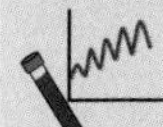

Pharmacokinetics

- Fluvoxamine is extensively metabolized in the liver and in children and

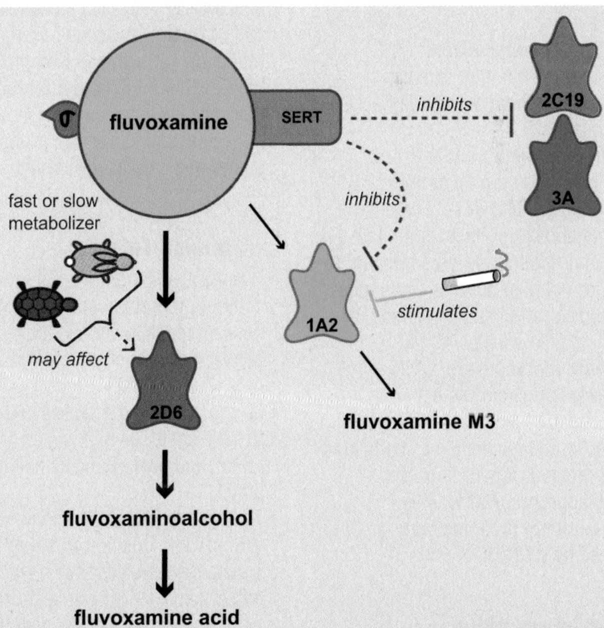

Figure 1 Fluvoxamine metabolism. Fluvoxamine is primarily metabolized by CYP2D6 and its major metabolite fluvoxamine acid (also called M1) represents around 30–60% of fluvoxamine urinary metabolites. None of its metabolites is pharmacologically active.

adolescents – like in adults – has on-linear pharmacokinetics. Also, in youth, fluvoxamine pharmacokinetics may be affected by the sex of the patient, with boys having lower peak concentrations (Cmax) and higher concentrations over time (AUC).

- Fluvoxamine is highly protein bound (80%), and most protein binding is to albumin
- In adults, the bioavailability is about 50%, although this is increased to 84% with the extended-release formulation
- Half-life elimination: ~14 to 16 hours in adults (not reported in pediatric patients)
- The time to peak plasma concentrations is 3 to 8 hours, although this has not been reported in youth
- Steady-state plasma concentrations are higher in children than in adolescents or adults
- Substrate for CYP2D6 (Figure 1)
- Inhibits CYP3A4, CYP1A2, and CYP2C9/2C19

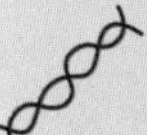

Pharmacogenetics

- There is a significant decrease in the clearance of fluvoxamine in CYP2D6 poor metabolizers compared to normal metabolizers
    - **CYP2D6 normal metabolizers:** CPIC strongly recommends that clinicians initiate therapy with recommended starting dose
    - **CYP2D6 intermediate metabolizers:** CPIC recommends starting at the recommended starting dose. There is reduced metabolism of fluvoxamine to less active compounds when compared to CYP2D6 normal metabolizers, and higher plasma concentrations may increase the probability of side effects.
    - **CYP2D6 poor metabolizers:** CPIC recommends that clinicians either consider a 25–50% lower starting dose and slower titration schedule as compared to normal metabolizers or consider a clinically appropriate alternative antidepressant not predominantly metabolized by CYP2D6

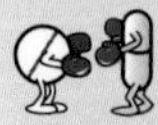

Drug Interactions

- Tramadol reported to increase the risk of seizures in adults taking an antidepressant
- Can increase tricyclic antidepressant (TCA) levels; use with caution with tricyclic antidepressants or when switching from a TCA to fluoxetine
- Can cause a fatal "serotonin syndrome" when combined with MAO inhibitors, so do not use with MAO inhibitors or for at least 14 days after MAOIs are stopped
- Do not start an MAO inhibitor for at least 5 half-lives (5 to 7 days for most drugs) after discontinuing fluvoxamine
- May displace highly protein-bound drugs (e.g., phenytoin, valproate)
- Possible increased risk of bleeding
- Via CYP1A2 inhibition, fluvoxamine may reduce clearance of theophylline and clozapine, thus raising their levels and requiring their dosing to be lowered
- Fluvoxamine administered with either caffeine or theophylline can thus cause jitteriness, excessive stimulation, or rarely seizures, so concomitant use should proceed cautiously
- Metabolism of fluvoxamine may be enhanced in smokers and thus its levels lowered, requiring higher dosing
- Via CYP3A4 inhibition, fluvoxamine may reduce clearance of carbamazepine and benzodiazepines such as alprazolam and triazolam, and thus require dosage reduction (Strawn and Stimpfl, 2023)
- Via CYP3A4 inhibition, fluvoxamine could theoretically increase the concentrations of pimozide, and cause QTc prolongation and dangerous cardiac arrhythmias

Dosing Tips

- Plasma levels are higher in lower-weight children; therefore, starting and target doses may be lower and longer intervals between dose increases may be needed (see How to Dose)
- 50 mg and 100 mg tablets are scored, so to save costs, give 25 mg as half of 50 mg tablet, and give 50 mg as half of 100 mg tablet
- To improve tolerability of immediate-release formulation, dosing can either be given once a day, usually all at night, or split either symmetrically or asymmetrically, usually with more of the dose given at night
- Some patients take more than 300 mg/day
- Controlled-release capsules should not be chewed or crushed

- The more anxious and agitated the patient, the lower the starting dose, the slower the titration
- If intolerable anxiety, insomnia, agitation, akathisia, or activation occurs either upon dosing initiation or discontinuation, consider the possibility of activated bipolar disorder and switch to an atypical antipsychotic or a mood stabilizer as an alternative to an SSRI. Importantly, the risk of activation with one SSRI does not predict the likelihood of activation with another SSRI.

How to Switch

- From another antidepressant to fluvoxamine:
  - When tapering a prior antidepressant, see its entry in this manual for how to stop and how to taper off that specific drug
  - In situations when there are antidepressant-related side effects, try to stop the first agent before starting fluvoxamine so that new side effects of fluvoxamine can be distinguished from withdrawal effects of the first agent
  - If urgent, cross taper
- Off fluvoxamine to another antidepressant:
  - Generally, try to stop fluvoxamine before starting another antidepressant
  - Taper to avoid withdrawal effects (dizziness, nausea, stomach cramps, sweating, tingling, dysesthesias)
  - Can reduce fluvoxamine dose by 50% every 7–10 days, or slower if this rate still causes withdrawal symptoms
  - If necessary, can cross taper off fluvoxamine this way while dosing up on another antidepressant simultaneously in urgent situations, being aware of all specific drug interactions to avoid

How to Stop

- Taper to avoid withdrawal effects (dizziness, nausea, stomach cramps, sweating, tingling, dysesthesias)
- Many patients tolerate 50% dose reduction for 7–10 days, then another 50% reduction for 7–10 days, then discontinuation. More recently however, hyperbolic discontinuation of SSRIs has been recommended in which the dose of the SSRI is halved every 4 weeks, and this may be a preferable strategy in youth (Strawn et al., 2023). Also, when SSRIs are stopped, the risk of relapse is highest during the first 8 weeks after discontinuation.
- If withdrawal symptoms emerge during discontinuation, raise dose to stop symptoms and then restart withdrawal much more slowly

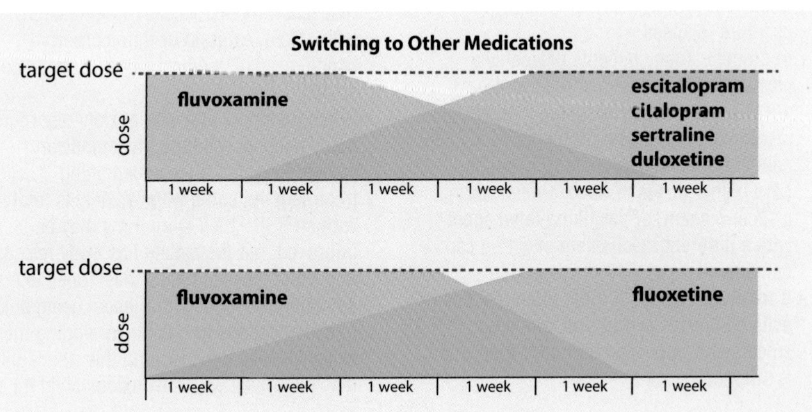

WHAT TO EXPECT

Onset of Action

- Some patients may experience increased energy or activation early after initiation of treatment
- Full onset of therapeutic actions is usually delayed by 2–4 weeks
- If it is not working within 6–8 weeks, it may require a dosage increase or it may not work at all

Duration of Action

- Effects are consistent over a 24-hour period
- May continue to work for many years to prevent relapse of symptoms

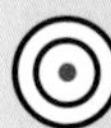

Primary Target Symptoms

- Depressed and/or irritable mood
- Obsessions, compulsions
- Anxiety (fear and worry are often target symptoms, but fluvoxamine can occasionally and transiently increase these symptoms short term before improving them)
- Prior to initiation of treatment, it is helpful to develop a list of target symptoms of OCD, depression, and/or anxiety to monitor during treatment to better assess treatment response. In a setting where OCD is the focus of fluvoxamine treatment, clinicians may consider using the Children's Yale–Brown Obsessive Compulsive Scale to assess symptoms over time.

What Is Considered a Positive Result?

- The goal of treatment is complete remission of current symptoms as well as prevention of future relapses
- In practice, many patients have only a partial response where some symptoms are improved but others persist (especially insomnia, fatigue, and problems concentrating in depression), in which case higher doses of fluvoxamine, adding a second agent, or switching to an agent with a different mechanism of action can be considered
- If treatment works, it most often reduces or even eliminates symptoms, but is not a cure since symptoms can recur after medicine is stopped

How Long to Treat

- For adolescents with depression, generally, 9–12 months of antidepressant treatment is recommended (Hathaway et al., 2018)
- For anxiety disorders, 6–9 months of antidepressant treatment may be sufficient, though many clinicians extend treatment to 12 months based on extrapolation of data from adults with anxiety disorders (Hathaway et al., 2018; Strawn et al., 2023)
- Extended treatment periods may decrease the risk of long-term morbidity and recurrence; however, the goal of treatment is ultimately remission, rather than duration of antidepressant pharmacotherapy (Hathaway et al., 2018)
- In terms of the length of antidepressant treatment, evidence-based guidelines represent a starting point; appropriate treatment duration varies, and patient-specific response, psychological factors, and timing of discontinuation must be considered for individual pediatric patients (Hathaway et al., 2018)

What If It Stops Working?

- Some patients who have an initial response may relapse even though they continue treatment, sometimes called "poop-out"
- Some patients may experience apparent lack of consistent efficacy due to activation syndrome or underlying or newly evolved bipolar disorder, or major depressive episodes with mixed features, and require antidepressant discontinuation and a switch to a second generation antipsychotic

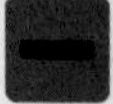

What If It Doesn't Work?

- Consider evaluation for another diagnosis (especially bipolar illness or depression with mixed features) or for a comorbid condition (e.g., medical illness, substance abuse)
- When treating youth with anxiety disorders, many patients will have had significant anxiety for years prior to beginning treatment. As such, when anxiety is treated with an SSRI, their symptoms may be improved, but the patient has likely missed important developmental milestones (e.g., spending the night with friends, being able to ask questions in class). Developing these skills will take time. Beyond this, the family may have lived with the anxious child for

years and following treatment of the child, the family may need to readjust.

- Be mindful of family conflict contributing to the presentation; sometimes treating parental depression or anxiety disorders improves psychiatric and social function without any treatment of youth. Also, accommodation is common in families of youth with anxiety disorders and may need to be addressed specifically, as it can perpetuate symptoms.
- Consider factors associated with poor response to SSRIs in treatment-resistant depression or anxiety disorders, such as severe symptoms, long-lasting symptoms, poor treatment adherence, prior nonresponse to other treatments, and the presence of comorbid disorders
- Consider other important potential factors such as ongoing conflicts, family psychopathology, and an adverse environment (e.g., poverty, chaos, violence, prior and ongoing psychological trauma, abuse, neglect). Additionally, when symptoms are prominent at school, consider the presence of a learning disorder.
- Institute trauma-informed care for appropriate children and adolescents
- A 2007 meta-analysis of published and unpublished trials in pediatric patients found that antidepressants had a number needed to treat (NNT) of 10 for depression, 6 for OCD, and 3 for anxiety disorders; thus, fluvoxamine may not work in all children, so consider switching to another antidepressant (Bridge et al., 2007)
- Consider a dose adjustment
- Consider augmenting options:
    - Cognitive behavioral therapy (CBT), interpersonal psychotherapy for adolescents (IPT-A), light therapy, family therapy, and exercise especially in adolescents
    - For partial response (depression): use caution when adding medications to fluvoxamine, especially in children since there are not sufficient studies of augmentation in children or adolescents; however, for the expert, consider bupropion, aripiprazole, or other atypical antipsychotics such as quetiapine; use combinations of antidepressants with caution as this may activate bipolar disorder and suicidal ideation
    - For insomnia: sleep hygiene, CBT for insomnia, melatonin, or alpha 2 agonists
    - For anxiety: buspirone, antihistamines
    - Add lithium or atypical antipsychotics for bipolar depression, psychotic depression, treatment-resistant depression, or treatment-resistant anxiety disorders
    - TMS (transcranial magnetic stimulation) may have a role although pediatric trials of TMS have been hampered by high sham response rates (Croarkin et al., 2021)
    - ECT (case studies show effectiveness; cognitive side effects are similar to those in adults; reserve for treatment-resistant cases)

TALKING TO PATIENTS AND CAREGIVERS

What to Tell Parents About Efficacy

- Doesn't work right away; full therapeutic benefits may take up to 8 weeks, yet parents and teachers might see improvement before the patient does
- While the medicine helps by reducing symptoms and improving function, it is not a cure, and it is therefore necessary to keep taking the medication to sustain its therapeutic effects
- Since every treatment consideration depends on a risk/benefit analysis, parents should fully understand short- and long-term risks as well as benefits
- One of the SSRIs specifically approved for children and adolescents with OCD (obsessive-compulsive disorder)
- After successful treatment, continuation of fluvoxamine may be necessary to prevent relapse, especially in those who have had more than one episode or a very severe episode. In general, when treating depression in children and adolescents, medications are continued for 12 months after symptoms have resolved, while for anxiety disorders, clinicians have generally treated for 6–9 months (Hathaway et al., 2018).
- Often a good idea to tell parents whether the medication chosen is specifically approved for the disorder being treated, or whether it is being given for "unapproved" or "off-label" reasons based on good clinical practice, expert consensus, and/or prudent extrapolation of controlled data from adults

What to Tell Children and Adolescents About Efficacy

- We are trying to make you feel better
- It may be a good idea to give the medication a try; if it's not working very well, we can stop the medication and try something else
- A good try takes 2 to 3 months or even longer
- If it does make you feel better, you cannot stop it right away or you may feel sad or worried again
- Medications don't change who you are as a person; they give you the opportunity to be the best person you can be

What to Tell Parents About Side Effects

- Explain that side effects are expected in many when starting and are most common in the first 2–3 weeks of starting or increasing the dose
- Some SSRI side effects emerge early and resolve quickly (e.g., activation, gastrointestinal symptoms). In contrast, other side effects are late-emerging (e.g., weight gain) or persistent (e.g., sexual dysfunction). Discussing the temporal course of the side effects and distinguishing between persistent and transient side effects is critical. Ensuring that patients are aware not only of side effects but the tendency of some side effects to be transient is important and should be part of discussions with patients and their families. For many, knowing that a side effect is likely transient, as opposed to persistent, may significantly influence the patient and family's anxiety or fears related to medication (Strawn et al., 2023).
- Tell parents many side effects go away and do so about the same time that therapeutic effects start
- Predict side effects in advance (you will look clever and competent to the parents, unless you scare them with too much information and cause nocebo effects, in which case you won't look so clever when the patient develops lots of side effects and stops medication; use your judgment here); a balanced but honest presentation is an art rather than a science
- Ask them to help monitor for increased suicidality and if present, report any such symptoms immediately
- Ask parents to support the patient while side effects are occurring
- Parents should fully understand short- and long-term risks as well as benefits
- Explaining to the parents what to expect from medication treatment, and especially potential side effects, can help prevent early termination of medication

What to Tell Children and Adolescents About Side Effects

- Even if you get side effects, most of them get better or go away in a few days to a few weeks
- Consider having a conversation about sexual side effects in some adolescents who can find these side effects confusing and especially burdensome
- Explaining to child/adolescent what to expect from medication treatment, and especially potential side effects, can help prevent early termination of medication
- Tell adolescents and children capable of understanding that some young patients, especially those who are depressed, may develop thoughts of hurting themselves, and if this happens, not to be alarmed but to tell their parents right away

What to Tell Teachers About the Medication (If Parents Consent)

- Fluvoxamine can make children/adolescents jittery or restless
- If the patient is sleepy, ask whether the medication is keeping them up at night
- It is not abusable
- Encourage dialogue with parents/guardians about any behavior or mood changes

SPECIAL POPULATIONS

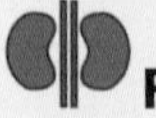

Renal Impairment

- Consider lower initial dose

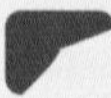

Hepatic Impairment

- Lower dose or give less frequently, perhaps by half; use slower titration

Cardiac Impairment

- Preliminary research suggests that fluvoxamine is safe in these patients

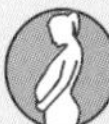

Pregnancy

- Controlled studies have not been conducted in pregnant women
- Not generally recommended for use during pregnancy, especially during first trimester
- Nonetheless, continuous treatment during pregnancy may be necessary and has not been proven to be harmful to the fetus
- At delivery there may be more bleeding in the mother and transient irritability or sedation in the newborn
- Must weigh the risk of treatment (first trimester fetal development, third trimester newborn delivery) to the child against the risk of no treatment (recurrence of depression, maternal health, infant bonding) to the mother and child
- For many patients this may mean continuing treatment during pregnancy
- Exposure to SSRIs early in pregnancy may be associated with increased risk of septal heart defects (absolute risk is small)
- SSRI use beyond the 20th week of pregnancy may be associated with increased risk of pulmonary hypertension in newborns, although this is not proven
- Exposure to SSRIs late in pregnancy may be associated with increased risk of gestational hypertension and preeclampsia
- Neonates exposed to SSRIs or SNRIs late in the third trimester have developed complications requiring prolonged hospitalization, respiratory support, and tube feeding; reported symptoms are consistent with either a direct toxic effect of SSRIs and SNRIs or, possibly, a drug discontinuation syndrome, and include respiratory distress, cyanosis, apnea, seizures, temperature instability, feeding difficulty, vomiting, hypoglycemia, hypotonia, hypertonia, hyperreflexia, tremor, jitteriness, irritability, and constant crying

Breast Feeding

- Some drug is found in breast milk
- Trace amounts may be present in nursing children whose mothers are on fluvoxamine
- If child becomes irritable or sedated, breast feeding or drug may need to be discontinued
- Immediate postpartum period is a high-risk time for depression, especially in women who have had prior depressive episodes, so drug may need to be reinstituted late in the third trimester or shortly after childbirth to prevent a recurrence during the postpartum period
- Must weigh benefits of breast feeding with risks and benefits of antidepressant treatment versus nontreatment to both the infant and the mother
- For many patients this may mean continuing treatment during breast feeding

THE ART OF PSYCHOPHARMACOLOGY

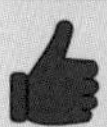

Potential Advantages

- In children:
  - One of only four agents specifically approved for OCD in children (also paroxetine, fluoxetine, and clomipramine). However, this medication was also one of the first SSRIs to be studied in pediatric anxiety disorders.
- In adolescents:
  - One of only four agents specifically approved for OCD in adolescents (also paroxetine, fluoxetine, and clomipramine)
- All ages:
  - Patients with mixed anxiety/depression

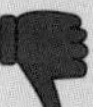

Potential Disadvantages

- In children and adolescents:
  - Those who are already psychomotor agitated, angry, or irritable, and who do not have a psychiatric diagnosis
  - Those who may possibly have a mood disorder with mixed or bipolar features, especially those with these features and a family history of bipolar disorder
- All ages:
  - Patients with irritable bowel or multiple gastrointestinal complaints
  - Can require dose titration and twice daily dosing

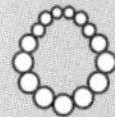

Pearls

- SSRIs show greater efficacy in pediatric anxiety disorders compared to depression
- Some withdrawal effects, especially gastrointestinal effects
- May have lower incidence of sexual dysfunction than other SSRIs

- May have higher incidence of nausea and sedation than other SSRIs
- In prospective studies of youth, higher fluvoxamine concentrations have been associated with greater activation-related side effects in youth (Reinblatt et al., 2009)
- Fluvoxamine has nonlinear kinetics in pediatric patients and this effect is greater in children compared to adolescents. In other words, the overall increase in fluvoxamine levels over time is disproportional to the dose increase. This likely relates to fluvoxamine inhibiting its own metabolism.
- Not FDA approved for depression, but used widely for depression in many countries
- CR formulation may be better tolerated than immediate-release formulation, particularly with less sedation; however, absorption of the CR formulation is greater than with the immediate-release formulation
- Actions at sigma 1 receptors may explain in part fluvoxamine's sometimes rapid onset effects in anxiety disorders and insomnia
- For treatment-resistant OCD, consider cautious combination of fluvoxamine and clomipramine by an expert:
    - Normally, clomipramine, a potent serotonin reuptake blocker, at steady state is metabolized extensively to its active metabolite desmethylclomipramine, a potent noradrenergic reuptake blocker. Thus, at steady state, plasma drug activity is generally more noradrenergic (with higher desmethylclomipramine levels) than serotonergic (with lower parent clomipramine levels).
    - Addition of fluvoxamine, a CYP1A2 inhibitor, blocks this conversion and results in higher clomipramine levels than desmethylclomipramine levels. Thus, adding fluvoxamine to clomipramine in treatment-resistant OCD can powerfully enhance serotonergic activity, not only due to the inherent serotonergic activity of fluvoxamine, but also due to a favorable pharmacokinetic interaction inhibiting CYP1A2 and thus converting clomipramine's metabolism to a more powerful serotonergic portfolio of parent drug.
- At therapeutic doses, fluvoxamine inhibits metabolism of caffeine (through CYP1A2) (Christensen et al., 2002)

SUGGESTED READING

Bridge JA, Iyengar S, Salary CB et al. Clinical response and risk for reported suicidal ideation and suicide attempts in pediatric antidepressant treatment: a meta-analysis of randomized controlled trials. JAMA 2007;297(15):1683–96.

Carrillo JA, Dahl ML, Svensson JO et al. Disposition of fluvoxamine in humans is determined by the polymorphic CYP2D6 and also by the CYP1A2 activity. Clin Pharmacol Ther 1996;60(2):183–190.

Christensen M, Tybring G, Mihara K et al. Low daily 10-mg and 20-mg doses of fluvoxamine inhibit the metabolism of both caffeine (cytochrome P4501A2) and omeprazole (cytochrome P4502C19). Clin Pharmacol Ther 2002;71(3):141–52.

Croarkin PE, Elmaadawi AZ, Aaronson ST et al. Left prefrontal transcranial magnetic stimulation for treatment-resistant depression in adolescents: a double-blind, randomized, sham-controlled trial. Neuropsychopharmacology 2021;46(2):462–9.

Fung R, Elbe D, Stewart SE. Retrospective review of fluvoxamine-clomipramine combination therapy in obsessive-compulsive disorder in children and adolescents. J Can Acad Child Adolesc Psychiatry 2021;30(3):150–5.

Hardy NE, Walkup JT. Clomipramine in combination with fluvoxamine: a potent medication combination for severe or refractory pediatric OCD. J Can Acad Child Adolesc Psychiatry 2021;30(4):273–7.

Hathaway EE, Walkup JT, Strawn JR. Antidepressant treatment duration in pediatric depressive and anxiety disorders: how long is long enough? Curr Probl Pediatr Adolesc Health Care 2018;48(2):31–9.

Labellarte M, Biederman J, Emslie G et al. Multiple-dose pharmacokinetics of fluvoxamine in children and adolescents. J Am Acad Child Adolesc Psychiatry 2004;43(12):1497–505.

Mulder H, Herder A, Wilmink FW et al. The impact of cytochrome P450-2D6 genotype on the use and interpretation of therapeutic drug monitoring in long-stay patients treated with antidepressant and antipsychotic drugs in daily psychiatric practice. Pharmacoepidemiol Drug Saf 2006;15(2):107–14.

Reinblatt SP, DosReis S, Walkup JT, Riddle MA. Activation adverse events induced by the selective serotonin reuptake inhibitor fluvoxamine in children and adolescents. J Child Adolesc Psychopharmacol 2009;19(2):119–26.

Riddle MA, Reeve EA, Yaryura-Tobias JA et al. Fluvoxamine for children and adolescents with obsessive-compulsive disorder: a randomized, controlled, multicenter trial. J Am Acad Child Adolesc Psychiatry 2001b;40(2):222–9.

RUPP. Fluvoxamine for the treatment of anxiety disorders in children and adolescents. The Research Unit on Pediatric Psychopharmacology Anxiety Study Group. N Engl J Med 2001;344(17):1279–85.

Strawn JR, Mills JA, Poweleit EA, Ramsey LB, Croarkin PE. Adverse effects of antidepressant medications and their management in children and adolescents. Pharmacotherapy 2023;43(7):675–90.

Strawn JR, Stimpfl J. Optimizing benzodiazepine treatment of anxiety disorders. Curr Psychiatry 2023;22(6):22–33, 39.

THERAPEUTICS

Brands

- Horizant
- Neurontin

Generic

Yes (not for extended-release)

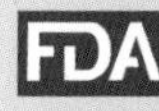

US FDA Approved for Pediatric Use

- Partial-onset seizures with and without secondary generalization (adjunctive, ages 3 and older)

Off-Label for Pediatric Use

- Approved in adults
  - Postherpetic neuralgia
  - Restless leg syndrome (extended-release)
- Other off-label uses
  - Neuropathic pain/chronic pain
  - Anxiety (adjunctive)

Class and Mechanism of Action

- Neuroscience-based Nomenclature: glutamate, voltage-gated calcium channel blocker (Glu-CB)
- Anticonvulsant, antineuralgic for chronic pain, alpha 2 delta ligand at voltage-sensitive calcium channels

SAFETY AND TOLERABILITY

Notable Side Effects

- Sedation (dose dependent), dizziness
- Ataxia (dose dependent), fatigue, nystagmus, tremor
- Peripheral edema
- Blurred vision
- Vomiting, dyspepsia, diarrhea, dry mouth, constipation, weight gain
- Additional effects in children under age 12: hostility, emotional lability, hyperkinesia, thought disorder, weight gain

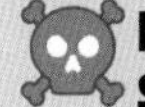

Life-Threatening or Dangerous Side Effects

- Anaphylaxis and angioedema
- Sudden unexplained deaths have occurred in epilepsy (unknown if related to gabapentin use)
- Rare activation of suicidal ideation and behavior (suicidality)

Growth and Maturation

- Not studied

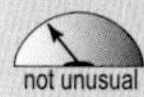

Weight Gain

- Occurs in some patients and may be dose related

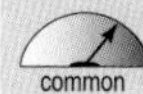

Sedation

- Many experience and/or can be significant in amount
- Dose related; can be problematic at high doses
- Can wear off with time, but may not wear off at high doses

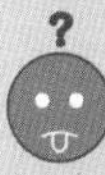

What to Do About Side Effects

- Wait
- Wait
- Wait
- Take more of the dose at night to reduce daytime sedation
- Lower the dose
- Switch to another agent

How Drug Causes Side Effects

- CNS side effects may be due to excessive blockade of voltage-sensitive calcium channels

Warnings and Precautions

- Depressive effects, including respiratory depression, may be increased by other CNS depressants (opioids, benzodiazepines, alcohol, MAOIs, other anticonvulsants, etc.)
- Use lowest possible dose of gabapentin and monitor for symptoms of respiratory depression if patient is taking concomitant CNS depressant, has underlying respiratory disease, or is elderly
- Dizziness and sedation could increase the chances of accidental injury (falls) in the elderly
- Pancreatic acinar adenocarcinomas have developed in male rats that were given gabapentin, but clinical significance is unknown
- Development of new tumors or worsening of tumors has occurred in humans

taking gabapentin; it is unknown whether gabapentin affected the development or worsening of tumors
- Warn patients and their caregivers about the possibility of activation of suicidal ideation and advise them to report such side effects immediately

When Not to Prescribe

- If there is a proven allergy to gabapentin or pregabalin

Long-Term Use

- Safe

Habit Forming

- No

Overdose

- Slurred speech, sedation, double vision, diarrhea

DOSING AND USE

Usual Dosage Range

- Ages 12 and older: 1,800 mg/day in 3 divided doses
- Ages 5–12: 25–35 mg/kg/day in 3 divided doses
- Ages 3–4: 40 mg/kg/day in 3 divided doses

Dosage Forms

- Capsule 100 mg, 300 mg, 400 mg
- Tablet 100 mg, 300 mg, 400 mg, 600 mg, 800 mg
- Tablet extended-release 300 mg, 600 mg
- Oral solution 250 mg/5 mL

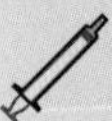

How to Dose

- Ages 12 and older: initial 900 mg/day in 3 doses; recommended dose generally 1,800 mg/day in 3 doses; maximum dose generally 3,600 mg/day; time between any 2 doses should usually not exceed 12 hours. However, when using for anxiety (off-label), may use lower doses and may start at 300 mg bid.
- Ages 5–12: initial 10–15 mg/kg per day in 3 doses; titrate over 3 days to 25–35 mg/kg per day given in 3 doses; maximum dose generally 50 mg/kg per day; time between any 2 doses should usually not exceed 12 hours. However, when using for anxiety (off-label), may use lower doses and may start at 150 mg bid.
- Ages 3–4: initial 10–15 mg/kg per day in 3 doses; titrate over 3 days to 40 mg/kg per day; maximum dose generally 50 mg/kg per day; time between any 2 doses should usually not exceed 12 hours. Generally, not used for anxiety or other psychiatric indications in the 3- to 4-year-old range.

Options for Administration

- Oral solution option for patients with difficulty swallowing pills

Tests

- None for healthy individuals
- False-positive readings with the Ames N-Multistix SG® dipstick test for urinary protein have been reported when gabapentin was administered with other anticonvulsants

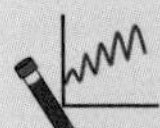

Pharmacokinetics

- Well absorbed from the gastrointestinal tract after oral administration. In pediatric patients, the time to peak plasma concentration (Tmax) is generally 2 to 3 hours (Figure 1).
- Absorption across the intestinal membrane depends on the neutral amino acid transporter system (system L); this is saturable and results in dose-dependent absorption
- Low plasma protein binding, which means a significant portion of the drug remains in its unbound, active form in the bloodstream. The volume of distribution in pediatric patients is similar to that in adults, indicating that gabapentin distributes relatively well throughout the body.
- Not significantly metabolized in the liver, it is primarily eliminated unchanged in the urine. This makes it easier to use in patients with hepatic impairment, as the risk of drug–drug interactions related to hepatic metabolism is low.
- Primarily eliminated through the kidneys via renal excretion. The elimination half-life in pediatric patients is similar to that in adults, typically ranging from 5 to 7 hours. However, in younger children, the half-life may be shorter compared to older children and adults due to increased renal clearance.

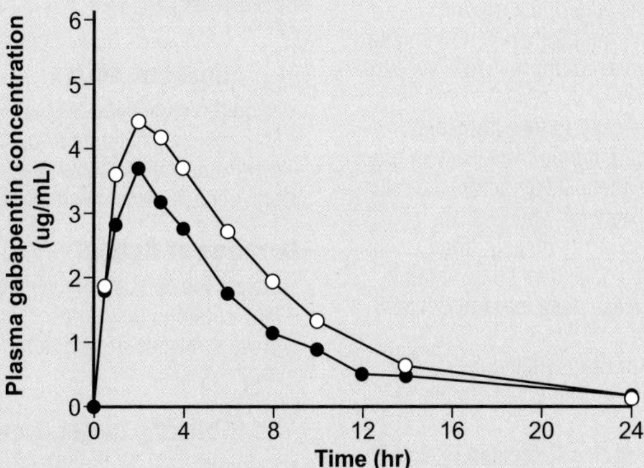

Figure 1 Gabapentin concentrations in pediatric patients. Patients younger than 5 years are shown by black circles, and open circles represent those between 5 and 12 years of age. Adapted from Haig et al., 2001.

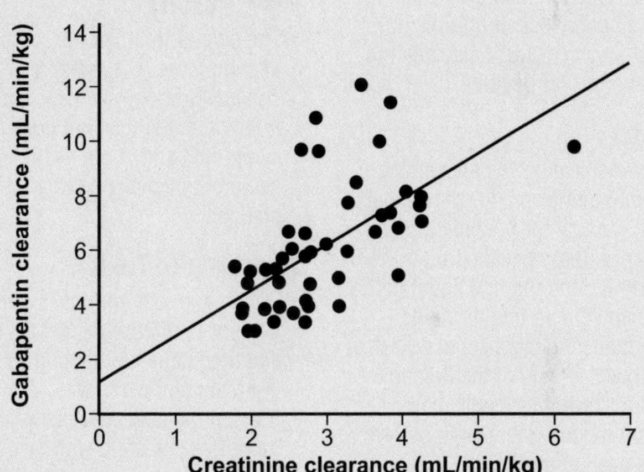

Figure 2 Relationship between gabapentin clearance and creatinine clearance in children up to age 12. Adapted from Haig et al., 2001.

- Renal excretion is directly proportional to CrCl in children. Thus, CrCl is an excellent predictor of gabapentin clearance in youth and adults (Haig et al., 2001) (Figure 2).

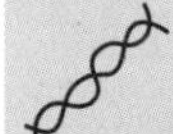

Pharmacogenetics

- No recommendations

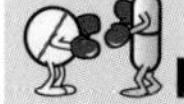

Drug Interactions

- Antacids may reduce the bioavailability of gabapentin, so gabapentin should be administered approximately 2 hours before antacids
- Naproxen may increase absorption of gabapentin
- Morphine and hydrocodone may increase gabapentin exposure [i.e., area under the curve (AUC)]

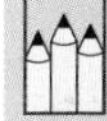

Dosing Tips

- Gabapentin should not be taken until 2 hours after an antacid

- If gabapentin is added to a second anticonvulsant, the titration period should be at least a week to improve tolerance to sedation
- Some patients need to take immediate-release gabapentin only twice daily in order to experience adequate symptomatic relief for pain or anxiety
- At the high end of the dosing range, tolerability may be enhanced by splitting immediate-release dose into more than 3 divided doses
- Half-tablets not used within several days of breaking the scored tablet should be discarded
- Do not break or chew extended-release tablets, as this could alter controlled-release properties
- Extended-release tablets should be taken with food
- For intolerable sedation, can give most of the dose at night and less during the day
- To improve slow-wave sleep, may need to take gabapentin only at bedtime

How to Switch

- From another medication to gabapentin:
  - When tapering a prior medication, see its entry in this manual for how to stop and how to taper off that specific drug
  - Generally, try to stop the first agent before starting gabapentin so that new side effects of gabapentin can be distinguished from withdrawal effects of the first agent
- Off gabapentin to another medication:
  - Generally, try to stop gabapentin before starting the new medication so that new side effects of the next drug can be distinguished from any withdrawal effects from gabapentin
  - Taper; may need to adjust dosage of concurrent medications as gabapentin is being discontinued

How to Stop

- Taper over a minimum of 1 week
- Epilepsy patients may seize upon withdrawal, especially if withdrawal is abrupt
- Rapid discontinuation may increase the risk of relapse in bipolar disorder
- Discontinuation symptoms uncommon

WHAT TO EXPECT

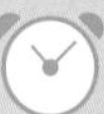

Onset of Action

- Should reduce seizures by 2 weeks
- May reduce pain in neuropathic pain syndromes within a few weeks
- May reduce anxiety within a week

Duration of Action

- Effects are consistent over a 24-hour period
- May continue to work for many years to prevent relapse of symptoms

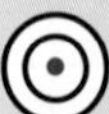

Primary Target Symptoms

- Seizures
- Pain
- Anxiety

What Is Considered a Positive Result?

- The goal of treatment is complete remission of symptoms (e.g., seizures)
- Treatment of chronic neuropathic pain most often reduces but does not eliminate symptoms and is not a cure since symptoms usually recur after medicine stopped

How Long to Treat

- Continue treatment until symptoms are gone or until improvement is stable and then continue treating as long as improvement persists
- If using for anxiety, treating for 9–12 months, consistent with recommendations for other pharmacotherapy in pediatric anxiety disorders, is reasonable

What If It Stops Working?

- Check for nonadherence and consider switching to another agent with fewer side effects
- If using for pain, consider adjunctive physical therapy interventions and psychosocial treatments for chronic pain in addition to consultation with pediatric pain specialists
- Consider evaluation for another diagnosis (e.g., autoimmune disorder or neuropathy, fibromyalgia contributing to pain symptoms)
- Screen for adverse changes in the home or school environment

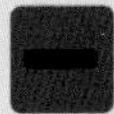

What If It Doesn't Work?

- If it is not reducing pain within 6–8 weeks, it may require a dosage increase or it may not work at all. Consider alternative agents with alternative mechanisms of action for neuropathic pain or other forms of chronic pain. Consider physical therapy interventions and psychosocial treatments for chronic pain in addition to consultation with pediatric pain specialists.
- Consider evaluation for another diagnosis (e.g., autoimmune disorder or neuropathy, fibromyalgia contributing to pain symptoms)
- If using for anxiety, consider a medication or psychosocial intervention with stronger evidence (e.g., CBT, SSRIs)
- Consider other important potential factors such as ongoing conflicts, family psychopathology, and an adverse environment (e.g., poverty, chaos, violence, prior and ongoing psychological trauma, abuse, neglect)

TALKING TO PATIENTS AND CAREGIVERS

What to Tell Parents About Efficacy

- For acute symptoms, it can work right away
- Explain which use gabapentin is being chosen for, how to tell if the drug is working by targeting specific symptoms, and why this is being done
- Since every treatment consideration depends on a risk/benefit analysis, parents should fully understand short- and long-term risks as well as benefits
- Often a good idea to tell parents whether the medication chosen is specifically approved for the disorder being treated, or whether it is being given for "unapproved" or "off-label" reasons based on good clinical practice, expert consensus, and/or prudent extrapolation of controlled data from adults

What to Tell Children and Adolescents About Efficacy

- Be specific about the symptoms being targeted: we are trying to help you …
- Give the medication a try; if it's not working very well, we can stop the medication and try something else
- A good try often takes 2 to 3 months
- If it does make you feel better, you cannot stop it right away or you may get sick again
- Medications don't change who you are as a person; they give you the opportunity to be the best person you can be

What to Tell Parents About Side Effects

- Explain that side effects are expected in many when starting
- Tell parents many side effects go away and do so about the same time that therapeutic effects start
- Predict side effects in advance (you will look clever and competent to the parents, unless you scare them with too much information and cause nocebo effects, in which case you won't look so clever when the patient develops lots of side effects and stops medication; use your judgment here); a balanced but honest presentation is an art rather than a science
- Ask parents to support the patient while side effects are occurring
- Parents should fully understand short- and long-term risks as well as benefits
- Explaining to the parents what to expect from medication treatment, and especially what potential side effects to expect, can help prevent early termination of medication

What to Tell Children and Adolescents About Side Effects

- Even if you get a side effect, we can usually reduce it over time
- If you have side effects that are bothering you, tell your parents and your parents should tell me
- Explaining to child/adolescent what to expect from medication treatment, and especially potential side effects, can help prevent early termination of medication

What to Tell Teachers About the Medication (If Parents Consent)

- Gabapentin can make children/adolescents sedated
- It is not abusable
- Encourage dialogue with parents/guardians about any behavior or mood changes

SPECIAL POPULATIONS

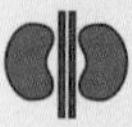

Renal Impairment

- Gabapentin is renally excreted, so the dose may need to be lowered
- Can be removed by hemodialysis; patients receiving hemodialysis may require supplemental doses of gabapentin
- Use in renal impairment has not been studied in children under age 12

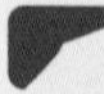

Hepatic Impairment

- No available data but not metabolized by the liver and clinical experience suggests normal dosing

Cardiac Impairment

- No specific recommendations

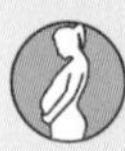

Pregnancy

- Controlled studies have not been conducted in pregnant women
- In animal studies, gabapentin was developmentally toxic (increased fetal skeletal and visceral abnormalities, and increased embryo-fetal mortality) when administered to pregnant animals at doses similar to or lower than those used clinically
- Use in women of childbearing potential requires weighing potential benefits to the mother against the risks to the fetus
- Antiepileptic Drug Pregnancy Registry: (888) 233-2334 or www.aedpregnancyregistry.org
- Taper drug if discontinuing
- Seizures, even mild seizures, may cause harm to the embryo/fetus

Breast Feeding

- Some drug is found in breast milk
- Recommended either to discontinue drug or formula feed
- If drug is continued while breast feeding, infant should be monitored for possible adverse effects
- If infant becomes irritable or sedated, breast feeding or drug may need to be discontinued

THE ART OF PSYCHOPHARMACOLOGY

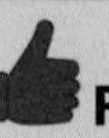

Potential Advantages

- Chronic neuropathic pain
- Has relatively mild side-effect profile
- Has few pharmacokinetic drug interactions

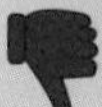

Potential Disadvantages

- Usually requires 3 times a day dosing

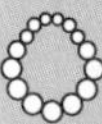

Pearls

- Gabapentin is generally well-tolerated, with only mild adverse effects
- Off-label use for treatment of neuropathic pain and anxiety may be justified, although the evidence for this is stronger in adults compared to youth
- Off-label use as an adjunct for bipolar disorder may not be justified based on studies in adults; there are essentially no data for this in youth
- May be useful for some patients in alcohol withdrawal
- If using for anxiety, ensure that you've tried a medication or psychosocial intervention with stronger evidence (e.g., CBT, SSRIs)
- One of the few agents that enhances slow-wave delta sleep, which may be helpful in chronic neuropathic pain syndromes
- Drug absorption and clinical efficacy may not necessarily be proportionately increased at high doses, and thus response to high doses may not be consistent

SUGGESTED READING

Brown S, Johnston B, Amaria K et al. A randomized controlled trial of amitriptyline versus gabapentin for complex regional pain syndrome type I and neuropathic pain in children. Scand J Pain 2016;13:156–63.

Haig GM, Bockbrader HN, Wesche DL et al. Single-dose gabapentin pharmacokinetics and safety in healthy infants and children. J Clin Pharmacol 2001;41(5):507–14.

Kuehn BM. New WHO guideline for treating chronic pain in children. JAMA 2021;325(11):1031.

THERAPEUTICS

Brands

- Intuniv
- Tenex, other

Generic

Yes

US FDA Approved for Pediatric Use

- Attention deficit hyperactivity disorder (Intuniv, ages 6 to 17, adjunct and monotherapy)

Off-Label for Pediatric Use

- Approved in adults
  - Hypertension (Tenex)
- Other off-label uses
  - Oppositional defiant disorder
  - Conduct disorder
  - Pervasive developmental disorders
  - Motor tics
  - Tourette syndrome

Class and Mechanism of Action

- Neuroscience-based Nomenclature: norepinephrine receptor agonist (N-RA)
- Centrally acting alpha 2A agonist; antihypertensive; nonstimulant for ADHD
- For ADHD, theoretically has central actions on postsynaptic alpha 2A receptors in the prefrontal cortex
- Guanfacine is 15–20 times more selective for alpha 2A receptors than for alpha 2B or alpha 2C receptors
- The prefrontal cortex is thought to be responsible for modulation of working memory, attention, impulse control, and planning
- For hypertension, stimulates alpha 2A adrenergic receptors in the brainstem, reducing sympathetic outflow from the CNS and decreasing peripheral resistance, renal vascular resistance, heart rate, and blood pressure

SAFETY AND TOLERABILITY

Notable Side Effects

- Sedation, dizziness
- Abdominal pain, nausea
- Fatigue, weakness
- Hypotension (dose related)
- Dry mouth, constipation

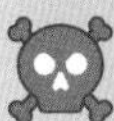

Life-Threatening or Dangerous Side Effects

- Sinus bradycardia

Growth and Maturation

- Existing data do not suggest that guanfacine has an adverse effect on growth

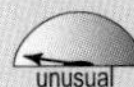

Weight Gain

- Reported but not expected

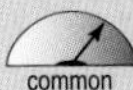

Sedation

- Many experience and/or can be significant in amount
- Some patients may not tolerate it
- Can abate with time
- May be less sedation with extended-release formulation

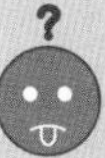

What to Do About Side Effects

- Wait, wait, wait: mild side effects are common, happen early, and usually improve with time, but treatment benefits can be delayed and often begin just as the side effects wear off
- Take larger dose at bedtime to avoid daytime sedation
- Often best to try another monotherapy prior to resorting to augmentation strategies to treat side effects
- Monitor side effects closely, especially when initiating treatment

How Drug Causes Side Effects

- Excessive actions on alpha 2A receptors, nonselective actions on alpha 2B and alpha 2C receptors

Warnings and Precautions

- In children and adolescents:

  - Safety and efficacy not established in children under age 6
  - Use in young children should be reserved for the expert
  - Consider distributing brochures provided by the FDA and the drug companies
- All ages:
  - Carefully weigh the risks and benefits of pharmacological treatment against the risks and benefits of nonpharmacological treatment and it is a good idea to document this in the patient's chart
  - Excessive heat (e.g., saunas) may exacerbate some of the side effects, such as dizziness and drowsiness
  - Titrate slowly and monitor vital signs frequently in patients at risk for hypotension, heart block, bradycardia, syncope, cardiovascular disease, vascular disease, cerebrovascular disease, or chronic renal failure

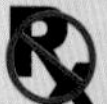

When Not to Prescribe

- If there is a proven allergy to guanfacine

Long-Term Use

- Shown to be safe and effective for treatment of hypertension
- Studies of up to 2 years in ADHD

Habit Forming

- No

Overdose

- Drowsiness, lethargy, bradycardia, hypotension

DOSING AND USE

Usual Dosage Range

- Extended-release: 1–7 mg once daily (0.08–0.12 mg/kg)
- Immediate-release: 1–2 mg bid

Dosage Forms

- Extended-release tablet 1 mg, 2 mg, 3 mg, 4 mg
- Immediate-release tablet 1 mg, 2 mg, 3 mg

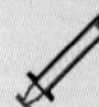

How to Dose

- Extended-release: initial 1 mg/day; can increase by 1 mg/week; 0.08–0.12 mg/kg target weight-based dose range; maximum dose generally 4 mg/day in children (ages 6 to 12) and 7 mg/day in adolescents (ages 13 to 17); dosed once daily either in the morning or evening; should be dosed at approximately the same time each day
- Immediate-release: initial 1 mg/day at bedtime; after 3–4 weeks can increase to 2 mg/day
- When converting from IR to extended-release formulations, use caution. The conversion between doses is NOT 1:1 (Figure 1).
- For PTSD symptoms in youth, begin guanfacine (extended-release) at 1 mg each evening and increase by 1 mg each week until effective (Strawn et al., 2023). The recommended target dose range is 0.08 to 0.12 mg/kg/day. In an uncontrolled trial, 19 children (ages 6 to 18 years) with symptoms of PTSD were treated with extended-release guanfacine 1 to 4 mg each evening (mean dose: 1.19 mg/0.03 mg/kg) (Connor et al., 2013). At 8 weeks, this reduced reexperiencing, avoidance, and hyperarousal as measured by the UCLA PTSD Reaction Index.

Options for Administration

- Oral extended-release formulation
- Oral immediate-release formulation

Tests

- Blood pressure (sitting and standing) and pulse should be measured at baseline and monitored following dose increases and periodically during treatment

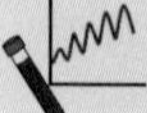

Pharmacokinetics

- Guanfacine is metabolized primarily in the liver through several pathways, including CYP3A4-mediated oxidative metabolism. The metabolites formed are pharmacologically inactive (Figure 2).
- The elimination half-life of guanfacine is approximately 14 hours in children and 18 hours in adolescents (Boellner et al., 2007)
- Maximum concentrations with extended release are reached in 5 hours in both children and adolescents
- Evening and morning dosing of extended-release guanfacine has been evaluated and there are no differences between efficacy or tolerability

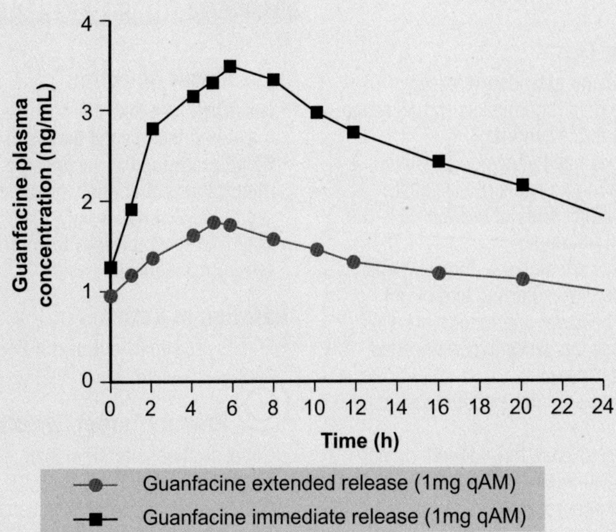

Figure 1 Guanfacine plasma concentrations over time in children and adolescents with extended- vs. immediate-release. Source: Guanfacine ER Package Insert.

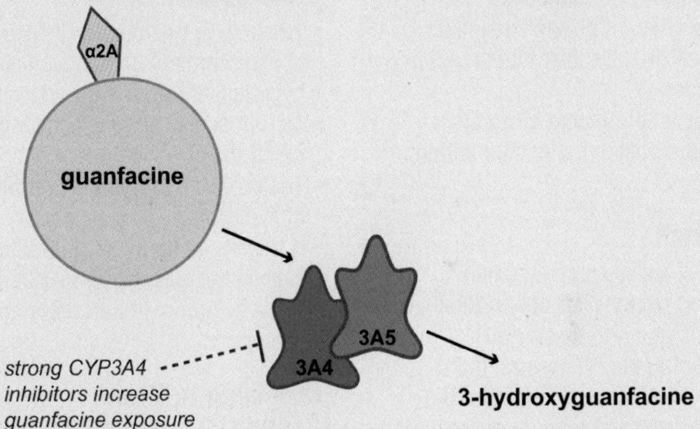

Figure 2 Guanfacine metabolism. Guanfacine is primarily metabolized by CYP3A4 and CYP3A5, and its metabolite is inactive. Additionally, strong CYP3A4 inhibitors increase guanfacine exposure (i.e., blood concentrations over time).

- Extended-release formulation should not be administered with a high-fat meal, as this increases exposure

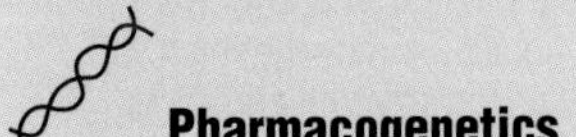

Pharmacogenetics

- No recommendations

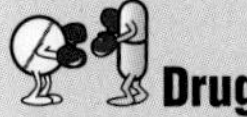

Drug Interactions

- CYP3A inhibitors such as fluoxetine, fluvoxamine, and ketoconazole may decrease clearance of guanfacine and raise guanfacine levels significantly
- CYP3A inducers may increase clearance of guanfacine and lower guanfacine levels significantly
- Combined use with valproate may increase plasma concentrations of valproate
- Increased depressive effects when taken with other CNS depressants
- Phenobarbital and phenytoin may reduce plasma concentrations of guanfacine

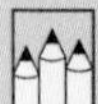

Dosing Tips

- Consider dosing extended-release formulation on a mg/kg basis (target range: 0.08 mg/kg to 0.12 mg/kg)
- Response has been shown to be dose related on a mg/kg basis (Sallee et al., 2009) with effect sizes of between 0.4–0.9 at doses > 0.08 mg/kg
- Plasma levels are higher in lower-weight children; therefore, starting and target doses may be lower and longer intervals between dose increases may be needed (see How to Dose)
- Adverse effects are dose related and usually transient
- For extended-release formulation, do not administer with high-fat meals because this increases exposure
- Extended-release tablets should not be crushed, chewed, or broken, as this could alter controlled-release properties
- Extended-release and immediate-release tablets have different pharmacokinetic properties, so do not substitute on a mg-per-mg basis
- If guanfacine is terminated abruptly, rebound hypertension may occur within 2–4 days

How to Switch

- Guanfacine is always tapered when discontinuing, whether or not another medication is going to be started
- Taper in decrements of no more than 1 mg every 3 to 7 days to minimize the risk of an increase in blood pressure upon discontinuation
- If switching from immediate-release guanfacine, discontinue that treatment and titrate with extended-release guanfacine as directed
- Discontinue clonidine before beginning guanfacine
- Be aware of drug interactions with other agents if cross tapering/combining with other agents

How to Stop

- Discontinuation reactions are common
- Taper in decrements of no more than 1 mg every 3 to 7 days to minimize the risk of an increase in blood pressure upon discontinuation

WHAT TO EXPECT

Onset of Action

- For ADHD, can take a few weeks to see maximum therapeutic benefits
- Blood pressure may be lowered 30–60 minutes after first dose; greatest reduction seen after 2–4 hours
- May take several weeks to control blood pressure adequately

Duration of Action

- Effects are consistent over a 24-hour period

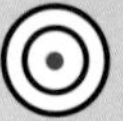

Primary Target Symptoms

- Concentration, attention span, distractibility
- Motor hyperactivity
- Oppositional and impulsive behavior
- High blood pressure

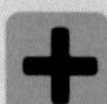

What Is Considered a Positive Result?

- The goal of treatment of ADHD is reduction of symptoms of inattentiveness, motor hyperactivity, and/or impulsiveness that disrupt social, school, and/or occupational functioning
- The goal of treatment is complete remission of symptoms
- If treatment works, it most often reduces or even eliminates symptoms, but is not a cure since symptoms often recur after medicine is stopped

How Long to Treat

- ADHD is typically a lifelong illness; if any symptoms improve, hyperactivity is more likely to improve than inattention
- Can tell parents there is some chance that their child can grow out of this in adulthood, but many adults continue to have symptoms of ADHD throughout adolescence and adulthood
- Tics are typically a lifelong illness
- However, oppositional and impulsive/aggressive behaviors may diminish with neurodevelopment from childhood to adolescence to adulthood
- Continue treatment until all symptoms are under control or improvement is stable and then continue treatment as long as improvement persists

- Reevaluate the need for treatment periodically; some clinicians advise to periodically taper ADHD medication in patients who are not severely symptomatic to observe how the patient responds, but not routinely done by most clinicians
- Treatment for ADHD begun in childhood may need to be continued into adolescence and adulthood if continued benefit is documented

What If It Stops Working?

- Consider titration of the medication. As patients gain weight, their weight-based dose has decreased!
- Consider using in combination with a stimulant medication; in some studies, combining a stimulant and an alpha 2 agonist is associated with greater tolerability and, in most studies, this is associated with improved efficacy

What If It Doesn't Work?

- In practice, many patients have only a partial response where some symptoms are improved but others persist, in which case higher doses of guanfacine, adding a second agent, or switching to an agent with a different mechanism of action can be considered
- Consider evaluation for another diagnosis or for a comorbid condition (e.g., medical illness, substance abuse). Also, when treating ADHD, consider the possibility of a learning disorder or learning weakness and consider school-based interventions.
- Consider adjusting dose or switching to another agent
- Consider the presence of nonadherence and counsel patient and parents
- Some ADHD patients may experience lack of consistent efficacy due to activation of latent or underlying bipolar disorder, and require either augmenting with a mood stabilizer or switching to a mood stabilizer
- Augmenting options:
  - Organizational skills training/executive function coaching
  - Exercise
  - Parent Management Training (PMT)
  - Coordinating with school for appropriate support
  - Augmentation with a stimulant is commonly used for treatment-resistant ADHD, particularly oppositional/aggressive/impulsive behaviors inadequately responding to stimulants alone
- Consider factors associated with poor response to any psychotropic medication in children and adolescents, such as severe symptoms, long-lasting symptoms, poor treatment adherence, prior nonresponse to other treatments, and the presence of comorbid psychiatric disorders or learning disorders
- Consider other important potential factors such as ongoing conflicts, family psychopathology, and an adverse environment (e.g., poverty, chaos, violence, prior and ongoing psychological trauma, abuse, bullying, less than ideal school placement, neglect)
- Institute trauma-informed care for appropriate children and adolescents

TALKING TO PATIENTS AND CAREGIVERS

What to Tell Parents About Efficacy

- It is a good idea to explain why this medication was chosen instead of a stimulant, or to use in combination with a stimulant, and if there are specific target symptoms for this medication compared to those for a stimulant
- Often works within several days once the dose is correct, although full therapeutic benefits may take a few weeks
- While the medicine helps ADHD by reducing symptoms and improving function, there are no cures for ADHD and it is therefore necessary to keep taking the medication to sustain its therapeutic effects
- Since every treatment consideration depends on a risk/benefit analysis, parents should fully understand short- and long-term risks as well as benefits compared to nontreatment of ADHD
- Often a good idea to tell parents whether the medication chosen is specifically approved for the disorder being treated, or whether it is being given for "unapproved" or "off-label" reasons based on good clinical practice, expert consensus, and/or prudent extrapolation of controlled data from adults

- The American Academy of Child & Adolescent Psychiatry (AACAP) has helpful handouts for parents

What to Tell Children and Adolescents About Efficacy

- Be specific about the symptoms being targeted: we are trying to help you remember things better, do your best at school, follow the rules, get into less trouble (as applicable)
- It may be a good idea to give the medication a try; if it's not working very well, we can stop the medication and try something else
- You can be part of a special plan to help us figure out if the medicine is helpful for you. Would you like to do that? (for the parents and prescriber, can consider here a trial both on and then off medication, and then on again to see if the effects are clear and thus worth continuing the medication)
- The medication often doesn't work right away, so a good try can take a few months to find the right dose and see if it works for you
- Even if it does make you feel better, it will wear off and no longer work shortly after you stop it
- The medication can help you decide what you want to do, like making good choices versus bad choices; the medicine does not make you do something you don't want to do
- Medications don't change who you are as a person; they give you the opportunity to be the best person you can be

What to Tell Parents About Side Effects

- Explain that side effects are expected in many when starting
- Tell parents many side effects often go away in a few days to weeks, but if they don't we will change the treatment
- Predict side effects in advance (you will look clever and competent to the parents, unless you scare them with too much information and cause nocebo effects, in which case you won't look so clever when the patient develops lots of side effects and stops medication; use your judgment here); a balanced but honest presentation is an art rather than a science
- Ask parents to support the patient while side effects are occurring
- Parents should fully understand short- and long-term risks as well as benefits
- Explaining to the parents what to expect from medication treatment, and especially what potential side effects to expect, can help prevent early termination
- Tell parents this medication – unlike stimulants – should be tapered rather than abruptly withdrawn when discontinuing it to avoid withdrawal side effects, some of which can be rarely dangerous; don't purposely skip a dose or stop over the weekend, for example, like you can do with stimulants

What to Tell Children and Adolescents About Side Effects

- When a medicine starts to work, your body can first experience this by giving you unpleasant sensations – just like if you take a cough medicine it may taste bad. So, just like with a cough medicine, the bad taste will often go away before the medicine begins to stop the cough – many medicines work like that. It's important for you to pay attention to what your body is telling you, and we'll go over some of the ways that can happen.
- Even if you get a side effect, it's not permanent (it won't last forever)
- Explaining to child/adolescent what to expect from medication treatment, and especially potential side effects, can help prevent early termination
- Make sure you tell your parents or your doctor if you decide to stop your medication, because stopping it all at once can cause you side effects, some of which can be dangerous

What to Tell Teachers About the Medication (If Parents Consent)

- Guanfacine can be helpful in improving the symptoms of ADHD: namely, inattention, impulsivity, and hyperactivity
- Some students will experience side effects from the medications that you may notice in or outside the classroom; many of these side effects can be modified
- Can make children/adolescents sleepy (often) or can make them dizzy or faint (not common)

SPECIAL POPULATIONS

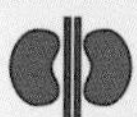

Renal Impairment

- Patients should receive lower doses

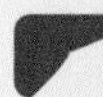

Hepatic Impairment

- Use with caution; may require lower dose

Cardiac Impairment

- Use with caution in patients at risk for hypotension, bradycardia, heart block, or syncope

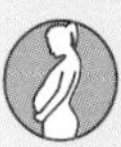

Pregnancy

- Controlled studies have not been conducted in pregnant women
- Animal studies do not show adverse effects
- Use in women of childbearing potential requires weighing potential benefits to the mother against potential risks to the fetus

Breast Feeding

- Unknown if guanfacine is secreted in human breast milk, but all psychotropics assumed to be secreted in breast milk
- Recommended either to discontinue drug or formula feed

THE ART OF PSYCHOPHARMACOLOGY

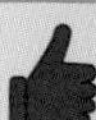

Potential Advantages

- In children:
  - For patients whose parents do not want them to take a stimulant or who cannot tolerate or do not respond to stimulants
  - For patients with co-occurring anxiety disorders or anxious youth who are SSRI-nonresponders
- In adolescents:
  - For patients who have a history of diverting or abusing stimulants
  - Can improve school performance and grades, especially if ADHD has been unrecognized and untreated prior to adolescence
- All ages:
  - No known abuse potential; not a controlled substance
  - Patients with co-occurring anxiety disorders or anxious youth who are SSRI-nonresponders
  - Patients with co-occurring tics and ADHD
  - For oppositional behavior associated with ADHD
  - Less sedation than clonidine

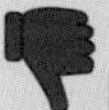

Potential Disadvantages

- All ages:
  - Some withdrawal reactions
  - Frequency and severity of withdrawal reactions may be less than for clonidine

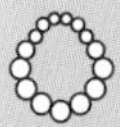

Pearls

- For children and adolescents with comorbid ADHD and Tourette syndrome, and whose tics worsen with stimulant treatment, guanfacine may improve both ADHD symptoms and tics
- Effects may be delayed and less robust on ADHD symptoms than stimulants; however, may add to the efficacy of stimulants when used in combination
- May be particularly helpful in targeting aggressive, impulsive, and oppositional behaviors associated with ADHD
- Unlike stimulants, guanfacine is not abusable and has little or no value to friends of adolescent patients who may otherwise divert stimulant medications, especially when responsible for self-administration of medications in college settings
- May have less sedation than clonidine
- May have less hypotension than clonidine in some patients
- May have less frequent and less severe withdrawal reactions than clonidine in some patients
- The extended-release formulation often is much more tolerable than the immediate-release formulation, especially for patients sensitive to peak dose sedation of the immediate-release formulation
- Guanfacine has been shown to be effective in both children and adults, and guanfacine extended-release formulation is approved for ADHD in children ages 6–17
- Guanfacine can also be used to treat tic disorders, including Tourette syndrome
- May be used as monotherapy or in combination with stimulants for the

treatment of oppositional behavior in children with or without ADHD
- Guanfacine may be helpful in reducing anxiety in some patients and has been evaluated in a double-blind, placebo-controlled trial of youth with generalized, separation and social anxiety disorders without ADHD (Strawn et al., 2017)
- Guanfacine is a related centrally active alpha 2 agonist also approved for ADHD, and may work better or be tolerated better than clonidine in some children/adolescents, although no head-to-head studies
- Although both guanfacine and clonidine are alpha 2 adrenergic agonists, guanfacine is relatively more selective for alpha 2A receptors, whereas clonidine binds not only alpha 2A, 2B, and 2C receptors, but also imidazoline receptors, hypothetically causing more sedation, hypotension, and side effects than guanfacine in some patients

SUGGESTED READING

Black BT, Soden SE, Kearns GL, Jones BL. Clinical and pharmacologic considerations for guanfacine use in very young children. J Child Adolesc Psychopharmacol 2016;26(6):498–504.

Boellner SW, Pennick M, Fiske K, Lyne A, Shojaei A. Pharmacokinetics of a guanfacine extended-release formulation in children and adolescents with attention-deficit-hyperactivity disorder. Pharmacotherapy 2007;27(9):1253–62.

Catalá-López F, Hutton B, Nuñez-Beltrán A et al. The pharmacological and non-pharmacological treatment of attention deficit hyperactivity disorder in children and adolescents: a systematic review with network meta-analyses of randomised trials. PLoS One. 2017;12(7):e0180355.

Connor DF, Grasso DJ, Slivinsky MD, et al. An open-label study of guanfacine extended release for traumatic stress related symptoms in children and adolescents. J Child Adolesc Psychopharmacol 2013; 23:244.

Kemper AR, Maslow GR, Hill S et al. Attention Deficit Hyperactivity Disorder: Diagnosis and Treatment in Children and Adolescents. Comparative Effectiveness Review No. 203. AHRQ Publication No. 18-EHC005-EF. Rockville, MD: Agency for Healthcare Research and Quality; January 2018.

Pliszka S ; AACAP Work Group on Quality Issues. Practice parameter for the assessment and treatment of children and adolescents with attention-deficit/hyperactivity disorder. J Am Acad Child Adolesc Psychiatry 2007;46(7):894–921.

Ruggiero S, Clavenna, Reale L et al. Guanfacine for attention deficit and hyperactivity disorder in pediatrics: a systematic review and meta-analysis. Eur Neuropsychopharmacol 2014;24(10):1589–90.

Sallee FR, McGough J, Wigal T et al.; SPD503 STUDY GROUP. Guanfacine extended release in children and adolescents with attention-deficit/hyperactivity disorder: a placebo-controlled trial. J Am Acad Child Adolesc Psychiatry 2009;48(2):155–65.

Sayer GR, McGough JJ, Levitt J et al. Acute and long-term cardiovascular effects of stimulant, guanfacine, and combination therapy for attention-deficit/ hyperactivity disorder. J Child Adolesc Psychopharmacol 2016;26(10):882–8.

Strawn JR, Compton SN, Robertson B et al. Extended release guanfacine in pediatric anxiety disorders: a pilot, randomized, placebo-controlled trial. J Child Adolesc Psychopharmacol 2017;27(1):29–37.

Strawn JR, Keeshin BR, Cohen JA. Posttraumatic stress disorder in children and adolescents: treatment and overview. UpToDate 2023. Last updated Sept. 6, 2023.

THERAPEUTICS

Brands

- Haldol

Generic

Yes

US FDA Approved for Pediatric Use

- Tics and vocal utterances in Tourette syndrome (oral, age not specified)
- Effective for second-line treatment of severe behavior problems in children of combative, explosive hyperexcitability (oral, age not specified)
- Effective for second-line short-term treatment of hyperactive children (oral, age not specified)

Off-Label for Pediatric Use

- Approved in adults
  - Tics and vocal utterances in Tourette syndrome (immediate-release injection)
  - Schizophrenia/manifestations of psychotic disorders (oral, immediate-release injection)
  - Treatment of schizophrenic patients who require prolonged parenteral antipsychotic therapy (depot intramuscular decanoate)
- Other off-label uses
  - Bipolar disorder
  - Delirium

Class and Mechanism of Action

- Neuroscience-based Nomenclature: dopamine receptor antagonist (D-RAn)
- Conventional antipsychotic (neuroleptic, butyrophenone, dopamine 2 antagonist)
- Blocks dopamine 2 receptors in the mesolimbic pathway, reducing positive symptoms of psychosis and possibly combative, explosive, and hyperactive behaviors
- Blocks dopamine 2 receptors in the nigrostriatal pathway, improving tics and other symptoms in Tourette syndrome

SAFETY AND TOLERABILITY

Notable Side Effects

- In adults:
  - Neuroleptic-induced deficit syndrome; in children and adolescents sometimes called the "zombie syndrome"
  - Akathisia
  - Drug-induced parkinsonism
  - Galactorrhea, amenorrhea (girls)
  - Gynecomastia (boys)
  - Sedation
  - Dizziness,
  - Dry mouth, constipation, blurred vision, urinary retention
  - Decreased sweating
  - Hypotension, hypertension
  - Tardive dyskinesia, tardive dystonia (risk is higher in children than in adults)
  - Risk of potentially irreversible, involuntary dyskinetic movements may increase with cumulative dose and treatment duration
  - Rare tachycardia

Life-Threatening or Dangerous Side Effects

- Rare neuroleptic malignant syndrome (NMS) may cause hyperpyrexia, muscle rigidity, delirium, and autonomic instability with elevated creatine phosphokinase, myoglobinuria (rhabdomyolysis), and acute renal failure
- Rare seizures
- Rare jaundice, agranulocytosis, leukopenia

Growth and Maturation

- Long-term effects are unknown

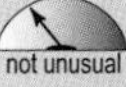

Weight Gain

- Occurs in significant minority
- May be more weight gain in children and adolescents than in adults

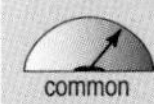

Sedation

- Sedation is usually transient

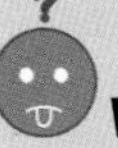

What to Do About Side Effects

- Wait, wait, wait: mild side effects are common, happen early, and usually

improve with time, but treatment benefits can be delayed
- Monitor side effects closely, especially when initiating treatment
- May wish to give at night if not tolerated during the day and doesn't disrupt sleep
- Often best to try another monotherapy trial of a different antipsychotic prior to resorting to augmentation strategies to treat side effects
- Exercise and diet programs and medical management for high BMI percentiles, diabetes, dyslipidemia. Also, randomized controlled trials in youth suggest that omega-3 fatty acids can reduce SGA-related hypertriglyceridemia.
- Reduce the dose, particularly for drug-induced parkinsonism, akathisia, sedation, and tremor
- For drug-induced parkinsonism: consider reducing dose or switching to another agent. Augmenting with diphenhydramine or benztropine is less preferred in youth.
- For akathisia: reduce the dose or add a beta blocker. If these are ineffective, raising the dose of the beta blocker may be helpful.
- Using a 5HT2A antagonist such as mirtazapine or cyproheptadine to treat drug-induced akathisia is less common in children and adolescents compared to adults

How Drug Causes Side Effects

- By blocking dopamine 2 receptors in the striatum, it can cause drug-induced parkinsonism and akathisia
- By blocking dopamine 2 receptors in the pituitary, it can cause elevations in prolactin
- By blocking dopamine 2 receptors excessively in the mesocortical and mesolimbic dopamine pathways, especially at high doses, it can cause worsening of negative and cognitive symptoms (neuroleptic-induced deficit syndrome)
- Blocking alpha 1 adrenergic receptors can cause dizziness, hypotension, and syncope
- Mechanism of any possible weight gain is unknown
- Mechanism of any possible increased incidence of diabetes or dyslipidemia is unknown

Warnings and Precautions

- Carefully weigh the risks and benefits of pharmacological treatment against the risks and benefits of treatment with a second generation atypical antipsychotic or even nontreatment with an antipsychotic and it is a good idea to document this in the patient's chart
- As with any antipsychotic, use with caution in patients with history of seizures
- If signs of neuroleptic malignant syndrome develop, treatment should be immediately discontinued
- Use with caution in patients with respiratory disorders
- Avoid extreme heat exposure
- If haloperidol is used to treat mania, patients may experience a rapid switch to depression
- Patients with thyrotoxicosis may experience neurotoxicity
- Higher doses and IV administration may be associated with increased risk of QTc prolongation and *torsades de pointes*; use particular caution if patient has a QT-prolonging condition, underlying cardiac abnormalities, hypothyroidism, familial long-QT syndrome, or is taking a drug known to prolong QTc interval

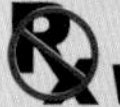

When Not to Prescribe

- If patient is in comatose state or has CNS depression
- If patient has Parkinson's disease
- If there is a proven allergy to haloperidol

Long-Term Use

- In adults, often used for long-term maintenance
- Should periodically reevaluate long-term usefulness in individual patients, but treatment may need to continue for many years

Habit Forming

- No

Overdose

- Fatalities have been reported; extrapyramidal symptoms, hypotension, sedation, respiratory depression, shock-like state

DOSING AND USE

Usual Dosage Range

- 0.05 mg/kg/day to 0.15 mg/kg/day for psychotic disorders (usually less than 5 mg/day)
- 0.05 mg/kg/day to 0.075 mg/kg/day for nonpsychotic behavior disorder and Tourette syndrome (usually less than 10 mg/day)

Dosage Forms

- Tablet 0.5 mg scored, 1 mg scored, 2 mg scored, 5 mg scored, 10 mg scored, 20 mg scored
- Concentrate 2 mg/mL
- Injection 5 mg/mL (immediate-release)
- Decanoate injection 50 mg haloperidol as 70.5 mg/mL haloperidol decanoate, 100 mg haloperidol as 141.04 mg/mL haloperidol decanoate

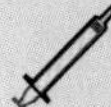

How to Dose

- Initiate treatment at the lowest possible dose (0.5 mg/day); can increase by 0.5 mg/day every 5–7 days as needed; dose may be divided in either 2 or 3 doses per day; dosing should be guided based on weight, tolerability, and clinical response
- Immediate-release injection: initial dose 2–5 mg; subsequent doses may be given as often as every hour; patient should be switched to oral administration as soon as possible

Options for Administration

- Solution available for patients with difficulty swallowing pills
- Long-acting injectable formulations not approved in children/adolescents and few studies; probably best not to use long-acting injectables in children at all, and only with caution off-label in adolescents who are older and have adult body weights and by experts in administering long-acting injectables

Tests

- Before starting haloperidol:
  - Plan to monitor weight and metabolic parameters more closely than in adults since children and adolescents may be more prone to these side effects than adults
  - Weigh all patients and monitor weight gain against that expected for normal growth, using the pediatric height/weight chart to monitor
  - Get baseline personal and family history of diabetes, obesity, dyslipidemia, hypertension, and cardiovascular disease
  - Obtain blood pressure, fasting plasma glucose (or hemoglobin A1C), and a lipid profile
- After starting haloperidol:
  - Monitor weight and BMI percentile
  - Consider monitoring fasting triglycerides monthly in patients at high risk for metabolic complications
  - Patients with low white blood cell count (WBC) or history of drug-induced leukopenia/neutropenia should have complete blood count (CBC) monitored frequently during the first few months and haloperidol should be discontinued at the first sign of decline of WBC in the absence of other causative factors
  - Patients should be monitored periodically for the development of abnormal movements of tardive dyskinesia using neurological exam and the Abnormal Involuntary Movement Scale (AIMS)
  - Monitoring elevated prolactin levels is of dubious clinical benefit
  - Consider monitoring plasma drug levels if not responding, or questions about compliance or side effects

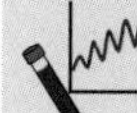

Pharmacokinetics

- Oral haloperidol is well absorbed from the gastrointestinal tract; however, it undergoes significant first-pass metabolism in the liver, resulting in a relatively low oral bioavailability of approximately 60–70%. By contrast, in adults, intramuscular haloperidol is rapidly absorbed and peak plasma concentrations are typically reached within 10 to 20 minutes after injection.
- Taking haloperidol with food may slightly delay its absorption but does not significantly affect the overall extent of absorption
- Haloperidol has a moderate to high protein binding of about 90–98%, primarily to albumin. The drug has a relatively large volume of distribution, indicating extensive tissue distribution throughout the body, including the central nervous system.

- Haloperidol is primarily metabolized by CYP3A4, with contributions from CYP2D6. The primary metabolite formed is reduced haloperidol (also known as reduced haloperidol hydroxylation); it is pharmacologically active but has lower potency compared to haloperidol.
- Haloperidol also inhibits CYP2D6 (Figure 1)
- Oral half-life is approximately 12–38 hours in adults
- Decanoate half-life is approximately 3 weeks in adults

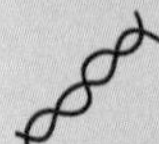

Pharmacogenetics

- No recommendations are available from CPIC; however, the Dutch Pharmacogenetics Working Group recommends that CYP2D6 poor metabolizers use 60% of the normal dose of haloperidol
- CYP2D6 ultrarapid metabolizers might be treated with 1.5 times the normal dose or choose an alternative to haloperidol

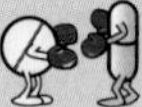

Drug Interactions

- May decrease the effects of levodopa, dopamine agonists
- May increase the effects of antihypertensive drugs except for guanethidine, whose antihypertensive actions haloperidol may antagonize
- Additive effects may occur if used with CNS depressants; dose of other agent should be reduced
- Some pressor agents (e.g., epinephrine) may interact with haloperidol to lower blood pressure
- Haloperidol and anticholinergic agents together may increase intraocular pressure
- Reduces effects of anticoagulants
- Plasma levels of haloperidol may be lowered by rifampin
- Some patients taking haloperidol and lithium have developed an encephalopathic syndrome similar to neuroleptic malignant syndrome (controversial)

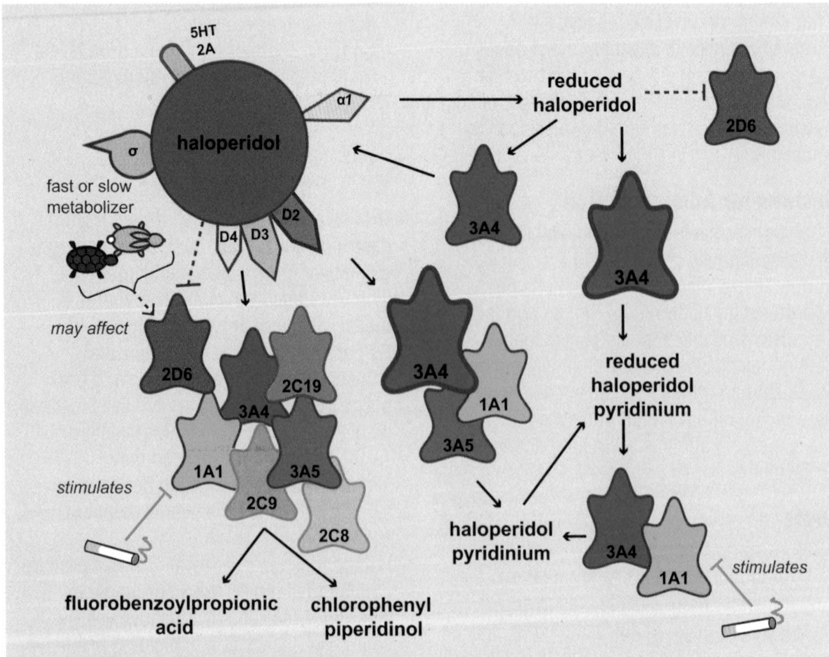

Figure 1 Metabolism of haloperidol.

Dosing Tips

- Children should generally be dosed at the lower end of the dosage spectrum when drug is initiated
- Little evidence to support additional efficacy beyond 6 mg/day for behavioral symptoms in children
- Unlike many antipsychotics, plasma drug levels are available to monitor compliance and to help set dose especially when not responding
- Haloperidol is frequently dosed too high
- Treatment should be suspended if absolute neutrophil count falls below 1,000/mm^3

How to Switch

- From another antipsychotic to haloperidol:
  - When tapering a prior antipsychotic, see its entry in this manual for how to stop and how to taper off that specific drug
  - Generally, try to stop the first agent before starting haloperidol so that new side effects of haloperidol can be distinguished from withdrawal effects of the first agent
  - If urgent, cross taper off the other antipsychotic while haloperidol is started at a low dose, with dose adjustments down of the other antipsychotic, and up for haloperidol, every 3 to 7 days
- Off haloperidol to another antipsychotic:
  - Generally, try to stop haloperidol before starting the new antipsychotic so that new side effects of the next drug can be distinguished from any withdrawal effects from haloperidol
  - If urgent, cross taper off haloperidol by cutting the dose in half as the new antipsychotic is also started with dose adjustments down of haloperidol and up for the new antipsychotic

How to Stop

- Slow down-titration of oral formulation (over 6–8 weeks), especially when simultaneously beginning a new antipsychotic while switching (i.e., cross-titration)
- Rapid oral discontinuation may lead to rebound psychosis and worsening of symptoms
- Rapid oral discontinuation may lead to withdrawal dyskinesias, sometimes reversible
- If antiparkinsonian agents are being used, they should be continued for a few weeks after haloperidol is discontinued

WHAT TO EXPECT

Onset of Action

- For all indications, symptoms can improve within 1 week of oral dosing, but it may take several weeks for full effect on behavior
- Not approved but effective for psychotic and manic behavior in schizophrenia and bipolar disorder in children and adolescents, but is considered a second-line treatment
- Formally effective for second-line treatment of severe behavior problems in children of combative, explosive hyperexcitability, but this use is controversial and based upon legacy studies done many years ago
- Effective for second-line short-term treatment of hyperactive children, but this use is also controversial and based upon legacy studies done many years ago when diagnostic criteria and clinical trial standards were different from what they are today
- If it is not working within 6–8 weeks, it may require a dosage increase or it may not work at all
- Acute intramuscular dosing for agitation can have onset within minutes to an hour, but not well studied or specifically approved for children/adolescents

Duration of Action

- Effects of oral medication are consistent over a 24-hour period
- Oral medication may continue to work for many years to prevent relapse of symptoms

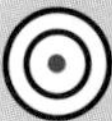

Primary Target Symptoms

- Motor and vocal tics
- Positive symptoms of psychosis
- Manic symptoms
- Violent or aggressive behavior
- Combative explosive hyperexcitability (now controversial)

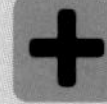

What Is Considered a Positive Result?

- In Tourette syndrome:
  - Reduction in the frequency and severity in both motor and vocal tics

- In schizophrenia:
  - Most often reduces positive symptoms but does not eliminate them
  - Can work for positive symptoms when other antipsychotics have failed
  - In children or adolescents with a first episode of psychosis, initial response may be greater than for recurrent episodes of psychosis in adults
- In mania:
  - Can significantly improve manic symptoms
  - Can improve acute agitation
- In hyperactive children or in severe behavioral problems in children:
  - Can improve these symptoms but is an outdated and controversial approach, especially if an accurate diagnostic evaluation of these symptoms and their comorbidities has not been done

How Long to Treat

- Continue treatment until reaching a plateau of improvement; however, haloperidol should generally not be used for first episodes of psychosis or mania
- After reaching a satisfactory plateau, continue treatment for at least a year after first episode of psychosis or mania
- For second and subsequent episodes of psychosis or mania, treatment may need to be indefinite

What If It Stops Working?

- Check for nonadherence, possibly by checking plasma drug level, and consider switching to another antipsychotic with fewer side effects
- Some patients who have an initial response may relapse even though they continue treatment, sometimes called "poop-out"
- Growth/developmental changes may contribute to apparent loss of efficacy as well as to new onset of side effects as metabolism slows and drug levels rise in transition from childhood to adolescence; dose adjustment (increase or decrease) should be considered
- Screen for the development of a new comorbid disorder, especially substance use
- Screen for adverse changes in the home or school environment

What If It Doesn't Work?

- Consider evaluation for another diagnosis (especially bipolar illness or depression with mixed features) or for a comorbid condition (e.g., medical illness, substance use)
- Consider obtaining plasma drug levels not only to rule out noncompliance but to assess for inadequate drug absorption/excessive drug metabolism
- Consider other important potential factors such as ongoing conflicts, family psychopathology, and an adverse environment (e.g., inadequate school placement or educational services, bullying, poverty, chaos, violence, prior and ongoing psychological trauma, abuse, neglect)
- Institute trauma-informed care for appropriate children and adolescents
- For behavioral symptoms, consider risperidone or aripiprazole

TALKING TO PATIENTS AND CAREGIVERS

What to Tell Parents About Efficacy

- Haloperidol is now considered a second-line therapy
- Since haloperidol was chosen, it is because other options have been tried and failed
- For acute symptoms, it can work right away
- Intramuscular haloperidol can be given by a healthcare professional on an as needed basis for some symptoms like agitation; oral haloperidol can be given by a parent under supervision by a healthcare professional off-label on an as needed basis as well
- Oral haloperidol is usually given every day
- Explain which use haloperidol is being chosen for, how to tell if the drug is working by targeting specific symptoms, and why this is being done
- Once the child/adolescent calms down, at some point after one dose or after several days of dosing or after long-term dosing, we should all assess whether the medication should be continued
- While the medicine helps by reducing symptoms and improving function, it is not a cure, and it therefore may be necessary

to keep taking the medication long term to sustain its therapeutic effects
- Since every treatment consideration depends on a risk/benefit analysis, parents should fully understand short- and long-term risks as well as benefits
- Often a good idea to tell parents whether the medication chosen is specifically approved for the disorder being treated, or whether it is being given for "unapproved" or "off-label" reasons based on good clinical practice, expert consensus, and/or prudent extrapolation of controlled data from adults

What to Tell Children and Adolescents About Efficacy
- Be specific about the symptoms being targeted: we are trying to help you ...
- Give the medication a try; if it's not working very well, we can stop the medication and try something else
- A good try often takes several weeks
- If it does make you feel better, you cannot stop it right away or you may get sick again
- Medications don't change who you are as a person; they give you the opportunity to be the best person you can be

What to Tell Parents About Side Effects
- Side effects (especially motor side effects) of haloperidol are generally expected to be more severe than with second generation atypical antipsychotics
- Explain that side effects are expected in many when starting
- Tell parents many side effects go away and do so about the same time that therapeutic effects start
- Predict side effects in advance (you will look clever and competent to the parents, unless you scare them with too much information and cause nocebo effects, in which case you won't look so clever when the patient develops lots of side effects and stops medication; use your judgment here); a balanced but honest presentation is an art rather than a science
- Ask parents to support the patient while side effects are occurring
- Parents should fully understand short- and long-term risks as well as benefits
- Explaining to the parents what to expect from medication treatment, and especially what potential side effects to expect, can help prevent early termination of medication
- Specifically, it may be prudent to warn that tardive dyskinesia can be more common after treatment with haloperidol than with second generation atypical antipsychotics

What to Tell Children and Adolescents About Side Effects
- Even if you get side effects, most of them get better or go away in a few weeks
- If you have side effects that are bothering you, tell your parents and your parents should tell me
- Consider having a conversation about sexual side effects in some adolescents who can find these side effects confusing and especially burdensome
- Explaining to child/adolescent what to expect from medication treatment, and especially potential side effects, can help prevent early termination of medication

What to Tell Teachers About the Medication (If Parents Consent)
- Haloperidol can make children/adolescents restless and have abnormal movements like tremor
- Haloperidol can make children/adolescents sedated
- It is not abusable
- Encourage dialogue with parents/guardians about any behavior or mood changes
- Notify the clinician of increased restlessness or akathisia symptoms, which may be apparent in the school setting

SPECIAL POPULATIONS

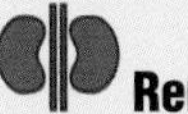

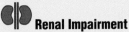

Renal Impairment
- Use with caution

Hepatic Impairment
- Use with caution

Cardiac Impairment
- Use in patients with cardiac impairment has not been studied; however, the risk of orthostatic hypotension in pediatric patients is less than in adults, as children rely less

on peripheral vasoconstriction to regulate blood pressure
- Possible increased risk of QTc prolongation or *torsades de pointes* at higher doses or with IV administration. However, meta-analyses in pediatric patients have not suggested an increased risk of QTc prolongation with oral haloperidol (Jensen et al., 2015).

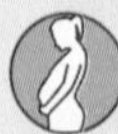

Pregnancy

- Controlled studies have not been conducted in pregnant women
- There is a risk of abnormal muscle movements and withdrawal symptoms in newborns whose mothers took an antipsychotic during the third trimester; symptoms may include agitation, abnormally increased or decreased muscle tone, tremor, sleepiness, severe difficulty breathing, and difficulty feeding
- Reports of extrapyramidal symptoms, jaundice, hyperreflexia, hyporeflexia in infants whose mothers took a conventional antipsychotic during pregnancy
- Reports of limb deformity in infants whose mothers took haloperidol during pregnancy
- Haloperidol should generally not be used during the first trimester
- Haloperidol should only be used during pregnancy if clearly needed
- Psychotic symptoms may worsen during pregnancy, and some form of treatment may be necessary
- Atypical antipsychotics may be preferable to conventional antipsychotics or anticonvulsant mood stabilizers if treatment is required during pregnancy

Breast Feeding

- Some drug is found in breast milk
- Recommended either to discontinue drug or formula feed

THE ART OF PSYCHOPHARMACOLOGY

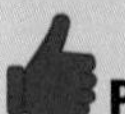

Potential Advantages

- In children and adolescents:
  - Approved for Tourette syndrome, severe combative behavior problems, and short-term treatment of hyperactivity, but used today as a second-line treatment of psychosis or mania when first-line treatment with atypical antipsychotics fails
- All ages:
  - Use of the intramuscular injection for patients requiring rapid onset of antipsychotic action without dosage titration orally or if an acute treatment is necessary (off-label in children and adolescents)
  - Low-cost, effective treatment

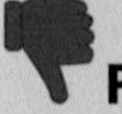

Potential Disadvantages

- In children and adolescents:
  - Many more side effects than numerous alternatives, including increased risk for drug-induced parkinsonism (extrapyramidal symptoms or EPS) as well as tardive dyskinesia
- All ages:
  - Patients in whom second generation atypical antipsychotics can be used with comparable efficacy and fewer side effects

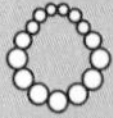

Pearls

- In the pre-atypical antipsychotic era, haloperidol was one of the most popular antipsychotics; however, use of haloperidol and other first generation antipsychotics has largely been supplanted by second generation antipsychotics, particularly given the decreased risk of drug-induced parkinsonism and akathisia in youth treated with SGAs compared to FGAs
- It is no longer acceptable to use haloperidol for behavioral control of children and adolescents or for nonspecific tranquilization
- Although FDA approved as effective for second-line treatment of severe behavior problems in children of combative, explosive hyperexcitability, it is no longer acceptable for haloperidol to be used for this unless these symptoms are part of a diagnosed psychiatric disorder, and trials of atypical antipsychotics have failed
- Effective for second-line short-term treatment of hyperactive children but rarely used for this indication
- When used second line, haloperidol can decrease motor tics and vocal utterances in Tourette syndrome; however, alpha 2 agonists and second generation antipsychotics should be attempted prior

to haloperidol and other first generation antipsychotics
- When discontinued, conventional antipsychotic haloperidol may cause more withdrawal dyskinesias than second generation agents, which may or may not reverse several weeks to months after discontinuation of haloperidol
- Low doses may not induce worsening of negative symptoms of schizophrenia, but high doses may

SUGGESTED READING

Carbon M, Kapoor S, Sheridan E, et al. Neuromotor adverse effects in 342 youth during 12 weeks of naturalistic treatment with 5 second-generation antipsychotics. J Am Acad Child Adolesc Psychiatry 2015;54(9):718–27.e3.

Fung LK, Mahajan R, Nozzolillo A et al. Pharmacologic treatment of severe irritability and problem behaviors in autism: a systematic review and meta-analysis. Pediatrics 2016;137(suppl 2):S124-35.

Jensen KG, Juul K, Fink-Jensen A, Correll CU, Pagsberg AK. Corrected QT changes during antipsychotic treatment of children and adolescents: a systematic review and meta-analysis of clinical trials. J Am Acad Child Adolesc Psychiatry 2015;54(1):25–36.

Lytle S, McVoy M, Sajatovic M. Long-acting injectable antipsychotics in children and adolescents. J Child Adolesc Psychopharmacol 2017;27(1):2–9.

McQuire C, Hassiotis A, Harrison B, Pilling S. Pharmacological interventions for challenging behaviour in children with intellectual disabilities: a systematic review and meta-analysis. BMS Psychiatry 2015;15:303.

Pillay J, Boylan K, Carrey N et al. First- and Second-Generation Antipsychotics in Children and Young Adults: Systematic Review Update [Internet]. Rockville, MD: Agency for Healthcare Research and Quality (US); 2017 Mar. Report No.: 17-EHC001-EF. AHRQ Comparative Effectiveness Reviews.

Pringsheim T, Hirsch L, Gardner D, Gorman DA. The pharmacological management of oppositional behaviour, conduct problems, and aggression in children and adolescents with attention-deficit hyperactivity disorder, oppositional defiant disorder, and conduct disorder: a systematic review and meta-analysis. Part 2: antipsychotics and traditional mood stabilizers. Can J Psychiatry 2015;60(2):52–61.

THERAPEUTICS

Brands

- Atarax
- Marax
- Vistaril, other

Generic

Yes

US FDA Approved for Pediatric Use

- Anxiety and tension associated with psychoneurosis
- Adjunct in organic disease states in which anxiety is manifested
- Pruritus due to allergic conditions
- Histamine-mediated pruritus
- Premedication sedation
- Sedation following general anesthesia
- Adjunct in pre/postoperative patients to allay anxiety, control emesis, and reduce narcotic dose (injection)
- Nausea and vomiting (injection)

Off-Label for Pediatric Use

- Approved in adults
  - Acute disturbance/hysteria (injection)
  - Anxiety withdrawal symptoms in alcoholics or patients with delirium tremens (injection)
  - Adjunct in pre/postpartum patients to allay anxiety, control emesis, and reduce narcotic dose (injection)
- Other off-label uses
  - Insomnia

Class and Mechanism of Action

- Neuroscience-based Nomenclature: histamine receptor antagonist (H-RAn)
- Antihistamine (anxiolytic, hypnotic, antiemetic)

SAFETY AND TOLERABILITY

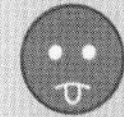

Notable Side Effects

- Sedation, dry mouth, headache
- Hyperactive children should be monitored for paradoxical effects

Life-Threatening or Dangerous Side Effects

- Rare tremor and convulsions (generally at high doses)
- QTc prolongation, *torsades de pointes*
- Acute generalized exanthematous pustulosis (AGEP)
- Rare cardiac arrest, death (intramuscular formulation combined with CNS depressants)
- Bronchodilation
- Respiratory depression (at high doses)

Growth and Maturation

- Not studied

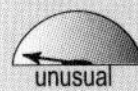

Weight Gain

- Reported but not expected
- Although histamine-1 antagonism may be associated with increased appetite/weight gain, this is not a common side effect with short-term use of hydroxyzine

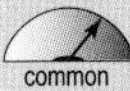

Sedation

- Many experience and/or can be significant in amount
- Sedation is usually transient

What to Do About Side Effects

- Wait; side effects are usually mild and short term
- If they persist or are intolerable, switch to another agent

How Drug Causes Side Effects

- Blocking histamine 1 receptors can cause sedation

Warnings and Precautions

- Hydroxyzine may potentiate the effects of CNS depressants, including alcohol
- Use with caution in patients with risk factors for QTc prolongation, congenital long QT syndrome, a family history of long QT syndrome, other conditions that predispose to QTc prolongation and ventricular arrhythmia, as well as recent myocardial infarction, uncompensated heart failure, and bradyarrhythmias
- Hydroxyzine may rarely cause AGEP, a serious skin reaction characterized by

fever and numerous small, superficial, nonfollicular, sterile pustules, arising within large areas of edematous erythema; discontinue hydroxyzine if signs of skin rash appear
- Antihistamines such as hydroxyzine may reduce mental alertness
- In younger children, antihistamines such as hydroxyzine may cause activation or excitation

When Not to Prescribe
- If patient is in early stages of pregnancy
- If patient has a prolonged QTc interval
- If there is a proven allergy to hydroxyzine, cetirizine hydrochloride, or levocetirizine hydrochloride

Long-Term Use
- Long-term effectiveness (greater than 4 months) for anxiety has not been evaluated
- Tolerance to sedation usually develops

Habit Forming
- No

Overdose
- Sedation, convulsions, stupor, nausea, and vomiting

DOSING AND USE

Usual Dosage Range
- Anxiety in children:
  - Ages 6 and older: 50–100 mg daily in divided doses
  - Under age 6: 50 mg/day in divided doses
- Sedative dosing in children: 0.6 mg/kg

Dosage Forms
- Tablet 10 mg, 25 mg, 50 mg
- Capsule 25 mg, 50 mg, 100 mg
- Oral syrup 10 mg/5 mL
- Intramuscular 25 mg/mL, 50 mg/mL

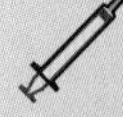

How to Dose
- Oral dosing does not require titration
- Hydroxyzine intramuscular injection should be given preferably in the mid-lateral muscles of the thigh

Options for Administration
- Oral solution can be beneficial for patients who cannot swallow tablets/capsules

Tests
- None for healthy individuals
- Hydroxyzine may cause falsely elevated urinary concentrations of 17-hydroxycorticosteroids in certain lab tests (e.g., Porter–Silber reaction, Glenn–Nelson method)

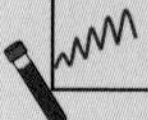

Pharmacokinetics
- Hydroxyzine is rapidly absorbed from the gastrointestinal tract after oral administration
- Peak concentrations occur approximately 2 hours after dose (Figure 1)
- Mean half-life is 7.1±2.3 hours; the half-life of hydroxyzine is also related to the age of the patient being treated (Figure 2)
- The metabolism of hydroxyzine occurs in the liver through hepatic microsomal enzymes, primarily CYP3A4.

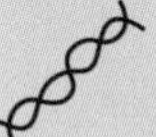

Pharmacogenetics
- No recommendations

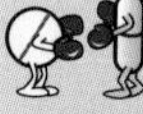

Drug Interactions
- If hydroxyzine is taken in conjunction with another CNS depressant, the dose of the CNS depressant should be reduced
- May enhance QTc prolongation of other drugs capable of prolonging QTc interval
- If anticholinergic agents are used with hydroxyzine, the anticholinergic effects may be enhanced
- Hydroxyzine may reverse the vasopressor effect of epinephrine; patients requiring a vasopressor agent should use norepinephrine or metaraminol instead

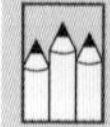

Dosing Tips
- In children, may consider starting at 10 mg bid prn or 10 mg bid
- In adolescents, consider starting at 25–50 mg bid or tid (either prn or scheduled)
- In both age groups, tachyphylaxis is common with repeated use, which results in decreased efficacy over time. Therefore, for antihistamines, prn use may be preferred.

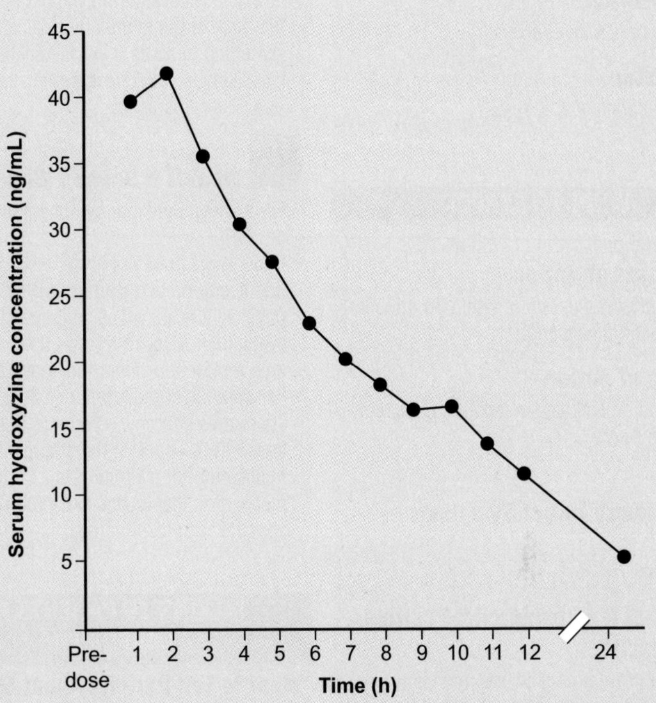

Figure 1 Hydroxyzine concentrations in children and adolescents following hydroxyzine liquid (0.7 mg/kg, n=12). Adapted from: Simons et al., The Journal of Pediatrics, 1984;104:123–127.

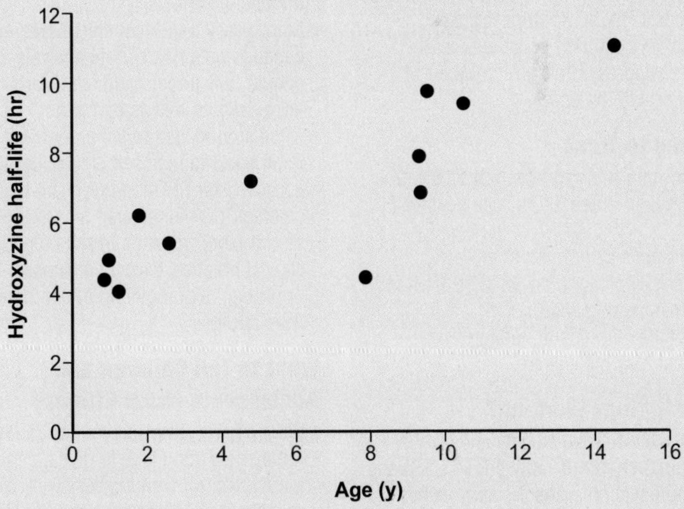

Figure 2 Hydroxyzine half-life versus age in children and adolescents ages 1 to 14 years. Adapted from: Simons et al., The Journal of Pediatrics, 1984;104:123–127.

How to Switch

- Taper generally not necessary

How to Stop

- Taper generally not necessary

WHAT TO EXPECT

Onset of Action

- Clinical effects can occur within 30 minutes after oral administration

Duration of Action

- Effects on anxiety and sleep are consistent over 4–6 hours

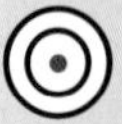

Primary Target Symptoms

- Anxiety
- Insomnia

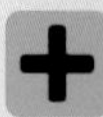

What Is Considered a Positive Result?

- The goal of treatment of insomnia is to improve the quality of sleep, including effects on total wake time and number of nighttime awakenings
- The goal of treatment for anxiety is complete remission of current symptoms as well as prevention of future relapses
- The goal of treatment in patients with appetite suppression is a restoration of normal growth trajectory

How Long to Treat

- For insomnia and short-term symptoms of anxiety: not intended for use beyond 2 weeks
- For long-term symptoms of anxiety, consider switching to an SSRI or SNRI for long-term maintenance
- For appetite stimulation, longer-term treatment may be needed

What If It Stops Working?

- If being used to treat anxiety and anxiety symptoms reemerge, consider an SSRI and re-trying psychotherapeutic approaches
- If the primary target symptom is insomnia, consider an alternative medication or melatonin and re-trying CBT-I
- If the primary symptom is appetite suppression, consider an alternative strategy, referral to nutritionist, lowering the dose of the stimulant medication, or switching to a stimulant medication that is less likely to produce appetite suppression (e.g., isomeric form)

What If It Doesn't Work?

- For anxiety, consider switching to an SSRI or SNRI
- If insomnia does not improve, it may be a manifestation of a primary psychiatric or physical illness, which requires independent evaluation. Also, re-trying other interventions for insomnia may be helpful.
- For appetite stimulation, consider an alternative strategy, referral to nutritionist, lowering the dose of the stimulant medication, or switching to a stimulant medication that is less likely to produce appetite suppression (e.g., isomeric form)

TALKING TO PATIENTS AND CAREGIVERS

What to Tell Parents About Efficacy

- While the medicine helps by reducing symptoms and improving function, it is not a cure, and it is therefore necessary to keep taking the medication to sustain its therapeutic effects
- Since every treatment consideration depends on a risk/benefit analysis, parents should fully understand short- and long-term risks as well as benefits
- Often a good idea to tell parents whether the medication chosen is specifically approved for the disorder being treated, or whether it is being given for “unapproved” or “off-label” reasons based on good clinical practice, expert consensus, and/or prudent extrapolation of controlled data from adults

What to Tell Children and Adolescents About Efficacy

- We are trying to make you feel better
- It may be a good idea to give the medication a try; if it's not working very well, we can stop the medication and try something else
- Medications don't change who you are as a person; they give you the opportunity to be the best person you can be

What to Tell Parents About Side Effects

- Explain that mild side effects are expected at initiation or when increasing the dose and are usually transitory
- Predict side effects in advance (you will look clever and competent to the parents, unless you scare them with too much information and cause nocebo effects, in which case you won't look so clever when the patient develops lots of side effects and stops medication; use your judgment here); a balanced but honest presentation is an art rather than a science
- Ask parents to support the patient while side effects are occurring
- Parents should fully understand short- and long-term risks as well as benefits
- Explaining to the parents what to expect from medication treatment, and especially potential side effects, can help prevent early termination of medication

What to Tell Children and Adolescents About Side Effects

- Even if you get side effects, most of them get better or go away in a few days to a few weeks; however, we will likely not use this medication for a long time
- Explaining to child/adolescent what to expect from medication treatment, and especially potential side effects, can help prevent early termination of medication

What to Tell Teachers About the Medication (If Parents Consent)

- Hydroxyzine can make children/adolescents sleepy
- It is not abusable
- Encourage dialogue with parents/guardians about any behavior or mood changes

SPECIAL POPULATIONS

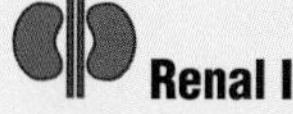

Renal Impairment

- Dosage adjustment may not be necessary

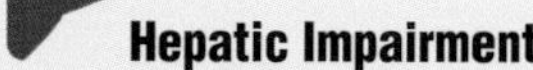

Hepatic Impairment

- Dosage adjustment may not be necessary

Cardiac Impairment

- Contraindicated in patients with a QTc prolongation

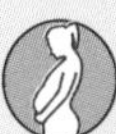

Pregnancy

- Hydroxyzine is contraindicated in early pregnancy

Breast Feeding

- Unknown if hydroxyzine is secreted in human breast milk, but all psychotropics assumed to be secreted in breast milk
- Recommended either to discontinue drug or formula feed

THE ART OF PSYCHOPHARMACOLOGY

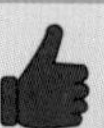

Potential Advantages

- Patients with dermatitis and itching
- No abuse liability, dependence, or withdrawal

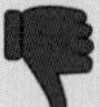

Potential Disadvantages

- Patients with severe anxiety

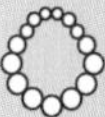

Pearls

- Anxiolytic actions may be proportional to sedating actions
- May be a preferred anxiolytic option for patients with dermatitis or skin symptoms such as pruritus
- A randomized, double-blind, placebo-controlled trial did not demonstrate efficacy of hydroxyzine for controlling preoperative anxiety in children

SUGGESTED READING

Aleo E, López Picado A, Joyanes Abancens B et al. Evaluation of the effect of hydroxyzine on preoperative anxiety and anesthetic adequacy in children: double blind randomized clinical trial. Biomed Res Int 2021;2021:7394042.

Guaiana G, Barbui C, Cipriani A. Hydroxyzine for generalised anxiety disorder. Cochrane Database Syst Rev 2010;(12):CD006815.

Simons FE, Simons KJ, Becker AB, Haydey RP. Pharmacokinetics and antipruritic effects of hydroxyzine in children with atopic dermatitis. J Pediatr 1984;104(1):123–7. doi:10.1016/s0022-3476(84)80608-3.

THERAPEUTICS

Brands
- Labileno
- Lamictal
- Lamictin

Generic
Yes

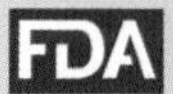

US FDA Approved for Pediatric Use
- Partial seizures (adjunctive; adults and children ages 2 and older)
- Generalized seizures of Lennox–Gastaut syndrome (adjunctive; adults and children ages 2 and older)
- Primary generalized tonic-clonic seizures (adjunctive; adults and children ages 2 and older)

Off-Label for Pediatric Use
- Approved in adults
  - Maintenance treatment of bipolar I disorder
  - Conversion to monotherapy in adults (ages 16 and older) with partial seizures who are receiving treatment with carbamazepine, phenytoin, phenobarbital, primidone, or valproate
- Other off-label uses
  - Bipolar depression
  - Bipolar mania (adjunctive and second line)
  - Psychosis, schizophrenia (adjunctive)
  - Major depressive disorder (adjunctive)
  - Other seizure types and as initial monotherapy for epilepsy

Class and Mechanism of Action
- Neuroscience-based Nomenclature: glutamate, voltage-gated sodium channel blocker (Glu-CB)
- Anticonvulsant, mood stabilizer, voltage-sensitive sodium channel antagonist
- Acts as a use-dependent blocker of voltage-sensitive sodium channels
- Interacts with the open channel conformation of voltage-sensitive sodium channels
- Interacts at a specific site of the alpha pore-forming subunit of voltage-sensitive sodium channels
- Inhibits release of glutamate and aspartate

SAFETY AND TOLERABILITY

Notable Side Effects
- Benign rash (approximately 10%)
- Dose dependent: blurred or double vision, dizziness, ataxia
- Sedation, headache, tremor, insomnia, poor coordination, fatigue
- Nausea (dose dependent), vomiting, dyspepsia, rhinitis
- Additional effects in pediatric patients with epilepsy: infection, pharyngitis, asthenia

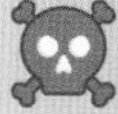

Life-Threatening or Dangerous Side Effects
- Rare serious rash (risk may be greater in pediatric patients but still rare)
- Rare multi-organ failure associated with Stevens–Johnson syndrome, toxic epidermal necrolysis, or drug hypersensitivity syndrome
- Rare blood dyscrasias
- Rare aseptic meningitis
- Rare hemophagocytic lymphohistiocytosis (HLH)
- Rare sudden unexplained deaths have occurred in epilepsy (unknown if related to lamotrigine use)
- Withdrawal seizures upon abrupt withdrawal
- Rare activation of suicidal ideation and behavior (suicidality)

Growth and Maturation
- Long-term effects are unknown

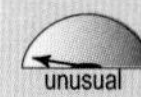

Weight Gain
- Reported but not expected

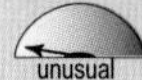

Sedation
- Reported but not expected
- Dose related
- Can wear off with time

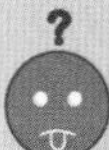

What to Do About Side Effects
- Wait
- Take at night to reduce daytime sedation
- Divide dosing to twice daily
- If patient develops signs of a rash with benign characteristics (i.e., a rash that

peaks within days, settles in 10–14 days, is spotty, nonconfluent, nontender, has no systemic features, and laboratory tests are normal):
  - Reduce lamotrigine dose or stop dosage increase
  - Warn patient to stop drug and contact physician if rash worsens or new symptoms emerge
  - Prescribe antihistamine and/or topical corticosteroid for pruritus
  - Monitor patient closely
- If patient develops signs of a rash with serious characteristics (i.e., a rash that is confluent and widespread, or purpuric or tender; with any prominent involvement of neck or upper trunk; any involvement of eyes, lips, mouth, etc.; any associated fever, malaise, pharyngitis, anorexia, or lymphadenopathy; abnormal laboratory tests for complete blood count, liver function, urea, creatinine):
  - Stop lamotrigine (and valproate if administered)
  - Monitor and investigate organ involvement (hepatic, renal, hematological)
  - Patient may require hospitalization
  - Monitor patient very closely

How Drug Causes Side Effects

- CNS side effects theoretically due to excessive actions at voltage-sensitive sodium channels

Warnings and Precautions

- Life-threatening rashes have developed in association with lamotrigine use; lamotrigine should generally be discontinued at the first sign of serious rash
- Risk of rash is increased in pediatric patients, especially in children under 12 and in children taking valproate
- Risk of rash may be increased with higher doses, faster dose escalation
- Patient should be instructed to report any symptoms of hypersensitivity immediately (fever; flu-like symptoms; rash; blisters on skin or in eyes, mouth, ears, nose, or genital areas; swelling of eyelids, conjunctivitis, lymphadenopathy)
- Aseptic meningitis has been reported rarely in association with lamotrigine use
- Patients should be advised to report any symptoms of aseptic meningitis immediately; these include headache, chills, fever, vomiting and nausea, a stiff neck, and sensitivity to light
- Lamotrigine may cause a rare but serious immune system reaction called hemophagocytic lymphohistiocytosis (HLH), which causes an uncontrolled immune system response
- Patient should be instructed to report any symptoms of HLH immediately (fever; rash; pain, swelling, or tenderness over the liver area; swollen lymph nodes; yellow skin or eyes; unusual bleeding; nervous system problems such as seizures, visual disturbance, or trouble walking)
- Depressive effects may be increased by other CNS depressants (alcohol, MAOIs, other anticonvulsants, etc.)
- A small number of people may experience a worsening of seizures
- May cause photosensitivity
- Lamotrigine binds to tissue that contains melanin, so for long-term treatment ophthalmological checks may be considered
- Warn patients and their caregivers about the possibility of activation of suicidal ideation and advise them to report such side effects immediately

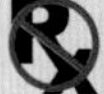

When Not to Prescribe

- If there is a proven allergy to lamotrigine

Long-Term Use

- Safe

Habit Forming

- No

Overdose

- Some fatalities have occurred; ataxia, nystagmus, seizures, coma, intraventricular conduction delay

DOSING AND USE

Usual Dosage Range

- Monotherapy for bipolar disorder (adults): 100–200 mg/day
- Adjunctive treatment for bipolar disorder (adults): 100 mg/day in combination with valproate; 400 mg/day in combination with enzyme-inducing antiepileptic drugs such as carbamazepine, phenobarbital, phenytoin, and primidone
- Monotherapy for seizures in patients over age 12: 300–500 mg/day in 2 doses
- Adjunctive treatment for seizures in patients over age 12: 100–400 mg/day for regimens containing valproate; 100–200 mg/day for valproate alone; 300–500 mg/day in 2 doses for regimens not containing valproate
- Patients ages 2–12 with epilepsy are dosed based on body weight and concomitant medications

Dosage Forms

- Tablet 25 mg, 50 mg, 100 mg, 150 mg, 200 mg, 250 mg
- Chewable tablet 2 mg, 5 mg, 25 mg
- Orally disintegrating tablet 25 mg, 50 mg, 100 mg, 200 mg
- Extended-release tablet 25 mg, 50 mg, 100 mg, 200 mg, 250 mg, 300 mg

How to Dose (Bipolar Disorder)

- When lamotrigine treatment does not include valproate or enzyme-inducing drugs (e.g., carbamazepine, others) (ages 10–12): for the first 2 weeks administer 0.3 mg/kg per day 2 divided doses rounded down to the nearest whole tablet; at week 3 increase to 0.6 mg/kg per day in 1–2 doses rounded down to the nearest whole tablet; every 1–2 weeks can increase by 0.6 mg/kg per day rounded down to the nearest whole tablet; usual maintenance dose 1–6 mg/kg per day in 1–2 doses (maximum generally 200 mg/day)
- When lamotrigine treatment does not include valproate or enzyme-inducing drugs (e.g., carbamazepine, others) (ages 13 and older): for the first 2 weeks administer 25 mg/day; at week 3 increase to 50 mg/day; every 1–2 weeks can increase by 50 mg/day; usual maintenance dose 200 mg/day; doses above 200 mg/day should be divided; maximum generally 300 mg/day
- When lamotrigine is added to treatment that includes valproate (ages 2–12): for the first 2 weeks administer 0.15 mg/kg per day in 2 divided doses rounded down to the nearest whole tablet; at week 3 increase to 0.3 mg/kg per day in 2 divided doses rounded down to the nearest whole tablet; every 1–2 weeks can increase by 0.3 mg/kg per day rounded down to the nearest whole tablet; usual maintenance dose 1–3 mg/kg per day in 2 divided doses (maximum generally 100 mg/day)
- When lamotrigine is added to treatment that includes valproate (ages 13 and older): for the first 2 weeks administer 25 mg every other day; at week 3 increase to 25 mg/day; every week can increase by 25 mg/day; usual maintenance dose 50–150 mg/day; maximum generally 150 mg/day
- When lamotrigine is added to treatment with carbamazepine, phenytoin, phenobarbital, or primidone (without valproate) (ages 2–12): for the first 2 weeks administer 0.6 mg/kg per day in 2 doses rounded down to the nearest whole tablet; at week 3 increase to 1.2 mg/kg per day in 2 doses rounded down to the nearest whole tablet; every 1–2 weeks can increase by 1.2 mg/kg per day rounded down to the nearest whole tablet; usual maintenance dose 5–12 mg/kg per day in 2 doses (maximum dose generally 300 mg per day)
- When lamotrigine is added to treatment that includes carbamazepine, phenytoin, phenobarbital, or primidone (without valproate) (ages 13 and older): for the first 2 weeks administer 50 mg/day; at week 3 increase to 100 mg/day in 2 doses; every week can increase by 50 mg/day; usual maintenance dose 200–400 mg/day in 2 doses; maximum generally 400 mg/day
- Clearance of lamotrigine may be influenced by weight, such that patients weighing less than 30 kg may require an increase of up to 50% for maintenance doses

Options for Administration

- Chewable and orally disintegrating tablet options for patients with difficulty swallowing pills

Tests

- None required

- The value of monitoring plasma concentrations of lamotrigine has not been established
- Because lamotrigine binds to melanin-containing tissues, ophthalmological checks may be considered

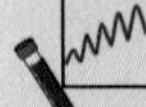

Pharmacokinetics

- Rapidly and completely absorbed; bioavailability not affected by food
- In healthy adults, the elimination half-life following single or multiple doses of immediate-release lamotrigine is approximately 33 or 25 hours, respectively
- After single or multiple doses of immediate-release lamotrigine in addition to valproate, elimination half-life was approximately 48 or 70 hours, respectively
- Elimination half-life in patients receiving concomitant enzyme-inducing antiepileptic drugs (such as carbamazepine, phenobarbital, phenytoin, and primidone) approximately 14 hours after a single dose of lamotrigine
- Clearance in children 2–18 years of age is influenced mainly by the patient's total body weight and concurrent anticonvulsant drug therapy. Children weighing < 30 kg have a higher weight-normalized lamotrigine clearance than those weighing > 30 kg; after accounting for body weight, lamotrigine clearance is not significantly influenced by age (Figure 1).
- Metabolized mainly by glucuronic acid conjugation; the major metabolite is an inactive 2-*N*-glucuronide conjugate
- Plasma protein binding is approximately 55% at plasma lamotrigine concentrations of 1–10 mcg/mL
- Lamotrigine inhibits dihydrofolate reductase and may therefore reduce folate concentrations

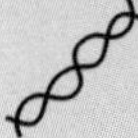

Pharmacogenetics

- No recommendations

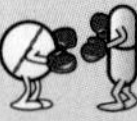

Drug Interactions

- Valproate increases plasma concentrations and half-life of lamotrigine, requiring lower doses of lamotrigine (half or less)

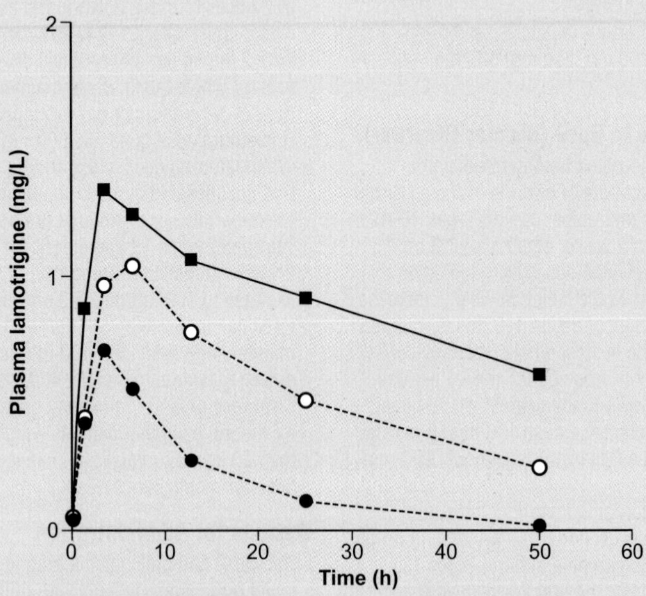

Figure 1 Lamotrigine plasma concentration over time in children (single 2 mg/kg oral dose). Closed circles represent patients treated with "inducers" while black squares represent patients treated with "inhibitors" and white circles represent patients treated with neither "inducers" nor "inhibitors." Data from Garnett, 1997.

- Use of lamotrigine with valproate may be associated with an increased incidence of rash
- Enzyme-inducing antiepileptic drugs (e.g., carbamazepine, phenobarbital, phenytoin, primidone) may increase the clearance of lamotrigine and lower its plasma levels
- Oral contraceptives may decrease plasma levels of lamotrigine
- No likely pharmacokinetic interactions of lamotrigine with lithium, oxcarbazepine, atypical antipsychotics, or antidepressants
- False-positive urine immunoassay screening tests for phencyclidine (PCP) have been reported in patients taking lamotrigine due to a lack of specificity of the screening tests

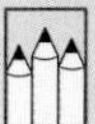

Dosing Tips

- Very slow dose titration may reduce the incidence of skin rash
- Therefore, dose should not be titrated faster than recommended because of possible risk of increased side effects, including rash
- If patient stops taking lamotrigine for 5 days or more it may be necessary to restart the drug with the initial dose titration, as rashes have been reported on re-exposure
- Advise patient to avoid new medications, foods, or products during the first 3 months of lamotrigine treatment in order to decrease the risk of unrelated rash; patient should also not start lamotrigine within 2 weeks of a viral infection, rash, or vaccination
- If lamotrigine is added to patients taking valproate, remember that valproate inhibits lamotrigine metabolism and therefore titration rate and ultimate dose of lamotrigine should be reduced by 50% to reduce the risk of rash
- Thus, if concomitant valproate is discontinued after lamotrigine dose is stabilized, then the lamotrigine dose should be cautiously doubled over at least 2 weeks in equal increments each week following discontinuation of valproate
- Also, if concomitant enzyme-inducing antiepileptic drugs such as carbamazepine, phenobarbital, phenytoin, and primidone are discontinued after lamotrigine dose is stabilized, then the lamotrigine dose should be maintained for 1 week following discontinuation of the other drug and then reduced by half over 2 weeks in equal decrements each week
- Since oral contraceptives and pregnancy can decrease lamotrigine levels, adjustments to the maintenance dose of lamotrigine are recommended in women taking, starting, or stopping oral contraceptives, becoming pregnant, or after delivery
- Chewable dispersible tablets should only be administered as whole tablets; dose should be rounded down to the nearest whole tablet
- Chewable dispersible tablets can be dispersed by adding the tablet to liquid (enough to cover the drug); after approximately 1 minute the solution should be stirred and then consumed immediately in its entirety
- Orally disintegrating tablet should be placed onto the tongue and moved around in the mouth; the tablet will disintegrate rapidly and can be swallowed with or without food or water
- Do not break or chew extended-release tablets, as this could alter controlled-release properties

How to Switch

- From another medication to lamotrigine:
  - When tapering a prior medication, see its entry in this manual for how to stop and how to taper off that specific drug
  - Generally, try to stop the first agent before starting lamotrigine so that new side effects of lamotrigine can be distinguished from withdrawal effects of the first agent
- Off lamotrigine to another medication:
  - Generally, try to stop lamotrigine before starting the new medication so that new side effects of the next drug can be distinguished from any withdrawal effects from lamotrigine
  - Taper; may need to adjust dosage of concurrent medications as lamotrigine is being discontinued

How to Stop

- Taper over at least 2 weeks
- Patients may seize upon withdrawal, especially if withdrawal is abrupt
- Rapid discontinuation increases the risk of relapse in bipolar disorder
- Discontinuation symptoms uncommon

WHAT TO EXPECT

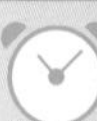

Onset of Action

- May take several weeks to improve bipolar depression
- May take several weeks to months to optimize an effect on mood stabilization
- Can reduce seizures by 2 weeks, but may take several weeks to months to reduce seizures

Duration of Action

- Effects are consistent over a 24-hour period
- May continue to work for many years to prevent relapse of symptoms

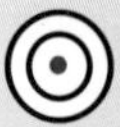

Primary Target Symptoms

- Incidence of seizures
- Unstable mood, especially depression, in bipolar disorder

What Is Considered a Positive Result?

- The goal of treatment is complete remission of symptoms (e.g., seizures, depression)

How Long to Treat

- Continue treatment until all symptoms are gone or until improvement is stable and then continue treating indefinitely as long as improvement persists
- Continue treatment indefinitely to avoid recurrence of mania, depression, and/or seizures

What If It Stops Working?

- Check for nonadherence and consider switching to another agent with fewer side effects
- Some patients who have an initial response may relapse even though they continue treatment, sometimes called "poop-out"
- Growth/developmental changes may contribute to apparent loss of efficacy as well as to new onset of side effects as metabolism slows and drug levels rise in transition from childhood to adolescence; dose adjustment (increase or decrease) should be considered
- Screen for the development of a new comorbid disorder, especially substance abuse
- Screen for adverse changes in the home or school environment

What If It Doesn't Work?

- Consider evaluation for another diagnosis or for a comorbid condition (e.g., medical illness, substance abuse)
- Consider other important potential factors such as ongoing conflicts, family psychopathology, and an adverse environment (e.g., poverty, chaos, violence, prior and ongoing psychological trauma, abuse, neglect)
- Institute trauma-informed care for appropriate children and adolescents
- Try one of the atypical antipsychotics or lithium
- Consider initiating rehabilitation and psychotherapy such as cognitive remediation, although these may be less well standardized for children/adolescents than for adults
- Consider presence of concomitant drug abuse
- Consider augmentation with lithium, an atypical antipsychotic, or an antidepressant (with caution because antidepressants can destabilize mood in some patients, including induction of rapid cycling or suicidal ideation; in particular, consider bupropion; also SSRIs, SNRIs, others; generally, avoid TCAs, MAOIs)

TALKING TO PATIENTS AND CAREGIVERS

What to Tell Parents About Efficacy

- Explain which use lamotrigine is being chosen for, how to tell if the drug is working by targeting specific symptoms, and why this is being done
- While the medicine helps by reducing symptoms and improving function, it is not a cure, and it therefore may be necessary to keep taking the medication long term to sustain its therapeutic effects
- Since every treatment consideration depends on a risk/benefit analysis, parents should fully understand short- and long-term risks as well as benefits
- Often a good idea to tell parents whether the medication chosen is specifically approved for the disorder being treated, or

whether it is being given for "unapproved" or "off-label" reasons based on good clinical practice, expert consensus, and/ or prudent extrapolation of controlled data from adults

What to Tell Children and Adolescents About Efficacy

- Be specific about the symptoms being targeted: we are trying to help you ...
- Give the medication a try; if it's not working very well, we can stop the medication and try something else
- A good try often takes 2 to 3 months
- If it does make you feel better, you cannot stop it right away or you may get sick again
- Medications don't change who you are as a person; they give you the opportunity to be the best person you can be

What to Tell Parents About Side Effects

- Explain that side effects are expected in many when starting
- Advise them their child should avoid new medications, foods, or products during the first 3 months to decrease the risk of unrelated rash
- Advise them to report any symptoms of hypersensitivity immediately (fever; flu-like symptoms; rash; any blisters; swelling of eyelids, conjunctivitis, lymphadenopathy)
- Tell parents many side effects go away and do so about the same time that therapeutic effects start
- Predict side effects in advance (you will look clever and competent to the parents, unless you scare them with too much information and cause nocebo effects, in which case you won't look so clever when the patient develops lots of side effects and stops medication; use your judgment here); a balanced but honest presentation is an art rather than a science
- Ask parents to support the patient while side effects are occurring
- Parents should fully understand short- and long-term risks as well as benefits
- Explaining to the parents what to expect from medication treatment, and especially what potential side effects to expect, can help prevent early termination of medication

What to Tell Children and Adolescents About Side Effects

- Even if you get a side effect, we can usually reduce it over time
- If you have side effects that are bothering you, tell your parents and your parents should tell me
- Avoid new medications, foods, or products during the first 3 months to decrease the risk of unrelated rash
- Report any symptoms of hypersensitivity immediately (fever; flu-like symptoms; rash; any blisters; swelling of eyelids, conjunctivitis, lymphadenopathy)
- Explaining to child/adolescent what to expect from medication treatment, and especially potential side effects, can help prevent early termination of medication

What to Tell Teachers About the Medication (If Parents Consent)

- It is not abusable
- Encourage dialogue with parents/guardians about any behavior or mood changes

SPECIAL POPULATIONS

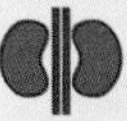

Renal Impairment

- Lamotrigine is renally excreted, so the maintenance dose may need to be lowered
- Mean plasma elimination half-life of immediate-release lamotrigine is approximately 43 hours in chronic renal failure (mean CrCl = 13 mL/minute; range: 6–23 mL/minute), 13 hours during hemodialysis session, and 57 hours between hemodialysis sessions, compared with 26 hours in healthy individuals
- On average, approximately 20% (range: 6–35%) of the amount of lamotrigine present in the body is eliminated during a 4-hour hemodialysis session

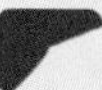

Hepatic Impairment

- Dose adjustment not necessary in mild impairment
- Initial, escalation, and maintenance doses should be reduced by 25% in patients with moderate and severe liver impairment without ascites and 50% in patients with severe liver impairment with ascites

Cardiac Impairment

- Clinical experience is limited
- Drug should be used with caution
- In vitro, lamotrigine exhibits Class 1B antiarrhythmic activity at therapeutically relevant concentrations, which prompted the FDA to warn against its use in patients with cardiac conduction disorders, ventricular arrhythmias, or cardiac disease

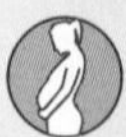

Pregnancy

- Controlled studies have not been conducted in pregnant women
- Use in women of childbearing potential requires weighing potential benefits to the mother against the risks to the fetus
- Pregnancy registry data show increased risk of isolated cleft palate or cleft lip deformity with first trimester exposure
- If treatment with lamotrigine is continued, plasma concentrations of lamotrigine may be reduced during pregnancy, possibly requiring increased doses with dose reduction following delivery
- Pregnancy exposure registry for lamotrigine: (800) 336-2176
- Taper drug if discontinuing
- Seizures, even mild seizures, may cause harm to the embryo/fetus
- Recurrent bipolar illness during pregnancy can be quite disruptive
- For bipolar patients, lamotrigine should generally be discontinued before anticipated pregnancies
- For bipolar patients in whom treatment is discontinued, given the risk of relapse in the postpartum period, lamotrigine should generally be restarted immediately after delivery
- Atypical antipsychotics may be preferable to lithium or anticonvulsants such as lamotrigine if treatment of bipolar disorder is required during pregnancy, but lamotrigine may be preferable to other anticonvulsants such as valproate if anticonvulsant treatment is required during pregnancy
- Bipolar symptoms may recur or worsen during pregnancy, and some form of treatment may be necessary

Breast Feeding

- Some drug is found in breast milk
- Generally recommended either to discontinue drug or formula feed
- If drug is continued while breast feeding, infant should be monitored for possible adverse effects
- If infant shows signs of irritability or sedation, drug may need to be discontinued
- Bipolar disorder may recur during the postpartum period, particularly if there is a history of prior postpartum episodes of either depression or psychosis
- Relapse rates may be lower in women who receive prophylactic treatment for postpartum episodes of bipolar disorder
- Atypical antipsychotics may be preferable to lithium or lamotrigine during the postpartum period when breast feeding

THE ART OF PSYCHOPHARMACOLOGY

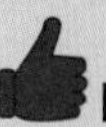

Potential Advantages

- Depressive stages of bipolar disorder (bipolar depression)
- To prevent recurrences of both depression and mania in bipolar disorder

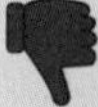

Potential Disadvantages

- May not be as effective in the manic stage of bipolar disorder

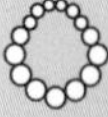

Pearls

- Efficacy of adjunctive lamotrigine in children and adolescents with bipolar disorder (n = ~300 patients ages 10–17) was assessed in a randomized placebo-controlled trial. After stabilization, lamotrigine was discontinued in a double-blind fashion with the primary outcome being time to occurrence of a bipolar event. In the whole sample, the difference between placebo and lamotrigine did not statistically significantly differ (although this was close to significance: $p = 0.07$). However, the details are very important in child and adolescent psychopharmacology. When the 10- to 12-year-olds were evaluated, there was no significant difference ($p = 0.877$) but in the adolescents ages 13–17, there was a large and significant effect (hazard ratio 46, $p = 0.015$) (Findling et al., 2015). Thus, lamotrigine may have value in older pediatric patients but not in those younger than 12 with bipolar disorder.

- Seems to be more effective in treating depressive episodes than manic episodes in bipolar disorder (treats from below better than it treats from above)
- Seems to be effective in preventing both manic relapses as well as depressive relapses (stabilizes both from above and from below) although it may be even better for preventing depressive relapses than for preventing manic relapses
- Rash, including serious rash, appears riskiest in younger children, in those who are receiving concomitant valproate, and/or in those receiving rapid lamotrigine titration and/or high dosing
- Risk of serious rash is less than 1% and has been declining since slower titration, lower dosing, adjustments to use of concomitant valproate administration, and limitations on use in children under 12 have been implemented
- Rashes that occur within the first 5 days or after 8–12 weeks of treatment are rarely drug related
- Benign rashes related to lamotrigine may affect up to 10% of patients and resolve rapidly with drug discontinuation

Suggested Reading

Findling RL, Chang K, Robb A et al. Adjunctive maintenance lamotrigine for pediatric bipolar I disorder: a placebo-controlled, randomized withdrawal study. J Am Acad Child Adolesc Psychiatry 2015;54(12):1020–31.e3.

Garnett WR. Lamotrigine: pharmacokinetics. J Child Neurol 1997;12(suppl 1):S10–15.

Kumar R, Garzon J, Yuruk D et al. Efficacy and safety of lamotrigine in pediatric mood disorders: a systematic review. Acta Psychiatr Scand 2023;147(3):248–56.

Wang Z, Gao K, Kemp DE et al. Lamotrigine adjunctive therapy to lithium and divalproex in depressed patients with rapid cycling bipolar disorder and a recent substance use disorder: a 12-week, double-blind, placebo-controlled pilot study. Psychopharmacol Bull 2010;43(4):5–21.

Zeng T, Long YS, Min FL, Liao WP, Shi YW, Association of HLA-B*1502 allele with lamotrigine-induced Stevens-Johnson syndrome and toxic epidermal necrolysis in Han Chinese subjects: a meta-analysis. Int J Dermatol 2015;54(4): 488–93.

THERAPEUTICS

Brands

- Vyvanse

Generic

No

US FDA Approved for Pediatric Use

- Attention deficit hyperactivity disorder (ages 6 and older)

Off-Label for Pediatric Use

- Approved in adults
  - Binge-eating disorder
- Other off-label uses
  - Narcolepsy
  - Treatment-resistant depression (rarely used for this in children)
  - Stimulants are sometimes used to augment antidepressants
  - Stimulants also sometimes used to treat amotivational or lethargic states in the elderly with dementia but rarely in children for these symptoms

Class and Mechanism of Action

- Neuroscience-based Nomenclature: dopamine, norepinephrine reuptake inhibitor and releaser (DN-RIRe)
- Stimulant
- Lisdexamfetamine is a prodrug of dextroamphetamine and is thus not active until after it has been absorbed by the intestinal tract and converted to dextroamphetamine (active component) and L-lysine
- Once converted to dextroamphetamine, it increases norepinephrine and especially dopamine actions by blocking their reuptake and facilitating their release
- Enhancement of dopamine and norepinephrine actions in certain brain regions (e.g., dorsolateral prefrontal cortex) may improve attention, concentration, executive dysfunction, wakefulness, and cortical inhibitory control of striatum (i.e., theoretically "tunes" inefficient information processing in cortical–striatal pathways, improving "top-down" regulation of striatal and other subcortical drives)
- Enhancement of dopamine actions in other brain regions (e.g., basal ganglia) may decrease hyperactivity
- Enhancement of dopamine and norepinephrine in yet other brain regions (e.g., medial prefrontal cortex, hypothalamus) may improve depressive symptoms as well as nondepression-associated fatigue and sleepiness
- Hypothetically rebalances signal to noise ratios of cortical neurons: enhances focus on importance tasks (signal), theoretically due to norepinephrine, and reduces awareness of background activity (noise), theoretically due to dopamine

SAFETY AND TOLERABILITY

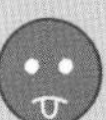

Notable Side Effects

- Anorexia and weight loss
- Nausea, abdominal pain
- Insomnia, headache, exacerbation of tics, tremor, dizziness, and possible irritability and anxiety. The risk of treatment-emergent irritability is higher with amphetamine-based stimulants compared to methylphenidate-based stimulants.
- Peripheral vasculopathy, including Raynaud's phenomenon
- Sexual dysfunction long term (impotence, libido changes) but can also improve sexual dysfunction short term

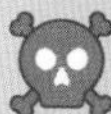

Life-Threatening or Dangerous Side Effects

- Psychosis
- Seizures
- Palpitations, tachycardia, hypertension
- Rare hypomania, mania, or suicidal ideation
- Cardiovascular adverse effects, death in patients with preexisting cardiac structural abnormalities often associated with a family history of cardiac disease

Growth and Maturation

- May temporarily slow normal growth in children (controversial): Multimodal Treatment of ADHD (MTA) study showed children/adolescents grew more slowly but eventually reached their expected adult height

- Controversy exists because theoretically stimulants might suppress appetite and reduce caloric intake, which could affect potential growth; also, dopaminergic actions of stimulants might suppress growth hormone secretion and affect height development. However, expected adult height is likely attained with a delay if stimulants are continued, and slowing of growth is likely reversible with withdrawal of treatment.

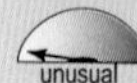

Weight Gain

- Patients may experience weight loss
- Weight gain is reported but not expected, rarely seen, controversial

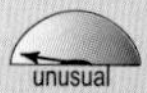

Sedation

- Activation much more common than sedation
- Sedation is reported but not expected, rarely seen, controversial

What to Do About Side Effects

- Wait, wait, wait: mild side effects are common, happen early, and usually improve with time, but treatment benefits can be delayed and often begin just as the side effects wear off
- Switch to a long-acting stimulant
- Switch to another agent
- For insomnia: avoid dosing in the midday, late afternoon, or evening
- However, insomnia is not always due to medication, but can be the result of relapse, rebound, and withdrawal effects from the daily dose, and in fact improves with additional late-day dosing of a short-acting stimulant
- Often best to try another monotherapy prior to resorting to augmentation strategies to treat side effects, with the exception of an early-evening dose of a stimulant
- Monitor side effects closely, especially when initiating treatment
- For persistent insomnia: consider adding melatonin or an alpha 2 agonist
- For loss of appetite or loss of weight:
  - Give medication after breakfast
  - Switch to a nonstimulant
  - Eat a high-protein, high-carbohydrate breakfast prior to taking medication or within 10–15 minutes of ingesting medication; snack on high-protein, densely caloric foods throughout the school day and after school; eat dinner and then a second dinner or very heavy snack at bedtime
  - Add "liquid calories" (i.e., smoothies made with whole milk or ice cream, fruit, and protein powder; Boost or Ensure shakes)
  - Introduce "fourth meal" in the evening
  - Add cyproheptadine

How Drug Causes Side Effects

- Increases in norepinephrine peripherally can cause autonomic side effects, including tremor, tachycardia, hypertension, and cardiac arrhythmias
- Increases in norepinephrine and dopamine centrally can cause CNS side effects such as insomnia, agitation, psychosis (rarely)

Warnings and Precautions

- Safety and efficacy not established in children under age 6
- Use in young children should be reserved for the expert
- Children who are not growing or gaining weight should stop treatment, at least temporarily
- Usual dosing has been associated with sudden death in children with structural cardiac abnormalities
- Stimulants used to treat ADHD are associated with peripheral vasculopathy, including Raynaud's phenomenon; careful observation for digital changes is necessary during treatment with ADHD stimulants
- Consider distributing brochures provided by the FDA and the drug companies
- Carefully weigh the risks and benefits of pharmacological treatment against the risks and benefits of nonpharmacological treatment and it is a good idea to document this in the patient's chart
- Use with caution in patients with any degree of hypertension, hyperthyroidism, or history of drug abuse
- Many believe tics may be worsened by stimulants, but evidence does not support this association. A meta-analysis of 22 studies, including 2,385 individuals in treatment, found that the rate of new onset or worsening tics was 5.7% for those on

stimulants versus 6.5% with placebo. In this analysis, there was no effect for type of stimulant, dose, duration of treatment, or age (Cohen et al., 2015). The presence of tics is not an absolute contraindication to use of stimulants.
- May worsen symptoms of thought disorder and behavioral disturbance in psychotic patients
- Stimulants have a high potential for abuse and must be used with caution in anyone with a current or past history of substance abuse or alcoholism, but stimulants for ADHD are less likely to be abused in terms of getting "high" and more likely to be used to stay awake, especially by college students. This misuse is the most common reason for diversion of prescription stimulants.
- Youth are neither more nor less likely to develop alcohol and substance use disorders as a result of being treated with stimulant medication. In fact, current data suggest that treating ADHD in children and adolescents decreases the likelihood of developing a substance use disorder.
- Adolescents and/or college students may divert/sell their medication to others for use in staying awake to study at the last minute, or to abuse; longer-acting preparations are harder to abuse than shorter-acting, immediate-release stimulants
- Particular attention should be paid to the possibility of adolescents you are seeing for the first time feigning ADHD in order to obtain stimulants for nontherapeutic use or distribution to others; the drugs should in general be prescribed sparingly with documentation of appropriate use, and if there is any doubt about the accuracy of their complaints, refer them for psychological-educational or neuropsychological testing
- Not an appropriate first-line treatment for depression or for normal fatigue
- May lower the seizure threshold; as long as seizures are well controlled, it is generally safe to use stimulants
- Emergence or worsening of activation and agitation may represent the induction of a bipolar state, especially a mixed dysphoric bipolar II condition sometimes associated with suicidal ideation, and may require the addition of lithium or an atypical antipsychotic, and/or discontinuation of lisdexamfetamine

When Not to Prescribe

- Treating ADHD comorbid with tics or Tourette syndrome is not contraindicated, but may be for the expert
- Patients with ADHD who are comorbid for motor or vocal tics of Tourette syndrome, or even with just a family history of Tourette syndrome, may experience worsening/onset of tics with stimulant treatment (controversial). Decision to use stimulants in such cases should weigh the potential benefits for ADHD against the risks of worsening tics, and may require expert referral or consultation.
- Should generally not be administered with an MAOI, including within 14 days of MAOI use, except in heroic circumstances and by an expert
- If patient has arteriosclerosis, cardiovascular disease, or severe hypertension
- If patient has glaucoma
- If patient has structural cardiac abnormalities
- If there is a proven allergy to any sympathomimetic agent
- If the patient has an eating disorder other than binge-eating disorder, be cautious

Long-Term Use

- Often used long-term for ADHD when ongoing monitoring documents continued efficacy
- Tolerance to therapeutic effects may develop in some patients
- Weight and height should be monitored during long-term treatment
- Periodic monitoring of blood pressure and heart rate
- For binge-eating disorder, lisdexamfetamine has demonstrated maintenance of efficacy in a 26-week double-blind randomized withdrawal-phase study

Habit Forming

- Paradoxically, stimulant abuse appears to be less likely in patients with ADHD than in those who do not have ADHD. In 2023, the FDA modified a boxed warning for stimulant medications, although they noted, "Our review found that nonmedical use has

remained relatively stable over the past two decades, despite the increasing number of prescription stimulants dispensed." The new warning notes that stimulants have a "high potential for abuse and misuse, which can lead to the development of a substance use disorder, including addiction." The new warning also notes that stimulant medications "can be diverted for non-medical use into illicit channels or distribution." They recommend:
  - Counsel patients not to give any of their medicine to anyone else
  - Monitor for signs and symptoms of diversion, such as requesting refills more frequently than needed
  - Regularly assess and monitor for signs and symptoms of nonmedical use and addiction
  - Keep careful records of prescribing information, including quantity, frequency, and renewal requests, as required by state and federal laws
- Stimulant abuse in ADHD patients more likely if there is a preexisting history of alcohol/drug abuse
- Tolerance to stimulants is surprisingly rare in ADHD; tolerance should not be confused with reduction of therapeutic effects over time due to growth: as youth grow, dose usually must be increased; otherwise, the appearance of tolerance occurs when in reality this is underdosing
- Theoretically less abuse potential than other stimulants when taken as directed because it is inactive until it reaches the gut and thus has delayed time to onset as well as long duration of action

Overdose

- Rarely fatal; panic, hyperreflexia, rhabdomyolysis, rapid respiration, confusion, coma, hallucination, convulsion, arrhythmia, change in blood pressure, circulatory collapse

DOSING AND USE

Usual Dosage Range

- ADHD (all ages): 30–70 mg/day
- Binge-eating disorder (adults): 50–70 mg/day

Dosage Forms

- Capsule 10 mg, 20 mg, 30 mg, 40 mg, 50 mg, 60 mg, 70 mg
- Chewable tablet 10 mg, 20 mg, 30 mg, 40 mg, 50 mg, 60 mg

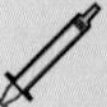

How to Dose

- ADHD (all ages): initial 30 mg/day in the morning; can increase by 10–20 mg each week; maximum dose generally 70 mg/day
- Binge-eating disorder (adults): initial 30 mg/day in the morning; can increase by 20 mg each week; maximum dose generally 70 mg/day

Options for Administration

- Chewable tablet can be beneficial for patients with difficulty swallowing pills

Tests

- Before treatment, assess for presence of cardiac disease (history, family history, physical exam); consider whether electrocardiogram (ECG) is indicated
- Blood pressure and heart should be monitored regularly, sitting and standing
- Monitor weight and height
- Current recommendations from the American Heart Association (AHA) are that it is reasonable but not mandatory to obtain an ECG prior to prescribing a stimulant to a child; the American Academy of Pediatrics (AAP) does not recommend an ECG prior to starting a stimulant for most children
- Document basic sleep patterns prior to starting a stimulant
- When necessary to rule out sleep apnea, nocturnal movements, or daytime sleepiness that may later be difficult to distinguish from side effects of stimulants, consider (rarely) a sleep study/polysomnogram (e.g., obese adolescents)

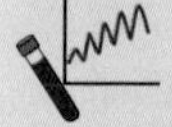

Pharmacokinetics

- Lisdexamfetamine is rapidly absorbed from the gastrointestinal tract. After oral ingestion, lisdexamfetamine is converted to dextroamphetamine primarily by enzymatic hydrolysis (Figure 1).
- 1 hour to maximum concentration of lisdexamfetamine, 3.5 hours to maximum concentration of dextroamphetamine
- Duration of clinical action 10–12 hours

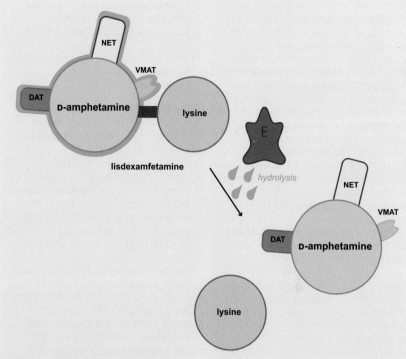

Figure 1 Lisdexamfetamine metabolism.

- Elimination half-life of dextroamphetamine is approximately 10 to 12 hours in adults
- Dextroamphetamine is primarily eliminated through renal excretion, both as unchanged drug and as metabolites
- Approximately 30% to 40% of the dose is excreted in urine as unchanged dextroamphetamine within 48 hours

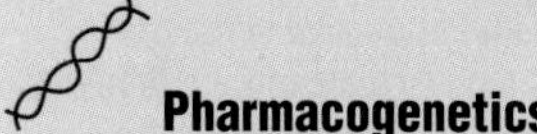

Pharmacogenetics

- No recommendations

Drug Interactions

- May affect blood pressure and should be used cautiously with agents used to control blood pressure
- Gastrointestinal acidifying agents (guanethidine, reserpine, glutamic acid, ascorbic acid, fruit juices, etc.) and urinary acidifying agents (ammonium chloride, sodium phosphate, etc.) lower amphetamine plasma levels, so such agents can be useful to administer after an overdose but may also lower therapeutic efficacy of amphetamines
- Gastrointestinal alkalinizing agents (sodium bicarbonate, etc.) and urinary alkalinizing agents (acetazolamide, some thiazides) increase amphetamine plasma levels and potentiate amphetamine's actions
- Desipramine and protriptyline can cause striking and sustained increases in brain concentrations of D-amphetamine and may also add to D-amphetamine's cardiovascular effects
- Theoretically, other agents with norepinephrine reuptake blocking properties, such as venlafaxine, duloxetine, atomoxetine, milnacipran, and reboxetine, could also add to amphetamine's CNS and cardiovascular effects
- Amphetamines may counteract the sedative effects of antihistamines
- Haloperidol, chlorpromazine, and lithium may inhibit stimulatory effects of amphetamines

- Theoretically, amphetamines could inhibit the antipsychotic actions of antipsychotics
- Theoretically, amphetamines could inhibit the mood-stabilizing actions of atypical antipsychotics in some patients; however, stimulants can be safely combined with atypical antipsychotics by experts
- Combinations of amphetamines with mood stabilizers (lithium, anticonvulsants, atypical antipsychotics) are generally something for experts only, when monitoring patients closely and when other options fail
- Absorption of phenobarbital, phenytoin, and ethosuximide is delayed by amphetamines
- Amphetamines inhibit adrenergic blockers and enhance adrenergic effects of norepinephrine
- MAOIs slow metabolism of amphetamines and thus potentiate their actions, which can cause headache, hypertension, and rarely hypertensive crisis and malignant hyperthermia, sometimes with fatal results
- Use with MAOIs, including within 14 days of MAOI use, is not advised, but this can sometimes be considered by experts who monitor depressed patients closely when other treatment options for depression fail

Dosing Tips

- Plasma levels are higher in lower-weight children; therefore, starting and target doses may be lower and longer intervals between dose increases may be needed (see How to Dose)
- Once-daily dosing can eliminate the hassle and pragmatic difficulties of lunchtime dosing at school, including storage problems, potential diversion, and the need for a medical professional to supervise dosing away from home
- Be aware that metabolism (and absorption) changes during puberty and entry into adolescence and becomes more like adults (i.e., slower than in children)
- If a child on a stable dose begins to lose tolerability with more side effects upon entering adolescence, this may signal the need for a dose reduction due to changing metabolism
- The duration of action is 10–12-hours
- Capsules can either be taken whole or they can be opened and the contents dissolved in water
- When taken in water, the entire solution should be consumed immediately
- Dose of a single capsule should not be divided
- Avoid dosing after the morning because of the risk of insomnia
- Can be taken with or without food

Drug Holidays

- Drug holidays were originally done in an attempt to avoid the possibility that stimulants may blunt height
- May be able to give drug holidays over the summer in order to reassess therapeutic utility and effects on growth and theoretically to allow catch-up from any growth suppression and assess any other side effects and the need to reinstitute stimulant treatment for the next school term
- However, most studies show that parental height is what determines a patient's final height, and that most children/adolescents taking stimulants reach their expected height, just more slowly than children/adolescents not exposed to stimulants
- May be possible to give weekend drug holidays and dose only during the school week for some ADHD patients, but there are risks as well:
  - Hyperactivity and impulsivity increase the chances of accidents (i.e., broken bones and head injuries) and illicit alcohol and drug abuse
  - Studies have shown that adolescents with ADHD who drive vehicles without their stimulants are much more likely to get into motor vehicle accidents and that the severity of the accident is much greater than would be expected
  - Hyperactive and impulsive children/adolescents tend to have more difficulties getting along with family members and friends, increasing the chances of developing low self-esteem and poor self-image
  - Social benefits can be lost over the summer if children/adolescents are taken off stimulants; social rejection by other children can lead to isolation and depression, increasing the chances of bullying, victimization, and further isolation and peer rejection
  - Inattention makes it harder for kids to learn the rules of life and pay attention

to what is going on around them (e.g., noticing when a peer is not being a true friend, when someone is starting to get annoyed, when a car is coming toward you and you're in the middle of the street)

How to Switch

- When switching from one stimulant to another, the first one can be abruptly stopped and the new one started the next morning. Side effects from abrupt discontinuation are not expected; however, some patients may experience marked fatigue and sleepiness for several days.
- See Appendix for approximate dosing equivalents when switching

How to Stop

- Taper not necessary, especially for patients who have only had short-term treatment or intermittent treatment
- However, if withdrawal symptoms develop, resume dosing the medication and then taper slowly over several days
- Withdrawal following chronic therapeutic use may unmask symptoms of the underlying disorder and may require follow-up and reinstitution of treatment
- Usually symptoms after discontinuation are return of symptoms of the underlying disorder rather than symptoms due to drug withdrawal
- Supervision during withdrawal is always recommended for any psychotropic medication

WHAT TO EXPECT

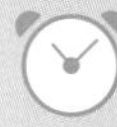

Onset of Action

- Some immediate effects can be seen with first dosing
- Takes a few days to attain therapeutic benefit generally

Duration of Action

- Clinical duration of action is 10–12 hours

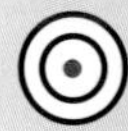

Primary Target Symptoms

- Concentration, attention span, distractibility
- Motor hyperactivity
- Impulsiveness
- Binge eating
- Physical and mental fatigue
- Daytime sleepiness

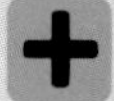

What Is Considered a Positive Result?

- The goal of treatment of ADHD is reduction of symptoms of inattentiveness, motor hyperactivity, and/or impulsiveness that disrupt social, school, and/or occupational functioning
- Can also improve oppositional and disruptive behaviors associated with ADHD
- The goal of treatment is complete remission of symptoms
- If treatment works, it most often reduces or even eliminates symptoms, but is not a cure since symptoms often recur after medicine is stopped

How Long to Treat

- ADHD is typically a lifelong illness; if any symptoms improve, hyperactivity is more likely to improve than inattention
- Can tell parents there is some chance that their child can grow out of this in adulthood, but many adults continue to have symptoms of ADHD throughout adolescence and adulthood
- Continue treatment until all symptoms are under control or improvement is stable and then continue treatment as long as improvement persists
- Reevaluate the need for treatment periodically; some clinicians advise to periodically stop stimulants in patients who are not severely symptomatic to observe how the patient responds, but not routinely done by most clinicians
- Treatment for ADHD begun in childhood may need to be continued into adolescence and adulthood if continued benefit is documented

What If It Stops Working?

- Some patients who have an initial response may relapse even though they continue treatment, sometimes called "poop-out"
- Growth/developmental changes may contribute to apparent loss of efficacy as well as to new onset of side effects as metabolism slows and drug levels rise in transition from childhood to adolescence; dose adjustment (increase or decrease) should be considered

- Some patients may experience apparent lack of consistent efficacy due to activation of latent or underlying or newly evolved bipolar disorder, major depressive episodes with mixed features of mania, new onset of major depression or an anxiety disorder (GAD, OCD, PD), and require stimulant discontinuation and a switch to the clinically appropriate medication(s)

What If It Doesn't Work?

- In practice, many patients have only a partial response where some symptoms are improved but others persist, in which case higher doses of amphetamine, adding a second agent, or switching to an agent with a different mechanism of action can be considered
- Consider evaluation for another diagnosis or for a comorbid condition (e.g., medical illness, substance abuse). Also, when treating ADHD, consider the possibility of a learning disorder or learning weakness and consider school-based interventions.
- Consider adjusting dose or switching to another formulation of amphetamine or to another agent
- Consider the presence of nonadherence and counsel patient and parents
- Some ADHD patients and some depressed patients may experience lack of consistent efficacy due to activation of latent or underlying bipolar disorder, and require either augmenting with a mood stabilizer or switching to a mood stabilizer
- Augmenting options:
  - Organizational skills training/executive function coaching
  - Exercise
  - Parent Management Training (PMT)
  - Coordinating with school for appropriate support
  - For the expert, can combine with viloxazine or atomoxetine for ADHD
  - For the expert, can occasionally combine with atypical antipsychotics in highly treatment-resistant cases of bipolar disorder or ADHD
  - For the expert, can combine with antidepressants to boost antidepressant efficacy in highly treatment-resistant cases of depression while carefully monitoring patient
  - Can combine with alpha 2 agonists such as guanfacine or clonidine
- Consider factors associated with poor response to any psychotropic medication in children and adolescents, such as severe symptoms, long-lasting symptoms, poor treatment adherence, prior nonresponse to other treatments, and the presence of comorbid psychiatric disorders or learning disorders
- Consider other important potential factors such as ongoing conflicts, family psychopathology, and an adverse environment (e.g., poverty, chaos, violence, prior and ongoing psychological trauma, abuse, bullying, less-than-ideal school placement, neglect)
- Institute trauma-informed care for appropriate children and adolescents

TALKING TO PATIENTS AND CAREGIVERS

What to Tell Parents About Efficacy

- Stimulant treatment for ADHD is one of the best studied of all medications in children and adolescents
- Often works right away once the dose is correct
- While the medicine helps ADHD by reducing symptoms and improving function, there are no cures for ADHD and it is therefore necessary to keep taking the medication to sustain its therapeutic effects
- It does not work that day if the child/adolescent has not taken their medication in the morning
- For longer-acting stimulants, be careful not to give too late (i.e., after 8 a.m.) because it can cause insomnia that night
- Does not stay in the body for a long time, so it stops working rapidly after you stop it
- Since every treatment consideration depends on a risk/benefit analysis, parents should fully understand short- and long-term risks as well as benefits compared to nontreatment of ADHD
- Although many stimulants are approved for ADHD, if using off-label, often a good idea to tell parents whether the medication chosen is specifically approved for the disorder being treated, or whether it is being given for "unapproved" or

"off-label" reasons based on good clinical practice, expert consensus, and/or prudent extrapolation of controlled data from adults
- Best results are often obtained when medications are combined with behavioral therapy
- Stimulants wear off after a number of hours and symptoms may return. Therefore, parents may complain that the medication isn't working if their child/adolescent is using a stimulant that lasts 8 hours, because it may have worn off after the patient has come home from school (and that is when the parents are seeing the child/adolescent) in comparison to a stimulant that lasts 10–12 hours and may keep working after the child/adolescent comes home from school.
- The American Academy of Child & Adolescent Psychiatry (AACAP) has helpful handouts for parents

What to Tell Children and Adolescents About Efficacy

- Be specific about the symptoms being targeted: we are trying to help you remember things better, do your best at school, follow the rules, get into less trouble (as applicable)
- It may be a good idea to give the medication a try; if it's not working very well, we can stop the medication and try something else
- You can be part of a special plan to help us figure out if the medicine is helpful for you. Would you like to do that? (for the parents and prescriber, can consider here a trial both on and then off medication, and then on again to see if the effects are clear and thus worth continuing the medication)
- The medication can work right away but a good try can take a few months to find the right dose
- Even if it does make you feel better, it will wear off and no longer work shortly after you stop it
- This medicine does not last very long in your body, so even if it does work, it won't work if you don't take it that day
- The medication can help you decide what you want to do, like making good choices versus bad choices; the medicine does not make you do something you don't want to do
- Medications don't change who you are as a person; they give you the opportunity to be the best person you can be

What to Tell Parents About Side Effects

- Explain that side effects are expected in many when starting
- Tell parents many side effects of stimulants often go away in a few days to weeks, especially nausea and insomnia, but if they don't we will change the treatment
- Predict side effects in advance (you will look clever and competent to the parents, unless you scare them with too much information and cause nocebo effects, in which case you won't look so clever when the patient develops lots of side effects and stops medication); a balanced but honest presentation is an art rather than a science
- Sometimes a trial off medication and then on again can clarify what the true therapeutic effects of the medication are
- Ask parents to support the patient while side effects are occurring
- Parents should fully understand short- and long-term risks as well as benefits
- Explaining to the parents what to expect from medication treatment, and especially what potential side effects to expect, can help prevent early termination

What to Tell Children and Adolescents About Side Effects

- When a medicine starts to work, your body can first experience this by giving you unpleasant sensations – just like if you take a cough medicine it may taste bad – these body sensations include loss of appetite and problems sleeping. So, just like with a cough medicine, the bad taste will often go away before the medicine begins to stop the cough – many medicines work like that. It's important for you to pay attention to what your body is telling you, and we'll go over some of the ways that can happen.
- Even if you get a side effect, it's not permanent (it won't last forever)
- Explaining to child/adolescent what to expect from medication treatment, and especially potential side effects, can help prevent early termination

What to Tell Teachers About the Medication (If Parents Consent)

- Stimulants can be very helpful in improving the symptoms of ADHD: namely, inattention, impulsivity, and hyperactivity
- It does not work if the child/adolescent has not taken their medication that morning
- If the patient is sleepy, ask whether the medication is keeping them up at night or if they are eating enough food
- If the patient won't eat lunch or snacks, ask whether the medication is making them lose their appetite
- Medically speaking, lisdexamfetamine is not a narcotic, because doctors define a narcotic as something that is sedating and sleep-inducing, like opioids such as heroin and Oxycontin and not stimulants like lisdexamfetamine
- Lisdexamfetamine should be kept in school under lock and key or at the nurse's office or not brought to school at all because it can be diverted and misused by those who do not have ADHD. Some schools will suspend students who are caught with medications on their person or in their backpacks; most schools know the misuse or even abuse potential of stimulants.

SPECIAL POPULATIONS

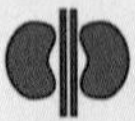

Renal Impairment

- Severe impairment: maximum dose 50 mg/day
- End-stage renal disease: maximum dose 30 mg/day

Hepatic Impairment

- Use with caution

Cardiac Impairment

- Do not use in patients with structural cardiac abnormalities without consultation with a cardiologist

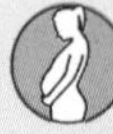

Pregnancy

- Controlled studies have not been conducted in pregnant women
- There is a greater risk of premature birth and low birth weight in infants whose mothers take D-amphetamine during pregnancy
- Infants whose mothers take D-amphetamine during pregnancy may experience withdrawal symptoms
- In animal studies, D-amphetamine caused delayed skeletal ossification and decreased postweaning weight gain in rats; no major malformations occurred in rat or rabbit studies
- Use in women of childbearing potential requires weighing potential benefits to the mother against potential risks to the fetus
- For ADHD patients, lisdexamfetamine should generally be discontinued before anticipated pregnancies
- National Pregnancy Registry for Psychiatric Medications: 1-866-961-2388 or https://womensmentalhealth.org/research/pregnancyregistry/

Breast Feeding

- Some drug is found in breast milk
- Recommended either to discontinue drug or formula feed
- If infant shows signs of irritability, drug may need to be discontinued

THE ART OF PSYCHOPHARMACOLOGY

Potential Advantages

- In children:
  - Stimulants are probably the best studied psychotropic medications for use in children
  - Amphetamine is one of the best studied stimulants in children
- In adolescents:
  - Can improve school performance and grades, especially if ADHD has been unrecognized and untreated prior to adolescence
  - Can improve performance in high school and college students whose ADHD is compromising academic performance due to the increased demands of higher levels of study
- All ages:
  - Although restricted as a Schedule II controlled substance like other stimulants, as a prodrug lisdexamfetamine may have less propensity for abuse, intoxication, or dependence than other stimulants

Potential Disadvantages

- Adolescents and especially college-age patients who divert their medication
- Patients with current substance abuse
- Patients with current manic or mixed symptoms associated with bipolar disorder or psychosis
- Patients with anorexia

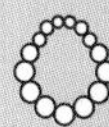

Pearls

- Half-life and duration of clinical action tend to be shorter in younger children than in adolescents and may require more frequent dosing or preferential use of long-acting preparations
- Drug abuse is no more likely and may even be lower (controversial) in ADHD adolescents treated with stimulants than in ADHD adolescents who are not treated with stimulants
- Stimulants have a moderate effect on decreasing ADHD symptoms and a moderate to large effect on decreasing aggression, oppositional behavior, and conduct problems in children with ADHD
- Some patients respond to or tolerate lisdexamfetamine better than methylphenidate or amphetamine and vice versa. However, recent meta-analyses suggest that amphetamine-based medications may work better in adults, while methylphenidate-based medications may work better in children and adolescents.
- Combinations of behavioral therapy or other nonmedication treatments along with stimulants may have better results than either treatment alone
- Rebound hyperactivity may occur in the afternoon and present with increased hyperactivity, restlessness, and irritability; if this occurs, can consider switching to a longer-acting agent or a nonstimulant or adding a short-acting stimulant
- On the other hand, too-high medication dosing may lead to cognitive rigidity, difficulty shifting attention, and seeming "spaced out" or "different"
- Many patients taking stimulants have early-morning ADHD symptoms and can be hard to get going, prepare for school, and be cooperative, especially for a few hours after awakening. In these patients, delayed-release/extended-release formulations may be especially helpful.
- Despite warnings, can be a useful adjunct to MAOIs for heroic treatment of highly refractory mood disorders when monitored with vigilance
- Can reverse sexual dysfunction caused by psychiatric illness and by some drugs such as SSRIs, including decreased libido, erectile dysfunction, delayed ejaculation, and anorgasmia
- Stimulants are a classic augmentation strategy for treatment-refractory depression, although this is most established in adults
- Interestingly, in some studies combining stimulants with alpha 2 agonists, decreased side effects are seen with the combination compared to either medication as monotherapy. This is likely because of complementary side effects.

SUGGESTED READING

Biederman J, Spencer TJ, Monuteaux MC, Faraone SV. A naturalistic 10-year prospective study of height and weight in children with attention-deficit hyperactivity disorder grown up: sex and treatment effects. J Pediatr 2010;157(4):635–40.

Cohen SC, Mulqueen JM, Ferracioli-Oda E et al. Meta-analysis: risk of tics associated with psychostimulant use in randomized, placebo-controlled trials. J Am Acad Child Adolesc Psychiatry 2015;54(9):728–36.

Cortese S, Adamo N, Del Giovane C et al. Comparative efficacy and tolerability of medications for attention-deficit hyperactivity disorder in children, adolescents, and adults: a systematic review and network meta-analysis. Lancet Psychiatry 2018;5(9):727–38.

Farhat LC, Flores JM, Behling E et al. The effects of stimulant dose and dosing strategy on treatment outcomes in attention-deficit/hyperactivity disorder in children and adolescents: a meta-analysis. Mol Psychiatry 2022;27(3):1562–72.

Jensen PS, Arnold LE, Swanson JM et al. 3-year follow-up of the NIMH MTA study. J Am Acad Child Adolesc Psychiatry 2007;46(8):989–1002.

Maneeton B, Maneeton N, Likhitsathian S et al. Comparative efficacy, acceptability, and tolerability of lisdexamfetamine in child and adolescent ADHD: a meta-analysis of randomized, controlled trials. Drug Dex Devel Ther 2015;9:1927–36.

Swanson JM, Arnold LE, Molina BSG et al. Young adult outcomes in the follow-up of the multimodal treatment study of attention-deficit/hyperactivity disorder: symptom persistence, source discrepancy, and height suppression. J Child Psychol Psychiatry 2017;58(6):663–78.

Zhang L, Yao H, Li L, et al. Risk of cardiovascular diseases associated with medications used in attention-deficit/hyperactivity disorder: a systematic review and meta-analysis. JAMA Netw Open 2022;5(11):e2243597.

THERAPEUTICS

Brands

- Eskalith
- Eskalith CR
- Lithium carbonate tablets
- Lithium citrate syrup
- Lithobid slow-release tablets
- Lithostat tablets

Generic

Yes

US FDA Approved for Pediatric Use

- Acute mania/mixed mania (ages 7 and older, monotherapy)
- Bipolar maintenance (ages 7 and older, monotherapy)

Off-Label for Pediatric Use

- Bipolar depression
- Major depressive disorder (adjunctive)

Class and Mechanism of Action

- Neuroscience-based Nomenclature: lithium enzyme interactions (Li-Eint)
- Mood stabilizer
- Lithium's mechanism of action is unknown and complex
- Lithium alters sodium transport across cell membranes in nerve and muscle cells
- Lithium alters metabolism of neurotransmitters including catecholamines and serotonin
- Lithium may alter intracellular signaling through actions on second messenger systems
- Specifically, lithium inhibits inositol monophosphatase, possibly affecting neurotransmission via phosphatidyl inositol second messenger system
- Lithium also reduces protein kinase C activity, possibly affecting genomic expression associated with neurotransmission
- Lithium increases cytoprotective proteins, activates signaling cascade utilized by endogenous growth factors, and increases gray matter content, possibly by activating neurogenesis and enhancing trophic actions that maintain synapses

SAFETY AND TOLERABILITY

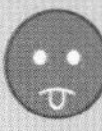

Notable Side Effects

- Ataxia, dysarthria, delirium, tremor, memory problems
- Polyuria, polydipsia (nephrogenic diabetes insipidus)
- Diarrhea, nausea
- Weight gain
- Euthyroid goiter or hypothyroid goiter, possibly with increased TSH and reduced thyroxine levels
- Acne, rash, alopecia, metallic taste
- Leukocytosis
- Side effects are typically dose related
- Younger children tend to have more frequent and severe side effects

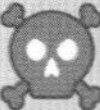

Life-Threatening or Dangerous Side Effects

- Lithium toxicity
- Renal impairment (interstitial nephritis)
- Nephrogenic diabetes insipidus
- Arrhythmia, cardiovascular changes, sick sinus syndrome, bradycardia, hypotension
- T-wave flattening and inversion
- Rare pseudotumor cerebri
- Rare seizures

Growth and Maturation

- Long-term effects are unknown

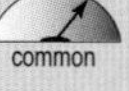

Weight Gain

- Many experience and/or can be significant in amount
- Can become a health problem in some
- May be associated with increased appetite

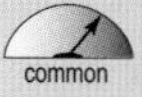

Sedation

- Many patients experience and/or can be significant in amount
- May wear off with time

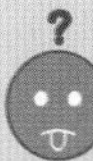

What to Do About Side Effects

- If signs of lithium toxicity occur, discontinue immediately
- For mild side effects, wait, wait, wait: mild side effects are common, happen early (often before therapeutic effects), and usually improve with time

- Monitor side effects closely, especially when initiating treatment
- For stomach upset, take with food
- Sustained-release formulation may reduce gastric irritation, lower peak lithium plasma levels, and diminish peak dose side effects
- For tremor, avoid caffeine; propranolol 20–30 mg 2–3 times/day may also reduce tremor
- For the expert, amiloride may reduce polydipsia and polyuria that does not go away with time alone. Amiloride blocks the epithelial sodium channel (ENaC) located in the apical membrane of principal cells within the nephron. This channel is thought to be the main entry site for lithium and the beneficial effect of amiloride may relate to the inhibition of lithium entry.
- Nearly 1 in 5 children and adolescents treated with lithium will have an increase in TSH. We recommend monitoring and in cases of treatment-emergent hypothyroidism, beginning L-thyroxine supplementation.
- Often best to try another monotherapy prior to resorting to augmentation strategies to treat side effects

How Drug Causes Side Effects

- Unknown and complex
- CNS side effects theoretically due to excessive actions at the same or similar sites that mediate its therapeutic actions
- Some renal side effects theoretically due to lithium's actions on ion transport and, in particular, chronic lithium therapy impair urinary concentrating ability in over half of patients, which likely underlie polyuria and polydipsia
- The effects of lithium on the thyroid are complex and relate to the accumulation of lithium within the thyroid gland, which may have effects on intercellular processes within thyrocytes and inhibits thyroid hormone release from the thyroid gland. Additionally, lithium increases thyroid autoimmunity if present before lithium treatment.

Warnings and Precautions

- Consider distributing brochures provided by the FDA and the drug companies or have the pharmacy do this for the parents
- Carefully weigh the risks and benefits of pharmacological treatment against the risks and benefits of nontreatment and it is a good idea to document this in the patient's chart
- Toxic levels are near therapeutic levels; signs of toxicity include tremor, ataxia, diarrhea, vomiting, sedation
- Monitor for dehydration; lower dose if patient exhibits signs of infection, excessive sweating, diarrhea
- Closely monitor patients with thyroid disorders
- Lithium may cause unmasking of Brugada syndrome; consultation with a cardiologist is recommended if patients develop unexplained syncope or palpitations after starting lithium

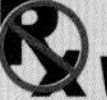

When Not to Prescribe

- If patient has severe kidney disease
- If patient has severe cardiovascular disease
- If patient has Brugada syndrome
- If patient has severe dehydration
- If patient has sodium depletion
- If there is a proven allergy to lithium

Long-Term Use

- Approved in adults for long-term prevention of relapse
- May cause reduced kidney function
- Requires regular therapeutic monitoring of lithium levels as well as of kidney function and thyroid function

Habit Forming

- No

Overdose

- Fatalities have occurred; tremor, dysarthria, delirium, coma, seizures, autonomic instability

DOSING AND USE

Usual Dosage Range

- Mania: recommended 1.0–1.5 mEq/L
- Depression: recommended 0.6–1.0 mEq/L
- Maintenance: recommended 0.7–1.0 mEq/L
- Liquid: 10 mL three times/day (acute mania); 5 mL 3–4 times/day (long-term)

Dosage Forms

- Tablet 300 mg (slow-release), 450 mg (controlled-release)
- Capsule 150 mg, 300 mg, 600 mg
- Liquid 8 mEq/5 mL

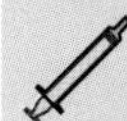

How to Dose

- In children and adolescents, water-soluble drugs like lithium have a proportionately larger volume of distribution and therefore a lower concentration, which may mean the need for a higher dose
- Children: in nonurgent situations, start with 150 mg at night; increase by 150–300 mg increments every few days as tolerated and as indicated by plasma levels until efficacy is achieved; can be given either as split doses or as one dose at night
- Adolescents: start 300 mg 2–3 times/day or as one dose at night; adjust dosage upward as indicated by plasma lithium levels

Options for Administration

- Sustained-release formulation may reduce gastric irritation, lower peak lithium plasma levels, and diminish peak dose side effects
- Oral solution can be beneficial for patients with difficulty swallowing pills
- In adults, compared with multiple-dose schedules, single-dose schedules have the same pharmacokinetic properties, the same brain lithium concentrations, increased adherence, less polyuria, and possibly less risk of renal damage
- If administered at night, single-dose schedules can also lower dose by 25%, which reduces peak-related and overall adverse effects

Tests

- Before initiating treatment, kidney function tests (including creatinine) and thyroid function tests; electrocardiogram for patients over age 50
- Repeat kidney function tests 1–2 times/year
- Frequent tests to monitor trough lithium plasma levels (about 12 hours after last dose; should generally be between 1.0 and 1.5 mEq/L for acute treatment, 0.6 and 1.2 mEq/L for chronic treatment)
- Initial monitoring: every 1–2 weeks until desired serum concentration is achieved, then every 2–3 months for the first 6 months
- Stable monitoring: every 6–12 months
- One-off monitoring after dose change, other medication change, illness change (not before 1 week)
- Since lithium is associated with weight gain in some patients, before starting treatment, weigh all patients and determine whether the patient is already overweight
- Before giving a drug that can cause weight gain to an overweight or obese patient, consider determining whether the patient already has pre-diabetes (fasting plasma glucose 100–125 mg/dL), diabetes (fasting plasma glucose > 126 mg/dL), or dyslipidemia (increased total cholesterol, LDL cholesterol, and triglycerides; decreased HDL cholesterol), and treat or refer such patients for treatment, including nutrition and weight management, physical activity counseling, smoking cessation, and medical management
- Monitor weight and BMI percentile during treatment
- While giving a drug to a patient who has gained >5% of initial weight, consider evaluating for the presence of pre-diabetes, diabetes, or dyslipidemia, or consider switching to a different agent

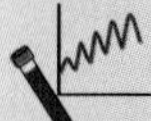

Pharmacokinetics

- Lithium is completely absorbed in the upper gastrointestinal tract
- Peak serum concentrations occur 15 minutes to 3 hours after oral administration of immediate-release formulations and 2–6 hours after sustained-release formulations
- Lithium is not metabolized; it is primarily excreted in urine
- Elimination half-life is approximately 18–36 hours in adults
- Lower absorption on empty stomach
- Average lithium concentration following a single 900 mg dose in youth varies considerably (Figure 1); this underscores the importance of obtaining true trough concentrations

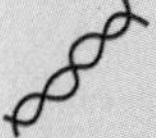

Pharmacogenetics

- No recommendations

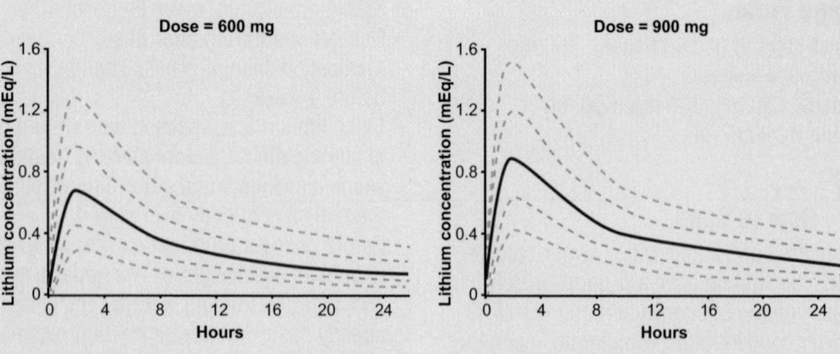

Figure 1 Pharmacokinetic single-dose modeling of pediatric lithium clearance from a sample of 39 youth with mean age 11.9 years. Adapted from Findling et al., 2011.

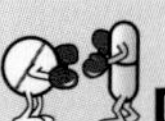

Drug Interactions

- Nonsteroidal anti-inflammatory agents, including ibuprofen and selective COX-2 inhibitors (cyclooxygenase 2), can increase plasma lithium concentrations; add with caution to patients stabilized on lithium
- Diuretics, especially thiazides, can increase plasma lithium concentrations; add with caution to patients stabilized on lithium
- Angiotensin-converting enzyme inhibitors can increase plasma lithium concentrations; add with caution to patients stabilized on lithium
- Metronidazole can lead to lithium toxicity through decreased renal clearance
- Acetazolamide, alkalizing agents, xanthine preparations, and urea may lower lithium plasma concentrations
- Carbamazepine and phenytoin may interact with lithium to increase its toxicity
- Use lithium cautiously with non-dihydropyridine calcium channel blockers, which may increase lithium toxicity
- Lithium may prolong effects of neuromuscular blocking agents
- No likely pharmacokinetic interactions of lithium with mood-stabilizing anticonvulsants or atypical antipsychotics

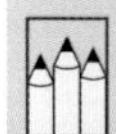

Dosing Tips

- In clinical trials of children and adolescents with bipolar disorder, average lithium levels were near 1.0 mEq/L and were relatively well tolerated (Findling et al., 2015, 2019)
- Data from CoLT1 provide weight-based dosing recommendations. As shown in Figure 2, (kinetic modeling simulation using the dosing recommendation of 25 mg/kg that best fits all of the parameters) optimizes the balance between efficacy and tolerability. From this dosing strategy of 25 mg/kg (administered as divided bid or tid doses) and the response of these manic patients to treatment, two important conclusions were reached.
    - The average lithium level required for a 50% reduction in Young Mania Rating Scale (YMRS) scores was 0.71 mEq/L, but with the caveat that the interindividual variance was very high (almost 60%)
    - A daily maintenance lithium carbonate dose of 25 mg/kg divided bid may achieve a ≥ 50% reduction in YMRS scores in approximately three-quarters of patients, with less than 1 in 10 patients expected to have supratherapeutic trough levels > 1.40 mEq/L
- As an adjunct to anticonvulsant mood stabilizers and/or atypical antipsychotics for the treatment of bipolar disorder, lithium can often be effective at doses at the lower end of the therapeutic plasma range and may also be better tolerated
- Toxic levels are near therapeutic levels; signs of toxicity include tremor, ataxia, diarrhea, vomiting, sedation
- If administered at night, single-dose schedules can also lower dose by 25%, which reduces peak-related and overall adverse effects
- Sustained-release formulation may reduce gastric irritation, lower peak lithium plasma

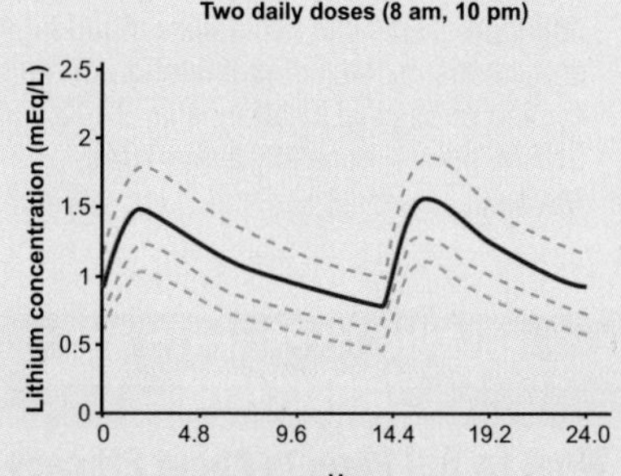

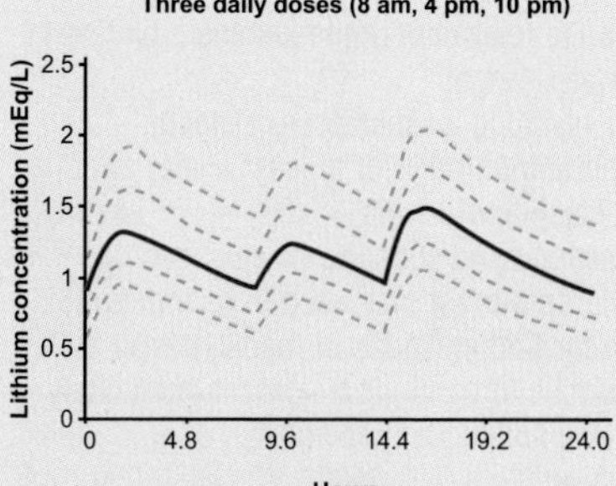

Figure 2 Monte Carlo simulations of lithium concentrations for a daily dosage of 25 mg/kg given in two or three divided doses. [NB: The doses administered were rounded to the nearest 300 mg lithium carbonate increment. Where applicable, the higher dose was given in the evening.] Adapted from Landersdorfer et al., 2017.

levels, and diminish peak dose side effects (i.e., side effects occurring 1–2 hours after each dose of standard lithium carbonate may be improved by sustained-release formulation)
- Use the lowest dose of lithium associated with adequate therapeutic response
- Rapid discontinuation increases the risk of relapse, so lithium may need to be tapered slowly over 3 months if it is to be discontinued after long-term maintenance

How to Switch

- From another medication to lithium:
  - When tapering a prior medication, see its entry in this manual or in the adult prescriber's guide for how to stop and how to taper off that specific drug
  - Generally, try to stop the first agent before starting lithium so that new side effects of lithium can be distinguished from withdrawal effects of the first agent
  - If urgent, cross taper
- Off lithium and onto another medication:
  - Generally, try to stop lithium before starting the new medication so that new side effects of the next drug can be distinguished from any withdrawal effects from lithium
  - If urgent, cross taper

How to Stop

- Taper gradually over 3 months to avoid relapse
- Rapid discontinuation increases the risk of relapse, and possibly suicide
- Discontinuation symptoms uncommon

WHAT TO EXPECT

Onset of Action

- Manic symptoms can improve within 1–3 weeks
- If it is not working within 6–8 weeks, it may require a dosage increase or it may not work at all

Duration of Action

- Effects are consistent over a 24-hour period
- May continue to work for many years to prevent relapse of symptoms

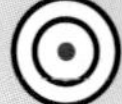

Primary Target Symptoms

- Unstable mood
- Mania

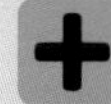

What Is Considered a Positive Result?

- Many patients may experience a reduction of symptoms by half or more

How Long to Treat

- Continue treatment until reaching a plateau of improvement
- After reaching a satisfactory plateau, continue treatment for at least a year after first episode of mania
- For second and subsequent episodes of mania, treatment may need to be indefinite
- Even for first episodes of mania, it may be preferable to continue treatment indefinitely to avoid subsequent episodes

What If It Stops Working?

- Check for nonadherence, possibly by checking plasma drug level, and consider switching to another agent with fewer side effects
- Some patients who have an initial response may relapse even though they continue treatment, sometimes called "poop-out"
- Growth/developmental changes may contribute to apparent loss of efficacy as well as to new onset of side effects as metabolism slows and drug levels rise in transition from childhood to adolescence; dose adjustment (increase or decrease) should be considered
- Screen for the development of a new comorbid disorder, especially substance use
- Screen for adverse changes in the home or school environment

What If It Doesn't Work?

- Consider evaluation for another diagnosis or for a comorbid condition (e.g., medical illness, substance use disorder, learning disorder)
- Consider other important potential factors such as ongoing conflicts, family psychopathology, and an adverse environment (e.g., poverty, chaos, violence, prior and ongoing psychological trauma, abuse, neglect)
- Institute trauma-informed care for appropriate children and adolescents
- Try one of the atypical antipsychotics
- Consider initiating psychotherapy, including family-focused therapy (FFT) in adolescents with bipolar disorder
- Consider presence of concomitant drug abuse
- Consider augmentation with an atypical antipsychotic, lamotrigine, or an antidepressant (with caution because antidepressants can destabilize mood in some patients, including induction of rapid cycling or suicidal ideation; also SSRIs, SNRIs, others; generally avoid TCAs, MAOIs)

TALKING TO PATIENTS AND CAREGIVERS

What to Tell Parents About Efficacy

- For acute symptoms, it can work right away
- Explain which use lithium is being chosen for, how to tell if the drug is working by targeting specific symptoms, and why this is being done
- Once the child/adolescent calms down, at some point after one dose or after several days of dosing or after long-term dosing, we should all assess whether the medication should be continued
- While the medicine helps by reducing symptoms and improving function, it is not a cure, and it therefore may be necessary to keep taking the medication long term to sustain its therapeutic effects
- Since every treatment consideration depends on a risk/benefit analysis, parents should fully understand short- and long-term risks as well as benefits
- Often a good idea to tell parents whether the medication chosen is specifically approved for the disorder being treated, or whether it is being given for "unapproved" or "off-label" reasons based on good clinical practice, expert consensus, and/or prudent extrapolation of controlled data from adults

What to Tell Children and Adolescents About Efficacy

- Be specific about the symptoms being targeted: we are trying to help you ...
- Give the medication a try; if it's not working very well, we can stop the medication and try something else
- A good try often takes 2 to 3 months
- If it does make you feel better, you cannot stop it right away or you may get sick again
- Medications don't change who you are as a person; they give you the opportunity to be the best person you can be

What to Tell Parents About Side Effects

- Explain that side effects are expected in many when starting
- Tell parents many side effects go away and do so about the same time that therapeutic effects start
- Predict side effects in advance (you will look clever and competent to the parents, unless you scare them with too much information and cause nocebo effects, in which case you won't look so clever when the patient develops lots of side effects and stops medication; use your judgment here); a balanced but honest presentation is an art rather than a science
- Helping parents understand when side effects first emerge and that they are transient can help reduce anxiety by decreasing uncertainty, which can help prevent early termination of medication
- Parents should fully understand short- and long-term risks as well as benefits

What to Tell Children and Adolescents About Side Effects

- Even if you get a side effect, we can usually reduce it over time
- If you have side effects that are bothering you, tell your parents and your parents should tell me
- Consider having a conversation about sexual side effects in some adolescents who can find these side effects confusing and especially burdensome
- Explaining to child/adolescent what to expect from medication treatment, and especially potential side effects, can help prevent early termination of medication

What to Tell Teachers About the Medication (If Parents Consent)

- Dehydration can increase lithium concentrations. Lithium-treated youth should have access to a water bottle at their desks and physical education teachers should minimize those activities that could lead to dehydration.
- Lithium-treated patients may have a fine tremor, which could interfere with fine motor skills and affect some schoolwork and school projects
- Lithium can make children/adolescents sedated
- It is not abusable
- Encourage dialogue with parents/guardians about any behavior or mood changes

SPECIAL POPULATIONS

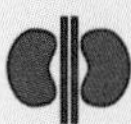

Renal Impairment

- Not recommended for use in patients with severe impairment

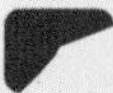

Hepatic Impairment

- No special indications

Cardiac Impairment

- Not recommended for use in patients with severe cardiac disease
- Lithium can cause reversible T-wave changes, sinus bradycardia, sick sinus syndrome, or heart block

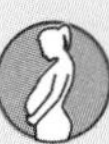

Pregnancy

- Evidence of increased risk of major birth defects (perhaps 2–3 times the general population), but probably lower than with some other mood stabilizers (e.g., valproate)
- Evidence of cardiac anomalies (especially Ebstein's anomaly) in infants whose mothers took lithium during pregnancy
- No long-term neurobehavioral effects of late-term neonatal lithium exposure have been observed
- If lithium is continued, monitor serum lithium levels every 4 weeks, then every week beginning at 36 weeks
- Dehydration due to morning sickness may cause rapid increases in lithium levels
- Lithium administration during delivery may be associated with hypotonia in the infant; most recommend withholding lithium for 24–48 hours before delivery
- Monitoring during delivery should include fluid balance
- After delivery, monitor for 48 hours for "floppy baby syndrome"
- Use in women of childbearing potential requires weighing potential benefits to the mother against the risks to the fetus
- Recurrent bipolar illness during pregnancy can be quite disruptive
- Taper drug if discontinuing

- Given the risk of bipolar relapse in the postpartum period, lithium should generally be restarted immediately after delivery
- This may mean no breast feeding, since lithium can be found in breast milk, possibly at full therapeutic levels
- Atypical antipsychotics may be preferable to lithium or anticonvulsants if treatment of bipolar disorder is required during pregnancy
- Bipolar symptoms may recur or worsen during pregnancy, and some form of treatment may be necessary

Breast Feeding

- Some drug is found in breast milk, possibly at full therapeutic levels since lithium is soluble in breast milk
- Recommended either to discontinue drug or formula feed

THE ART OF PSYCHOPHARMACOLOGY

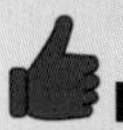

Potential Advantages

- In children and adolescents:
  - Clinical studies in pediatric patients suggest efficacy in managing mania and for maintenance treatment in youth with bipolar disorder
  - Some clinical data suggest efficacy in managing aggression in patients with conduct disorder
- All ages:
  - Euphoric mania
  - Treatment-resistant depression
  - Reduces suicide risk
  - Works well in combination with atypical antipsychotics

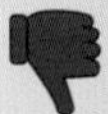

Potential Disadvantages

- In children and adolescents:
  - Efficacy not established for treating depressive symptoms of bipolar disorder, and studies do not support efficacy in unipolar depression and severe mood dysregulation
  - Younger children tend to have more frequent and severe side effects
- All ages:
  - Dysphoric mania
  - Mixed mania, rapid-cycling mania
  - Depressed phase of bipolar disorder
  - Patients unable to tolerate weight gain, sedation, gastrointestinal effects, renal effects, and other side effects
  - Requires blood monitoring

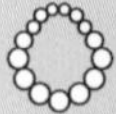

Pearls

- Twice-daily or tid lithium regimens are more common in pediatric populations compared to adults. However, as patients approach adulthood, the lithium dose could be consolidated to qHS starting initially by converting tid to bid dosing, and then slowly transitioning to qHS. The eventual goal by early adulthood is qHS dosing with a 12 h trough of 0.6–0.8 ideally, but up to 1.0 as needed. The rationale for this approach, as described in detail in Meyer and Stahl's *Lithium Handbook*, is that high lithium concentrations over time are nephrotoxic and that it may be advantageous to avoid excursions above 1 to 1.2 mEq/L.
- In adults, two patterns of lithium treatment are associated with significantly increased renal disease risk: use of lithium more than once daily, and having even one lithium level > 1.2 mEq/L (Meyer and Stahl, 2023)
- In adults, the debate over the renoprotective effect of once-daily lithium dosing originated in the early 1980s, with papers noting a greater degree of polyuria in patients receiving bid dosing compared to those on qHS dosing. It later became clear that polyuria is the earliest clinical manifestation of intracellular lithium accumulation in collecting duct principal cells and of the ensuing processes that combine with chronic kidney disease risks to accelerate age-related GFR declines (Meyer and Stahl, 2023).
- The underlying reason for the association between once-daily dosing in adults and decreased renal dysfunction risk is unknown, but two plausible hypotheses are advanced (Meyer and Stahl, 2023):
  - The first rests on the concept that many clinicians may unwittingly expose patients to more lithium when it is prescribed bid due to the distorting effect on morning trough values from divided dosages

  - The second hypothesis is that prolonged higher trough lithium levels from divided daily dosing may lead to a sufficiently high lithium concentration in tubular fluid
- Most pediatric patients receiving lithium will develop elevated thyroid-stimulating hormone concentrations; therefore, screening and monitoring are very helpful, particularly when signs of hypothyroidism (increased weight, decreased energy) are reported
- May also be more effective in preventing manic relapses than in preventing depressive episodes (stabilizes from above better than it stabilizes from below)
- May decrease suicide and suicide attempts not only in bipolar I disorder but also in bipolar II disorder and in unipolar depression
- Due to its narrow therapeutic index, lithium's toxic side effects occur at doses close to its therapeutic effects
- Close therapeutic monitoring of plasma drug levels is required during lithium treatment; lithium is the first psychiatric drug that required blood-level monitoring
- Probably less effective than atypical antipsychotics for severe, excited, disturbed, hyperactive, or psychotic patients with mania
- Due to delayed onset of action, lithium monotherapy may not be the first choice in acute mania, but rather may be used as an adjunct to second generation antipsychotics
- After acute symptoms of mania are controlled, some patients can be maintained on lithium monotherapy
- Lithium is not a convincing augmentation agent to atypical antipsychotics for the treatment of schizophrenia
- Lithium may be useful for a number of patients with episodic, recurrent symptoms with or without affective illness, including episodic rage, anger or violence, and self-destructive behavior; such symptoms may be associated with psychotic or nonpsychotic illnesses, personality disorders, organic disorders, or mental retardation
- Lithium is better tolerated during acute manic phases than when manic symptoms have abated
- Adverse effects generally increase in incidence and severity as lithium serum levels increase

SUGGESTED READING

Baldessarini RJ, Tondo L, Davis P et al. Decreased risk of suicides and attempts during long-term lithium treatment: a meta-analytic review. Bipolar Disord 2006;8(5 Pt 2):625–39.

Findling RL, Kafantaris V, Pavuluri M et al. Dosing strategies for lithium monotherapy in children and adolescents with bipolar I disorder. J Child Adolesc Psychopharmacol 2011;21(3):195–205.

Findling RL, Robb A, McNamara NK et al. Lithium in the acute treatment of bipolar I disorder: a double-blind, placebo-controlled study. Pediatrics 2015;136(5):885–94.

Findling RL, McNamara NK, Pavuluri M et al. Lithium for the maintenance treatment of bipolar I disorder: a double-blind, placebo-controlled discontinuation study. J Am Acad Child Adolesc Psychiatry 2019;58(2):287–96.e4.

Geller B, Luby JL, Joshi P et al. A randomized controlled trial of risperidone, lithium, or divalproex sodium for initial treatment of bipolar I disorder, manic or mixed phase, in children and adolescents. Arch Gen Psychiatry 2012;69(5):515–28.

Landersdorfer CB, Findling RL, Frazier JA, Kafantaris V, Kirkpatrick CM. Lithium in paediatric patients with bipolar disorder: implications for selection of dosage regimens via population pharmacokinetics/pharmacodynamics. Clin Pharmacokinet 2017;56(1):77–90.

Meyer JM, Stahl SM. The Lithium Handbook: Stahl's Handbooks. New York: Cambridge University Press, 2023.

Pisano S, Pozzi M, Catone G et al. Putative mechanisms of action and clinical use of lithium in children and adolescents: a critical review. Curr Neuropharmacol 2019;17(4):318–41.

THERAPEUTICS

Brands

- Ativan
- Loreev XR

Generic

Yes (not for extended-release)

FDA US FDA Approved for Pediatric Use

- Short-term treatment of anxiety or anxiety associated with depressive symptoms (oral, ages 12 and older)

Off-Label for Pediatric Use

- Approved in adults
  - Initial treatment of status epilepticus (injection)
  - Preanesthetic (injection)
- Other off-label uses
  - Insomnia
  - Muscle spasm
  - Alcohol withdrawal psychosis
  - Headache
  - Panic disorder
  - Acute mania (adjunctive)
  - Acute psychosis (adjunctive)
  - Delirium (with haloperidol)
  - Catatonia

Class and Mechanism of Action

- Neuroscience-based Nomenclature: GABA positive allosteric modulator (GABA-PAM)
- Benzodiazepine (anxiolytic, anticonvulsant)
- As positive allosteric modulators of GABA-A receptors, benzodiazepines (in the presence of GABA) increase the frequency of opening of the inhibitory chloride channels (although it does not increase the conductance of chloride across the individual channels or the time that the channel is open). This enhances the inhibitory effects of GABA.
- Inhibits neuronal activity presumably in amygdala-centered fear circuits to provide therapeutic benefits in anxiety disorders
- Inhibiting actions in the cerebral cortex may provide therapeutic benefits in seizure disorders

SAFETY AND TOLERABILITY

Notable Side Effects

- Sedation, fatigue, depression
- Dizziness, ataxia, slurred speech, weakness
- Forgetfulness, confusion
- Agitation and irritability
- Sialorrhea, dry mouth
- Rare hallucinations, mania
- Rare hypotension
- Pain at injection site

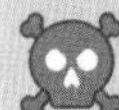

Life-Threatening or Dangerous Side Effects

- Respiratory depression, especially when taken with CNS depressants in overdose
- Rare hepatic dysfunction, renal dysfunction, blood dyscrasias

Growth and Maturation

- Not studied

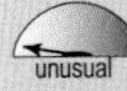

Weight Gain

- Reported but not expected

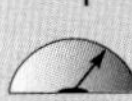

Sedation

- Many experience and/or can be significant in amount
- Especially at initiation of treatment or when dose increases
- Tolerance often develops over time

What to Do About Side Effects

- Wait
- Wait
- Wait
- Lower the dose
- Take largest dose at bedtime to avoid sedative effects during the day
- Switch to another agent
- Administer flumazenil if side effects are severe or life-threatening

How Drug Causes Side Effects

- Same mechanism for side effects as for therapeutic effects – namely due to excessive actions at benzodiazepine receptors
- Long-term adaptations in benzodiazepine receptors may explain the development of dependence, tolerance, and withdrawal

- Side effects are generally immediate, but immediate side effects often disappear in time

Warnings and Precautions

- Boxed warning regarding the increased risk of CNS depressant effects when benzodiazepines and opioid medications are used together, including specifically the risk of slowed or difficulty breathing and death
- If alternatives to the combined use of benzodiazepines and opioids are not available, clinicians should limit the dosage and duration of each drug to the minimum possible while still achieving therapeutic efficacy
- Patients and their caregivers should be warned to seek medical attention if unusual dizziness, lightheadedness, sedation, slowed or difficulty breathing, or unresponsiveness occur
- Dosage changes should be made in collaboration with prescriber
- Use with caution in patients with pulmonary disease; rare reports of death after initiation of benzodiazepines in patients with severe pulmonary impairment
- History of drug or alcohol abuse often creates greater risk for dependency
- Use oral formulation only with extreme caution if patient has obstructive sleep apnea; injection is contraindicated in patients with sleep apnea
- Some depressed patients may experience a worsening of suicidal ideation
- Some patients may exhibit abnormal thinking or behavioral changes similar to those caused by other CNS depressants (i.e., either depressant actions or disinhibiting actions)

When Not to Prescribe

- If patient has angle-closure glaucoma
- If patient has sleep apnea (injection)
- Must not be given intra-arterially because it may cause arteriospasm and result in gangrene
- If there is a proven allergy to lorazepam or any benzodiazepine

Long-Term Use

- Evidence of efficacy up to 16 weeks
- Risk of dependence, particularly for treatment periods longer than 12 weeks and especially in patients with past or current polysubstance abuse

Habit Forming

- Lorazepam is a Schedule IV drug
- Patients may develop dependence and/or tolerance with long-term use

Overdose

- Fatalities can occur; hypotension, tiredness, ataxia, confusion, coma

DOSING AND USE

Usual Dosage Range

- Oral: 1–4 mg/day in divided doses, largest dose at bedtime
- Injection: 1 mg administered slowly
- Catatonia: 1–2 mg per dose

Dosage Forms

- Tablet 0.5 mg, 1 mg, 2 mg
- Extended-release capsule 1 mg, 1.5 mg, 2 mg, 3 mg
- Oral concentrate 2 mg/mL
- Injection 2 mg/mL, 4 mg/mL

How to Dose

- Oral: initial 0.5–1 mg/day in 2–3 doses; increase as needed, starting with evening dose; maximum generally 6 mg/day. May convert to extended-release once dose is stable.
- Injection: initial 1–2 mg administered slowly; after 60 minutes may administer again
- Take liquid formulation with water, soda, applesauce, or pudding
- Catatonia: initial 1–2 mg; can repeat in 3 hours and then again in another 3 hours if necessary

Options for Administration

- Available in an oral liquid formulation

Tests

- In patients with seizure disorders, concomitant medical illness, and/or those with multiple concomitant long-term medications, periodic liver tests and blood counts may be prudent

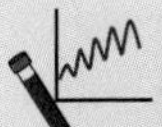

Pharmacokinetics

- After oral administration, lorazepam is rapidly and well absorbed from the gastrointestinal tract
- Peak plasma concentrations are generally reached within 2 hours, although this is longer with the extended-release formulation (not studied in children or adolescents). Also, mucosal atomization devices have been used to administer lorazepam in the pediatric acute care setting and may produce faster onset and faster peak concentrations than IM administration.
- In adults, extended-release lorazepam produces similar concentrations over time compared to tid dosing (Figure 1), which may be clinically helpful as some adverse effects of benzodiazepines are related to peak levels (i.e., Cmax)
- Food intake does not significantly affect the absorption of lorazepam
- Lorazepam is extensively distributed throughout the body, including the CNS
- Readily crosses the blood–brain barrier, leading to its sedative and anxiolytic effects
- Highly protein bound, primarily to albumin
- Lorazepam undergoes extensive hepatic metabolism, primarily via glucuronidation, and the major metabolite formed is lorazepam glucuronide, which is pharmacologically inactive
- The elimination half-life of lorazepam in children and adolescents ranges from approximately 10±2 hours and does not significantly differ from adults (Relling et al., 1989)

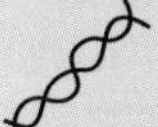

Pharmacogenetics

- No recommendations

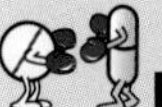

Drug Interactions

- Increased depressive effects when taken with other CNS depressants
- Valproate and probenecid may reduce clearance and raise plasma concentrations of lorazepam
- Flumazenil (used to reverse the effects of benzodiazepines) may precipitate seizures and should not be used in patients treated for seizure disorders with lorazepam

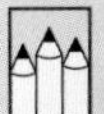

Dosing Tips

- For anxiety disorders, use lowest possible effective dose for the shortest possible period of time (a benzodiazepine sparing strategy). In adolescents, these medications

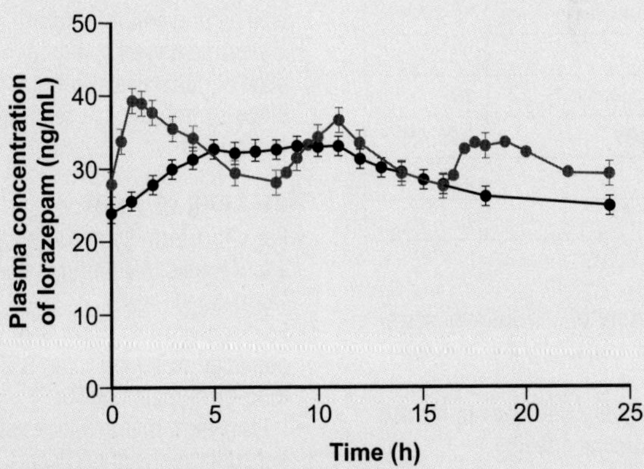

Figure 1 Concentration–time curve for immediate-release and extended-release lorazepam in adults. Source: Lorazepam ER package insert. Note: Cmax is lower with the extended-release formulation.

may be administered prior to some anxiety-producing situations and can help to facilitate returning to school in patients with school refusal.

- Assess need for continuous treatment regularly
- Risk of dependence may increase with dose and duration of treatment and with more lipophilic benzodiazepines (e.g., alprazolam)
- For interdose symptoms of anxiety, can either increase dose or maintain same daily dose but divide into more frequent doses
- One of the few benzodiazepines available in an oral liquid formulation
- One of the few benzodiazepines available in an injectable formulation
- Lorazepam injection is intended for acute use; patients who require long-term treatment should be switched to the oral formulation
- Because panic disorder can require doses higher than 6 mg/day, the risk of dependence may be greater in these patients
- Frequency of dosing in practice is often different than predicted from half-life, as duration for benzodiazepines is often related to redistribution (Stimpfl et al., 2023)

How to Switch

- Use the accompanying equivalence table to convert from the lorazepam dose to the dose of the new benzodiazepine

Approximate equivalent dosage (mg)	
Alprazolam (Xanax)	0.5
Chlordiazepoxide (Librium)	25
Clonazepam (Klonopin)	0.25–0.5
Diazepam (Valium)	5
Lorazepam (Ativan)	1

How to Stop

- Patients with history of seizure may seize upon withdrawal, especially if withdrawal is abrupt
- Taper by 0.5 mg every 5–7 days to reduce chances of withdrawal effects
- For difficult to taper cases, consider reducing dose much more slowly once reaching 3 mg/day, perhaps by as little as 0.25 mg per week or less
- Be sure to differentiate the reemergence of symptoms requiring reinstitution of treatment from withdrawal symptoms
- Benzodiazepine-dependent anxiety patients and insulin-dependent diabetics are not addicted to their medications. When benzodiazepine-dependent patients stop their medication, disease symptoms can reemerge, disease symptoms can worsen (rebound), and/or withdrawal symptoms can emerge.

WHAT TO EXPECT

Onset of Action

- Some immediate relief with first dosing is common; can take several weeks with daily dosing for maximal therapeutic benefit

Duration of Action

- Duration of action varies for benzodiazepines, including lorazepam, in pediatric patients, but is generally considered to be between 10 and 12 hours

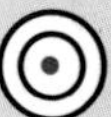

Primary Target Symptoms

- Panic attacks
- Anxiety
- Incidence of seizures (adjunct)

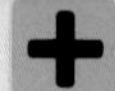

What Is Considered a Positive Result?

- The goal of treatment for anxiety is complete remission of current symptoms as well as prevention of future relapses
- If treatment works, it most often reduces or even eliminates symptoms, but is not a cure since symptoms can recur after medicine is stopped

How Long to Treat

- For short-term symptoms of anxiety – after a few weeks, discontinue use or use on an "as-needed" basis
- For long-term symptoms of anxiety, consider switching to an SSRI or SNRI for long-term maintenance
- If long-term maintenance with a benzodiazepine is necessary, continue treatment for 6 months after symptoms resolve, and then taper dose slowly

What If It Stops Working?

- If anxiety symptoms reemerge, consider an SSRI, and re-trying psychotherapeutic approaches

What If It Doesn't Work?

- Consider a trial of an SSRI
- When treating youth with anxiety disorders, many patients will have had significant anxiety for years prior to beginning treatment. As such, when anxiety is treated with lorazepam, their symptoms may be improved, but the patient has likely missed important developmental milestones (e.g., spending the night with friends, being able to ask questions in class). Developing these skills will take time. Beyond this, the family may have lived with the anxious child for years and following treatment of the child, the family may need to readjust.
- Be mindful of family conflict contributing to the presentation; sometimes treating parental depression or anxiety disorders improves psychiatric and social function without any treatment of youth. Also, accommodation is common in families of youth with anxiety disorders and may need to be addressed specifically, as it can perpetuate symptoms.

TALKING TO PATIENTS AND CAREGIVERS

What to Tell Parents About Efficacy

- While the medicine helps by reducing symptoms and improving function, it is not a cure, and it is therefore necessary to keep taking the medication to sustain its therapeutic effects
- Since every treatment consideration depends on a risk/benefit analysis, parents should fully understand short- and long-term risks as well as benefits
- Often a good idea to tell parents whether the medication chosen is specifically approved for the disorder being treated, or whether it is being given for "unapproved" or "off-label" reasons based on good clinical practice, expert consensus, and/or prudent extrapolation of controlled data from adults

What to Tell Children and Adolescents About Efficacy

- We are trying to make you feel better
- It may be a good idea to give the medication a try; if it's not working very well, we can stop the medication and try something else
- Medications don't change who you are as a person; they give you the opportunity to be the best person you can be

What to Tell Parents About Side Effects

- Explain that mild side effects are expected at initiation or when increasing the dose and are usually transitory
- Predict side effects in advance (you will look clever and competent to the parents, unless you scare them with too much information and cause nocebo effects, in which case you won't look so clever when the patient develops lots of side effects and stops medication; use your judgment here); a balanced but honest presentation is an art rather than a science
- Ask parents to support the patient while side effects are occurring
- Parents should fully understand short- and long-term risks as well as benefits
- Explaining to the parents what to expect from medication treatment, and especially potential side effects, can help prevent early termination of medication

What to Tell Children and Adolescents About Side Effects

- Even if you get side effects, most of them get better or go away in a few days to a few weeks; however, we will likely not use this medication for a long time
- Explaining to child/adolescent what to expect from medication treatment, and especially potential side effects, can help prevent early termination of medication

What to Tell Teachers About the Medication (If Parents Consent)

- Lorazepam can make children/adolescents sleepy and make it difficult for children or adolescents to pay attention. In these situations, it is important to notify the clinician so that the dose can be decreased
- Lorazepam may interfere with children's ability to engage in some activities at recess and in physical education class
- Encourage dialogue with parents/guardians about any behavior or mood changes

SPECIAL POPULATIONS

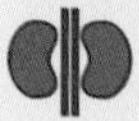

Renal Impairment

- 1–2 mg/day in 2–3 doses

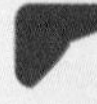

Hepatic Impairment

- 1–2 mg/day in 2–3 doses
- Because of its short half-life and inactive metabolites, lorazepam may be a preferred benzodiazepine in some patients with liver disease

Cardiac Impairment

- Rare reports of QTc prolongation in patients with underlying arrhythmia
- Lorazepam may be used as an adjunct during cardiovascular emergencies

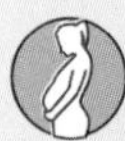

Pregnancy

- Possible increased risk of birth defects when benzodiazepines taken during pregnancy
- Because of the potential risks, lorazepam is not generally recommended as treatment for anxiety during pregnancy, especially during the first trimester
- Drug should be tapered if discontinued
- Infants whose mothers received a benzodiazepine late in pregnancy may experience withdrawal effects
- Neonatal flaccidity has been reported in infants whose mothers took a benzodiazepine during pregnancy
- Seizures, even mild seizures, may cause harm to the embryo/fetus

Breast Feeding

- Some drug is found in breast milk
- Recommended either to discontinue drug or formula feed
- Effects on infant have been observed and include feeding difficulties, sedation, and weight loss

THE ART OF PSYCHOPHARMACOLOGY

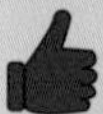

Potential Advantages

- Rapid onset of action
- Availability of oral liquid and injectable dosage formulations
- Can be used intranasally in the inpatient setting

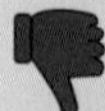

Potential Disadvantages

- Abuse especially risky in past or present substance users

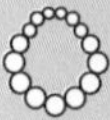

Pearls

- Despite trials of benzodiazepines in adults with anxiety disorders consistently demonstrating benefit, trials of benzodiazepines in pediatric patients have produced mixed results:
  - Small double-blind placebo-controlled trials and meta-analyses do not reveal differences between benzodiazepines and placebo for the management of anxiety disorders. However, these studies were small and included very young children and high doses of short-acting benzodiazepines (e.g., alprazolam).
  - By contrast, for acute anxiety in children and adolescents, a meta-analysis of nearly 1,500 patients suggests that benzodiazepines are more effective than placebo in treating acute anxiety; in this meta-analysis, there was no significant difference in the risk of developing irritability or behavioral changes between benzodiazepine and control groups (Kuang et al., 2017)
- In the pediatric benzodiazepine trials, the poor tolerability – particularly in younger patients – may relate to age-related pharmacodynamic factors (Strawn and Stahl, 2023)
- The pharmacodynamics of the GABA receptor in children and adolescents differ from adults, with adult expression/function not being achieved until ages 14–17½ years for subcortical regions and 18–22 years for cortical regions, although girls reach adult expression of GABA receptors slightly earlier than boys (Chugani et al., 2001)
- The neuropsychological effects of lorazepam have been evaluated in children

ages 3–14 years. In this study, lorazepam (0.03 mg/kg), did not affect long-term memory or attention but significantly decreased affective symptoms and anxiety. One-third of youth had a selective anterograde amnestic effect (Relling et al., 1989).

- In adults with anxiety disorders, benzodiazepines may be a very useful adjunct to SSRIs and SNRIs in the treatment of numerous anxiety disorders; however, the evidence for this is limited in children and adolescents
- May both cause depression and treat depression in different patients
- Clinical duration of action may be shorter than plasma half-life, leading to dosing more frequently than 2–3 times daily in some patients
- When using to treat insomnia, remember that insomnia may be a symptom of some other primary disorder itself, and thus warrant evaluation for comorbid psychiatric and/or medical conditions
- Though not systematically studied, benzodiazepines, and lorazepam in particular, have been used effectively to treat catatonia and are the initial recommended treatment
- Because of its short half-life and inactive metabolites, lorazepam may be preferred over some benzodiazepines for patients with liver disease
- Lorazepam may be preferred over other benzodiazepines for the treatment of delirium
- When treating delirium, lorazepam is often combined with haloperidol, with the haloperidol dose two times the lorazepam dose
- Lorazepam is often used to induce preoperative anterograde amnesia to assist in anesthesiology

SUGGESTED READING

Chugani DC, Muzik O, Juhász C et al. Postnatal maturation of human GABAA receptors measured with positron emission tomography. Ann Neurol 2001;49(5):618–26.

Kuang H, Johnson JA, Mulqueen JM, Bloch MH. The efficacy of benzodiazepines as acute anxiolytics in children: a meta-analysis. Depress Anxiety 2017;34(10):888–96.

Mathew SJ, Jean-Lys S, Phull R, Yarasani R. Characterization of extended-release lorazepam: pharmacokinetic results across phase 1 clinical studies. J Clin Psychopharmacol 2023;43(4):350–60.

Nicotra CM, Strawn JS. Advances in pharmacotherapy for pediatric anxiety disorders. Child Adolesc Psychiatr Clin N Am 2023;32(3):573–87.

Relling MV, Mulhern RK, Dodge RK et al. Lorazepam pharmacodynamics and pharmacokinetics in children. J Pediatr 1989;114(4 Pt 1):641–6.

Sidorchuk A, Isomura K, Molero Y et al. Benzodiazepine prescribing for children, adolescents, and young adults from 2006 through 2013: a total population register-linkage study. PLoS Med 2018;15(8):e1002635.

Stimpfl JN, Mills JA, Strawn JR. Pharmacologic predictors of benzodiazepine response trajectory in anxiety disorders: a Bayesian hierarchical modeling meta-analysis. CNS Spectr 2023;28(1):53–60.

Strawn JR, Lu L, Peris TS, Levine A, Walkup JT. Research review: pediatric anxiety disorders – what have we learnt in the last 10 years? J Child Psychol Psychiatry 2021;62(2):114–39.

Strawn JR, Stahl SM. Case Studies: Stahl's Essential Psychopharmacology: Volume 4: Children and Adolescents. New York: Cambridge University Press, 2023.

THERAPEUTICS

Brands

- Latuda

Generic

Yes

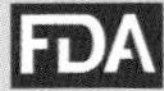

US FDA Approved for Pediatric Use

- Schizophrenia (ages 13 and older)
- Bipolar depression (ages 10 and older, monotherapy)

Off-Label for Pediatric Use

- Approved in adults
  - Bipolar depression (adjunct)
- Other off-label uses
  - Acute mania/mixed mania
  - Other psychotic disorders
  - Bipolar maintenance
  - Treatment-resistant depression
  - Behavioral disturbances in children and adolescents
  - Disorders associated with problems with impulse control
  - Unipolar and bipolar depression with mixed features

Class and Mechanism of Action

- Neuroscience-based Nomenclature: dopamine, serotonin receptor partial agonist (DS-RPA)
- Atypical antipsychotic (serotonin-dopamine antagonist; second generation antipsychotic; also a mood stabilizer)
- Blocks dopamine 2 receptors, reducing positive symptoms of psychosis and stabilizing affective symptoms
- Blockade of serotonin type 2A receptors may also contribute at clinical doses to the enhancement of dopamine release in certain brain regions, thus theoretically reducing motor side effects
- Interactions at a myriad of other neurotransmitter receptors may contribute to lurasidone's efficacy
- Potently blocks serotonin 7 receptors, which may be beneficial for mood, sleep, cognitive impairment, and negative symptoms in schizophrenia, and also in bipolar disorder and major depressive disorder
- Partial agonist at 5HT1A receptors, and antagonist actions at serotonin 7 and alpha 2A and alpha 2C receptors, which may be beneficial for mood, anxiety, and cognition in a number of disorders
- Lacks potent actions at dopamine D1, muscarinic M1, and histamine H1 receptors, theoretically suggesting less propensity for inducing cognitive impairment, weight gain, or sedation compared to other agents with these properties

SAFETY AND TOLERABILITY

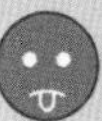

Notable Side Effects

- May increase risk for diabetes and dyslipidemia
- Dose-dependent sedation, dizziness
- Akathisia, extrapyramidal symptoms (EPS, also called drug-induced parkinsonism)
- Nausea, vomiting
- Hyperprolactinemia (in children and adolescents, serum prolactin levels tend to rise and peak within the first 1 to 2 months and then steadily decline to values within or very close to the normal range within 6 months)
- Risk of drug-induced parkinsonism and dystonic reactions may be higher in children than it is in adults
- Risk of withdrawal dyskinesias

Life-Threatening or Dangerous Side Effects

- Tachycardia, first-degree AV block
- Hyperglycemia, in some cases extreme and associated with ketoacidosis or hyperosmolar coma or death, has been reported in patients taking atypical antipsychotics
- Rare neuroleptic malignant syndrome (NMS) may cause hyperpyrexia, muscle rigidity, delirium, and autonomic instability with elevated creatine phosphokinase, myoglobinuria (rhabdomyolysis), and acute renal failure
- Rare seizures

Growth and Maturation

- Long-term effects are unknown

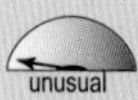

Weight Gain

- Little or no weight gain documented in long-term studies up to 2 years
- Appears to be less weight gain than observed with some antipsychotics

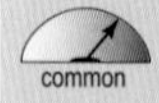

Sedation

- Some patients experience and/or can be significant in amount
- May be higher in short-term trials than in long-term use

What to Do About Side Effects

- Wait, wait, wait: mild side effects are common, happen early, and usually improve with time, but treatment benefits can be delayed
- Monitor side effects closely, especially when initiating treatment
- May wish to give at night if not tolerated during the day and doesn't disrupt sleep
- Often best to try another monotherapy trial of a different antipsychotic prior to resorting to augmentation strategies to treat side effects
- Exercise and diet programs and medical management for high BMI percentiles, diabetes, dyslipidemia. Also, randomized controlled trials in youth suggest that omega-3 fatty acids can reduce SGA-related hypertriglyceridemia.
- Reduce the dose, particularly for drug-induced parkinsonism, akathisia, sedation, and tremor
- For drug-induced parkinsonism: consider reducing dose or switching to another agent. Augmenting with diphenhydramine or benztropine is less preferred in youth.
- For akathisia: reduce the dose or add a beta blocker. If these are ineffective, raising the dose of the beta blocker may be helpful.
- Using a 5HT2A antagonist such as mirtazapine or cyproheptadine to treat drug-induced akathisia is less common in children and adolescents compared to adults

How Drug Causes Side Effects

- By blocking dopamine 2 receptors in the striatum, it can cause drug-induced parkinsonism, especially at high doses
- By blocking dopamine 2 receptors in the pituitary, it can cause elevations in prolactin
- Mechanism of any possible weight gain is unknown
- Mechanism of any possible increased incidence of diabetes or dyslipidemia is unknown

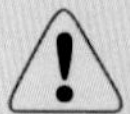

Warnings and Precautions

- Consider distributing brochures provided by the FDA and the drug companies or have the pharmacy do this for the parents
- When lurasidone is used to treat depressive mood disorders off-label in children, either as a monotherapy or an augmenting agent to an SSRI/SNRI, it is a good idea to warn patients and their caregivers about the possibility of activating side effects and suicidality as for any antidepressant in this age group and advise them to report such symptoms immediately
- Carefully weigh the risks and benefits of pharmacological treatment against the risks and benefits of nontreatment with an antipsychotic and it is a good idea to document this in the patient's chart
- Use with caution in patients with conditions that predispose to hypotension (dehydration, overheating)
- Atypical antipsychotics have the potential for cognitive and motor impairment, especially related to sedation
- Atypical antipsychotics can cause body temperature dysregulation; use caution in patients who may experience conditions that increase body temperature (e.g., strenuous exercise, saunas, extreme heat, dehydration, or concomitant anticholinergic medication)
- As with any antipsychotic, use with caution in patients with history of seizures

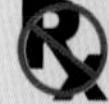

When Not to Prescribe

- If patient is taking a strong CYP3A4 inhibitor (e.g., ketoconazole) or inducer (e.g., rifampin)
- In patients with a history of angioedema
- If there is a proven allergy to lurasidone

Long-Term Use

- Should periodically reevaluate long-term usefulness in individual patients, but treatment may need to continue for many years

Habit Forming

- No

Overdose

- Limited data

DOSING AND USE

Usual Dosage Range

- 40–80 mg/day for schizophrenia
- 20–80 mg/day for bipolar depression

Dosage Forms

- Tablet 20 mg, 40 mg, 60 mg, 80 mg, 120 mg

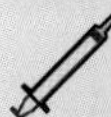

How to Dose

- Schizophrenia: initial 40 mg once daily with food; maximum recommended dose 80 mg/day; often a good idea to initiate at 20 mg to test for tolerability before raising dose to 40 mg, especially in children and in small body weight adolescents; can dose up to 160 mg/day for difficult cases if tolerated
- Bipolar depression: initial 20 mg once daily with food; can increase after 1 week; maximum recommended dose 80 mg/day

Options for Administration

- Oral tablet only option

Tests

- Before starting lurasidone:
  - Plan to monitor weight and metabolic parameters more closely than in adults since children and adolescents may be more prone to metabolic side effects than adults
  - Weigh all patients and monitor weight gain against that expected for normal growth, using the pediatric height/weight chart to monitor. In particular, monitor BMI percentiles.
  - Get baseline personal and family history of diabetes, obesity, dyslipidemia, hypertension, and cardiovascular disease
  - Obtain blood pressure, fasting plasma glucose (or hemoglobin A1C), and a lipid profile
- After starting lurasidone:
  - BMI percentile monthly for 3 months, then quarterly
  - Consider monitoring fasting triglycerides monthly in patients at high risk for metabolic complications
  - Blood pressure, fasting plasma glucose (or hemoglobin A1C), lipid profile within 3 months and then annually
  - Treat or refer for treatment and consider switching to another atypical antipsychotic for patients who become overweight, obese, pre-diabetic, diabetic, or dyslipidemic while receiving an atypical antipsychotic
  - Even in patients without known diabetes, be vigilant for the rare but life-threatening onset of diabetic ketoacidosis, which always requires immediate treatment, by monitoring for the rapid onset of polyuria, polydipsia, weight loss, nausea, vomiting, dehydration, rapid respiration, weakness, and clouding of sensorium, even coma
  - Patients with low white blood cell count (WBC) or history of drug-induced leukopenia/neutropenia should have complete blood count (CBC) monitored frequently during the first few months and lurasidone should be discontinued at the first sign of decline of WBC in the absence of other causative factors
  - Therapeutic drug levels not widely available for monitoring
  - Patients should be monitored periodically for the development of abnormal movements using neurological exam and the Abnormal Involuntary Movement Scale (AIMS)

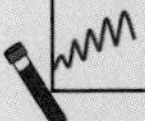

Pharmacokinetics

- Lurasidone is rapidly absorbed from the gastrointestinal tract. However, it undergoes significant first-pass metabolism, resulting in low oral bioavailability of approximately 9–19%. Administration with food increases its bioavailability, so it is generally recommended to take lurasidone with a meal.
- Lurasidone has a high protein binding of approximately 99% and primarily binds to albumin and α1-acid glycoprotein
- Lurasidone undergoes extensive hepatic metabolism, primarily via CYP3A4, with

minor contributions from CYP2D6 and CYP1A2
- In children and adolescents, peak concentrations are achieved within approximately 2 hours of oral administration (Figure 1) and the half-life is approximately 16–24 hours (Findling et al., 2015)
- In pediatric clinical trials (ages 10 to 17), the exposure of lurasidone was similar to that in adults, without adjusting for body weight

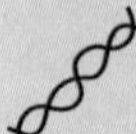

Pharmacogenetics

- No recommendations

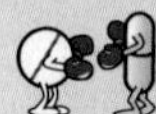

Drug Interactions

- Inhibitors of CYP3A4 (e.g., nefazodone, fluvoxamine, fluoxetine, ketoconazole) may increase plasma levels of lurasidone
- Coadministration of lurasidone with a strong CYP3A4 inhibitor (e.g., ketoconazole) or with a strong CYP3A4 inducer (e.g., rifampin) is contraindicated
- Coadministration of lurasidone with moderate CYP3A4 inhibitors can be considered; recommended starting dose is 20 mg/day; recommended maximum dose is 80 mg/day
- Moderate inducers of CYP3A4 may decrease plasma levels of lurasidone
- May increase effect of antihypertensive agents

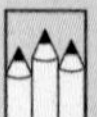

Dosing Tips

- Use lower starting dose in children and adolescents without prior exposure to antipsychotics, especially if not switching from another antipsychotic
- In patients who have no prior exposure to antipsychotics, there may be more nausea than in those who have been exposed
- Give lurasidone in most cases at night for best tolerability
- Lurasidone absorption can be decreased by up to 50% on an empty stomach, and more consistent efficacy will be seen if dosing is done regularly with food (i.e., at least a small meal of a minimum of 350 calories)
- Although generally dosed once daily, some children benefit from twice-daily dosing, mostly to improve tolerability
- For schizophrenia, the starting dose (40 mg/day) may be an adequate dose for some patients, especially first-episode and early-onset psychosis cases

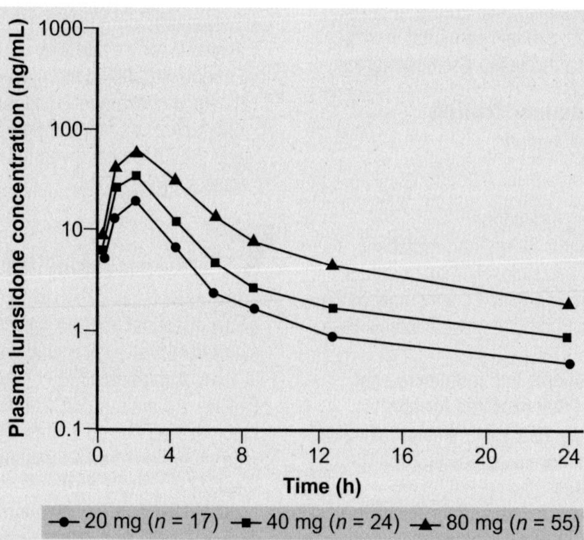

Figure 1 Mean lurasidone concentration over time in children and adolescents 30 minutes after a breakfast of at least 350 kcal. Adapted from Findling et al., Pharmacokinetics and Tolerability of Lurasidone in Children and Adolescents With Psychiatric Disorders. Clinical Therapeutics; 2015;37:2788–2797.

- Treatment should be suspended if absolute neutrophil count falls below 1,000/mm³
- Studies in adults show side effects less frequent when given at night than when given during the day

How to Switch

- From another antipsychotic to lurasidone:
  - When tapering a prior antipsychotic, see its entry in this manual for how to stop and how to taper off that specific drug
  - Generally, try to stop the first agent before starting lurasidone so that new side effects of lurasidone can be distinguished from withdrawal effects of the first agent
  - If urgent, cross taper off the other antipsychotic while lurasidone is started at a low dose, with dose adjustments down of the other antipsychotic, and up for lurasidone every 3 to 7 days
- Off lurasidone to another antipsychotic:
  - Generally, try to stop lurasidone before starting the new antipsychotic so that new side effects of the next drug can be distinguished from any withdrawal effects from lurasidone
  - If urgent, cross taper off lurasidone by cutting the dose in half as the new antipsychotic is also started with dose adjustments down of lurasidone and up for the new antipsychotic

How to Stop

- Slow down-titration of oral formulation (over 6–8 weeks), especially when simultaneously beginning a new antipsychotic while switching (i.e., cross-titration)
- Make down-titration even slower if any signs of anticholinergic rebound such as tachycardia, tremor, gastrointestinal symptoms
- Rapid oral discontinuation may lead to withdrawal dyskinesias, which are generally reversible in the pediatric population. Of note, withdrawal dyskinesias are more common in pediatric patients than in adults.
- If antiparkinsonian agents are being used, they should be continued for a few weeks after lurasidone is discontinued

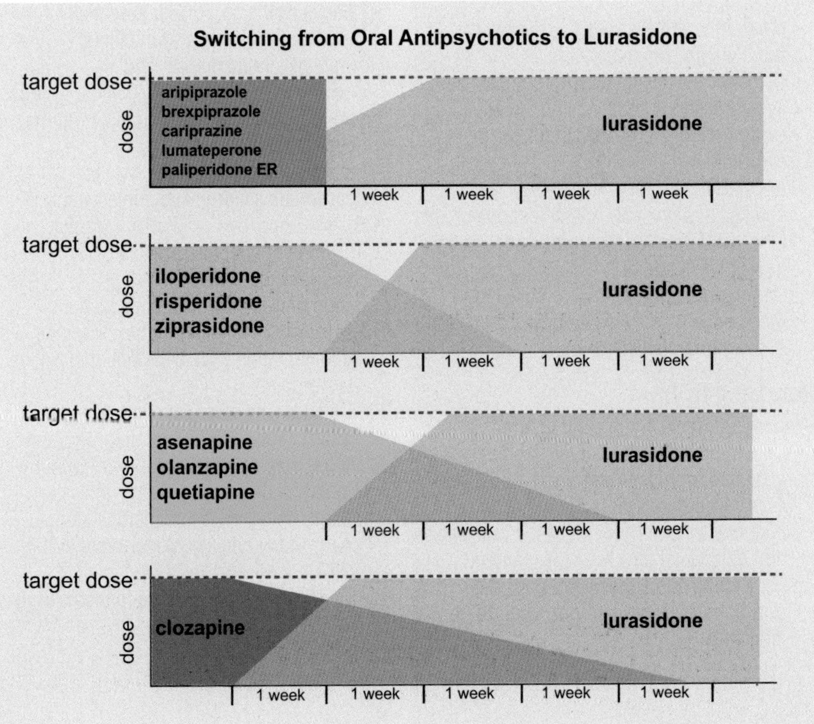

WHAT TO EXPECT

Onset of Action

- Psychotic and manic symptoms can improve within 1 week, but it may take several weeks for full effect on behavior as well as on cognition and affective stabilization
- If it is not working within 6–8 weeks, it may require a dosage increase or it may not work at all

Duration of Action

- Effects are consistent over a 24-hour period
- Oral medication may continue to work for many years to prevent relapse of symptoms

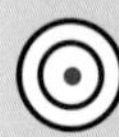

Primary Target Symptoms

- Positive symptoms of psychosis
- Negative symptoms of psychosis
- Cognitive symptoms
- Unstable mood and depression
- Aggressive symptoms

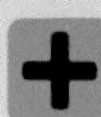

What Is Considered a Positive Result?

- In schizophrenia:
  - Most often reduces positive symptoms but does not eliminate them
  - Can improve negative symptoms, as well as aggressive, cognitive, and affective symptoms but less so than for positive symptoms
  - In children or adolescents with a first episode of psychosis, initial response may be greater than for recurrent episodes of psychosis in adults
- In bipolar disorder:
  - Many patients may experience a reduction of symptoms by half or more

How Long to Treat

- In schizophrenia and bipolar disorder:
  - Continue treatment until reaching a plateau of improvement
  - After reaching a satisfactory plateau, continue treatment for at least a year after first episode of psychosis or mania
  - For second and subsequent episodes of psychosis, treatment may need to be indefinite

What If It Stops Working?

- Check for nonadherence, possibly by checking plasma drug level, and consider switching to another antipsychotic with fewer side effects
- Some patients who have an initial response may relapse even though they continue treatment, sometimes called "poop-out"
- Growth/developmental changes may contribute to apparent loss of efficacy as well as to new onset of side effects as metabolism slows and drug levels rise in transition from childhood to adolescence; dose adjustment (increase or decrease) should be considered
- Screen for the development of a new comorbid disorder, especially substance use
- Screen for adverse changes in the home or school environment

What If It Doesn't Work?

- Consider evaluation for another diagnosis (especially bipolar illness or depression with mixed features) or for a comorbid condition (e.g., medical illness, substance use)
- Consider other important potential factors such as ongoing conflicts, family psychopathology, and an adverse environment (e.g., poverty, chaos, violence, prior and ongoing psychological trauma, abuse, neglect)
- Institute trauma-informed care for appropriate children and adolescents
- For schizophrenia or bipolar disorder:
  - Try one of the other atypical antipsychotics
  - If no first-line atypical antipsychotic is effective, consider higher doses or augmentation with valproate, lithium, or lamotrigine
  - Consider initiating psychotherapy. In adolescents with bipolar disorder (and those with affective symptoms who are at risk of developing bipolar disorder), family-focused psychotherapy can be particularly helpful (Miklowitz et al., 2020).
  - Consider presence of concomitant drug abuse

TALKING TO PATIENTS AND CAREGIVERS

What to Tell Parents About Efficacy

- For acute symptoms, it can work right away
- Lurasidone is usually given every day
- Explain which use lurasidone is being chosen for, how to tell if the drug is working by targeting specific symptoms, and why this is being done
- Once the child/adolescent calms down, at some point after one dose or after several days of dosing or after long-term dosing, we should all assess whether the medication should be continued
- While the medicine helps by reducing symptoms and improving function, it is not a cure, and it therefore may be necessary to keep taking the medication long term to sustain its therapeutic effects
- Since every treatment consideration depends on a risk/benefit analysis, parents should fully understand short- and long-term risks as well as benefits
- Often a good idea to tell parents whether the medication chosen is specifically approved for the disorder being treated, or whether it is being given for "unapproved" or "off-label" reasons based on good clinical practice, expert consensus, and/or prudent extrapolation of controlled data from adults

What to Tell Children and Adolescents About Efficacy

- Be specific about the symptoms being targeted: we are trying to help you …
- Give the medication a try; if it's not working very well, we can stop the medication and try something else
- A good try often takes many months
- If it does make you feel better, you cannot stop it right away or you may get sick again
- Medications don't change who you are as a person; they give you the opportunity to be the best person you can be

What to Tell Parents About Side Effects

- Explain that side effects are expected in many when starting
- Tell parents many side effects go away and do so about the same time that therapeutic effects start
- Predict side effects in advance (you will look clever and competent to the parents, unless you scare them with too much information and cause nocebo effects, in which case you won't look so clever when the patient develops lots of side effects and stops medication; use your judgment here); a balanced but honest presentation is an art rather than a science
- Ask parents to support the patient while side effects are occurring
- Parents should fully understand short- and long-term risks as well as benefits
- Explaining to the parents what to expect from medication treatment, and especially what potential side effects to expect, can help prevent early termination of medication

What to Tell Children and Adolescents About Side Effects

- Even if you get side effects, most of them get better or go away in a few weeks
- If you have side effects that are bothering you, tell your parents and your parents should tell me
- Consider having a conversation about sexual side effects in some adolescents who can find these side effects confusing and especially burdensome
- Explaining to child/adolescent what to expect from medication treatment, and especially potential side effects, can help prevent early termination of medication

What to Tell Teachers About the Medication (If Parents Consent)

- Lurasidone can make children/adolescents sedated
- Lurasidone can cause nausea
- It is not abusable
- Encourage dialogue with parents/guardians about any behavior or mood changes
- Notify the clinician of increased restlessness or akathisia symptoms, which may be apparent in the school setting

SPECIAL POPULATIONS

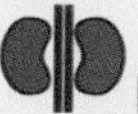

Renal Impairment

- In adults, moderate and severe impairment: initial 20 mg/day; maximum dose 80 mg/day
- Possibly reduce these doses by half in children and adolescents

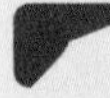

Hepatic Impairment

- In adults, moderate impairment: initial 20 mg/day; maximum dose 80 mg/day
- In adults, severe impairment: initial 20 mg/day; maximum dose 40 mg/day
- Possibly reduce these doses by half in children and adolescents

Cardiac Impairment

- Use in patients with cardiac impairment has not been studied; however, the risk of orthostatic hypotension in pediatric patients is less than in adults, as children rely less on peripheral vasoconstriction to regulate blood pressure
- Lurasidone is one of the few antipsychotics that does not have a warning for QTc prolongation

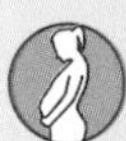

Pregnancy

- Controlled studies have not been conducted in pregnant women
- There is a risk of abnormal muscle movements and withdrawal symptoms in newborns whose mothers took an antipsychotic during the third trimester; symptoms may include agitation, abnormally increased or decreased muscle tone, tremor, sleepiness, severe difficulty breathing, and difficulty feeding
- Animal studies do not show adverse effects; not teratogenic in rats and rabbits at doses up to 1.5–6 times the maximum recommended human dose
- Psychotic symptoms may worsen during pregnancy, and some form of treatment may be necessary
- Lurasidone may be preferable to anticonvulsant mood stabilizers if treatment is required during pregnancy
- National Pregnancy Registry for Atypical Antipsychotics: 1-866-961-2388 or http://womensmentalhealth.org/clinical-and-research-programs/pregnancyregistry/

Breast Feeding

- Unknown if lurasidone is secreted in human breast milk, but all psychotropics assumed to be secreted in breast milk
- Recommended either to discontinue drug or formula feed
- Infants of women who choose to breast feed while on lurasidone should be monitored for possible adverse effects; sedation, failure to thrive, jitteriness, tremor, and abnormal muscle movements have been reported

THE ART OF PSYCHOPHARMACOLOGY

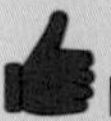

Potential Advantages

- In children:
  - Approved for bipolar depression (ages 10 and older)
- In adolescents:
  - Approved for schizophrenia
  - Approved for bipolar depression
- All ages:
  - Patients requiring rapid onset of antipsychotic action without dosage titration
  - Off-label for those who may possibly have major depressive episodes with mixed features off-label, especially those with these features and a family history of bipolar disorder
  - Major depressive episodes with mixed features may be even more common in adolescents than in adults
  - Patients concerned about gaining weight
  - Patients with diabetes mellitus, obesity, and/or dyslipidemia

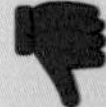

Potential Disadvantages

- In children and adolescents:
  - May be more susceptible to side effects
  - Efficacy was not demonstrated in a 6-week study evaluating lurasidone for the treatment of irritability in autism in children ages 6–17
- All ages:
  - Patients who cannot take a medication consistently with food

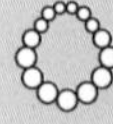

Pearls

- One of the few "metabolically friendly" antipsychotics, with clinical trials suggesting a lack of weight gain and neutral effects on lipids and glucose in both adults and adolescents
- Only atypical antipsychotic documented not to cause QTc prolongation, and one of the

few atypical antipsychotics without a QTc warning
- Somnolence and akathisia are the most common side effects in short-term clinical trials of schizophrenia that dosed lurasidone in the daytime, but these adverse effects were reduced in an adult controlled study of lurasidone administered at night with food
- Nausea and occasional vomiting occurred in bipolar depression studies especially at higher doses
- Nausea and vomiting generally rapidly abates within a few days or can be avoided by slow dose titration and giving lower doses
- Prolactin elevations low and generally transient
- Agitation experienced by some patients
- Receptor binding profile suggests favorable potential as an antidepressant
- 5HT7 antagonism is antidepressant in animal models and has pro-cognitive actions in animal models
- 5HT7 antagonism and 5HT1A partial agonism enhance serotonin levels in animals treated with SSRIs/SNRIs, suggesting use for lurasidone as an augmenting agent to SSRIs/SNRIs in depression
- 5HT7 antagonism plus the absence of D1, H1, and M1 antagonism suggest potential for cognitive improvement
- Lack of D1 antagonist, anticholinergic, and antihistamine properties may explain relative lack of cognitive side effects in most patients
- In pediatric trials of bipolar depression, meta-analyses suggest that lurasidone and olanzapine fluoxetine combination (OFC), but not quetiapine, were efficacious for the treatment of bipolar depression compared to placebo. However, lurasidone was associated with less weight gain and smaller impacts on cholesterol and triglycerides compared with quetiapine and OFC (DelBello et al., 2021)
- Recent post-hoc analyses suggest that in children and adolescents, lurasidone may improve mixed (subsyndromal hypomanic) features (Singh et al., 2020)
- Not approved for mania, but almost all atypical antipsychotics approved for acute treatment of schizophrenia have proven effective in the acute treatment of mania as well

SUGGESTED READING

DelBello MP, Goldman R, Phillips D et al. Efficacy and safety of lurasidone in children and adolescents with bipolar I depression: a double-blind, placebo-controlled study. J Am Acad Child Adolesc Psychiatry 2017;56(12):1015–25.

DelBello MP, Tocco M, Pikalov A, Deng L, Goldman R. Tolerability, safety, and effectiveness of two years of treatment with lurasidone in children and adolescents with bipolar depression. J Child Adolesc Psychopharmacol 2021;31(7):494–503.

DelBello MP, Kadakia A, Heller V et al. Systematic review and network meta-analysis: efficacy and safety of second-generation antipsychotics in youths with bipolar depression. J Am Acad Child Adolesc Psychiatry 2022;61(2):243–54.

Findling RL, Goldman R, Chiu YY et al. Pharmacokinetics and tolerability of lurasidone in children and adolescents with psychiatric disorders. Clin Ther 2015;37(12):2788–97.

Goldman R, Loebel A, Cucchiaro J, Deng L, Findling RL. Efficacy and safety of lurasidone in adolescents with schizophrenia: a 6-weeks, randomized placebo-controlled study. J Child Adolesc Psychopharmacol 2017;27(6):516–25.

Loebel A, Brams M, Goldman RS et al. Lurasidone for the treatment of irritability associated with autistic disorder. J Autism Dev Disord 2016;46(4):1153–63.

McQuire C, Hassiotis A, Harrison B, Pilling S. Pharmacological interventions for challenging behaviour in children with intellectual disabilities: a systematic review and meta-analysis. BMS Psychiatry 2015;15:303.

Miklowitz DJ, Schneck CD, Walshaw PD et al. Effects of family-focused therapy vs enhanced usual care for symptomatic youths at high risk for bipolar disorder: a randomized clinical trial. JAMA Psychiatry 2020;77(5):455–63.

Pillay J, Boylan K, Carrey N et al. First- and Second-Generation Antipsychotics in Children and Young Adults: Systematic Review Update [Internet]. Rockville, MD: Agency for Healthcare Research and Quality (US); 2017 Mar. Report No.: 17-EHC001-EF. AHRQ Comparative Effectiveness Reviews.

Singh MK, Pikalov A, Siu C, Tocco M, Loebel A. Lurasidone in children and adolescents with bipolar depression presenting with mixed (subsyndromal hypomanic) features: *post hoc* analysis of a randomized placebo-controlled trial. J Child Adolesc Psychopharmacol 2020;30(10):590–8.

THERAPEUTICS

Brands

- Focalin
- Focalin XR

Generic

Yes

US FDA Approved for Pediatric Use

- Attention deficit hyperactivity disorder (Focalin, ages 6–17)
- Attention deficit hyperactivity disorder (Focalin XR, ages 6 and older)

Off-Label for Pediatric Use

- Approved in adults
  - None
- Other off-label uses
  - Narcolepsy
  - Treatment-resistant depression (rarely used for this in children)
  - Stimulants are sometimes used to augment antidepressants
  - Stimulants also sometimes used to treat amotivational or lethargic states in the elderly with dementia but rarely in children for these symptoms

Class and Mechanism of Action

- Neuroscience-based Nomenclature: dopamine, norepinephrine multimodal
- Stimulant
- Increases norepinephrine and especially dopamine actions by blocking their reuptake
- Enhancement of dopamine and norepinephrine actions in certain brain regions (e.g., dorsolateral prefrontal cortex) may improve attention, concentration, executive dysfunction, wakefulness, and cortical inhibitory control of striatum (i.e., theoretically "tunes" inefficient information processing in cortical–striatal pathways, improving "top-down" regulation of striatal and other subcortical drives)
- Enhancement of dopamine actions in other brain regions (e.g., basal ganglia) may decrease hyperactivity
- Enhancement of dopamine and norepinephrine in yet other brain regions (e.g., medial prefrontal cortex, hypothalamus) may improve depressive symptoms as well as nondepression-associated fatigue and sleepiness
- Hypothetically rebalances signal to noise ratios of cortical neurons: enhances focus on importance tasks (signal), theoretically due to norepinephrine, and reduces awareness of background activity (noise), theoretically due to dopamine

SAFETY AND TOLERABILITY

Notable Side Effects

- Anorexia and weight loss
- Nausea, abdominal pain
- Insomnia, headache, exacerbation of tics, tremor, dizziness, and possible irritability and anxiety. The risk of treatment-emergent irritability is lower with methylphenidate-based stimulants compared to amphetamine-based stimulants.
- Peripheral vasculopathy, including Raynaud's phenomenon

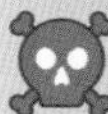

Life-Threatening or Dangerous Side Effects

- Psychosis
- Seizures
- Palpitations, tachycardia, hypertension
- Rare hypomania, mania, or suicidal ideation
- Cardiovascular adverse effects, death in patients with preexisting cardiac structural abnormalities often associated with a family history of cardiac disease

Growth and Maturation

- May temporarily slow normal growth in children (controversial): Multimodal Treatment of ADHD (MTA) study showed children/adolescents grew more slowly but eventually reached their expected adult height
- Controversy exists because theoretically stimulants might suppress appetite and reduce caloric intake, which could affect potential growth; also, dopaminergic actions of stimulants might suppress growth hormone secretion and affect height development. However, expected adult height is likely attained with a delay if stimulants are continued, and slowing of growth is likely reversible with withdrawal of treatment.

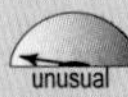

Weight Gain

- Patients may experience weight loss
- Weight gain is reported but not expected, rarely seen, controversial

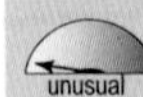

Sedation

- Activation much more common than sedation
- Sedation is reported but not expected, rarely seen, controversial

What to Do About Side Effects

- Wait, wait, wait: mild side effects are common, happen early, and usually improve with time, but treatment benefits can be delayed and often begin just as the side effects wear off
- Adjust dose
- Switch to a formulation of D,L-methylphenidate
- Switch to another agent
- For insomnia: avoid dosing in the midday, late afternoon, or evening
- However, insomnia is not always due to medication, but can be the result of relapse, rebound, and withdrawal effects from the daily dose, and in fact improves with additional late-day dosing of a short-acting stimulant
- Use beta blockers for peripheral autonomic side effects
- Often best to try another monotherapy prior to resorting to augmentation strategies to treat side effects, with the exception of an early-evening dose of a stimulant
- Monitor side effects closely, especially when initiating treatment
- For persistent insomnia: consider adding melatonin, or an alpha 2 agonist
- For loss of appetite or loss of weight:
  - Give medication after breakfast
  - Switch to a nonstimulant
  - Eat a high-protein, high-carbohydrate breakfast prior to taking medication or within 10–15 minutes of ingesting medication; snack on high-protein, densely caloric foods throughout the school day and after school; eat dinner and then a second dinner or very heavy snack at bedtime
  - Add "liquid calories" (i.e., smoothies made with whole milk or ice cream, fruit, and protein powder; Boost or Ensure shakes)
  - Introduce "fourth meal" in the evening
  - Add cyproheptadine

How Drug Causes Side Effects

- Increases in norepinephrine peripherally can cause autonomic side effects, including tremor, tachycardia, hypertension, and cardiac arrhythmias
- Increases in norepinephrine and dopamine centrally can cause CNS side effects such as insomnia, agitation, psychosis (rarely)

Warnings and Precautions

- In children and adolescents:
  - Safety and efficacy not established in children under age 6
  - Use in young children should be reserved for the expert
  - Children who are not growing or gaining weight should stop treatment, at least temporarily
  - Usual dosing has been associated with sudden death in children with structural cardiac abnormalities
  - Consider distributing brochures provided by the FDA and the drug companies
- All ages:
  - Stimulants used to treat ADHD are associated with peripheral vasculopathy, including Raynaud's phenomenon; careful observation for digital changes is necessary during treatment with ADHD stimulants
  - Carefully weigh the risks and benefits of pharmacological treatment against the risks and benefits of nonpharmacological treatment and it is a good idea to document this in the patient's chart
  - Use with caution in patients with any degree of hypertension, hyperthyroidism, or history of drug abuse
  - Many believe tics may be worsened by stimulants, but evidence does not support this association. A meta-analysis of 22 studies, including 2,385 individuals in treatment, found that the rate of new onset or worsening tics was 5.7% for those on stimulants versus 6.5% with placebo. In this analysis, there was no effect for type of stimulant, dose, duration of treatment, or age (Cohen et al., 2015).

The presence of tics is not an absolute contraindication to use of stimulants.
- May worsen symptoms of thought disorder and behavioral disturbance in psychotic patients
- Stimulants have a high potential for abuse and must be used with caution in anyone with a current or past history of substance abuse or alcoholism, but stimulants for ADHD are less likely to be abused in terms of getting "high" and more likely to be used to stay awake, especially by college students. This misuse is the most common reason for diversion of prescription stimulants.
- Youth are neither more nor less likely to develop alcohol and substance use disorders as a result of being treated with stimulant medication. In fact, current data suggest that treating ADHD in children and adolescents decreases the likelihood of developing a substance use disorder.
- Adolescents and/or college students may divert/sell their medication to others for use in staying awake to study at the last minute, or to abuse; longer-acting preparations are harder to abuse than shorter-acting, immediate-release stimulants
- Particular attention should be paid to the possibility of adolescents you are seeing for the first time feigning ADHD in order to obtain stimulants for nontherapeutic use or distribution to others; the drugs should in general be prescribed sparingly with documentation of appropriate use, and if there is any doubt about the accuracy of their complaints, refer them for psychological-educational or neuropsychological testing
- Not an appropriate first-line treatment for depression or for normal fatigue
- May lower the seizure threshold; as long as seizures are well controlled, it is generally safe to use stimulants
- Emergence or worsening of activation and agitation may represent the induction of a bipolar state, especially a mixed dysphoric bipolar II condition sometimes associated with suicidal ideation, and may require the addition of lithium or an atypical antipsychotic, and/or discontinuation of D-methylphenidate

When Not to Prescribe

- Treating ADHD comorbid with tics or Tourette syndrome is not contraindicated, but may be for the expert
- Patients with ADHD who are comorbid for motor or vocal tics of Tourette syndrome, or even with just a family history of Tourette syndrome, may experience worsening/ onset of tics with stimulant treatment (controversial). Decision to use stimulants in such cases should weigh the potential benefits for ADHD against the risks of worsening tics, and may require expert referral or consultation.
- Should generally not be administered with an MAOI, including within 14 days of MAOI use, except in heroic circumstances and by an expert
- If patient has glaucoma
- If patient has structural cardiac abnormalities
- If there is a proven allergy to methylphenidate
- If the patient has an eating disorder other than binge-eating disorder, be very cautious

Long-Term Use

- Often used long-term for ADHD when ongoing monitoring documents continued efficacy
- Tolerance to therapeutic effects may develop in some patients
- Weight and height should be monitored during long-term treatment
- Periodic monitoring of blood pressure and heart rate

Habit Forming

- Paradoxically, stimulant abuse appears to be less likely in patients with ADHD than in those who do not have ADHD. In 2023, the FDA modified a boxed warning for stimulant medications, although they noted, "Our review found that nonmedical use has remained relatively stable over the past two decades, despite the increasing number of prescription stimulants dispensed." The new warning notes that stimulants have a "high potential for abuse and misuse, which can lead to the development of a substance use disorder, including addiction." The new warning also notes that stimulant medications "can be diverted

for non-medical use into illicit channels or distribution." They recommend:
  - Counsel patients not to give any of their medicine to anyone else
  - Monitor for signs and symptoms of diversion, such as requesting refills more frequently than needed
  - Regularly assess and monitor for signs and symptoms of nonmedical use and addiction
  - Keep careful records of prescribing information, including quantity, frequency, and renewal requests, as required by state and federal laws
- Stimulant abuse in ADHD patients more likely if there is a preexisting history of alcohol/drug abuse
- Tolerance to stimulants is surprisingly rare in ADHD; tolerance should not be confused with reduction of therapeutic effects over time due to growth: as youth grow, dose usually must be increased; otherwise, the appearance of tolerance occurs when this in reality is underdosing
- Misuse may be more likely with immediate-release stimulants than with controlled-release stimulants

Overdose

- Vomiting, tremor, coma, convulsion, hyperreflexia, euphoria, confusion, hallucination, tachycardia, flushing, palpitations, sweating, hyperpyrexia, hypertension, arrhythmia, mydriasis, agitation, delirium, headache

DOSING AND USE

Usual Dosage Range

- ADHD: 2.5–10 mg twice per day
- Extended-release: up to 30 mg once per day

Dosage Forms

- Immediate-release tablet 2.5 mg, 5 mg, 10 mg
- Extended-release capsule 5 mg, 10 mg, 15 mg, 20 mg, 25 mg, 30 mg, 35 mg, 40 mg

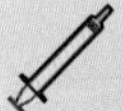

How to Dose

- Immediate-release (for patients who are not taking racemic D,L-methylphenidate): initial 2.5 mg twice per day in 4-hour intervals; may adjust dose in weekly intervals by 2.5–5 mg/day; maximum dose generally 10 mg twice per day
- Extended-release (for patients who are not taking racemic D,L-methylphenidate): initial 5 mg/day in the morning; may adjust dose in weekly intervals by 5 mg/day; maximum dose 30 mg/day. Some patients may ultimately require bid dosing of extended-release formulations.
- For patients already using methylphenidate, initiate treatment at half the current total daily dose of methylphenidate

Options for Administration

- Extended-release capsule may have sufficient duration of action to eliminate the need for lunchtime dosing

Tests

- Before treatment, assess for presence of cardiac disease (history, family history, physical exam); consider whether electrocardiogram (ECG) is indicated
- Blood pressure and heart rate should be monitored regularly, sitting and standing
- Monitor weight and height
- Periodic complete blood cell and platelet counts may be considered during prolonged therapy (rare leukopenia and/or anemia)
- Current recommendations from the American Heart Association (AHA) are that it is reasonable but not mandatory to obtain an ECG prior to prescribing a stimulant to a child; the American Academy of Pediatrics (AAP) does not recommend an ECG prior to starting a stimulant for most children
- Document basic sleep patterns prior to starting a stimulant
- When necessary to rule out sleep apnea, nocturnal movements, or daytime sleepiness that may later be difficult to distinguish from side effects of stimulants, consider (rarely) a sleep study/ polysomnogram (e.g., obese adolescents)

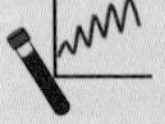

Pharmacokinetics

- D-threo-enantiomer of racemic D,L-methylphenidate
- Mean plasma elimination half-life approximately 2.2 hours (same as D,L-methylphenidate)
- Does not inhibit CYP450 enzymes

- Taking with food may delay peak actions for 2–3 hours
- Dexmethylphenidate plasma concentrations increase rapidly with immediate-release formulations (open circles in Figure 1) and the extended-release formulation mirrors the release properties of two doses of immediate-release dexmethylphenidate

Pharmacogenetics

- Methylphenidate is not metabolized by CYP450 isoenzymes to a clinically relevant extent and therefore there are no pharmacogenetic recommendations related to methylphenidate based on pharmacokinetic genes. Additionally, there are no recommendations related to pharmacodynamic genes and stimulant selection.

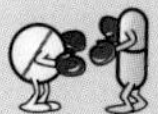

Drug Interactions

- May affect blood pressure and should be used cautiously with agents used to control blood pressure
- Methylphenidate is metabolized by carboxylesterase 1 and is not a substrate or inhibitor of the CYP450 drug-metabolizing system
- Most drug interactions are pharmacodynamic rather than pharmacokinetic
- CNS and cardiovascular actions of D-methylphenidate could theoretically be enhanced by combination with agents that block norepinephrine reuptake, such as the tricyclic antidepressants desipramine or protriptyline, venlafaxine, duloxetine, atomoxetine, milnacipran, and reboxetine
- Theoretically, D-methylphenidate could inhibit the antipsychotic actions of antipsychotics
- Theoretically, D-methylphenidate could inhibit the mood-stabilizing actions of atypical antipsychotics in some patients; however, stimulants can be safely combined with atypical antipsychotics by experts
- Combinations of D-methylphenidate with mood stabilizers (lithium, anticonvulsants, atypical antipsychotics) are generally something for experts only when monitoring patients closely and when other options fail
- Antacids or acid suppressants could alter the release of extended-release formulation
- Use with MAOIs, including within 14 days of MAOI use, is not advised, but this can sometimes be considered by experts who

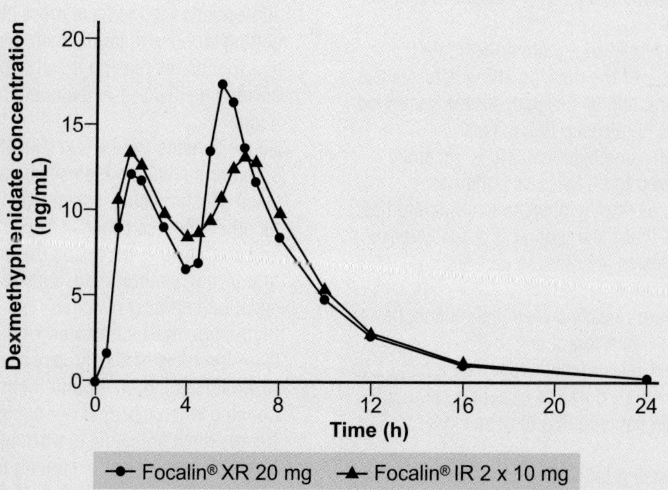

Figure 1 Mean dexmethylphenidate plasma concentration–time profiles. Adapted from the Focalin package insert.

monitor depressed patients closely when other treatment options for depression fail

Dosing Tips

- Plasma levels are higher in lower-weight children; therefore, starting and target doses may be lower and longer intervals between dose increases may be needed (see How to Dose)
- The extended-release formulation can eliminate the hassle and pragmatic difficulties of lunchtime dosing at school, including storage problems, potential diversion, and the need for a medical professional to supervise dosing away from home
- If there are concerns about diversion or abuse, longer-acting stimulant preparations are much harder to abuse than immediate-release preparations
- Be aware that metabolism (and absorption) changes during puberty and entry into adolescence and becomes more like adults (i.e., slower than in children)
- If a child on a stable dose begins to lose tolerability with more side effects upon entering adolescence, this may signal the need for a dose reduction due to changing metabolism
- Immediate-release D-methylphenidate has the same onset of action and duration of action as immediate-release racemic D,L-methylphenidate (i.e., 2–4 hours) but at half the dose
- Extended-release D-methylphenidate contains half the dose as immediate-release beads and half as delayed-release beads, so the dose is released in 2 pulses
- Although D-methylphenidate is generally considered to be twice as potent as racemic D,L-methylphenidate, some studies suggest that the D-isomer is actually more than twice as effective as racemic D,L-methylphenidate
- Immediate-release D-methylphenidate has a 4–6-hour duration of action
- Extended-release methylphenidate has up to an 8–10-hour duration of action, although for some patients this may be closer to 6 hours
- Avoid dosing late in the day because of the risk of insomnia
- Off-label uses are dosed the same as for ADHD
- Side effects are generally dose related

Drug Holidays

- Drug holidays were originally done in an attempt to avoid the possibility that stimulants may blunt height
- May be able to give drug holidays over the summer in order to reassess therapeutic utility and effects on growth and theoretically to allow catch-up from any growth suppression and assess any other side effects and the need to reinstitute stimulant treatment for the next school term
- However, most studies show that parental height is what determines a patient's final height, and that most children/adolescents taking stimulants reach their expected height, just more slowly than children/adolescents not exposed to stimulants
- May be possible to give weekend drug holidays and dose only during the school week for some ADHD patients, but there are risks as well:
  - Hyperactivity and impulsivity increase the chances of accidents (i.e., broken bones and head injuries) and illicit alcohol and drug abuse
  - Studies have shown that adolescents with ADHD who drive vehicles without their stimulants are much more likely to get into motor vehicle accidents and that the severity of the accident is much greater than would be expected
  - Hyperactive and impulsive children/adolescents tend to have more difficulties getting along with family members and friends, increasing the chances of developing low self-esteem and poor self-image
  - Social benefits can be lost over the summer if children/adolescents are taken off stimulants; social rejection by other children can lead to isolation and depression, increasing the chances of bullying, victimization, and further isolation and peer rejection
  - Inattention makes it harder for kids to learn the rules of life and pay attention to what is going on around them (e.g., noticing when a peer is not being a true friend, when someone is starting to get annoyed, when a car is coming toward you and you're in the middle of the street)

How to Switch

- When switching from one stimulant to another, the first one can be abruptly stopped and the new one started the next morning. Side effects from abrupt discontinuation are not expected; however, some patients may experience marked fatigue and sleepiness for several days.
- See Appendix for approximate dosing equivalents when switching

How to Stop

- Taper not necessary, especially for patients who have only had short-term treatment or intermittent treatment
- However, if withdrawal symptoms develop, resume dosing the medication and then taper slowly over several days
- Withdrawal following chronic therapeutic use may unmask symptoms of the underlying disorder and may require follow-up and reinstitution of treatment
- Usually symptoms after discontinuation are return of symptoms of the underlying disorder rather than symptoms due to drug withdrawal
- Supervision during withdrawal is always recommended for any psychotropic medication

WHAT TO EXPECT

Onset of Action

- Onset of action can occur 20–30 minutes post-administration; however, food may slow absorption and decrease the peak concentration of stimulants
- Takes a few days to attain therapeutic benefit generally

Duration of Action

- Immediate-release: 4–6-hour duration, early peak
- Extended-release: 8–10-hour duration, two peaks (after 1.5 and 6.5 hours)

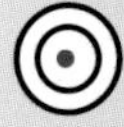

Primary Target Symptoms

- Concentration, attention span, distractibility
- Motor hyperactivity
- Impulsiveness
- Physical and mental fatigue
- Daytime sleepiness

What Is Considered a Positive Result?

- The goal of treatment of ADHD is reduction of symptoms of inattentiveness, motor hyperactivity, and/or impulsiveness that disrupt social, school, and/or occupational functioning
- Can also improve oppositional and disruptive behaviors associated with ADHD
- The goal of treatment is complete remission of symptoms
- If treatment works, it most often reduces or even eliminates symptoms, but is not a cure since symptoms often recur after medicine is stopped

How Long to Treat

- ADHD is typically a lifelong illness; if any symptoms improve, hyperactivity is more likely to improve than inattention
- Can tell parents there is some chance that their child can grow out of this in adulthood, but many adults continue to have symptoms of ADHD throughout adolescence and adulthood
- Continue treatment until all symptoms are under control or improvement is stable and then continue treatment as long as improvement persists
- Reevaluate the need for treatment periodically; some clinicians advise to periodically stop stimulants in patients who are not severely symptomatic to observe how the patient responds, but not routinely done by most clinicians
- Treatment for ADHD begun in childhood may need to be continued into adolescence and adulthood if continued benefit is documented

What If It Stops Working?

- Some patients who have an initial response may relapse even though they continue treatment, sometimes called "poop-out"
- Growth/developmental changes may contribute to apparent loss of efficacy as well as to new onset of side effects as metabolism slows and drug levels rise in transition from childhood to adolescence; dose adjustment (increase or decrease) should be considered
- Some patients may experience apparent lack of consistent efficacy due to activation of latent or underlying or newly evolved bipolar disorder, major depressive episodes

with mixed features of mania, new onset of major depression or an anxiety disorder (GAD, OCD, PD), and require stimulant discontinuation and a switch to the clinically appropriate medication(s)

What If It Doesn't Work?

- In practice, many patients have only a partial response where some symptoms are improved but others persist, in which case higher doses of methylphenidate, adding a second agent, or switching to an agent with a different mechanism of action can be considered
- Consider evaluation for another diagnosis or for a comorbid condition (e.g., medical illness, substance abuse). Also, when treating ADHD, consider the possibility of a learning disorder or learning weakness and consider school-based interventions.
- Consider adjusting dose or switching to another formulation of D-methylphenidate or to another agent
- Consider the presence of nonadherence and counsel patient and parents
- Some ADHD patients and some depressed patients may experience lack of consistent efficacy due to activation of latent or underlying bipolar disorder, and require either augmenting with a mood stabilizer or switching to a mood stabilizer
- Augmenting options:
  - Organizational skills training/executive function coaching
  - Exercise
  - Parent Management Training (PMT)
  - Coordinating with school for appropriate support
  - For the expert, can combine with modafinil, atomoxetine, or viloxazine for ADHD
  - For the expert, can occasionally combine with atypical antipsychotics in highly treatment-resistant cases of bipolar disorder or ADHD
  - For the expert, can combine with antidepressants to boost antidepressant efficacy in highly treatment-resistant cases of depression while carefully monitoring patient
  - Can combine with alpha 2 agonists such as guanfacine or clonidine
- Consider factors associated with poor response to any psychotropic medication in children and adolescents, such as severe symptoms, long-lasting symptoms, nonadherence, prior nonresponse to other treatments, and the presence of comorbid psychiatric disorders or learning disorders
- Consider other important potential factors such as ongoing conflicts, family psychopathology, and an adverse environment (e.g., poverty, chaos, violence, prior and ongoing psychological trauma, abuse, bullying, less-than-ideal school placement, neglect)
- Institute trauma-informed care for appropriate children and adolescents

TALKING TO PATIENTS AND CAREGIVERS

What to Tell Parents About Efficacy

- Stimulant treatment for ADHD is one of the best studied of all medications in children and adolescents
- Often works right away once the dose is correct
- While the medicine helps ADHD by reducing symptoms and improving function, there are no cures for ADHD and it is therefore necessary to keep taking the medication to sustain its therapeutic effects
- It does not work that day if the child/adolescent has not taken their medication in the morning
- For longer-acting stimulants, be careful not to give too late (i.e., after 11 a.m.) because it can cause insomnia that night
- Does not stay in the body for a long time, so it stops working rapidly after you stop it
- Since every treatment consideration depends on a risk/benefit analysis, parents should fully understand short- and long-term risks as well as benefits compared to nontreatment of ADHD
- Although many stimulants are approved for ADHD, if using off-label, often a good idea to tell parents whether the medication chosen is specifically approved for the disorder being treated, or whether it is being given for "unapproved" or "off-label" reasons based on good clinical practice, expert consensus, and/or prudent extrapolation of controlled data from adults
- Best results are often obtained when medications are combined with behavioral therapy

- Stimulants wear off after a number of hours and symptoms may return. Therefore, parents may complain that the medication isn't working if their child/adolescent is using a stimulant that lasts 8 hours, because it may have worn off after the patient has come home from school (and that is when the parents are seeing the child/adolescent) in comparison to a stimulant that lasts 10–12 hours and may keep working after the child/adolescent comes home from school.
- The American Academy of Child & Adolescent Psychiatry (AACAP) has helpful handouts for parents

What to Tell Children and Adolescents About Efficacy

- Be specific about the symptoms being targeted: we are trying to help you remember things better, do your best at school, follow the rules, get into less trouble (as applicable)
- It may be a good idea to give the medication a try; if it's not working very well, we can stop the medication and try something else
- You can be part of a special plan to help us figure out if the medicine is helpful for you. Would you like to do that? (for the parents and prescriber, can consider here a trial both on and then off medication, and then on again to see if the effects are clear and thus worth continuing the medication)
- The medication can work right away but a good try can take a few months to find the right dose
- Even if it does make you feel better, it will wear off and no longer work shortly after you stop it
- This medicine does not last very long in your body, so even if it does work, it won't work if you don't take it that day
- The medication can help you decide what you want to do, like making good choices versus bad choices; the medicine does not make you do something you don't want to do
- Medications don't change who you are as a person; they give you the opportunity to be the best person you can be

What to Tell Parents About Side Effects

- Explain that side effects are expected in many when starting
- Tell parents many side effects of stimulants often go away in a few days to weeks, especially nausea and insomnia, but if they don't we will change the treatment
- Predict side effects in advance (you will look clever and competent to the parents, unless you scare them with too much information and cause nocebo effects, in which case you won't look so clever when the patient develops lots of side effects and stops medication; use your judgment here); a balanced but honest presentation is an art rather than a science
- Sometimes a trial off medication and then on again can clarify what the true therapeutic effects of the medication are
- Ask parents to support the patient while side effects are occurring
- Parents should fully understand short- and long-term risks as well as benefits
- Explaining to the parents what to expect from medication treatment, and especially what potential side effects to expect, can help prevent early termination

What to Tell Children and Adolescents About Side Effects

- When a medicine starts to work, your body can first experience this by giving you unpleasant sensations – just like if you take a cough medicine it may taste bad – these body sensations include loss of appetite and problems sleeping. So, just like with a cough medicine, the bad taste will often go away before the medicine begins to stop the cough – many medicines work like that. It's important for you to pay attention to what your body is telling you, and we'll go over some of the ways that can happen.
- Even if you get a side effect, it's not permanent (it won't last forever)
- In a way, a side effect tells you the medication is working on your body and good effects should come soon
- Explaining to child/adolescent what to expect from medication treatment, and especially potential side effects, can help prevent early termination

What to Tell Teachers About the Medication (If Parents Consent)

- Stimulants can be very helpful in improving the symptoms of ADHD: namely, inattention, impulsivity, and hyperactivity

- It does not work if the child/adolescent has not taken their medication that morning
- If the patient is sleepy, ask whether the medication is keeping them up at night or if they are eating enough food
- If the patient won't eat lunch or snacks, ask whether the medication is making them lose their appetite
- Medically speaking, methylphenidate is not a narcotic, because doctors define a narcotic as something that is sedating and sleep-inducing, like opioids such as heroin and Oxycontin and not stimulants like methylphenidate
- Methylphenidate should be kept in school under lock and key or at the nurse's office or not brought to school at all because it can be diverted and misused by those who do not have ADHD. Some schools will suspend students who are caught with medications on their person or in their backpacks; most schools know the misuse or even abuse potential of stimulants.

SPECIAL POPULATIONS

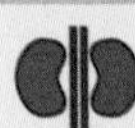

Renal Impairment

- No dose adjustment necessary

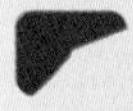

Hepatic Impairment

- No dose adjustment necessary

Cardiac Impairment

- Use with caution, particularly in patients with recent myocardial infarction or other conditions that could be negatively affected by increased blood pressure
- Do not use in patients with structural cardiac abnormalities without consultation with a cardiologist

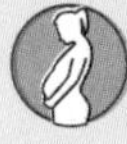

Pregnancy

- Controlled studies have not been conducted in pregnant women
- Infants whose mothers took methylphenidate during pregnancy may experience withdrawal symptoms
- Racemic methylphenidate has been shown to have teratogenic effects in rabbits when given in doses of 200 mg/kg/day throughout organogenesis
- Use in women of childbearing potential requires weighing potential benefits to the mother against potential risks to the fetus
- For ADHD patients, methylphenidate should generally be discontinued before anticipated pregnancies
- National Pregnancy Registry for Psychiatric Medications: 1-866-961-388 or https://womensmentalhealth.org/research/pregnancyregistry/

Breast Feeding

- Unknown if methylphenidate is secreted in human breast milk, but all psychotropics assumed to be secreted in breast milk
- Recommended either to discontinue drug or formula feed
- If infant shows signs of irritability, drug may need to be discontinued

THE ART OF PSYCHOPHARMACOLOGY

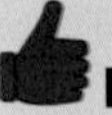

Potential Advantages

- In children:
  - Stimulants are probably the best studied psychotropic medications for use in children
  - Methylphenidate is one of the best studied stimulants in children
- In adolescents:
  - Can improve school performance and grades, especially if ADHD has been unrecognized and untreated prior to adolescence
  - Can improve performance in high school and college students whose ADHD is compromising academic performance due to the increased demands of higher levels of study
- All ages:
  - Methylphenidate has established long-term efficacy as a first-line treatment for ADHD
  - The active d enantiomer of methylphenidate may be slightly more than twice as efficacious as racemic D,L-methylphenidate

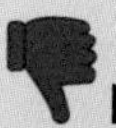

Potential Disadvantages

- Adolescents and especially college-age patients who divert their medication
- Patients with current substance abuse
- Patients with current manic or mixed symptoms associated with bipolar disorder or psychosis
- Patients with anorexia

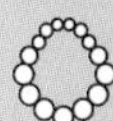

Pearls

- Half-life and duration of clinical action tend to be shorter in younger children than in adolescents and may require more frequent dosing or preferential use of long-acting preparations
- Preschool ADHD Treatment Study (PATS) is one of the very few studies of stimulant treatment for preschool children with ADHD; PATS showed that preschoolers may benefit from low doses of stimulants when closely monitored, but the positive effects are less evident and the side effects somewhat greater than in older children
- Drug abuse is no more likely and may even be lower (controversial) in ADHD adolescents treated with stimulants than in ADHD adolescents who are not treated with stimulants
- Stimulants have a moderate effect on decreasing ADHD symptoms and a moderate to large effect on decreasing aggression, oppositional behavior, and conduct problems in children with ADHD
- Meta-analyses suggest that when taking into account both efficacy and safety, methylphenidate is the best first-line stimulant in children and adolescents, whereas amphetamine is best in adults (Cortese et al., 2018)
- Stimulant dosing and titration are critical to optimizing response. Meta-analyses involving nearly 8,000 children/adolescents show that both methylphenidate and amphetamine salts have increased efficacy (but increased likelihood of discontinuation due to side effects) with higher doses (Farhat et al., 2022). In general, goal doses are often in the range of 0.8 mg/kg for methylphenidate and 0.5 mg/kg for amphetamine salts. However, these are rough guides that may not always be applicable depending on the formulation used and how completely (or incompletely) it's absorbed.
- Combinations of behavioral therapy or other nonmedication treatments along with stimulants may have better results than either treatment alone
- Extended-release capsule can be sprinkled over applesauce for patients unable to swallow the capsule
- Some patients may benefit from an occasional addition of an immediate-release dose of D-methylphenidate as an afternoon "booster" to their extended-release D-methylphenidate
- Rebound hyperactivity may occur in the afternoon and present with increased hyperactivity, restlessness, and irritability; if this occurs, can consider switching to a longer-acting agent or a nonstimulant or adding a short-acting stimulant
- On the other hand, too-high medication dosing may lead to cognitive rigidity, difficulty shifting attention, and seeming "spaced out" or "different"
- Many patients taking stimulants have early-morning ADHD symptoms and can be hard to get going, prepare for school, and be cooperative, especially for a few hours after awakening. In these patients, delayed-release/extended-release formulations may be especially helpful.
- Stimulants are a classic augmentation strategy for treatment-refractory depression, although this is most established in adults
- Interestingly, in some studies combining stimulants with alpha 2 agonists, decreased side effects are seen with the combination compared to either medication as monotherapy. This is likely because of complementary side effects.

SUGGESTED READING

Biederman J, Spencer TJ, Monuteaux MC, Faraone SV. A naturalistic 10-year prospective study of height and weight in children with attention-deficit hyperactivity disorder grown up: sex and treatment effects. J Pediatr 2010 Oct;157(4):635–40.

Cohen SC, Mulqueen JM, Ferracioli-Oda E et al. Meta-analysis: risk of tics associated with psychostimulant use in randomized, placebo-controlled trials. J Am Acad Child Adolesc Psychiatry 2015;54(9):728–36.

Cortese S, Adamo N, Del Giovane C et al. Comparative efficacy and tolerability of medications for attention-deficit hyperactivity disorder in children, adolescents, and adults: a systematic review and network meta-analysis. Lancet Psychiatry 2018;5(9):727–38.

Farhat LC, Flores JM, Behling E et al. The effects of stimulant dose and dosing strategy on treatment outcomes in attention-deficit/hyperactivity disorder in children and adolescents: a meta-analysis. Mol Psychiatry 2022;27(3):1562–72.

Jensen PS, Arnold LE, Swanson JM et al. 3-year follow-up of the NIMH MTA study. J Am Acad Child Adolesc Psychiatry 2007;46(8):989–1002.

The MTA Cooperative Group. A 14-month randomized clinical trial of treatment strategies for attention-deficit/hyperactivity disorder. The MTA Cooperative Group. Multimodal Treatment Study of Children with ADHD. Arch Gen Psychiatry 1999;56(12):1073–86.

Po MD, Gomeni R, Incledon B. Quantitative characterization of the smoothness of extended-release methylphenidate pharmacokinetic profiles. Innov Clin Neurosci 2022;19(7–9):32–7.

Posner K, Melvin GA, Murray DW et al. Clinical presentation of attention-deficit/hyperactivity disorder in preschool children: the Preschoolers with Attention-Deficit/Hyperactivity Disorder Treatment Study (PATS). J Child Adolesc Psychopharmacol 2007;17(5):547–62.

Riddle MA, Yershova K, Lazzaretto D et al. The Preschool Attention-Deficit/Hyperactivity Disorder Treatment Study (PATS) 6-year follow-up. J Am Acad Child Adolesc Psychiatry 2013;52(3):264–78.

Swanson JM, Arnold LE, Molina BSG et al. Young adult outcomes in the follow-up of the multimodal treatment study of attention-deficit/hyperactivity disorder: symptom persistence, source discrepancy, and height suppression. J Child Psychol Psychiatry 2017;58(6):663–78.

Zhang L, Yao H, Li L et al. Risk of cardiovascular diseases associated with medications used in attention-deficit/hyperactivity disorder: a systematic review and meta-analysis. JAMA Netw Open 2022;5(11):e2243597.

THERAPEUTICS

Brands

- Aptensio XR
- Concerta
- Cotempla XR-ODT
- Daytrana
- Jornay PM
- Metadate CD
- Methylin
- Methylin ER
- QuilliChew ER
- Quillivant XR
- Relexxii
- Ritalin
- Ritalin LA

Generic

Yes

US FDA Approved for Pediatric Use

- Attention deficit hyperactivity disorder (Ritalin, Methylin, ages 6 to 12 and adults)
- Attention deficit hyperactivity disorder (Ritalin LA, ages 6 to 12)
- Attention deficit hyperactivity disorder (Metadate CD, Daytrana, Cotempla XR-ODT, ages 6 to 17)
- Attention deficit hyperactivity disorder (Methylin ER, Concerta, QuilliChew ER, Aptensio XR, Quillivant XR, Jornay PM, Relexxii, ages 6 and older)

Off-Label for Pediatric Use

- Approved in adults
  - Narcolepsy (Methylin ER, Ritalin)
- Other off-label uses
  - Treatment-resistant depression (rarely used for this in children)
  - Stimulants are sometimes used to augment antidepressants
  - Stimulants also sometimes used to treat amotivational or lethargic states in the elderly with dementia but rarely in children for these symptoms

Class and Mechanism of Action

- Neuroscience-based Nomenclature: dopamine, norepinephrine multimodal
- Stimulant
- Increases norepinephrine and especially dopamine actions by blocking their reuptake
- Enhancement of dopamine and norepinephrine actions in certain brain regions (e.g., dorsolateral prefrontal cortex) may improve attention, concentration, executive dysfunction, wakefulness, and cortical inhibitory control of striatum (i.e., theoretically "tunes" inefficient information processing in cortical–striatal pathways, improving "top-down" regulation of striatal and other subcortical drives)
- Enhancement of dopamine actions in other brain regions (e.g., basal ganglia) may decrease hyperactivity
- Enhancement of dopamine and norepinephrine in yet other brain regions (e.g., medial prefrontal cortex, hypothalamus) may improve depressive symptoms as well as nondepression-associated fatigue and sleepiness
- Hypothetically rebalances signal to noise ratios of cortical neurons: enhances focus on importance tasks (signal), theoretically due to norepinephrine, and reduces awareness of background activity (noise), theoretically due to dopamine

SAFETY AND TOLERABILITY

Notable Side Effects

- Anorexia and weight loss
- Nausea, abdominal pain
- Insomnia, headache, exacerbation of tics, tremor, dizziness, and possible irritability and anxiety. The risk of treatment-emergent irritability is lower with methylphenidate-based stimulants compared to amphetamine-based stimulants.
- Peripheral vasculopathy, including Raynaud's phenomenon
- Blurred vision
- Transdermal: application site reactions, including contact sensitization (erythema, edema, papules, vesicles) and chemical leukoderma

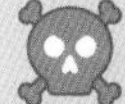

Life-Threatening or Dangerous Side Effects

- Psychosis
- Seizures
- Palpitations, tachycardia, hypertension
- Rare hypomania, mania, or suicidal ideation

- Cardiovascular adverse effects, death in patients with preexisting cardiac structural abnormalities often associated with a family history of cardiac disease

Growth and Maturation

- May temporarily slow normal growth in children (controversial): Multimodal Treatment of ADHD (MTA) study showed children/adolescents grew more slowly but eventually reached their expected adult height
- Controversy exists because theoretically stimulants might suppress appetite and reduce caloric intake, which could affect potential growth; also, dopaminergic actions of stimulants might suppress growth hormone secretion and affect height development. However, expected adult height is likely attained with a delay if stimulants are continued, and slowing of growth is likely reversible with withdrawal of treatment.

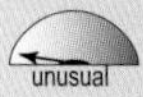

Weight Gain

- Patients may experience weight loss
- Weight gain is reported but not expected, rarely seen, controversial

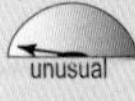

Sedation

- Activation much more common than sedation
- Sedation is reported but not expected, rarely seen, controversial

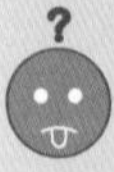

What to Do About Side Effects

- Wait, wait, wait: mild side effects are common, happen early, and usually improve with time, but treatment benefits can be delayed and often begin just as the side effects wear off
- Adjust dose
- Switch to another formulation of D,L-methylphenidate
- Switch to another agent
- For insomnia: avoid dosing in the midday, late afternoon, or evening
- However, insomnia is not always due to medication, but can be the result of relapse, rebound, and withdrawal effects from the daily dose, and in fact improves with additional late-day dosing of a short-acting stimulant
- Use beta blockers for peripheral autonomic side effects
- Often best to try another monotherapy prior to resorting to augmentation strategies to treat side effects, with the exception of an early-evening dose of a stimulant
- Monitor side effects closely, especially when initiating treatment
- For persistent insomnia: consider adding melatonin or an alpha 2 agonist
- For loss of appetite or loss of weight:
  - Give medication after breakfast
  - Switch to a nonstimulant
  - Eat a high-protein, high-carbohydrate breakfast prior to taking medication or within 10–15 minutes of ingesting medication; snack on high-protein, densely caloric foods throughout the school day and after school; eat dinner and then a second dinner or very heavy snack at bedtime
  - Add "liquid calories" (i.e., smoothies made with whole milk or ice cream, fruit, and protein powder; Boost or Ensure shakes)
  - Introduce "fourth meal" in the evening
  - Add cyproheptadine

How Drug Causes Side Effects

- Increases in norepinephrine peripherally can cause autonomic side effects, including tremor, tachycardia, hypertension, and cardiac arrhythmias
- Increases in norepinephrine and dopamine centrally can cause CNS side effects such as insomnia, agitation, psychosis (rarely)

Warnings and Precautions

- In children and adolescents:
  - Safety and efficacy not established in children under age 6
  - Use in young children should be reserved for the expert
  - Children who are not growing or gaining weight should stop treatment, at least temporarily
  - Usual dosing has been associated with sudden death in children with structural cardiac abnormalities
  - Consider distributing brochures provided by the FDA and the drug companies

- All ages:
  - Stimulants used to treat ADHD are associated with peripheral vasculopathy, including Raynaud's phenomenon; careful observation for digital changes is necessary during treatment with ADHD stimulants
  - Carefully weigh the risks and benefits of pharmacological treatment against the risks and benefits of nonpharmacological treatment and it is a good idea to document this in the patient's chart
  - Use with caution in patients with any degree of hypertension, hyperthyroidism, or history of drug abuse
  - Many believe tics may be worsened by stimulants, but evidence does not support this association. A meta-analysis of 22 studies, including 2,385 individuals in treatment, found that the rate of new onset or worsening tics was 5.7% for those on stimulants versus 6.5% with placebo. In this analysis, there was no effect for type of stimulant, dose, duration of treatment, or age (Cohen et al., 2015). The presence of tics is not an absolute contraindication to use of stimulants.
  - May worsen symptoms of thought disorder and behavioral disturbance in psychotic patients
  - Stimulants have a high potential for abuse and must be used with caution in anyone with a current or past history of substance abuse or alcoholism, but stimulants for ADHD are less likely to be abused in terms of getting "high" and more likely to be used to stay awake, especially by college students. This misuse is the most common reason for diversion of prescription stimulants.
  - Youth are neither more nor less likely to develop alcohol and substance use disorders as a result of being treated with stimulant medication. In fact, current data suggest that treating ADHD in children and adolescents decreases the likelihood of developing a substance use disorder.
  - Adolescents and/or college students may divert/sell their medication to others for use in staying awake to study at the last minute, or to abuse; longer-acting preparations are harder to abuse than shorter-acting, immediate-release stimulants
  - Particular attention should be paid to the possibility of adolescents you are seeing for the first time feigning ADHD in order to obtain stimulants for nontherapeutic use or distribution to others; the drugs should in general be prescribed sparingly with documentation of appropriate use, and if there is any doubt about the accuracy of their complaints, refer them for psychological-educational or neuropsychological testing
  - Not an appropriate first-line treatment for depression or for normal fatigue
  - May lower the seizure threshold; as long as seizures are well controlled, it is generally safe to use stimulants
  - Emergence or worsening of activation and agitation may represent the induction of a bipolar state, especially a mixed dysphoric bipolar II condition sometimes associated with suicidal ideation, and may require the addition of lithium or an atypical antipsychotic, and/or discontinuation of D,L-methylphenidate
  - Permanent skin color loss, known as chemical leukoderma, may occur with use of the transdermal Daytrana patch; patients should be advised to watch for signs of skin color changes and, if they occur, alternative treatment options should be considered
  - Certain transdermal patches containing even small traces of aluminum or other metals in the adhesive backing can cause skin burns if worn during magnetic resonance imaging (MRI), so warn patients taking the transdermal formulation about this possibility and advise them to disclose this information if they need an MRI

When Not to Prescribe

- Treating ADHD comorbid with tics or Tourette syndrome is not contraindicated, but may be for the expert
- Patients with ADHD who are comorbid for motor or vocal tics of Tourette syndrome, or even with just a family history of Tourette syndrome, may experience worsening/onset of tics with stimulant treatment (controversial). Decision to use stimulants in such cases should weigh the potential benefits for ADHD against the risks of worsening tics, and may require expert referral or consultation.

- Should generally not be administered with an MAOI, including within 14 days of MAOI use, except in heroic circumstances and by an expert
- If patient has glaucoma
- If patient has structural cardiac abnormalities
- If there is a proven allergy to methylphenidate
- If the patient has an eating disorder other than binge-eating disorder, be very cautious

Long-Term Use

- Often used long term for ADHD when ongoing monitoring documents continued efficacy
- Tolerance to therapeutic effects may develop in some patients
- Weight and height should be monitored during long-term treatment
- Periodic monitoring of blood pressure and heart rate

Habit Forming

- Paradoxically, stimulant abuse appears to be less likely in patients with ADHD than in those who do not have ADHD. In 2023, the FDA modified a boxed warning for stimulant medications, although they noted, "Our review found that nonmedical use has remained relatively stable over the past two decades, despite the increasing number of prescription stimulants dispensed." The new warning notes that stimulants have a "high potential for abuse and misuse, which can lead to the development of a substance use disorder, including addiction." The new warning also notes that stimulant medications "can be diverted for non-medical use into illicit channels or distribution." They recommend:
    - Counsel patients not to give any of their medicine to anyone else
    - Monitor for signs and symptoms of diversion, such as requesting refills more frequently than needed
    - Regularly assess and monitor for signs and symptoms of nonmedical use and addiction
    - Keep careful records of prescribing information, including quantity, frequency, and renewal requests, as required by state and federal laws
- Stimulant abuse in ADHD patients more likely if there is a preexisting history of alcohol/drug abuse
- Tolerance to stimulants is surprisingly rare in ADHD; tolerance should not be confused with reduction of therapeutic effects over time due to growth: as youth grow, dose usually must be increased; otherwise, the appearance of tolerance occurs when this in reality is underdosing
- Misuse may be more likely with immediate-release stimulants than with controlled-release stimulants

Overdose

- Vomiting, tremor, coma, convulsion, hyperreflexia, euphoria, confusion, hallucination, tachycardia, flushing, palpitations, sweating, hyperpyrexia, hypertension, arrhythmia, mydriasis

DOSING AND USE

Usual Dosage Range

- ADHD (all ages, oral): varies by formulation; see How to Dose section
- ADHD (all ages, transdermal): 10–30 mg/9 hours
- Narcolepsy (all ages): 20–60 mg/day in 2–3 divided doses

Dosage Forms

- Ritalin, generic methylphenidate (immediate-release tablet) 5 mg, 10 mg, 20 mg
- Generic methylphenidate (immediate-release chewable tablet) 2.5 mg, 5 mg, 10 mg
- Methylin (oral solution) 5 mg/5 mL, 10 mg/5 mL
- Ritalin LA (sustained-release capsule) 10 mg, 20 mg, 30 mg, 40 mg
- Methylin ER (sustained-release tablet) 10 mg, 20 mg
- Metadate CD (sustained-release capsule) 10 mg, 20 mg, 30 mg, 40 mg, 50 mg, 60 mg
- Concerta (sustained-release tablet) 18 mg, 27 mg, 36 mg, 54 mg
- Relexxii (extended-release tablet) 18 mg, 27 mg, 36 mg, 45 mg, 54 mg, 63 mg, 72 mg

- QuilliChew ER (sustained-release chewable tablet) 20 mg scored, 30 mg, 40 mg
- Quillivant XR (extended-release oral suspension) 5 mg/mL
- Aptensio XR (extended-release capsule, multi-layer release) 10 mg, 15 mg, 20 mg, 30 mg, 40 mg, 50 mg, 60 mg
- Cotempla-XR-ODT (extended-release orally disintegrating tablet) 8.6 mg, 17.3 mg, 25.9 mg
- Jornay PM (extended-release capsule) 20 mg, 40 mg, 60 mg, 80 mg, 100 mg
- Daytrana (transdermal patch) 27 mg/12.5 cm^2 (10 mg/9 hr; 1.1 mg/hr), 41.3 mg/18.75 cm^2 (15 mg/9 hr; 1.6 mg/hr), 55 mg/25 cm^2 (20 mg/9 hr; 2.2 mg/hr), 82.5 mg/37.5 cm^2 (30 mg/9 hr; 3.3 mg/hr)

How to Dose (in ADHD)

- Immediate-release Ritalin, Methylin (ages 6 and older): initial 5 mg in morning, 5 mg at lunch, 5 mg after school; can increase by 5–10 mg/day each week; maximum daily dose generally 60 mg/day, given in divided doses every 4 hours, up to three times a day
- Ritalin LA (ages 6 to 12): initial 20 mg once daily; dosage may be adjusted in weekly increments of 10 mg to a maximum of 60 mg/day taken in the morning
- Methylin ER (ages 6 and older): average dose is 20–30 mg/day, usually in 2 divided doses
- Metadate CD (ages 6 to 17): initial 20 mg once daily; dosage may be adjusted in weekly increments of 10 mg to a maximum of 60 mg/day taken in the morning
- Concerta (ages 6 and older): initial 18 mg/day in morning; can increase by 18 mg each week; maximum dose generally 72 mg/day
- QuilliChew ER (ages 6 and older): initial 20 mg once daily; dosage may be adjusted in weekly increments of 10 mg or 20 mg (QuilliChew ER only) to a maximum of 60 mg/day taken in the morning
- Quillivant XR (ages 6 and older): initial 20 mg once daily; dosage may be adjusted in weekly increments of 10–20 mg to a maximum of 60 mg/day taken in the morning
- Aptensio XR (ages 6 and older): initial 10 mg once daily; dosage may be adjusted in weekly increments of 10 mg to a maximum of 60 mg/day taken in the morning
- Cotempla XR-ODT (ages 6 to 17): initial dose 17.3 mg once daily in the morning; can increase weekly in increments of 8.6 mg to 17.3 mg per day; maximum recommended dose 51.8 mg; should be taken consistently either with or without food
- Jornay PM (ages 6 and older): initial dose 20 mg once in the evening at 8 p.m.; can increase weekly in increments of 20 mg per day; maximum daily dose 100 mg; can adjust administration time between 6:30 and 9:30 p.m., depending on optimal efficacy and tolerability; once optimal administration time is set it should remain consistent; if the evening dose is missed and not remembered until the next morning, then the patient should wait until their next scheduled evening administration
- Transdermal Daytrana (ages 6 to 17): initial 10 mg/9 hours; can increase by 5 mg/9 hours every week; maximum dose generally 30 mg/9 hours; higher doses such as 40 mg in the morning can be given off-label by experts; patch should be applied 2 hours before effect is needed and should be worn for 9 hours

Options for Administration

- Multiple formulation alternatives for patients with difficulty swallowing pills, including: oral solution; small beads that can be mixed with yogurt, applesauce, or pudding; chewable tablet; and orally disintegrating tablet
- Several extended-release formulations have sufficient duration of action to eliminate the need for lunchtime dosing

Tests

- Before treatment, assess for presence of cardiac disease (history, family history, physical exam); consider whether electrocardiogram (ECG) is indicated
- Blood pressure and heart rate should be monitored regularly, sitting and standing
- Monitor weight and height
- Current recommendations from the American Heart Association (AHA) are that it is reasonable but not mandatory to obtain an ECG prior to prescribing a stimulant to a child; the American Academy of Pediatrics

(AAP) does not recommend an ECG prior to starting a stimulant for most children
- Document basic sleep patterns prior to starting a stimulant
- When necessary to rule out sleep apnea, nocturnal movements, or daytime sleepiness that may later be difficult to distinguish from side effects of stimulants, consider (rarely) a sleep study/polysomnogram (e.g., obese adolescents)

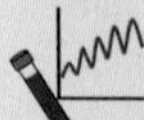

Pharmacokinetics

- Average half-life in adults is 3.5 hours (1.3–7.7 hours)
- Average half-life in children is 2.5 hours (1.5–5 hours); however, biological activity and clinical duration of action are often longer, up to 3.5–4 hours
- Clinical duration of action often differs from pharmacokinetic half-life and can be longer for any formulation
- Taking oral formulations with food may delay peak actions for 2–3 hours
- First-pass metabolism is not extensive with transdermal dosing, thus resulting in notably higher exposure to methylphenidate and lower exposure to metabolites as compared to oral dosing

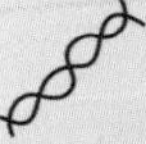

Pharmacogenetics

- Methylphenidate is not metabolized by CYP450 isoenzymes to a clinically relevant extent and therefore there are no pharmacogenetic recommendations related to methylphenidate based on pharmacokinetic genes. Additionally, there are no recommendations related to pharmacodynamic genes and stimulant selection.

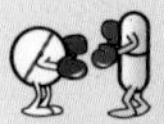

Drug Interactions

- May affect blood pressure and should be used cautiously with agents used to control blood pressure
- Methylphenidate is metabolized by carboxylesterase 1 and is not a substrate or inhibitor of the CYP450 drug-metabolizing system
- Most drug interactions are pharmacodynamic rather than pharmacokinetic
- CNS and cardiovascular actions of D,L-methylphenidate could theoretically be enhanced by combination with agents that block norepinephrine reuptake, such as the tricyclic antidepressants desipramine or protriptyline, venlafaxine, duloxetine, atomoxetine, milnacipran, and reboxetine
- Theoretically, D,L-methylphenidate could inhibit the antipsychotic actions of antipsychotics
- Theoretically, D,L-methylphenidate could inhibit the mood-stabilizing actions of atypical antipsychotics in some patients; however, stimulants can be safely combined with atypical antipsychotics by experts
- Combinations of D,L-methylphenidate with mood stabilizers (lithium, anticonvulsants, atypical antipsychotics) are generally something for experts only, when monitoring patients closely and when other options fail
- Use with MAOIs, including within 14 days of MAOI use, is not advised, but this can sometimes be considered by experts who monitor depressed patients closely when other treatment options for depression fail

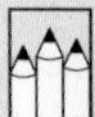

Dosing Tips

- Plasma levels are higher in lower-weight children; therefore, starting and target doses may be lower and longer intervals between dose increases may be needed (see How to Dose)
- The newer extended-release formulations can eliminate the hassle and pragmatic difficulties of lunchtime dosing at school, including storage problems, potential diversion, and the need for a medical professional to supervise dosing away from home
- If the patient is doing well on a stimulant that lasts 10–12 hours during the week, but wakes up later on the weekends and has insomnia with later dosing, can either (1) have the child/adolescent take the medication at the same time as during the week and let them go back to sleep; or (2) use a stimulant with a shorter duration of action (i.e., 8 hours) or Daytrana transdermal patch
- If there are concerns about diversion or abuse, longer-acting stimulant preparations are much harder to abuse than immediate-release preparations
- Be aware that metabolism (and absorption) changes during puberty and entry into

adolescence and becomes more like adults (i.e., slower than in children)
- If a child on a stable dose begins to lose tolerability with more side effects upon entering adolescence, this may signal the need for a dose reduction due to changing metabolism
- Do not substitute methylphenidate products on a mg-per-mg basis due to differing methylphenidate base compositions and pharmacokinetic profiles (see Appendix)
- Immediate-release formulations (Ritalin, Methylin, generic methylphenidate) have 3–4-hour durations of action
- Methylin ER has an early peak and approximately 3–8-hour durations of clinical action, which for most patients is generally not long enough for once-daily dosing in the morning and thus generally requires lunchtime dosing at school
- Metadate CD and QuilliChew ER have 8-hour durations of action
- Sustained-release Ritalin LA has two strong peaks (immediately and at 4 hours) and a 6–8-hour duration of action
- Concerta, Cotempla XR-ODT, Quillivant XR, Aptensio XR, and Daytrana have 12-hour durations of action
- Jornay PM has both delayed- and extended-release properties and is taken the evening before
- Concerta tablet does not change shape in the GI tract and may be excreted in the stool; it generally should not be used in patients with gastrointestinal narrowing because of the risk of intestinal obstruction
- Most sustained-release formulations should not be chewed but rather should only be swallowed whole
- QuilliChew ER is a chewable tablet and can be taken with or without food
- Jornay PM can be taken with or without food, but should be consistent; the capsule can be opened and sprinkled on applesauce
- Ritalin LA, Metadate CD, and Aptensio XR capsules can all be taken apart and the contents put into pudding, yogurt, or applesauce
- Avoid dosing late in the day because of the risk of insomnia (except for Jornay PM)
- Off-label uses are dosed the same as for ADHD
- Side effects are generally dose related
- Transdermal Daytrana (ages 6 to 17) can be dosed (off-label) as high as 40 mg in the morning
- Transdermal patch should be applied to dry, intact skin on the hip
- New application site should be selected for each day; only one patch should be applied at a time; patches should not be cut
- Avoid touching the exposed (sticky) side of the patch, and after application, wash hands with soap and water; do not touch eyes until after hands have been washed
- Heat can increase the amount of methylphenidate absorbed from the transdermal patch, so patients should avoid exposing the application site to external source of direct heat (e.g., heating pads, prolonged direct sunlight)
- If a patch comes off a new patch may be applied at a different site; total daily wear time should remain 9 hours regardless of number of patches used
- Early removal of transdermal patch can be useful to terminate drug action when desired

Drug Holidays

- Drug holidays were originally done in an attempt to avoid the possibility that stimulants may blunt height
- May be able to give drug holidays over the summer in order to reassess therapeutic utility and effects on growth and theoretically to allow catch-up from any growth suppression and assess any other side effects and the need to reinstitute stimulant treatment for the next school term
- However, most studies show that parental height is what determines a patient's final height, and that most children/adolescents taking stimulants reach their expected height, just more slowly than children/adolescents not exposed to stimulants
- May be possible to give weekend drug holidays and dose only during the school week for some ADHD patients, but there are risks as well:
  - Hyperactivity and impulsivity increase the chances of accidents (i.e., broken bones and head injuries) and illicit alcohol and drug abuse
  - Studies have shown that adolescents with ADHD who drive vehicles without their stimulants are much more likely to get into motor vehicle accidents and that the

severity of the accident is much greater than would be expected
- Hyperactive and impulsive children/adolescents tend to have more difficulties getting along with family members and friends, increasing the chances of developing low self-esteem and poor self-image
- Social benefits can be lost over the summer if children/adolescents are taken off stimulants; social rejection by other children can lead to isolation and depression, increasing the chances of bullying, victimization, and further isolation and peer rejection
- Inattention makes it harder for kids to learn the rules of life and pay attention to what is going on around them (e.g., noticing when a peer is not being a true friend, when someone is starting to get annoyed, when a car is coming toward you and you're in the middle of the street)

How to Switch

- When switching from one stimulant to another, the first one can be abruptly stopped and the new one started the next morning. Side effects from abrupt discontinuation are not expected; however, some patients may experience marked fatigue and sleepiness for several days.
- See Appendix for approximate dosing equivalents when switching

How to Stop

- Taper not necessary, especially for patients who have only had short-term treatment or intermittent treatment
- However, if withdrawal symptoms develop, resume dosing the medication and then taper slowly over several days
- Withdrawal following chronic therapeutic use may unmask symptoms of the underlying disorder and may require follow-up and reinstitution of treatment
- Usually symptoms after discontinuation are return of symptoms of the underlying disorder rather than symptoms due to drug withdrawal
- Supervision during withdrawal is always recommended for any psychotropic medication

WHAT TO EXPECT

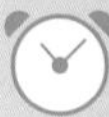

Onset of Action

- Some immediate effects can be seen with first dosing
- Takes a few days to attain therapeutic benefit generally

Duration of Action

Formulation	Brand names	Duration
Immediate-release tablet	Ritalin	3–4-hr duration, early peak
Immediate-release oral solution	Methylin	3–4-hr duration, early peak
Extended-release tablet	Methylin ER	3–8-hr duration, early peak
Extended-release tablet	Concerta	12-hr duration, small early peak
Extended-release chewable tablet	QuilliChew ER	8-hr duration, peak at 5 hr
Extended-release capsule	Metadate CD	8-hr duration, strong early peak
Extended-release capsule	Ritalin LA	6–8-hr duration, two strong peaks (early and at 4 hr)
Extended-release capsule	Aptensio XR	Up to 12-hr duration
Extended-release oral suspension	Quillivant XR	12-hr duration, peak at 5 hr
Extended-release transdermal patch	Daytrana	12-hr duration, peak at 7–10 hr
Orally disintegrating tablet	Cotempla XR-ODT	12-hour duration
Extended-release capsule	Jornay PM	Initial absorption delayed by 10 hr, single peak at 14 hr

- The pharmacokinetic curves for methylphenidate-based medications vary considerably based on their release properties (Figure 1).

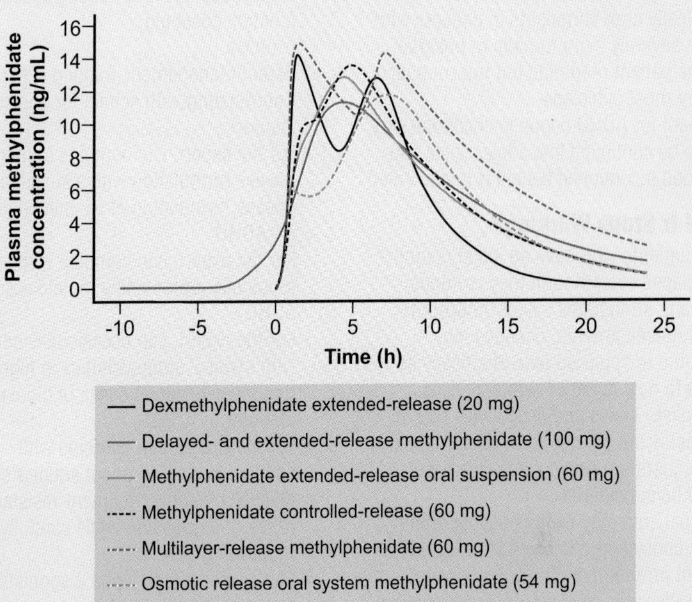

Figure 1 Methylphenidate concentrations over time with six preparations of methylphenidate. Adapted from Po et al., 2022.

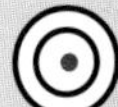

Primary Target Symptoms

- Concentration, attention span, distractibility
- Motor hyperactivity
- Impulsiveness
- Physical and mental fatigue
- Daytime sleepiness

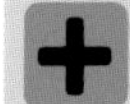

What Is Considered a Positive Result?

- The goal of treatment of ADHD is reduction of symptoms of inattentiveness, motor hyperactivity, and/or impulsiveness that disrupt social, school, and/or occupational functioning
- Can also improve oppositional and disruptive behaviors associated with ADHD
- The goal of treatment is complete remission of symptoms
- If treatment works, it most often reduces or even eliminates symptoms, but is not a cure since symptoms often recur after medicine is stopped

How Long to Treat

- ADHD is typically a lifelong illness; if any symptoms improve, hyperactivity is more likely to improve than inattention
- Can tell parents there is some chance that their child can grow out of this in adulthood, but many adults continue to have symptoms of ADHD throughout adolescence and adulthood
- Continue treatment until all symptoms are under control or improvement is stable and then continue treatment as long as improvement persists

- Reevaluate the need for treatment periodically; some clinicians advise to periodically stop stimulants in patients who are not severely symptomatic to observe how the patient responds but not routinely done by most clinicians
- Treatment for ADHD begun in childhood may need to be continued into adolescence and adulthood if continued benefit is documented

What If It Stops Working?

- Some patients who have an initial response may relapse even though they continue treatment, sometimes called "poop-out"
- Growth/developmental changes may contribute to apparent loss of efficacy as well as to new onset of side effects as metabolism slows and drug levels rise in transition from childhood to adolescence; dose adjustment (increase or decrease) should be considered
- Some patients may experience apparent lack of consistent efficacy due to activation of latent or underlying or newly evolved bipolar disorder, major depressive episodes with mixed features of mania, new onset of major depression or an anxiety disorder (GAD, OCD, PD), and require stimulant discontinuation and a switch to the clinically appropriate medication(s)

What If It Doesn't Work?

- In practice, many patients have only a partial response where some symptoms are improved but others persist, in which case higher doses of methylphenidate or adding a second agent, or switching to an agent with a different mechanism of action can be considered
- Consider evaluation for another diagnosis or for a comorbid condition (e.g., medical illness, substance abuse). Also, when treating ADHD, consider the possibility of a learning disorder or learning weakness and consider school-based interventions.
- Consider the presence of nonadherence and counsel patient and parents
- Consider a dose adjustment
- Some ADHD patients and some depressed patients may experience lack of consistent efficacy due to activation of latent or underlying bipolar disorder, and require either augmenting with a mood stabilizer or switching to a mood stabilizer
- Augmenting options:
  - Organizational skills training/executive function coaching
  - Exercise
  - Parent Management Training (PMT)
  - Coordinating with school for appropriate support
  - For the expert, can combine immediate-release formulation with a sustained-release formulation of D,L-methylphenidate for ADHD
  - For the expert, can combine with modafinil, atomoxetine, or viloxazine for ADHD
  - For the expert, can occasionally combine with atypical antipsychotics in highly treatment-resistant cases of bipolar disorder or ADHD
  - For the expert, can combine with antidepressants to boost antidepressant efficacy in highly treatment-resistant cases of depression while carefully monitoring patient
  - Can combine with alpha 2 agonists such as guanfacine or clonidine
- Consider factors associated with poor response to any psychotropic medication in children and adolescents, such as severe symptoms, long-lasting symptoms, nonadherence, prior nonresponse to other treatments, and the presence of comorbid psychiatric disorders or learning disorders
- Consider other important potential factors such as ongoing conflicts, family psychopathology, and an adverse environment (e.g., poverty, chaos, violence, prior and ongoing psychological trauma, abuse, bullying, less-than-ideal school placement, neglect)
- Institute trauma-informed care for appropriate children and adolescents

TALKING TO PATIENTS AND CAREGIVERS

What to Tell Parents About Efficacy

- Stimulant treatment for ADHD is one of the best studied of all medications in children and adolescents
- Often works right away once the dose is correct
- While the medicine helps ADHD by reducing symptoms and improving function, there are no cures for ADHD and it is therefore

necessary to keep taking the medication to sustain its therapeutic effects
- It does not work that day if the child/adolescent has not taken their medication in the morning
- For longer-acting stimulants, be careful not to give too late (i.e., after 11 a.m.) because it can cause insomnia that night
- Does not stay in the body for a long time, so it stops working rapidly after you stop it
- Since every treatment consideration depends on a risk/benefit analysis, parents should fully understand short- and long-term risks as well as benefits compared to nontreatment of ADHD
- Although many stimulants are approved for ADHD, if using off-label, often a good idea to tell parents whether the medication chosen is specifically approved for the disorder being treated, or whether it is being given for "unapproved" or "off-label" reasons based on good clinical practice, expert consensus, and/or prudent extrapolation of controlled data from adults
- Best results are often obtained when medications are combined with behavioral therapy
- Stimulants wear off after a number of hours and symptoms may return. Therefore, parents may complain that the medication isn't working if their child/adolescent is using a stimulant that lasts 8 hours, because it may have worn off after the patient has come home from school (and that is when the parents are seeing the child/adolescent) in comparison to a stimulant that lasts 10–12 hours and may keep working after the child/adolescent comes home from school.
- The American Academy of Child & Adolescent Psychiatry (AACAP) has helpful handouts for parents

What to Tell Children and Adolescents About Efficacy

- Be specific about the symptoms being targeted: we are trying to help you remember things better, do your best at school, follow the rules, get into less trouble (as applicable)
- It may be a good idea to give the medication a try; if it's not working very well, we can stop the medication and try something else
- You can be part of a special plan to help us figure out if the medicine is helpful for you. Would you like to do that? (for the parents and prescriber, can consider here a trial both on and then off medication, and then on again to see if the effects are clear and thus worth continuing the medication)
- The medication can work right away but a good try can take a few months to find the right dose
- Even if it does make you feel better, it will wear off and no longer work shortly after you stop it
- This medicine does not last very long in your body, so even if it does work, it won't work if you don't take it that day
- The medication can help you decide what you want to do, like making good choices versus bad choices; the medicine does not make you do something you don't want to do
- Medications don't change who you are as a person; they give you the opportunity to be the best person you can be

What to Tell Parents About Side Effects

- Explain that side effects are expected in many when starting
- Tell parents many side effects of stimulants often go away in a few days to weeks, especially nausea and insomnia, but if they don't we will change the treatment
- Predict side effects in advance (you will look clever and competent to the parents unless you scare them with too much information and cause nocebo effects, in which case you won't look so clever when the patient develops lots of side effects and stops medication; use your judgment here); a balanced but honest presentation is an art rather than a science
- Sometimes a trial off medication and then on again can clarify what the true therapeutic effects of the medication are
- Ask parents to support the patient while side effects are occurring
- Parents should fully understand short- and long-term risks as well as benefits
- Explaining to the parents what to expect from medication treatment, and especially potential side effects can help prevent early termination

What to Tell Children and Adolescents About Side Effects

- When a medicine starts to work, your body can first experience this by giving you unpleasant sensations – just like if you take a cough medicine it may taste bad – these body sensations include loss of appetite and problems sleeping. So, just like with a cough medicine, the bad taste will often go away before the medicine begins to stop the cough – many medicines work like that. It's important for you to pay attention to what your body is telling you, and we'll go over some of the ways that can happen.
- Even if you get a side effect, it's not permanent (it won't last forever)
- Explaining to child/adolescent what to expect from medication treatment, and especially potential side effects, can help prevent early termination

What to Tell Teachers About the Medication (If Parents Consent)

- Stimulants can be very helpful in improving the symptoms of ADHD: namely, inattention, impulsivity, and hyperactivity
- It does not work if the child/adolescent has not taken their medication that morning
- If the patient is sleepy, ask whether the medication is keeping them up at night or if they are eating enough food
- If the patient won't eat lunch or snacks, ask whether the medication is making them lose their appetite
- Medically speaking, methylphenidate is not a narcotic because doctors define narcotics as something that is sedating and sleep-inducing like opioids such as heroin and Oxycontin and not stimulants like methylphenidate
- Methylphenidate should be kept in school under lock and key or at the nurse's office or not brought to school at all because it can be diverted and misused by those who do not have ADHD. Some schools will suspend students who are caught with medications on their person or in their backpacks; most schools know the misuse or even abuse potential of stimulants.

SPECIAL POPULATIONS

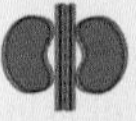

Renal Impairment

- No dose adjustment necessary

Hepatic Impairment

- No dose adjustment necessary

Cardiac Impairment

- Use with caution, particularly in patients with recent myocardial infarction or other conditions that could be negatively affected by increased blood pressure
- Do not use in patients with structural cardiac abnormalities without consultation with a cardiologist

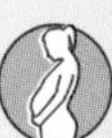

Pregnancy

- Controlled studies have not been conducted in pregnant women
- Infants whose mothers took methylphenidate during pregnancy may experience withdrawal symptoms
- Racemic methylphenidate has been shown to have teratogenic effects in rabbits when given in doses of 200 mg/kg/day throughout organogenesis
- Use in women of childbearing potential requires weighing potential benefits to the mother against potential risks to the fetus
- For ADHD patients, methylphenidate should generally be discontinued before anticipated pregnancies
- National Pregnancy Registry for Psychiatric Medications: 1-866-961-2388 or https://womensmentalhealth.org/research/pregnancyregistry/

Breast Feeding

- Unknown if methylphenidate is secreted in human breast milk, but all psychotropics assumed to be secreted in breast milk
- Recommended either to discontinue drug or formula feed
- If infant shows signs of irritability, drug may need to be discontinued

THE ART OF PSYCHOPHARMACOLOGY

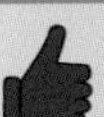

Potential Advantages

- In children:
  - Stimulants are probably the best studied psychotropic medications for use in children
  - Methylphenidate is one of the best studied stimulants in children
- In adolescents:
  - Can improve school performance and grades, especially if ADHD has been unrecognized and untreated prior to adolescence
  - Can improve performance in high school and college students whose ADHD is compromising academic performance due to the increased demands of higher levels of study
- All ages:
  - Methylphenidate has established long-term efficacy as a first-line treatment for ADHD
  - Multiple options for drug delivery, peak actions, and duration of action

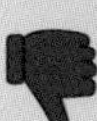

Potential Disadvantages

- Adolescents and especially college-age patients who divert their medication
- Patients with current substance abuse
- Patients with current manic or mixed symptoms associated with bipolar disorder or psychosis
- Patients with anorexia

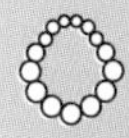

Pearls

- Half-life and duration of clinical action tend to be shorter in younger children than in adolescents and may require more frequent dosing or preferential use of long-acting preparations
- Drug abuse is no more likely and may even be lower (controversial) in ADHD adolescents treated with stimulants than in ADHD adolescents who are not treated with stimulants
- Stimulants have a moderate effect on decreasing ADHD symptoms and a moderate to large effect in decreasing aggression, oppositional behavior, and conduct problems in children with ADHD
- Meta-analyses suggest that when taking into account both efficacy and safety, methylphenidate is the best first-line stimulant in children and adolescents, whereas amphetamine is best in adults (Cortese et al., 2018)
- Stimulant dosing and titration are critical to optimizing response. Meta-analyses involving nearly 8,000 children/adolescents show that both methylphenidate and amphetamine salts have increased efficacy (but increased likelihood of discontinuation due to side effects) with higher doses (Farhat et al., 2022). In general, goal doses are often in the range of 0.8 mg/kg for methylphenidate and 0.5 mg/kg for amphetamine salts. However, these are rough guides that may not always be applicable depending on the formulation used and how completely (or incompletely) it's absorbed.
- Combinations of behavioral therapy or other nonmedication treatments along with stimulants may have better results than either treatment alone
- Newer sustained-release technologies are truly once-a-day dosing systems, with many options in terms of duration, timing of peak actions, and type of administration (Figure 1)
- Formulation options with a duration of action up to 12 hours may be preferable for those ADHD patients who do homework in the evening, have after-school jobs or extracurricular activities, including sports, or whose symptoms affect their family and/or social life
- Formulations with 8-hour-durations of action may be preferable for those ADHD patients who lose their appetite for dinner or have insomnia
- Some patients may benefit from an occasional addition of 5–10 mg of immediate-release methylphenidate as an afternoon "booster" to their sustained-release methylphenidate
- Rebound hyperactivity may occur in the afternoon and present with increased hyperactivity, restlessness, and irritability; if this occurs, can consider switching to a longer-acting agent or a nonstimulant or adding a short-acting stimulant
- On the other hand, too-high medication dosing may lead to cognitive rigidity,

difficulty shifting attention, and seeming "spaced out" or "different"

- Many patients taking stimulants have early-morning ADHD symptoms and can be hard to get going, prepare for school and be cooperative, especially for a few hours after awakening. In these patients, delayed-release/extended-release formulations may be especially helpful.
- Transdermal formulation may enhance adherence to treatment compared to some oral formulations because it allows once-daily application with all-day efficacy, has a smoother absorption curve, and allows for daily customization of treatment (i.e., it can be removed early if desired)
- On the other hand, the transdermal formulation has slower onset than oral formulations, requires a specific removal time, can cause skin sensitization, can be large depending on dose, and may lead to reduced efficacy if removed prematurely; also a risk if transdermal patch transferred to another child
- Stimulants are a classic augmentation strategy for treatment-refractory depression, although this is most established in adults
- Interestingly, in some studies combining stimulants with alpha 2 agonists, decreased side effects are seen with the combination compared to either medication as monotherapy. This is likely because of complementary side effects.

SUGGESTED READING

Biederman J, Spencer TJ, Monuteaux MC, Faraone SV. A naturalistic 10-year prospective study of height and weight in children with attention-deficit hyperactivity disorder grown up: sex and treatment effects. J Pediatr 2010;157(4):635–40.

Cohen SC, Mulqueen JM, Ferracioli-Oda E et al. Meta-analysis: risk of tics associated with psychostimulant use in randomized, placebo-controlled trials. J Am Acad Child Adolesc Psychiatry 2015;54(9):728–36.

Cortese S, Adamo N, Del Giovane C et al. Comparative efficacy and tolerability of medications for attention-deficit hyperactivity disorder in children, adolescents, and adults: a systematic review and network meta-analysis. Lancet Psychiatry 2018;5(9):727–38.

Farhat LC, Flores JM, Behling E et al. The effects of stimulant dose and dosing strategy on treatment outcomes in attention-deficit/hyperactivity disorder in children and adolescents: a meta-analysis. Mol Psychiatry 2022;27(3):1562–72.

Jensen PS, Arnold LE, Swanson JM et al. 3-year follow-up of the NIMH MTA study. J Am Acad Child Adolesc Psychiatry 2007;46(8):989–1002.

The MTA Cooperative Group. A 14-month randomized clinical trial of treatment strategies for attention-deficit/hyperactivity disorder. The MTA Cooperative Group. Multimodal Treatment Study of Children with ADHD. Arch Gen Psychiatry 1999;56(12):1073–86.

Po MD, Gomeni R, Incledon B. Quantitative characterization of the smoothness of extended-release methylphenidate pharmacokinetic profiles. Innov Clin Neurosci 2022;19(7–9):32–7.

Posner K, Melvin GA, Murray DW et al. Clinical presentation of attention-deficit/hyperactivity disorder in preschool children: the Preschoolers with Attention-Deficit/Hyperactivity Disorder Treatment Study (PATS). J Child Adolesc Psychopharmacol 2007;17(5):547–62.

Riddle MA, Yershova K, Lazzaretto D et al. The Preschool Attention-Deficit/Hyperactivity Disorder Treatment Study (PATS) 6-year follow-up. J Am Acad Child Adolesc Psychiatry 2013;52(3):264–78.

Swanson JM, Arnold LE, Molina BSG et al. Young adult outcomes in the follow-up of the multimodal treatment study of attention-deficit/hyperactivity disorder: symptom persistence, source discrepancy, and height suppression. J Child Psychol Psychiatry 2017;58(6):663–78.

Zhang L, Yao H, Li L, et al. Risk of cardiovascular diseases associated with medications used in attention-deficit/hyperactivity disorder: a systematic review and meta-analysis. JAMA Netw Open 2022;5(11):e2243597.

THERAPEUTICS

Brands

- Remeron, other

Generic

Yes

US FDA Approved for Pediatric Use

- None

Off-Label for Pediatric Use

- Approved in adults
  - Major depressive disorder
- Other off-label uses
  - Panic disorder
  - Generalized anxiety disorder
  - Posttraumatic stress disorder

Class and Mechanism of Action

- Neuroscience-based Nomenclature: serotonin, norepinephrine receptor antagonist (SN-RAn)
- Alpha 2 antagonist; NaSSA (noradrenaline and specific serotonergic agent); dual serotonin and norepinephrine agent; antidepressant
- Boost neurotransmitters serotonin and norepinephrine/noradrenaline
- Antagonism at presynaptic α2-receptors results in central disinhibition of serotonin and norepinephrine release
- When mirtazapine disinhibits serotonin release by the α2-antagonist mechanism, it causes serotonin to be released onto all serotonin receptors; however, mirtazapine simultaneously blocks the actions of serotonin at 5HT2A, 5HT2C, and 5HT3 receptors, leaving net stimulation of only 5HT1A receptors
- Blocks H1 histamine receptors

SAFETY AND TOLERABILITY

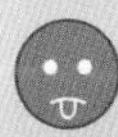

Notable Side Effects

- Dry mouth, constipation
- Increased appetite, weight gain
- Sedation, dizziness, abnormal dreams, confusion
- Flu-like symptoms (may indicate low white blood cell or granulocyte count)
- Change in urinary function
- Hypotension is less common in youth compared to adults and in pediatric trials occurred in 1.3% versus 1.1% of patients receiving mirtazapine versus placebo, respectively
- Note: patients with diagnosed or undiagnosed bipolar or psychotic disorders may be more vulnerable to CNS-activating actions of serotonergic agents like mirtazapine; pay particular attention to signs of activation in children with developmental disorders or autism spectrum disorders
- Treatment-emergent activation syndrome (TEAS) includes agitation, anxiety, panic attacks, irritability, aggression, impulsivity, and insomnia
- TEAS can represent side effects but should not be confused with bipolar mania or the onset of suicidality and should be monitored and investigated with consideration of discontinuing or decreasing the dose of mirtazapine or addition of another agent or switching to another agent to reduce these symptoms

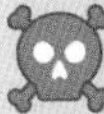

Life-Threatening or Dangerous Side Effects

- Rare seizures
- Rare induction of mania
- Rare suicidal ideation and behavior (suicidality) (short-term regulatory studies did not show any actual suicides in any age group and also did not show an increase in the risk of suicidality with antidepressants compared to placebo beyond age 24)

Growth and Maturation

- Growth should be monitored; long-term effects are unknown

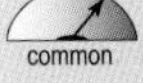

Weight Gain

- Many experience and/or can be significant in amount and in pediatric trials half of patients gained > 7% of their body weight

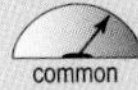

Sedation

- Many experience and/or can be significant in amount

What to Do About Side Effects

- Wait, wait, wait: mild side effects are common, happen early, and usually improve with time, but treatment benefits can be delayed and often begin just as the side effects wear off. However, some side effects may emerge later, such as weight gain.
- Monitor side effects closely, especially when initiating treatment
- May wish to give in the evening or at bedtime, particularly if the medication is associated with sedation
- For activation (jitteriness, anxiety, insomnia):
  - Consider a temporary dose reduction or a more gradual up-titration
  - Administer dose in the morning
  - Consider switching to an SSRI or potentially an SNRI (other than venlafaxine)
  - Optimize psychotherapeutic interventions
  - Activation and agitation may represent the induction of a bipolar state, especially a mixed dysphoric bipolar II condition sometimes associated with suicidal ideation, and may require the addition of lithium, or an atypical antipsychotic, and/or discontinuation of mirtazapine
- Often best to try another monotherapy prior to resorting to augmentation strategies to treat side effects
- For insomnia: consider adding melatonin

How Drug Causes Side Effects

- Histamine 1 receptor antagonism may explain sedative effects
- Histamine 1 receptor antagonism plus 5HT2C antagonism may explain some aspects of weight gain
- Alpha 2 receptors mediate peripheral vasoconstriction, and blockade of these receptors by mirtazapine may relate to (orthostatic) hypotension

Warnings and Precautions

- Consider distributing the brochures provided by the FDA and the drug companies as well as the medication guides from the American Academy of Child & Adolescent Psychiatry (AACAP)
- Carefully consider monitoring patients regularly and within the practical limits, particularly during the first several weeks of treatment
- Warn patients and their caregivers when possible about the possibility of activating side effects and advise them to report such symptoms
- Carefully weigh the risks and benefits of pharmacological treatment against the risks and benefits of nontreatment with antidepressants and make sure to document this in the patient's chart
- As with any antidepressant, use with caution in patients with history of seizure
- As with any antidepressant, use with caution in patients with bipolar disorder unless treated with concomitant mood-stabilizing agent
- Monitor patients for activation and suicidal ideation and involve parents/guardians
- Drug may lower white blood cell count (rare; may not be increased compared to other antidepressants but controlled studies lacking; not a common problem reported in postmarketing surveillance)
- Drug may increase cholesterol
- May cause photosensitivity
- Avoid alcohol, which may increase sedation and cognitive and motor effects

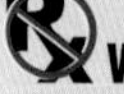

When Not to Prescribe

- If patient is taking an MAO inhibitor
- If there is a proven allergy to mirtazapine

Long-Term Use

- Growth should be monitored; long-term effects are unknown

Habit Forming

- No

Overdose

- Rarely lethal; all fatalities have involved other medications; symptoms include sedation, disorientation, memory impairment, rapid heartbeat

DOSING AND USE

Usual Dosage Range

- 15–45 mg at night

Dosage Forms

- Tablet 7.5 mg, 15 mg scored, 30 mg scored, 45 mg

- SolTab disintegrating tablet 15 mg, 30 mg, 45 mg

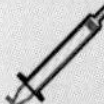

How to Dose

- Initial 15 mg/day in the evening; increase every 1–2 weeks until desired efficacy is reached; maximum generally 45 mg/day

Options for Administration

- Disintegrating tablet option for patients who have difficulty swallowing pills

Tests

- None for healthy individuals
- May need liver function tests for those with hepatic abnormalities before initiating treatment
- May need to monitor blood count during treatment for those with blood dyscrasias, leukopenia, or granulocytopenia
- Monitor weight and BMI percentiles during treatment

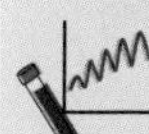

Pharmacokinetics

- Absorption is rapid and its bioavailability is approximately 50%
- Its protein binding is approximately 85%
- Half-life is 20–40 hours in adults and is significantly shorter in pediatric patients. In children, its half-life is approximately 23–24 hours and in adolescents (ages 12–17 years), its half-life is 32–35 hours.
- In general, by age 14 (male) or 15 (female), plasma concentrations become similar to those of an adult
- In children ages 7–17 years, the time to maximum concentration (Tmax) is 1.5–2.5 hours
- CYP2D6 and CYP1A2 are involved in the formation of the 8-hydroxy metabolite of mirtazapine, whereas CYP3A4 is responsible for the formation of the *N*-demethyl and *N*-oxide metabolites (Figure 1)
- Demethyl metabolite is pharmacologically active and appears to have the same pharmacokinetic profile as the parent compound in pediatric populations
- Food does not affect absorption

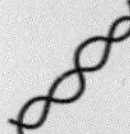

Pharmacogenetics

- The Clinical Pharmacogenetics Implementation Consortium does not provide dosing recommendations for mirtazapine

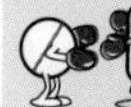

Drug Interactions

- Tramadol increases the risk of seizures in adults taking an antidepressant

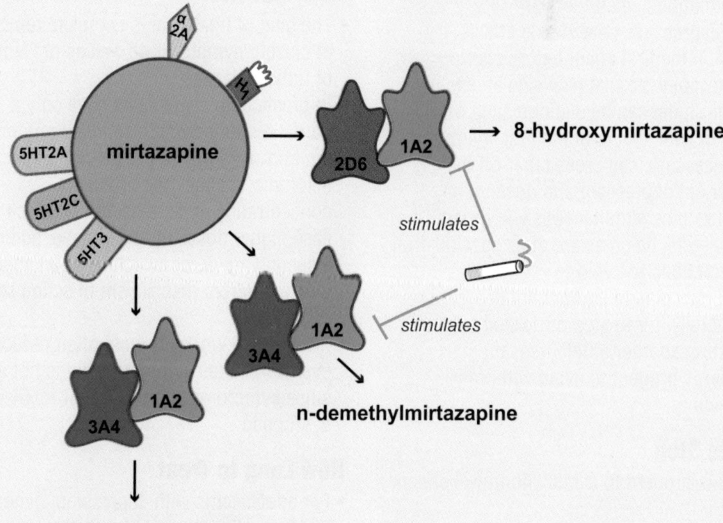

Figure 1 Mirtazapine metabolism.

- Can cause a fatal "serotonin syndrome" when combined with MAO inhibitors, so do not use with MAO inhibitors or for at least 14 days after MAOIs are stopped
- Do not start an MAO inhibitor for at least 5 half-lives (5 to 7 days for most drugs) after discontinuing mirtazapine
- No significant pharmacokinetic drug interactions

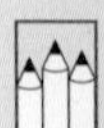

Dosing Tips

- Sedation may not worsen as dose increases
- Breaking a 15 mg tablet in half and administering 7.5 mg dose may actually increase sedation
- The more anxious and agitated the patient, the lower the starting dose, the slower the titration
- If intolerable anxiety, insomnia, agitation, akathisia, or activation occurs either upon dosing initiation or discontinuation, consider an alternative antidepressant. Importantly, the risk of activation with one antidepressant does not predict the likelihood of activation with another antidepressant.

How to Switch

- From another antidepressant to mirtazapine:
  - When tapering a prior antidepressant, see its entry in this manual for how to stop and how to taper off that specific drug
  - In situations when there are antidepressant-related side effects, try to stop the first agent before starting mirtazapine so that new side effects of mirtazapine can be distinguished from withdrawal effects of the first agent
  - If necessary, can cross taper off the prior antidepressant and dose up on mirtazapine simultaneously in urgent situations, being aware of all specific drug interactions to avoid
- Off mirtazapine to another antidepressant
  - Generally, try to stop mirtazapine before starting another antidepressant
  - Taper is prudent to avoid withdrawal effects

How to Stop

- Taper is prudent to avoid withdrawal effects

WHAT TO EXPECT

Onset of Action

- Actions on insomnia and anxiety can start shortly after initiation of dosing
- Full onset of therapeutic actions in depression is usually delayed by 2–4 weeks
- If it is not working within 6–8 weeks, it may require a dosage increase or it may not work at all

Duration of Action

- Effects are consistent over a 24-hour period
- May continue to work for many years to prevent relapse of symptoms

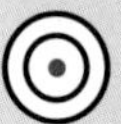

Primary Target Symptoms

- Depressed and/or irritable mood
- Anxiety (fear and worry are often target symptoms, but mirtazapine can occasionally and transiently increase these symptoms short term before improving them)
- Insomnia
- Prior to initiation of treatment, it is helpful to develop a list of target symptoms of depression and/or anxiety to monitor during treatment to better assess treatment response

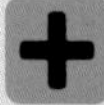

What Is Considered a Positive Result?

- The goal of treatment is complete remission of current symptoms as well as prevention of future relapses
- In practice, many patients have only a partial response where some symptoms are improved but others persist (especially insomnia, fatigue, and problems concentrating in depression), in which case higher doses of mirtazapine, adding a second agent, or switching to an agent with a different mechanism of action can be considered
- If treatment works, it most often reduces or even eliminates symptoms, but is not a cure since symptoms can recur after medicine is stopped

How Long to Treat

- For adolescents with depression, generally, 9–12 months of antidepressant treatment is recommended (Hathaway et al., 2018)

- For anxiety disorders, 6–9 months of antidepressant treatment may be sufficient, though many clinicians extend treatment to 12 months based on extrapolation of data from adults with anxiety disorders (Hathaway et al., 2018; Strawn et al., 2023)
- Extended treatment periods may decrease the risk of long-term morbidity and recurrence; however, the goal of treatment is ultimately remission, rather than duration of antidepressant pharmacotherapy (Hathaway et al., 2018)
- In terms of the length of antidepressant treatment, evidence-based guidelines represent a starting point; appropriate treatment duration varies, and patient-specific response, psychological factors, and timing of discontinuation must be considered for individual pediatric patients (Hathaway et al., 2018)

What If It Stops Working?

- Some patients who have an initial response may relapse even though they continue treatment, sometimes called "poop-out"
- Some patients may experience apparent lack of consistent efficacy due to activation syndrome or latent or underlying or newly evolved bipolar disorder, or major depressive episodes with mixed features, and require antidepressant discontinuation and a switch to a second generation antipsychotic

What If It Doesn't Work?

- Consider evaluation for another diagnosis (especially bipolar illness or depression with mixed features) or for a comorbid condition (e.g., medical illness, substance abuse)
- When treating youth with anxiety disorders, many patients will have had significant anxiety for years prior to beginning treatment. As such, when anxiety is treated with an SRI, their symptoms may be improved, but the patient has likely missed important developmental milestones (e.g., spending the night with friends, being able to ask questions in class). Developing these skills will take time. Beyond this, the family may have lived with the anxious child for years and following treatment of the child, the family may need to readjust.
- Be mindful of family conflict contributing to the presentation; sometimes treating parental depression or anxiety disorders improves psychiatric and social function without any treatment of youth. Also, accommodation is common in families of youth with anxiety disorders and may need to be addressed specifically, as it can perpetuate symptoms.
- Consider factors associated with poor response to medications in treatment-resistant depression or anxiety disorders, such as severe symptoms, long-lasting symptoms, poor treatment adherence, prior nonresponse to other treatments, and the presence of comorbid disorders
- Consider other important potential factors such as ongoing conflicts, family psychopathology, and an adverse environment (e.g., poverty, chaos, violence, prior and ongoing psychological trauma, abuse, neglect). Additionally, when symptoms are prominent at school, consider the presence of a learning disorder.
- Institute trauma-informed care for appropriate children and adolescents
- A 2007 meta-analysis of published and unpublished trials in pediatric patients found that antidepressants had a number needed to treat (NNT) of 10 for depression, 6 for OCD, and 3 for anxiety disorders; thus, mirtazapine may not work in all children, so consider switching to another antidepressant (Bridge et al., 2007)
- Consider a dose adjustment
- Consider augmenting options:
  - Cognitive behavioral therapy (CBT), interpersonal psychotherapy for adolescents (IPT-A), light therapy, family therapy, and exercise especially in adolescents
  - For partial response (depression): use caution when adding medications to mirtazapine, especially in children, since there are not sufficient studies of augmentation in children or adolescents; however, for the expert, consider bupropion, aripiprazole, or other atypical antipsychotics such as quetiapine; use combinations of antidepressants with caution as this may activate bipolar disorder and suicidal ideation
  - For insomnia: sleep hygiene, CBT for insomnia, melatonin

- For anxiety: buspirone, antihistamines
- Add lithium or atypical antipsychotics for bipolar depression, psychotic depression, treatment-resistant depression, or treatment-resistant anxiety disorders
- TMS (transcranial magnetic stimulation) may have a role although pediatric trials of TMS have been hampered by high sham response rates (Croarkin et al., 2021)
- ECT (case studies show effectiveness; cognitive side effects are similar to those in adults; reserve for treatment-resistant cases)

TALKING TO PATIENTS AND CAREGIVERS

What to Tell Parents About Efficacy

- Doesn't work right away; full therapeutic benefits may take up to 8 weeks, yet parents and teachers might see improvement before the patient does
- While the medicine helps by reducing symptoms and improving function, it is not a cure, and it is therefore necessary to keep taking the medication to sustain its therapeutic effects
- Since every treatment consideration depends on a risk/benefit analysis, parents should fully understand short- and long-term risks as well as benefits
- After successful treatment, continuation of mirtazapine may be necessary to prevent relapse, especially in those who have had more than one episode or a very severe episode. In general, when treating depression in children and adolescents, medications are continued for 12 months after symptoms have resolved, while for anxiety disorders, clinicians have generally treated for 6–9 months (Hathaway et al., 2017).
- Often a good idea to tell parents whether the medication chosen is specifically approved for the disorder being treated, or if it is "unapproved" or "off-label" but nevertheless good clinical practice and based upon prudent extrapolation of controlled data from adults and from experience in children and adolescents instead of formal FDA approval

What to Tell Children and Adolescents About Efficacy

- We are trying to make you feel better
- It may be a good idea to give the medication a try; if it's not working very well, we can stop the medication and try something else
- A good try takes 2 to 3 months or even longer
- If it does make you feel better, you cannot stop it right away or you may feel sad or worried again
- Medications don't change who you are as a person; they give you the opportunity to be the best person you can be

What to Tell Parents About Side Effects

- Explain that side effects are expected in many when starting and are most common in the first 2–3 weeks of starting or increasing the dose
- Some side effects emerge early and resolve quickly (e.g., activation, gastrointestinal symptoms). In contrast, other side effects are late-emerging (e.g., weight gain) or persistent (e.g., sexual dysfunction). Discussing the temporal course of the side effects and distinguishing between persistent and transient side effects is critical. Ensuring that patients are aware not only of side effects but the tendency of some side effects to be transient is important and should be part of discussions with patients and their families. For many, knowing that a side effect is likely transient, as opposed to persistent, may significantly influence the patient and family's anxiety or fears related to medication (Strawn et al., 2023).
- Tell parents many side effects go away and do so about the same time that therapeutic effects start
- Predict side effects in advance (you will look clever and competent to the parents, unless you scare them with too much information and cause nocebo effects, in which case you won't look so clever when the patient develops lots of side effects and stops medication; use your judgment here); a balanced but honest presentation is an art rather than a science
- Ask them to help monitor for increased suicidality and if present, report any such symptoms immediately
- Ask parents to support the patient while side effects are occurring

- Parents should fully understand short- and long-term risks as well as benefits
- Explaining to the parents what to expect from medication treatment, and especially potential side effects, can help prevent early termination of medication

What to Tell Children and Adolescents About Side Effects

- Even if you get side effects, most of them get better or go away in a few days to a few weeks
- Explaining to child/adolescent what to expect from medication treatment, and especially potential side effects, can help prevent early termination of medication
- Tell adolescents and children capable of understanding that some young patients, especially those who are depressed, may develop thoughts of hurting themselves, and if this happens, not to be alarmed but to tell their parents right away

What to Tell Teachers About the Medication (If Parents Consent)

- It is not abusable
- Encourage dialogue with parents/guardians about any behavior or mood changes

SPECIAL POPULATIONS

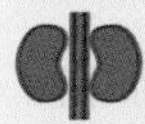

Renal Impairment

- Drug should be used with caution

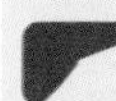

Hepatic Impairment

- Drug should be used with caution
- May require lower dose

Cardiac Impairment

- Should be used with caution, although in pediatric trials mirtazapine did not induce clinically relevant QTc interval changes compared to placebo
- The potential risk of hypotension should be considered, although this appears to be less common in pediatric patients than adults

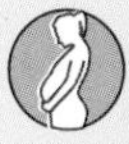

Pregnancy

- Controlled studies have not been conducted in pregnant women
- Increased risk of major neonatal malformations has not been reported
- Not generally recommended for use during pregnancy, especially during first trimester
- Must weigh the risk of treatment (first trimester fetal development, third trimester newborn delivery) to the child against the risk of no treatment (recurrence of depression, maternal health, infant bonding) to the mother and child
- For many patients, this may mean continuing treatment during pregnancy
- National Pregnancy Registry for Psychiatric Medications: 1-866-961-2388 or https://womensmentalhealth.org/research/pregnancyregistry/

Breast Feeding

- Unknown if mirtazapine is secreted in human breast milk, but all psychotropics assumed to be secreted in breast milk
- Trace amounts may be present in nursing children whose mothers are on mirtazapine
- If child becomes irritable or sedated, breast feeding or drug may need to be discontinued
- Immediate postpartum period is a high-risk time for depression, especially in women who have had prior depressive episodes, so drug may need to be reinstituted late in the third trimester or shortly after childbirth to prevent a recurrence during the postpartum period
- Must weigh benefits of breast feeding with risks and benefits of antidepressant treatment versus nontreatment to both the infant and the mother
- For many patients, this may mean continuing treatment during breast feeding

THE ART OF PSYCHOPHARMACOLOGY

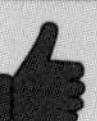

Potential Advantages

- Patients who wish to avoid sexual dysfunction
- Patients with symptoms of anxiety
- Patients on concomitant medications

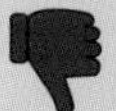

Potential Disadvantages

- Double-blind, randomized, placebo-controlled trial of mirtazapine for anxiety in children and adolescents with autism

spectrum disorder did not demonstrate efficacy
- Patients particularly concerned about gaining weight
- Patients with low energy

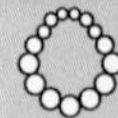

Pearls

- Adding alpha 2 antagonism to agents that block serotonin and/or norepinephrine reuptake may be synergistic for severe depression
- Two randomized, double-blind, placebo-controlled trials in children ages 7–18 years with major depressive disorder ($n = 259$) failed to demonstrate significant differences between mirtazapine and placebo (the studies used a flexible dose for the first 4 weeks (15–45 mg mirtazapine) followed by a fixed dose (15, 30, or 45 mg mirtazapine) for another 4 weeks
- In prospective trials of mirtazapine in youth, significant weight gain (≥7%) was observed in 49% of the mirtazapine-treated youth compared to 6% of those receiving placebo. Also, in these studies, youth experienced more urticaria (12% vs. 7%) and hypertriglyceridemia (3% vs. 0%).
- Does not affect the CYP system, and so may be preferable in patients requiring concomitant medications
- May cause sexual dysfunction only infrequently
- Patients can have carryover sedation and intoxicated-like feeling if particularly sensitive to sedative side effects when initiating dosing
- Rarely, patients may complain of visual "trails" or after-images on mirtazapine

Suggested Reading

Bridge JA, Iyengar S, Salary CB et al. Clinical response and risk for reported suicidal ideation and suicide attempts in pediatric antidepressant treatment: a meta-analysis of randomized controlled trials. JAMA 2007;297(15):1683–96.

Croarkin PE, Elmaadawi AZ, Aaronson ST et al. Left prefrontal transcranial magnetic stimulation for treatment-resistant depression in adolescents: a double-blind, randomized, sham-controlled trial. Neuropsychopharmacology 2021;46(2):462–9.

Haapasalo-Pesu K-M et al. Mirtazapine in the treatment of adolescents with major depression: an open-label, multicenter pilot study. J Child Adol Psychopharmacol 2004;14(2):175–84.

Hathaway EE, Walkup JT, Strawn JR. Antidepressant treatment duration in pediatric depressive and anxiety disorders: how long is long enough? Curr Probl Pediatr Adolesc Health Care 2018;48(2):31–9.

McDougle CJ, Thom R, Ravichandran CT et al. A randomized double-blind, placebo-controlled pilot trial of mirtazapine for anxiety in children and adolescents with autism spectrum disorder. Neuropsychopharmacology 2022;47(6):1263–70.

Smit M, Dolman KM, Honig A. Mirtazapine in pregnancy and lactation – a systematic review. Eur Neuropsychopharmacol 2016;26(1):126–35.

Strawn JR, Mills JA, Poweleit EA, Ramsey LB, Croarkin PE. Adverse effects of antidepressant medications and their management in children and adolescents. Pharmacotherapy 2023;43(7):675–90.

THERAPEUTICS

Brands

- Relprevv
- Symbyax (olanzapine–fluoxetine combination)
- Zydis
- Zyprexa

Generic

Yes

US FDA Approved for Pediatric Use

- Schizophrenia (Zyprexa, ages 13 and older)
- Acute mania/mixed mania (Zyprexa, ages 13 and older, monotherapy)
- Bipolar depression [in combination with fluoxetine (Symbyax), ages 10 and older]

Off-Label for Pediatric Use

- Approved in adults
  - Maintaining response in schizophrenia (Relprevv)
  - Acute mania/mixed mania (Zyprexa, adjunct)
  - Bipolar maintenance (Zyprexa, monotherapy)
  - Acute agitation associated with schizophrenia and bipolar I mania (intramuscular)
  - Treatment-resistant depression [in combination with fluoxetine (Symbyax)]
- Other off-label uses
  - Other psychotic disorder
  - Behavioral disturbances in children and adolescents
  - Disorders associated with problems with impulse control
  - Borderline personality disorder
  - Posttraumatic stress disorder
  - Appetite stimulation in adolescents with anorexia nervosa and some additional eating disorders

Class and Mechanism of Action

- Neuroscience-based Nomenclature: dopamine and serotonin receptor antagonist (DS-RAn)
- Atypical antipsychotic (serotonin-dopamine antagonist; second generation antipsychotic; also a mood stabilizer)
- Blocks dopamine 2 receptors, reducing positive symptoms of psychosis and stabilizing affective symptoms
- Blockade of serotonin type 2A receptors may also contribute at clinical doses to the enhancement of dopamine release in certain brain regions, thus theoretically reducing motor side effects
- Interactions at a myriad of other neurotransmitter receptors may contribute to olanzapine's efficacy
- Specifically, antagonist actions at 5HT2C receptors may contribute to efficacy for cognitive and affective symptoms in some patients
- 5HT2C antagonist actions plus serotonin reuptake blockade of fluoxetine add to the actions of olanzapine when given as Symbyax (olanzapine–fluoxetine combination)

SAFETY AND TOLERABILITY

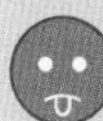

Notable Side Effects

- Probably increases risk for diabetes and dyslipidemia
- Drug-induced parkinsonism
- Dizziness, sedation, headache
- Abdominal pain, extremity pain
- Dry mouth
- Liver enzymes increased
- Weight gain, increased appetite
- Hyperprolactinemia: in a naturalistic inception cohort study of 396 children and adolescents, risperidone, and, to a lesser extent, olanzapine were associated with prolactin elevation and hyperprolactinemia, whereas quetiapine and aripiprazole were not; peak prolactin levels with olanzapine were observed between 4–5 weeks (Koch et al., 2023)
- Risk of drug-induced parkinsonism and dystonic reactions may be higher in children than it is in adults
- Risk of withdrawal dyskinesias

Life-Threatening or Dangerous Side Effects

- Hyperglycemia, in some cases extreme and associated with ketoacidosis or hyperosmolar coma or death, has been reported in patients taking atypical antipsychotics
- Rare but serious skin condition known as Drug Reaction with Eosinophilia and Systemic Symptoms (DRESS)

- Rare neuroleptic malignant syndrome (NMS) may cause hyperpyrexia, muscle rigidity, delirium, and autonomic instability with elevated creatine phosphokinase, myoglobinuria (rhabdomyolysis), and acute renal failure
- Rare seizures
- As a class, antidepressants have been reported to increase the risk of suicidal thoughts and behaviors in children and young adults

Growth and Maturation

- Long-term effects are unknown

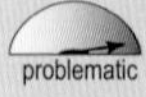

Weight Gain

- Frequent and can be significant in amount
- Can become a health problem in some
- May be even more risk of weight gain and metabolic effects in children than in adults

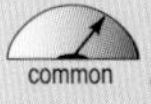

Sedation

- Many patients experience and/or can be significant in amount

What to Do About Side Effects

- Wait, wait, wait: mild side effects are common, happen early, and usually improve with time, but treatment benefits can be delayed. However, weight gain and metabolic disturbance can emerge at any point (although they are more common earlier).
- Monitor side effects closely, especially when initiating treatment
- May wish to give at night if not tolerated during the day and doesn't disrupt sleep
- Often best to try another monotherapy trial of a different antipsychotic prior to resorting to augmentation strategies to treat side effects
- Exercise and diet programs and medical management for high BMI percentiles, diabetes, dyslipidemia. Also, randomized controlled trials in youth suggest that omega-3 fatty acids can reduce SGA-related hypertriglyceridemia.
- Reduce the dose, particularly for drug-induced parkinsonism, akathisia, sedation, and tremor
- For drug-induced parkinsonism: consider reducing dose or switching to another agent. Augmenting with diphenhydramine or benztropine is less preferred in youth.
- For akathisia: reduce the dose or add a beta blocker. If these are ineffective, raising the dose of the beta blocker may be helpful.
- Using a 5HT2A antagonist such as mirtazapine or cyproheptadine to treat drug-induced akathisia is less common in children and adolescents compared to adults

How Drug Causes Side Effects

- By blocking histamine 1 receptors in the brain, it can cause sedation and possibly weight gain
- Blocking alpha 1 adrenergic receptors can cause dizziness, hypotension, and syncope
- Blocking muscarinic cholinergic receptors can cause dry mouth, blurred vision, urinary retention, constipation, and paralytic ileus
- By blocking dopamine 2 receptors in the striatum, it can cause drug-induced parkinsonism and akathisia as well as hyperprolactinemia
- Mechanism of any possible weight gain is unknown but may relate to effects at 5HT2C receptors
- Mechanism of any possible increased incidence of diabetes or dyslipidemia is unknown

Warnings and Precautions

- Consider distributing brochures provided by the FDA and the drug companies or have the pharmacy do this for the parents
- When olanzapine is used to treat depressive mood disorders off-label in children, either as a monotherapy or an augmenting agent to an SSRI/SNRI, it is a good idea to warn patients and their caregivers about the possibility of activating side effects and suicidality as for any antidepressant in this age group and advise them to report such symptoms immediately
- Carefully weigh the risks and benefits of pharmacological treatment against the risks and benefits of nontreatment with an antipsychotic and it is a good idea to document this in the patient's chart
- Olanzapine is associated with a rare but serious skin condition known as Drug Reaction with Eosinophilia and Systemic Symptoms (DRESS). DRESS may begin as

a rash but can progress to other parts of the body and can include symptoms such as fever, swollen lymph nodes, swollen face, inflammation of organs, and an increase in white blood cells known as eosinophilia. In some cases, DRESS can lead to death. Clinicians prescribing olanzapine should inform patients about the risk of DRESS; patients who develop a fever with rash and swollen lymph nodes or swollen face should seek medical care. Patients are not advised to stop their medication without consulting their prescribing clinician.
- Use with caution in patients with conditions that predispose to hypotension (dehydration, overheating)
- Use with caution in patients with prostatic hypertrophy, angle-closure glaucoma, paralytic ileus
- Atypical antipsychotics have the potential for cognitive and motor impairment, especially related to sedation
- Atypical antipsychotics can cause body temperature dysregulation; use caution in patients who may experience conditions that increase body temperature (e.g., strenuous exercise, saunas, extreme heat, dehydration, or concomitant anticholinergic medication)
- Patients receiving the intramuscular formulation of olanzapine should be observed closely for hypotension
- Intramuscular formulation is not generally recommended to be administered with parenteral benzodiazepines; if patient requires a parenteral benzodiazepine, it should be given at least 1 hour after intramuscular olanzapine
- As with any antipsychotic, use with caution in patients with history of seizures
- Dose-dependent hyperprolactinemia (in children and adolescents, serum prolactin levels tend to rise and peak within the first 1 to 2 months and then steadily decline to values within or very close to the normal range within 6 months)

When Not to Prescribe

- If there is a proven allergy to olanzapine
- Intramuscular formulation only: if there is a known risk of angle-closure glaucoma or if the patient has an unstable medical condition (e.g., acute myocardial infarction, unstable angina pectoris, severe hypotension and/or bradycardia, sick sinus syndrome, recent heart surgery)

Long-Term Use

- Approved in adults for long-term maintenance in bipolar disorder
- Approved in adults to maintain response in long-term treatment of schizophrenia
- Often used for long-term maintenance in various behavioral disorders

Habit Forming

- No

Overdose

- Rarely lethal in monotherapy overdose; sedation, slurred speech

DOSING AND USE

Usual Dosage Range

- Bipolar mania and schizophrenia: 10 mg/day
- Bipolar depression: 3 mg/25 mg–12 mg/50 mg once daily in the evening

Dosage Forms

- Tablet 2.5 mg, 5 mg, 7.5 mg, 10 mg, 15 mg, 20 mg
- Orally disintegrating tablet 5 mg, 10 mg, 15 mg, 20 mg
- Intramuscular formulation 5 mg/mL, each vial contains 10 mg (available in some countries)
- Depot 210 mg, 300 mg, 405 mg
- Olanzapine–fluoxetine combination capsule (mg equivalent olanzapine/mg equivalent fluoxetine) 3 mg/25 mg, 6 mg/25 mg, 6 mg/50 mg, 12 mg/25 mg, 12 mg/50 mg

How to Dose

- Bipolar depression: initial 2.5 mg olanzapine/20 mg fluoxetine once daily in the evening; adjust based on tolerability/efficacy; usual dose 3 mg/25 mg–12 mg/50 mg once daily in the evening
- Bipolar mania and schizophrenia: initial 2.5–5 mg once daily; increase by 2.5–5 mg/day once a week until desired efficacy is reached; target dose is 10 mg/day; maximum dose studied in clinical trials is 20 mg/day

Options for Administration

- Orally disintegrating tablet provides an alternative for patients who have difficulty swallowing pills
- Long-acting injectable formulations not approved in children/adolescents and few studies; probably best not to use long-acting injectables in children at all, and only with caution off-label in adolescents who are older and have adult body weights

Tests

- Before starting olanzapine:
  - Plan to monitor weight and metabolic parameters more closely than in adults since children and adolescents may be more prone to metabolic side effects than adults
  - Weigh all patients and monitor weight gain against that expected for normal growth, using the pediatric height/weight chart to monitor. In particular, monitor BMI percentiles.
  - Get baseline personal and family history of diabetes, obesity, dyslipidemia, hypertension, and cardiovascular disease
  - Obtain blood pressure, fasting plasma glucose (or hemoglobin A1C), and a lipid profile
- After starting olanzapine:
  - BMI percentile monthly for 3 months, then quarterly
  - Consider monitoring fasting triglycerides monthly in patients at high risk for metabolic complications
  - Blood pressure, fasting plasma glucose (or hemoglobin A1C), lipid profile within 3 months and then annually
  - Treat or refer for treatment and consider switching to another atypical antipsychotic for patients who become overweight, obese, pre-diabetic, diabetic, or dyslipidemic while receiving an atypical antipsychotic
  - Even in patients without known diabetes, be vigilant for the rare but life-threatening onset of diabetic ketoacidosis, which always requires immediate treatment, by monitoring for the rapid onset of polyuria, polydipsia, weight loss, nausea, vomiting, dehydration, rapid respiration, weakness, and clouding of sensorium, even coma
  - Patients with low white blood cell count (WBC) or history of drug-induced leukopenia/neutropenia should have complete blood count (CBC) monitored frequently during the first few months and olanzapine should be discontinued at the first sign of decline of WBC in the absence of other causative factors
  - Consider monitoring plasma drug levels of olanzapine if not responding, or questions about compliance or side effects
  - Patients should be monitored periodically for the development of abnormal movements using neurological exam and the Abnormal Involuntary Movement Scale (AIMS)

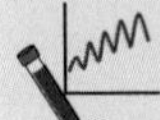

Pharmacokinetics

- Olanzapine is highly lipophilic and absorbed from the gastrointestinal tract, although ~40% of the drug is metabolized prior to reaching the systemic circulation, which results in 60% bioavailability
- Olanzapine is extensively metabolized in the liver through the CYP1A2 and CYP2D6 enzymes (Strawn and DelBello, 2008) (Figure 1)
- Food does not significantly affect absorption in clinical studies of adults
- Peak plasma concentrations in adults are observed within 6 hours of oral administration, although because of the long half-life of olanzapine (21–54 hours), steady-state concentrations are not reached until ~7 days
- In children and adolescents, the half-life is slightly lower than in adults. This lower half-life, as well as findings of increased clearance in children and adolescents, was thought to be related to a reduced first-pass effect and higher bioavailability. Alternatively, these pharmacokinetic differences may also be related to lower rates of cigarette smoking in children and adolescents.
- Olanzapine is highly (93%) protein bound and has a large volume of distribution (1,000 L in adults)
- In pediatric patients, olanzapine's pharmacokinetics are linear over a dosage range of 2.5–20 mg

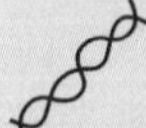

Pharmacogenetics

- No recommendations

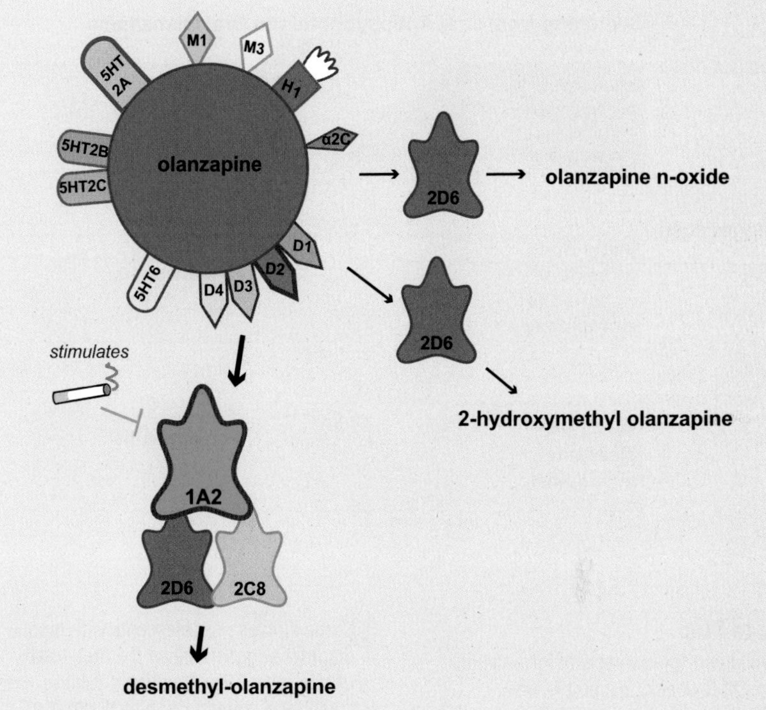

Figure 1 Metabolism of olanzapine.

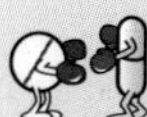

Drug Interactions

- Dose may need to be lowered if given with CYP1A2 inhibitors (e.g., fluvoxamine); raised if given in conjunction with CYP1A2 inducers (e.g., cigarette smoke, carbamazepine)
- Parenteral olanzapine should not be administered within 1 hour of benzodiazepines

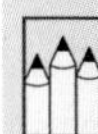

Dosing Tips

- Intramuscular formulation has not been studied in patients under 18 and is not recommended for use in this population
- Orally disintegrating tablet can be administered with or without liquid
- For treatment resistance, consider obtaining plasma drug levels to guide dosing above recommended levels
- Treatment should be suspended if absolute neutrophil count falls below 1,000/mm³

How to Switch

- From another antipsychotic to olanzapine:
  - When tapering a prior antipsychotic, see its entry in this manual for how to stop and how to taper off that specific drug
  - Generally, try to stop the first agent before starting olanzapine so that new side effects of olanzapine can be distinguished from withdrawal effects of the first agent
  - If urgent, cross taper off the other antipsychotic while olanzapine is started at a low dose, with dose adjustments down of the other antipsychotic, and up for olanzapine every 3 to 7 days
- Off olanzapine to another antipsychotic:
  - Generally, try to stop olanzapine before starting the new antipsychotic so that new side effects of the next drug can be distinguished from any withdrawal effects from olanzapine
  - If urgent, cross taper off olanzapine by cutting the dose in half as the new antipsychotic is also started with dose adjustments down of olanzapine and up for the new antipsychotic

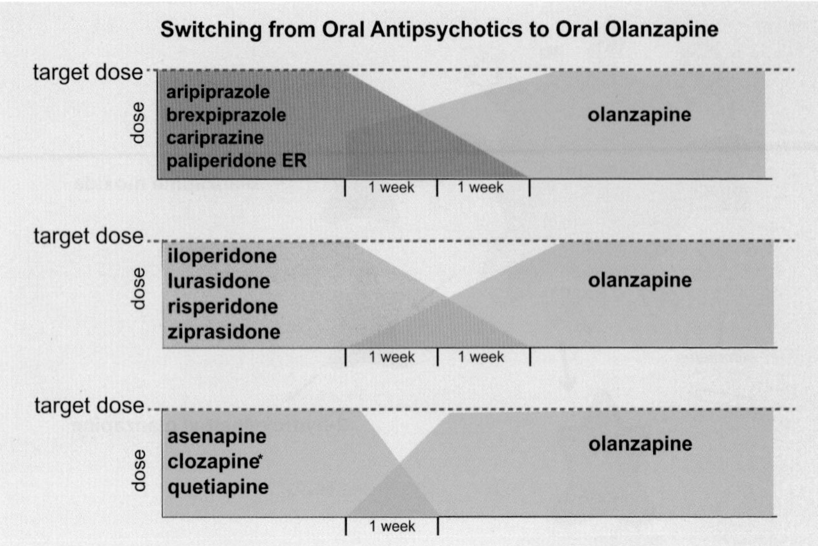

How to Stop

- Slow down-titration of oral formulation (over 6–8 weeks), especially when simultaneously beginning a new antipsychotic while switching (i.e., cross-titration)
- Make down-titration even slower if any signs of anticholinergic rebound such as tachycardia, tremor, gastrointestinal symptoms
- Rapid oral discontinuation may lead to rebound psychosis and worsening of symptoms
- Rapid oral discontinuation may lead to withdrawal dyskinesias, which are generally reversible in the pediatric population. Of note, withdrawal dyskinesias are more common in pediatric patients than in adults.
- If antiparkinsonian agents are being used, they should be continued for a few weeks after olanzapine is discontinued

WHAT TO EXPECT

Onset of Action

- Psychotic and manic symptoms can improve within 1 week of oral dosing, but it may take several weeks for full effect on behavior as well as on cognition and affective stabilization
- Some studies in adolescents with bipolar disorder suggest that by the first week of treatment 70% of patients achieve "response" criteria (Xiao et al., 2017)
- If it is not working within 6–8 weeks, it may require a dosage increase or it may not work at all
- Acute intramuscular dosing for agitation can have onset within minutes to an hour, but not well studied or specifically approved for children/adolescents

Duration of Action

- Effects of oral medication are consistent over a 24-hour period
- However, in children with rapid drug metabolism, two divided doses may be necessary for consistent effects over 24 hours
- Oral medication may continue to work for many years to prevent relapse of symptoms

Primary Target Symptoms

- Positive symptoms of psychosis
- Negative symptoms of psychosis
- Cognitive symptoms
- Unstable mood (both depressed mood and mania)
- Aggressive symptoms
- Appetite stimulation in patients with anorexia nervosa or other eating disorders

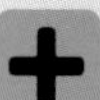

What Is Considered a Positive Result?

- In schizophrenia:
  - Most often reduces positive symptoms but does not eliminate them
  - Can improve negative symptoms, as well as aggressive, cognitive, and affective symptoms but less so than for positive symptoms
  - Can improve acute agitation
  - In children or adolescents with a first episode of psychosis, initial response may be greater than for recurrent episodes of psychosis in adults
- In bipolar disorder:
  - Many patients may experience a reduction of symptoms by half or more
  - Can improve agitation in bipolar mania
- In depression:
  - Full elimination of depressed mood, anxiety, and other symptoms of depression is the goal

How Long to Treat

- In schizophrenia and bipolar disorder:
  - Continue treatment until reaching a plateau of improvement
  - After reaching a satisfactory plateau, continue treatment for at least a year after first episode of psychosis or mania
  - For second and subsequent episodes of psychosis or mania, treatment may need to be indefinite
- In depression:
  - If it is the first episode, continue for 6–12 months after reaching full remission
  - If it is the second episode, continue for 12–24 months after reaching full remission
  - If it is the third or greater episode, continue treatment indefinitely

What If It Stops Working?

- Check for nonadherence, possibly by checking plasma drug level, and consider switching to another antipsychotic with fewer side effects
- Some patients who have an initial response may relapse even though they continue treatment, sometimes called "poop-out"
- Screen for the development of a new comorbid disorder, especially substance use
- Screen for adverse changes in the home or school environment

What If It Doesn't Work?

- Consider evaluation for another diagnosis (especially bipolar illness or depression with mixed features) or for a comorbid condition (e.g., medical illness, substance use)
- Consider other important potential factors such as ongoing conflicts, family psychopathology, and an adverse environment (e.g., poverty, chaos, violence, prior and ongoing psychological trauma, abuse, neglect)
- Institute trauma-informed care for appropriate children and adolescents
- For schizophrenia or bipolar disorder:
  - Try one of the other atypical antipsychotics
  - If no first-line atypical antipsychotic is effective, consider higher doses or augmentation with valproate, lithium, or lamotrigine
  - Consider initiating psychotherapy. In adolescents with bipolar disorder (and those with affective symptoms who are at risk of developing bipolar disorder), family-focused psychotherapy can be particularly helpful (Miklowitz et al., 2020).
  - Consider presence of concomitant drug abuse
- Fluoxetine and other antidepressants may be effective augmenting agents to olanzapine for bipolar depression, psychotic depression, and for unipolar depression not responsive to antidepressants alone (e.g., olanzapine–fluoxetine combination)

TALKING TO PATIENTS AND CAREGIVERS

What to Tell Parents About Efficacy

- For acute symptoms, it can work right away
- Intramuscular olanzapine can be given by a healthcare professional on an as needed basis for some symptoms like agitation; oral olanzapine can be given by a parent under supervision by a healthcare professional off-label on an as needed basis as well
- Oral olanzapine is usually given every day
- Explain which use olanzapine is being chosen for, how to tell if the drug is working

by targeting specific symptoms, and why this is being done
- Once the child/adolescent calms down, at some point after one dose or after several days of dosing or after long-term dosing, we should all assess whether the medication should be continued
- While the medicine helps by reducing symptoms and improving function, it is not a cure, and it therefore may be necessary to keep taking the medication long term to sustain its therapeutic effects
- Since every treatment consideration depends on a risk/benefit analysis, parents should fully understand short- and long-term risks as well as benefits
- Often a good idea to tell parents whether the medication chosen is specifically approved for the disorder being treated, or whether it is being given for "unapproved" or "off-label" reasons based on good clinical practice, expert consensus, and/or prudent extrapolation of controlled data from adults

What to Tell Children and Adolescents About Efficacy

- Be specific about the symptoms being targeted: we are trying to help you …
- Give the medication a try; if it's not working very well, we can stop the medication and try something else
- A good try often takes several weeks
- If it does make you feel better, you cannot stop it right away or you may get sick again
- Medications don't change who you are as a person; they give you the opportunity to be the best person you can be

What to Tell Parents About Side Effects

- Explain that side effects are expected in many when starting
- Tell parents many side effects go away and do so about the same time that therapeutic effects start
- Predict side effects in advance (you will look clever and competent to the parents, unless you scare them with too much information and cause nocebo effects, in which case you won't look so clever when the patient develops lots of side effects and stops medication; use your judgment here); a balanced but honest presentation is an art rather than a science
- Ask parents to support the patient while side effects are occurring
- Parents should fully understand short- and long-term risks as well as benefits
- Explaining to the parents what to expect from medication treatment, and especially what potential side effects to expect, can help prevent early termination of medication

What to Tell Children and Adolescents About Side Effects

- Even if you get side effects, most of them get better or go away in a few weeks
- If you have side effects that are bothering you, tell your parents and your parents should tell me
- Consider having a conversation about sexual side effects in some adolescents who can find these side effects confusing and especially burdensome
- Explaining to child/adolescent what to expect from medication treatment, and especially potential side effects, can help prevent early termination of medication

What to Tell Teachers About the Medication (If Parents Consent)

- Olanzapine can make children/adolescents sedated
- It is not abusable
- Encourage dialogue with parents/guardians about any behavior or mood changes
- Notify the clinician of increased restlessness or akathisia symptoms, which may be apparent in the school setting

SPECIAL POPULATIONS

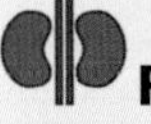

Renal Impairment

- No dose adjustment required for oral formulation
- Not removed by hemodialysis

Hepatic Impairment

- May need to lower dose
- Patients with liver disease should have liver function tests a few times a year

Cardiac Impairment

- Use in patients with cardiac impairment has not been studied; however, the risk of orthostatic hypotension in pediatric patients is less than in adults, as children rely less on peripheral vasoconstriction to regulate blood pressure

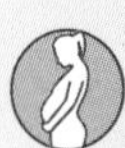

Pregnancy

- Controlled studies have not been conducted in pregnant women
- There is a risk of abnormal muscle movements and withdrawal symptoms in newborns whose mothers took an antipsychotic during the third trimester; symptoms may include agitation, abnormally increased or decreased muscle tone, tremor, sleepiness, severe difficulty breathing, and difficulty feeding
- Psychotic symptoms may worsen during pregnancy, and some form of treatment may be necessary
- Early findings of infants exposed to olanzapine in utero currently do not show adverse consequences
- When administered to pregnant rats and rabbits, olanzapine was not teratogenic at doses that are 9- and 30-times the maximum recommended human dose; some fetal toxicities were observed at these doses
- Olanzapine may be preferable to anticonvulsant mood stabilizers if treatment is required during pregnancy
- National Pregnancy Registry for Atypical Antipsychotics: 1-866-961-2388 or http://womensmentalhealth.org/clinical-and-research-programs/pregnancyregistry/

Breast Feeding

- Some drug is found in breast milk
- Recommended either to discontinue drug or formula feed
- Infants of women who choose to breast feed while on olanzapine should be monitored for possible adverse effects; sedation, failure to thrive, jitteriness, tremor, and abnormal muscle movements have been reported

THE ART OF PSYCHOPHARMACOLOGY

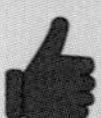

Potential Advantages

- In children:
  - Can provide more sedation than some other atypical antipsychotics if that is desired for symptom control
- In adolescents:
  - Approved for schizophrenia and manic/mixed episodes
- All ages:
  - Some cases of psychosis and bipolar disorder refractory to treatment with other antipsychotics
  - Often a preferred augmenting agent in bipolar depression or treatment-resistant unipolar depression

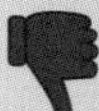

Potential Disadvantages

- In children and adolescents:
  - Can provide more sedation than some other atypical antipsychotics if that is NOT desired for symptom control
  - May be more susceptible to side effects, including sedation and weight gain
- All ages:
  - Patients concerned about gaining weight
  - Patients with diabetes mellitus, obesity, and/or dyslipidemia

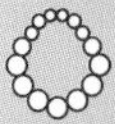

Pearls

- Often considered an atypical antipsychotic with "more efficacy but also more side effects"
- May cause more metabolic disturbances and weight gain than most other atypical antipsychotics; however, metformin (Ellul et al., 2018) or topiramate (DelBello et al., 2023) could decrease – but not eliminate – this risk
- Patients with inadequate responses to olanzapine may benefit either from switching to another atypical antipsychotic, or for experts, determination of plasma drug levels of olanzapine to guide dosage increase even beyond the usual prescribing limits
- Well accepted for use in schizophrenia and bipolar disorder, including difficult cases
- Documented utility in treatment-refractory cases, especially at higher doses

- Documented efficacy as augmenting agent to SSRIs (fluoxetine) in nonpsychotic treatment-resistant major depressive disorder in adults
- Documented efficacy and FDA approval in children and adolescents with bipolar I depression (ages 10–17) in combination with fluoxetine; however, in the clinical trials OFC was associated with very significant weight gain and hyperlipidemia (Detke et al., 2015)
- Motor side effects unusual at low- to mid-doses
- Cigarette smoke can decrease olanzapine levels and patients may require a dose increase if they begin or increase smoking

SUGGESTED READING

DelBello MP, Bruns KM, Bloom T et al. A double-blind placebo-controlled pilot study of topiramate in manic adolescents treated with olanzapine. J Child Adolesc Psychopharmacol 2023;33(4):126–33.

Detke HC, DelBello MP, Landry J, Usher RW. Olanzapine/fluoxetine combination in children and adolescents with bipolar I depression: a randomized, double-blind, placebo-controlled trial. J Am Acad Child Adolesc Psychiatry 2015;54(3):217–24.

Ellul P, Delorme R, Cortese S. Metformin for weight gain associated with second-generation antipsychotics in children and adolescents: a systematic review and meta-analysis. CNS Drugs 2018;32(12):1103–12.

Han R, Bian Q, Chen H. Effectiveness of olanzapine in the treatment of anorexia nervosa: A systematic review and meta-analysis. Brain Behav 2022;12(2):e2498.

Koch MT, Carlson HE, Kazimi MM, Correll CU. Antipsychotic-related prolactin levels and sexual dysfunction in mentally ill youth: a 3-month cohort-study. J Am Acad Child Adolesc Psychiatry 2023 ;62(9): 1021–50.

Kryzhanovskaya L, Schulz SC, McDougle C et al. Olanzapine versus placebo in adolescents with schizophrenia: a 6-week, randomized, double-blind, placebo-controlled trial. J Am Acad Child Adolesc Psychiatry 2009;48(1):60–70.

Lytle S, McVoy M, Sajatovic M. Long-acting injectable antipsychotics in children and adolescents. J Child Adolesc Psychopharmacol 2017;27(1):2–9.

Miklowitz DJ, Schneck CD, Walshaw PD et al. Effects of family-focused therapy vs enhanced usual care for symptomatic youths at high risk for bipolar disorder: a randomized clinical trial. JAMA Psychiatry 2020;77(5):455–63.

Pillay J, Boylan K, Carrey N et al. First- and Second-Generation Antipsychotics in Children and Young Adults: Systematic Review Update [Internet]. Rockville, MD: Agency for Healthcare Research and Quality (US); 2017 Mar. Report No.: 17-EHC001-EF. AHRQ Comparative Effectiveness Reviews.

Stentebjerg-Olesen M, Ganocy SJ, Findling RL et al. Early response or nonresponse at week 2 and week 3 predict ultimate response or nonresponse in adolescents with schizophrenia treated with olanzapine: results from a 6-week randomized, placebo-controlled trial. Eur Child Adolesc Psychiatry 2015;24(12):1485–96.

Strawn JR, Delbello MP. Olanzapine for the treatment of bipolar disorder in children and adolescents. Expert Opin Pharmacother 2008;9(3):467–74.

Xiao L, Ganocy SJ, Findling RL, et al. Baseline characteristics and early response at week 1 predict treatment outcome in adolescents with bipolar manic or mixed episode treated with olanzapine: results from a 3-week, randomized, placebo-controlled trial. J Clin Psychiatry 2017;78(9):e1158-66.

THERAPEUTICS

Brands
- Oxtellar XR
- Trileptal

Generic
Yes

US FDA Approved for Pediatric Use
- Monotherapy treatment for partial seizures in children ages 4–16 with epilepsy (immediate-release) (also approved for this use in adults)
- Adjunctive therapy for partial seizures in children ages 2–16 with epilepsy (immediate-release) (also approved for this use in adults)
- Treatment of partial-onset seizures in patients ages 6 years and older (extended-release)

Off-Label for Pediatric Use
- Approved in adults
  - None
- Other off-label uses
  - Bipolar disorder

Class and Mechanism of Action
- Anticonvulsant, voltage-sensitive sodium channel modulator
- Acts as a use-dependent blocker of voltage-sensitive sodium channels
- Interacts with the open channel conformation of voltage-sensitive sodium channels
- Interacts at a specific site of the alpha pore-forming subunit of voltage-sensitive sodium channels
- Inhibits release of glutamate

SAFETY AND TOLERABILITY

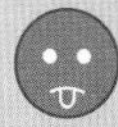

Notable Side Effects
- Sedation (dose dependent), dizziness (dose dependent), headache, ataxia (dose dependent), nystagmus, abnormal gait, confusion, nervousness, fatigue
- Nausea (dose dependent), vomiting, abdominal pain, dyspepsia
- Diplopia (dose dependent), vertigo, abnormal vision
- Rash

Life-Threatening or Dangerous Side Effects
- Hyponatremia
- Rare activation of suicidal ideation and behavior (suicidality)

Growth and Maturation
- Not studied

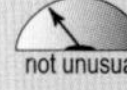

Weight Gain
- Occurs in significant minority
- Some patients experience increased appetite

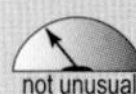

Sedation
- Occurs in significant minority
- Dose related
- Less than carbamazepine
- More when combined with other anticonvulsants
- Can wear off with time, but may not wear off at high doses

What to Do About Side Effects
- Wait
- Wait
- Wait
- Switch to another agent

How Drug Causes Side Effects
- CNS side effects theoretically due to excessive actions at voltage-sensitive sodium channels

Warnings and Precautions
- Because oxcarbazepine has a tricyclic chemical structure, it is not recommended to be taken with MAOIs, including 14 days after MAOIs are stopped; do not start an MAOI until 2 weeks after discontinuing oxcarbazepine
- Because oxcarbazepine can lower plasma levels of hormonal contraceptives, it may also reduce their effectiveness
- May exacerbate angle-closure glaucoma
- May need to restrict fluids and/or monitor sodium because of risk of hyponatremia

- Use cautiously in patients who have demonstrated hypersensitivity to carbamazepine
- Warn patients and their caregivers about the possibility of activation of suicidal ideation and advise them to report such side effects immediately

When Not to Prescribe

- If patient is taking an MAOI
- If there is a proven allergy to any tricyclic compound
- If there is a proven allergy to oxcarbazepine

Long-Term Use

- Monitoring of sodium may be required, especially during the first 3 months

Habit Forming

- No

Overdose

- Nausea, vomiting, somnolence, aggression, agitation, hypotension, and tremor

DOSING AND USE

Usual Dosage Range

- 1,200–2,400 mg/day

Dosage Forms

- Tablet 150 mg, 300 mg, 600 mg
- Extended-release tablet 150 mg, 300 mg, 600 mg
- Oral solution 300 mg/5 mL

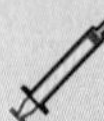

How to Dose

- Ages 4–16 (adjunctive): initial 8–10 mg/kg per day or less than 600 mg/day in 2 doses; increase over 2 weeks to 900 mg/ day (20–29 kg), 1,200 mg/day (29.1–39 kg), or 1,800 mg/day (>39 kg)
- For children ages 2 to < 4 years and under 20 kg: can consider a starting dose of 16–20 mg/kg/day; maximum maintenance dose should be achieved over 2 to 4 weeks and should not exceed 60 mg/kg/day
- When converting from adjunctive to monotherapy, titrate concomitant drug down over 3–6 weeks while titrating oxcarbazepine up by no more than 10 mg/kg per day each week, with an initial daily oxcarbazepine dose of 8–10 mg/kg per day divided in 2 doses
- Monotherapy: initial 8–10 mg/kg per day in 2 doses (immediate-release) or 1 dose (extended-release); increase every 3 days by 5 mg/kg per day; recommended maintenance dose dependent on weight
- 0–20 kg (600–900 mg/day); 21–30 kg (900–1,200 mg/day); 31–40 kg (900–1,500 mg/day); 41–45 kg (1,200–1,500 mg/day); 46–55 kg (1,200–1,800 mg/day); 56–65 kg (1,200–2,100 mg/day); over 65 kg (1,500–2,100 mg/day)
- Children below age 8 may have increased clearance compared to adults
- Extended-release: initial 8–10 mg/kg once per day, not to exceed 600 mg/day in the first week; can increase dose weekly by 8–10 mg/kg/day (not to exceed 600 mg/day); recommended maintenance dose is based on weight:

Weight	Target daily dose
20–29 kg	900 mg/day
29.1–39 kg	1,200 mg/day
>39 kg	1,800 mg/day

Options for Administration

- Immediate- and extended-release options

Tests

- Consider monitoring serum sodium because of possibility of hyponatremia, especially during the first 3 months

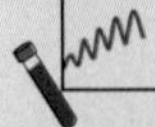

Pharmacokinetics

- Food does not affect absorption
- Oxcarbazepine and its metabolites have a moderate to high distribution throughout the body
- Relatively low plasma protein binding of about 40–42%
- Extensively metabolized in the liver, and the main metabolite is the active compound monohydroxy derivative (MHD, also known as licarbazepine). CrCl correlates with the clearance of MHD in pediatric patients.
- Elimination half-life of oxcarbazepine is relatively short, ranging from 2 to 9 hours, while the half-life of MHD is slightly longer, typically between 8 and 15 hours, but

this may be shorter in youth because of increased CrCl
- Metabolites are eliminated mainly through the kidneys. A small amount of unchanged oxcarbazepine is excreted in the urine as well.
- Oxcarbazepine and its active metabolite, MHD, have the potential to induce certain drug-metabolizing enzymes in the liver, notably CYP3A4 and UDP-glucuronosyltransferases (UGTs). This induction can lead to increased metabolism and decreased plasma concentrations of other medications coadministered with oxcarbazepine, potentially reducing their effectiveness.

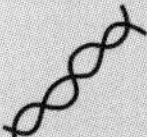

Pharmacogenetics

- Before starting: individuals with ancestry across broad areas of Asia consider screening for the HLAB*1502 allele (see accompanying table)

Genotype	Risk implication	Recommendation
HLAB*1502 negative	Normal risk of oxcarbazepine-induced SJS/TEN	Standard dosing guidelines
HLAB*1502 positive	Greater risk of oxcarbazepine-induced SJS/TEN	Oxcarbazepine-naïve patients: do not use For patients previously treated with oxcarbazepine for > 3 months without cutaneous reactions, cautiously consider

Abbreviations: SJS/TEN: Stevens–Johnson syndrome; TEN: toxic epidermal necrolysis.

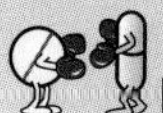

Drug Interactions

- Depressive effects may be increased by other CNS depressants (alcohol, MAOIs, other anticonvulsants, etc.)
- Strong inducers of CYP (e.g., carbamazepine, phenobarbital, phenytoin, and primidone) can decrease plasma levels of the active metabolite MHD
- Verapamil may decrease plasma levels of the active metabolite MHD
- Oxcarbazepine can decrease plasma levels of hormonal contraceptives and dihydropyridine calcium antagonists
- Oxcarbazepine at doses greater than 1,200 mg/day may increase plasma levels of phenytoin, possibly requiring dose reduction of phenytoin

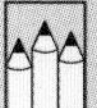

Dosing Tips

- Doses of oxcarbazepine need to be about one-third higher than those of carbamazepine for similar results
- Usually administered as adjunctive medication to other anticonvulsants, lithium, or atypical antipsychotics for bipolar disorder
- Side effects may increase with dose
- Although increased efficacy for seizures is seen at 2,400 mg/day compared to 1,200 mg/day, CNS side effects may be intolerable at the higher dose
- Liquid formulation can be administered mixed in a glass of water or directly from the oral dosing syringe supplied
- Slow dose titration may delay onset of therapeutic action but enhance tolerability to sedating side effects
- Should titrate slowly in the presence of other sedating agents, such as other anticonvulsants, in order to best tolerate additive sedative side effects
- When converting from immediate-release to extended-release, higher doses may be necessary

How to Switch

- From another medication to oxcarbazepine:
  - When tapering a prior medication, see its entry in this manual for how to stop and how to taper off that specific drug
  - Generally, try to stop the first agent before starting oxcarbazepine so that new side effects of oxcarbazepine can be distinguished from withdrawal effects of the first agent
- Off oxcarbazepine to another medication:
  - Generally, try to stop oxcarbazepine before starting the new medication so that new side effects of the next drug can be distinguished from any withdrawal effects from oxcarbazepine
  - Taper; may need to adjust dosage of concurrent medications as oxcarbazepine is being discontinued

How to Stop

- Taper
- Epilepsy patients may seize upon withdrawal, especially if withdrawal is abrupt
- Rapid discontinuation may increase the risk of relapse in bipolar disorder
- Discontinuation symptoms uncommon

WHAT TO EXPECT

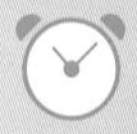

Onset of Action

- Should reduce seizures by 2 weeks

Duration of Action

- Effects are consistent over a 24-hour period
- May continue to work for many years to prevent relapse of symptoms

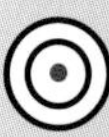

Primary Target Symptoms

- Incidence of seizures
- Severity of seizures

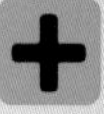

What Is Considered a Positive Result?

- The goal of treatment is complete remission of symptoms

How Long to Treat

- Continue treatment until all symptoms are gone or until improvement is stable and then continue treating indefinitely as long as improvement persists
- Continue treatment indefinitely to avoid the recurrence of mania and seizures

What If It Stops Working?

- Check for nonadherence, possibly by checking plasma drug level, and consider switching to another agent with fewer side effects
- Screen for the development of a new comorbid disorder, especially substance abuse
- Screen for adverse changes in the home or school environment

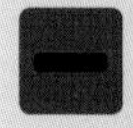

What If It Doesn't Work?

- Consider evaluation for another diagnosis or for a comorbid condition (e.g., medical illness, substance abuse)
- Consider other important potential factors such as ongoing conflicts, family psychopathology, and an adverse environment (e.g., poverty, chaos, violence, prior and ongoing psychological trauma, abuse, neglect)
- Institute trauma-informed care for appropriate children and adolescents
- Consider initiating rehabilitation and psychotherapy such as cognitive remediation, although these may be less well standardized for children/adolescents than for adults
- Consider presence of concomitant drug abuse

TALKING TO PATIENTS AND CAREGIVERS

What to Tell Parents About Efficacy

- For acute symptoms, it can work right away
- Explain which use oxcarbazepine is being chosen for, how to tell if the drug is working by targeting specific symptoms, and why this is being done
- Once the child/adolescent calms down, at some point after one dose or after several days of dosing or after long term dosing, we should all assess whether the medication should be continued
- While the medicine helps by reducing symptoms and improving function, it is not a cure, and it therefore may be necessary to keep taking the medication long term to sustain its therapeutic effects
- Since every treatment consideration depends on a risk/benefit analysis, parents should fully understand short- and long-term risks as well as benefits
- Often a good idea to tell parents whether the medication chosen is specifically approved for the disorder being treated, or whether it is being given for "unapproved" or "off-label" reasons based on good clinical practice, expert consensus, and/or prudent extrapolation of controlled data from adults

What to Tell Children and Adolescents About Efficacy

- Be specific about the symptoms being targeted: we are trying to help you …

- Give the medication a try; if it's not working very well, we can stop the medication and try something else
- A good try often takes 2 to 3 months
- If it does make you feel better, you cannot stop it right away or you may get sick again
- Medications don't change who you are as a person; they give you the opportunity to be the best person you can be

What to Tell Parents About Side Effects

- Explain that side effects are expected in many when starting
- Tell parents many side effects go away and do so about the same time that therapeutic effects start
- Predict side effects in advance (you will look clever and competent to the parents, unless you scare them with too much information and cause nocebo effects, in which case you won't look so clever when the patient develops lots of side effects and stops medication; use your judgment here); a balanced but honest presentation is an art rather than a science
- Ask parents to support the patient while side effects are occurring
- Parents should fully understand short- and long-term risks as well as benefits
- Explaining to the parents what to expect from medication treatment, and especially what potential side effects to expect, can help prevent early termination of medication

What to Tell Children and Adolescents About Side Effects

- Even if you get a side effect, we can usually reduce it over time
- If you have side effects that are bothering you, tell your parents and your parents should tell me
- Consider having a conversation about sexual side effects in some adolescents who can find these side effects confusing and especially burdensome
- Explaining to child/adolescent what to expect from medication treatment, and especially potential side effects, can help prevent early termination of medication

What to Tell Teachers About the Medication (If Parents Consent)

- Oxcarbazepine can make children/adolescents sedated
- It is not abusable
- Encourage dialogue with parents/guardians about any behavior or mood changes

SPECIAL POPULATIONS

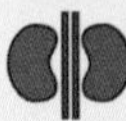

Renal Impairment

- Oxcarbazepine is renally excreted
- Elimination half-life of active metabolite MHD is increased
- Reduce initial dose by half; may need to use slower titration

Hepatic Impairment

- No dose adjustment recommended for mild to moderate hepatic impairment
- Use with caution in patients with severe impairment

Cardiac Impairment

- No dose adjustment recommended

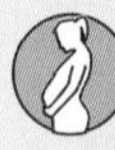

Pregnancy

- Controlled studies have not been conducted in pregnant women
- Oxcarbazepine is structurally similar to carbamazepine, which is thought to be teratogenic in humans
- Use during first trimester may raise risk of neural tube defects (e.g., spina bifida) or other congenital anomalies
- Use in women of childbearing potential requires weighing potential benefits to the mother against the risks to the fetus
- If drug is continued, perform tests to detect birth defects
- If drug is continued, start on folate 1 mg/day to reduce risk of neural tube defects
- Antiepileptic Drug Pregnancy Registry: (888) 233-2334 or www.aedpregnancyregistry.org
- Taper drug if discontinuing
- For bipolar patients, oxcarbazepine should generally be discontinued before anticipated pregnancies
- Seizures, even mild seizures, may cause harm to the embryo/fetus
- Recurrent bipolar illness during pregnancy can be quite disruptive
- For bipolar patients, given the risk of relapse in the postpartum period, some

form of mood stabilizer treatment may need to be restarted immediately after delivery if patient is unmedicated during pregnancy

- Atypical antipsychotics may be preferable to lithium or anticonvulsants such as oxcarbazepine if treatment of bipolar disorder is required during pregnancy
- Bipolar symptoms may recur or worsen during pregnancy, and some form of treatment may be necessary

Breast Feeding

- Some drug is found in breast milk
- Recommended either to discontinue drug or formula feed
- If drug is continued while breast feeding, infant should be monitored for possible adverse effects, including hematological effects
- If infant shows signs of irritability or sedation, drug may need to be discontinued
- Bipolar disorder may recur during the postpartum period, particularly if there is a history of prior postpartum episodes of either depression or psychosis
- Relapse rates may be lower in women who receive prophylactic treatment for postpartum episodes of bipolar disorder
- Atypical antipsychotics and anticonvulsants such as valproate may be safer than oxcarbazepine during the postpartum period when breast feeding

THE ART OF PSYCHOPHARMACOLOGY

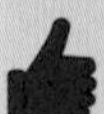

Potential Advantages

- Those who responded to but did not tolerate carbamazepine

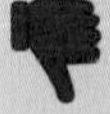

Potential Disadvantages

- Patients at risk for hyponatremia

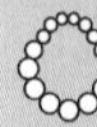

Pearls

- In pediatric trials of bipolar disorder, oxcarbazepine has not separated from placebo
- Oxcarbazepine is the 10-keto analog of carbamazepine, but not a metabolite of carbamazepine
- Oxcarbazepine seems to have the same mechanism of therapeutic action as carbamazepine but with fewer side effects
- Specifically, risk of leukopenia, aplastic anemia, agranulocytosis, elevated liver enzymes, or Stevens–Johnson syndrome and serious rash associated with carbamazepine does not seem to be associated with oxcarbazepine
- Skin rash reactions to carbamazepine may resolve in 75% of patients with epilepsy when switched to oxcarbazepine; thus, 25% of patients who experience rash with carbamazepine may also experience it with oxcarbazepine
- Oxcarbazepine has much less prominent actions on CYP enzyme systems than carbamazepine, and thus fewer drug–drug interactions
- Specifically, oxcarbazepine and its active metabolite, the monohydroxy derivative (MHD), cause less enzyme induction of CYP 3A4 than the structurally related carbamazepine
- The active metabolite MHD, also called licarbazepine, is a racemic mixture of 80% S-MHD (active) and 20% R-MHD (inactive)
- Most significant risk of oxcarbazepine may be clinically significant hyponatremia (sodium level < 125 m mol/L), most likely occurring within the first 3 months of treatment, and occurring in 2–3% of patients
- Unknown if this risk is higher than for carbamazepine
- Since SSRIs can sometimes also reduce sodium due to syndrome of inappropriate antidiuretic hormone production (SIADH), patients treated with combinations of oxcarbazepine and SSRIs should be carefully monitored, especially in the early stages of treatment

SUGGESTED READING

Hobbs E, Reed R, Lorberg B, Robb AS, Dorfman J. Psychopharmacological treatment algorithms of manic/mixed and depressed episodes in pediatric bipolar disorder. J Child Adolesc Psychopharmacol 2022;32(10):507–21.

Li X, Wei S, Wu H et al. Population pharmacokinetics of oxcarbazepine active metabolite in Chinese children with epilepsy. Eur J Pediatr 2023;182(10):4509–21.

Phillips EJ, Sukasem C, Whirl-Carrillo M et al. Clinical Pharmacogenetics Implementation Consortium guideline for HLA genotype and use of carbamazepine and oxcarbazepine: 2017 update. Clin Pharmacol Ther 2018 103(4):574–81.

Wagner KD, Kowatch RA, Emslie GJ et al. A double-blind, randomized, placebo-controlled trial of oxcarbazepine in the treatment of bipolar disorder in children and adolescents. Am J Psychiatry 2006;163(7):1179–86.

THERAPEUTICS

Brands

- Invega
- Invega Hafyera
- Invega Sustenna
- Invega Trinza
- Trevicta
- Xeplion

Generic

Yes

US FDA Approved for Pediatric Use

- Schizophrenia (Invega, ages 12 and older)

Off-Label for Pediatric Use

- Approved in adults
  - Schizophrenia (Invega Sustenna, Invega Trinza)
  - Maintaining response in schizophrenia (Invega)
  - Schizoaffective disorder (Invega, Invega Sustenna; monotherapy and adjunct)
- Other off-label uses
  - Other psychotic disorders
  - Acute mania / mixed mania
  - Bipolar maintenance
  - Bipolar depression
  - Behavioral disturbances in children and adolescents
  - Disorders associated with problems with impulse control

Class and Mechanism of Action

- Neuroscience-based Nomenclature: dopamine, serotonin receptor antagonist (DS-RAn)
- Atypical antipsychotic (serotonin-dopamine antagonist; second generation antipsychotic; also a mood stabilizer)
- Blocks dopamine 2 receptors, reducing positive symptoms of psychosis and stabilizing affective symptoms
- Blockade of serotonin type 2A receptors may also contribute at clinical doses to the enhancement of dopamine release in certain brain regions, thus theoretically reducing motor side effects
- Serotonin 7 antagonist properties may contribute to antidepressant actions
- Paliperidone is the 9-hydroxy active metabolite of risperidone

SAFETY AND TOLERABILITY

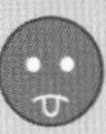

Notable Side Effects

- May increase risk for diabetes and dyslipidemia
- Extrapyramidal symptoms (EPS, also called drug-induced parkinsonism)
- Hyperprolactinemia (in children and adolescents, serum prolactin levels tend to rise and peak within the first 1 to 2 months and then steadily decline to values within or very close to the normal range within 6 months)
- Tachycardia, sedation, tremor, akathisia
- Weight gain
- Risk of drug-induced parkinsonism and dystonic reactions may be higher in children than it is in adults
- Risk of withdrawal dyskinesias
- Galactorrhea/amenorrhea (girls)
- Gynecomastia (boys)

Life-Threatening or Dangerous Side Effects

- Hyperglycemia, in some cases extreme and associated with ketoacidosis or hyperosmolar coma or death, has been reported in patients taking atypical antipsychotics
- Rare neuroleptic malignant syndrome (NMS) may cause hyperpyrexia, muscle rigidity, delirium, and autonomic instability with elevated creatine phosphokinase, myoglobinuria (rhabdomyolysis), and acute renal failure
- Rare seizures

Growth and Maturation

- Retrospective analyses have not shown a clinically significant growth failure or delay in pubertal onset or progression in children treated for up to 1 year with risperidone, which is the parent drug of paliperidone

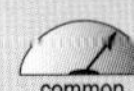

Weight Gain

- Many patients experience and/or can be significant. In pediatric samples, higher plasma concentrations of paliperidone's parent compound (risperidone) are associated with more weight gain (Kloosterboer et al., 2021).
- May be more weight gain in children and adolescents than in adults. Current practice

often includes adding metformin in pediatric patients who experience early weight gain (or are at high risk of antipsychotic weight gain, that is, greater than 85%ile for BMI).
- Can become a health problem in some

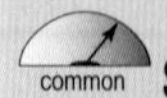

Sedation

- Many patients experience and/or can be significant. In pediatric samples, higher plasma concentrations of paliperidone's parent compound (risperidone) are associated with more sedation (Kloosterboer et al., 2021).
- In randomized controlled trials of paliperidone in adolescents, sedation is dose related (6% at low doses, 15% at medium doses, and 21% at high doses)

What to Do About Side Effects

- Wait, wait, wait: mild side effects are common, happen early, and usually improve with time, but treatment benefits can be delayed
- Monitor side effects closely, especially when initiating treatment
- May wish to give at night if not tolerated during the day and doesn't disrupt sleep
- Often best to try another monotherapy trial of a different antipsychotic prior to resorting to augmentation strategies to treat side effects
- Exercise and diet programs and medical management for high BMI percentiles, diabetes, dyslipidemia. Also, randomized controlled trials in youth suggest that omega-3 fatty acids can reduce SGA-related hypertriglyceridemia.
- Reduce the dose, particularly for drug-induced parkinsonism, akathisia, sedation, and tremor
- For drug-induced parkinsonism: consider reducing dose or switching to another agent. In adolescents, the percentage of patients experiencing dystonia was 2% for low and medium doses and quadrupled to more than 8% in patients receiving high doses (no subjects receiving placebo reported dystonia). Augmenting with diphenhydramine or benztropine is less preferred in youth.
- For akathisia: reduce the dose [in clinical trials of adolescents with schizophrenia, paliperidone produced akathisia in 4% of patients receiving low doses, 8% of those receiving medium doses and 17% of those receiving high doses (compared to 0% of adolescents receiving placebo)] or add a beta blocker. If these are ineffective, raising the dose of the beta blocker may be helpful. Using a 5HT2A antagonist such as mirtazapine or cyproheptadine to treat drug-induced akathisia is less common in children and adolescents compared to adults.

How Drug Causes Side Effects

- Blocking alpha 1 adrenergic receptors can cause dizziness, hypotension, and syncope. However, these effects may be less commonly seen as side effects in pediatric patients compared to adults.
- By blocking dopamine 2 receptors in the striatum, it can cause drug-induced parkinsonism, especially at high doses
- By blocking dopamine 2 receptors in the pituitary, it can cause elevations in prolactin
- Mechanism of any possible weight gain is unknown but may relate to effects at 5HT2C receptors
- Mechanism of any possible increased incidence of diabetes or dyslipidemia is unknown

Warnings and Precautions

- Carefully weigh the risks and benefits of pharmacological treatment against the risks and benefits of nontreatment with an antipsychotic and it is a good idea to document this in the patient's chart
- Use with caution in patients with conditions that predispose to hypotension (dehydration, overheating)
- Atypical antipsychotics have the potential for cognitive and motor impairment, especially related to sedation
- Atypical antipsychotics can cause body temperature dysregulation; use caution in patients who may experience conditions that increase body temperature (e.g., strenuous exercise, saunas, extreme heat, dehydration, or concomitant anticholinergic medication)
- Paliperidone prolongs QTc interval more than some other antipsychotics
- Priapism has been reported with other antipsychotics, including risperidone (the parent drug of paliperidone)

- As with any antipsychotic, use with caution in patients with history of seizures

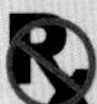

When Not to Prescribe

- If there is a proven allergy to paliperidone and risperidone
- Avoid use if patient is taking agents capable of significantly prolonging QTc interval (e.g., pimozide, thioridazine, selected antiarrhythmics, moxifloxacin, sparfloxacin)
- Avoid use if there is a history of QTc prolongation or cardiac arrhythmia
- Avoid use if patient has a preexisting severe gastrointestinal narrowing

Long-Term Use

- In adults, oral paliperidone is approved for maintenance treatment of schizophrenia
- Tolerability and efficacy have been demonstrated in an open-label, 2-year, flexible-dose trial in adolescents with schizophrenia

Habit Forming

- No

Overdose

- Drug-induced parkinsonism, gait unsteadiness, sedation, tachycardia, hypotension, QTc prolongation

DOSING AND USE

Usual Dosage Range

- Schizophrenia (patients weighing less than 51 kg): 3–6 mg/day
- Schizophrenia (patients weighing at least 51 kg): 3–12 mg/day

Dosage Forms

- Tablet (extended-release) 1.5 mg, 3 mg, 6 mg, 9 mg
- 1-month injection 39 mg, 78 mg, 117 mg, 156 mg, 234 mg
- 3-month injection 273 mg, 410 mg, 546 mg, 819 mg

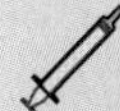

How to Dose

- Schizophrenia (patients weighing less than 51 kg): initial dose 3 mg/day; after 5 days can increase to 6 mg/day if needed
- Schizophrenia (patients weighing at least 51 kg): initial dose 3 mg/day; can increase 3 mg/day increments every 5 days as needed; maximum dose 12 mg/day
- If clinical effects wear off with once-daily administration, give as twice a day dosing, especially in children

Options for Administration

- Long-acting injectable formulations not approved in children/adolescents and few studies; probably best not to use long-acting injectables in children at all, and only with caution off-label in adolescents who are older and have adult body weights

Tests

- Before starting paliperidone:
  - Plan to monitor weight and metabolic parameters more closely than in adults since children and adolescents may be more prone to metabolic side effects than adults
  - Weigh all patients and monitor weight gain against that expected for normal growth, using the pediatric height/weight chart to monitor. In particular, monitor BMI percentiles.
  - Get baseline personal and family history of diabetes, obesity, dyslipidemia, hypertension, and cardiovascular disease
  - Obtain blood pressure, fasting plasma glucose (or hemoglobin A1C), and a lipid profile
- After starting paliperidone:
  - BMI percentile monthly for 3 months, then quarterly
  - Consider monitoring fasting triglycerides in patients at high risk for metabolic complications
  - Blood pressure, fasting plasma glucose (or hemoglobin A1C), lipid profile within 3 months and then annually
  - Treat or refer for treatment and consider switching to another atypical antipsychotic for patients who become overweight, obese, pre-diabetic, diabetic, or dyslipidemic while receiving an atypical antipsychotic
  - Even in patients without known diabetes, be vigilant for the rare but life-threatening onset of diabetic ketoacidosis, which always requires immediate treatment, by monitoring for the rapid onset of polyuria, polydipsia, weight loss, nausea, vomiting,

dehydration, rapid respiration, weakness, and clouding of sensorium, even coma
  - Patients with low white blood cell count (WBC) or history of drug-induced leukopenia/neutropenia should have complete blood count (CBC) monitored frequently during the first few months and paliperidone should be discontinued at the first sign of decline of WBC in the absence of other causative factors
  - Monitoring elevated prolactin levels is of dubious clinical benefit, although paliperidone is known to increase prolactin levels and cause galactorrhea and amenorrhea in girls and gynecomastia in boys. Prolactin levels should be obtained in female patients with secondary amenorrhea.
  - Consider monitoring plasma levels of paliperidone (i.e., 9-hydroxyrisperidone) if not responding, or questions about compliance or side effects
  - Patients should be monitored periodically for the development of abnormal movements using neurological exam and the Abnormal Involuntary Movement Scale (AIMS)

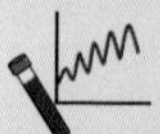

Pharmacokinetics

- Active metabolite of risperidone
- Plasma concentrations of paliperidone rise steadily to reach peak plasma concentration approximately 24 hours after dosing in adolescents
- Half-life approximately 24 hours in adolescents
- In adolescent clinical trials, the paliperidone systemic exposure was similar to that in adults and steady-state drug concentrations are attained within 4–5 days of daily dosing
- Can be taken with or without food

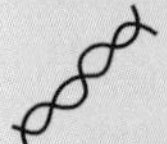

Pharmacogenetics

- No recommendations

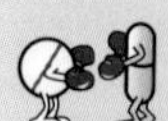

Drug Interactions

- May increase effect of antihypertensive agents
- May enhance QTc prolongation of other drugs capable of prolonging QTc interval

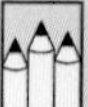

Dosing Tips

- In pediatric clinical trials, no additional benefit was observed above 6 mg per day (patients weighing less than 51 kg) or 12 mg (patients weighing at least 51 kg), while adverse event were dose related
- Tablet should not be divided or chewed, but rather should only be swallowed whole
- Tablet does not change shape in the GI tract and generally should not be used in patients with gastrointestinal narrowing because of the risk of intestinal obstruction
- A common dosage error is to assume the paliperidone ER oral dose is the same as the risperidone oral dose in mg
- For treatment resistance, consider obtaining plasma drug levels to guide dosing above recommended levels
- Treatment should be suspended if absolute neutrophil count falls below 1,000/mm^3

How to Switch

- From another antipsychotic to paliperidone:
  - When tapering a prior antipsychotic, see its entry in this manual for how to stop and how to taper off that specific drug
  - Generally, try to stop the first agent before starting paliperidone so that new side effects of paliperidone can be distinguished from withdrawal effects of the first agent
  - If urgent, cross taper off the other antipsychotic while paliperidone is started at a low dose, with dose adjustments down of the other antipsychotic, and up for paliperidone, every 5 to 7 days
- Off paliperidone to another antipsychotic:
  - Generally, try to stop paliperidone before starting the new antipsychotic so that new side effects of the next drug can be distinguished from any withdrawal effects from paliperidone. However, withdrawal dyskinesias are very common with paliperidone discontinuation in pediatric patients and should not be mistaken for tardive dyskinesia.
  - If urgent, cross taper off paliperidone by cutting the dose in half as the new antipsychotic is also started with dose adjustments down of paliperidone and up for the new antipsychotic

Switching from Oral Antipsychotics to Paliperidone ER

target dose
dose
aripiprazole
brexpiprazole
cariprazine
paliperidone ER
1 week | 1 week | 1 week | 1 week

target dose
dose
iloperidone
lurasidone
risperidone*
ziprasidone
paliperidone ER
1 week | 1 week | 1 week | 1 week

target dose
dose
asenapine
olanzapine
quetiapine
paliperidone ER
1 week | 1 week | 1 week | 1 week

target dose
dose
clozapine
paliperidone ER
1 week | 1 week | 1 week | 1 week

How to Stop

- Slow down-titration of oral formulation (over 6–8 weeks), especially when simultaneously beginning a new antipsychotic while switching (i.e., cross-titration)
- Rapid oral discontinuation may lead to rebound psychosis and worsening of symptoms
- Rapid oral discontinuation may lead to withdrawal dyskinesias, which are generally reversible in the pediatric population. Of note, withdrawal dyskinesias are more common in pediatric patients than in adults.
- If antiparkinsonian agents are being used, they should be continued for a few weeks after paliperidone is discontinued

WHAT TO EXPECT

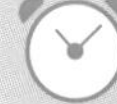

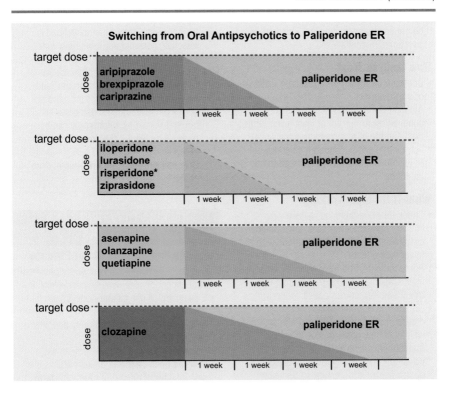

Onset of Action

- Psychosis can improve within 1 week of oral dosing, but it may take several weeks for full effect on behavior as well as on cognition and affective stabilization
- If it is not working within 6–8 weeks, it may require a dosage increase or it may not work at all

Duration of Action

- Effects of oral medication are consistent over a 24-hour period
- Oral medication may continue to work for many years to prevent relapse of symptoms

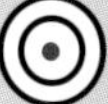

Primary Target Symptoms

- Positive symptoms of psychosis
- Negative symptoms of psychosis
- Unstable mood and depression
- Aggressive symptoms

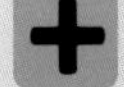

What Is Considered a Positive Result?

- Most often reduces positive symptoms but does not eliminate them
- Can improve negative symptoms, as well as aggressive, cognitive, and affective symptoms but less so than for positive symptoms
- In children or adolescents with a first episode of psychosis, initial response may

be greater than for recurrent episodes of psychosis in adults

How Long to Treat

- Continue treatment until reaching a plateau of improvement
- After reaching a satisfactory plateau, continue treatment for at least a year after first episode of psychosis or mania
- For second and subsequent episodes of psychosis, treatment may need to be indefinite

What If It Stops Working?

- Check for nonadherence, possibly by checking plasma drug level, and consider switching to another antipsychotic with fewer side effects
- Some patients who have an initial response may relapse even though they continue treatment, sometimes called "poop-out"
- Growth/developmental changes may contribute to apparent loss of efficacy as well as to new onset of side effects as metabolism slows and drug levels rise in transition from childhood to adolescence; dose adjustment (increase or decrease) should be considered
- Screen for the development of a new comorbid disorder, especially substance use
- Screen for adverse changes in the home or school

What If It Doesn't Work?

- Consider evaluation for another diagnosis (especially bipolar illness or depression with mixed features) or for a comorbid condition (e.g., medical illness, substance use)
- Consider other important potential factors such as ongoing conflicts, family psychopathology, and an adverse environment (e.g., poverty, chaos, violence, prior and ongoing psychological trauma, abuse, neglect)
- Institute trauma-informed care for appropriate children and adolescents
- For schizophrenia or bipolar disorder:
  - Try one of the other atypical antipsychotics
  - If no first-line atypical antipsychotic is effective, consider higher doses guided by plasma drug levels
  - If no first-line atypical antipsychotic is effective, consider augmentation with valproate, lithium, or lamotrigine
  - Consider initiating psychotherapy. In adolescents with bipolar disorder (and those with affective symptoms who are at risk of developing bipolar disorder), family-focused psychotherapy can be particularly helpful (Miklowitz et al., 2020).
  - Consider presence of concomitant drug abuse

TALKING TO PATIENTS AND CAREGIVERS

What to Tell Parents About Efficacy

- For acute symptoms, it can work right away
- Oral paliperidone is usually given every day
- Explain which use paliperidone is being chosen for, how to tell if the drug is working by targeting specific symptoms, and why this is being done
- Once the child/adolescent calms down, at some point after one dose or after several days of dosing or after long-term dosing, we should all assess whether the medication should be continued
- While the medicine helps by reducing symptoms and improving function, it is not a cure, and it therefore may be necessary to keep taking the medication long term to sustain its therapeutic effects
- Since every treatment consideration depends on a risk/benefit analysis, parents should fully understand short- and long-term risks as well as benefits
- Often a good idea to tell parents whether the medication chosen is specifically approved for the disorder being treated, or whether it is being given for "unapproved" or "off-label" reasons based on good clinical practice, expert consensus, and/or prudent extrapolation of controlled data from adults

What to Tell Children and Adolescents About Efficacy

- Be specific about the symptoms being targeted: we are trying to help you ...
- Give the medication a try; if it's not working very well, we can stop the medication and try something else
- A good try often takes several weeks

- If it does make you feel better, you cannot stop it right away or you may get sick again
- Medications don't change who you are as a person; they give you the opportunity to be the best person you can be

What to Tell Parents About Side Effects

- Explain that side effects are expected in many when starting
- Tell parents many side effects go away and do so about the same time that therapeutic effects start
- Predict side effects in advance (you will look clever and competent to the parents, unless you scare them with too much information and cause nocebo effects, in which case you won't look so clever when the patient develops lots of side effects and stops medication; use your judgment here); a balanced but honest presentation is an art rather than a science
- Ask parents to support the patient while side effects are occurring
- Parents should fully understand short- and long-term risks as well as benefits
- Explaining to the parents what to expect from medication treatment, and especially what potential side effects to expect, can help prevent early termination of medication

What to Tell Children and Adolescents About Side Effects

- Even if you get side effects, most of them get better or go away in a few weeks
- If you have side effects that are bothering you, tell your parents and your parents should tell me
- Consider having a conversation about sexual side effects in some adolescents who can find these side effects confusing and especially burdensome
- Explaining to child/adolescent what to expect from medication treatment, and especially potential side effects, can help prevent early termination of medication

What to Tell Teachers About the Medication (If Parents Consent)

- Paliperidone can make children/adolescents restless and have abnormal movements like tremor
- Paliperidone can make children/adolescents sedated
- It is not abusable
- Encourage dialogue with parents/guardians about any behavior or mood changes
- Notify the clinician of increased restlessness or akathisia symptoms, which may be apparent in the school setting

SPECIAL POPULATIONS

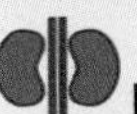

Renal Impairment

- In adults:
  - For mild impairment, maximum recommended dose 6 mg/day
  - For moderate impairment, initial and maximum recommended dose 3 mg/day
  - For severe impairment, initial dose 1.5 mg/day; maximum recommended dose 3 mg/day

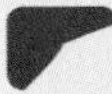

Hepatic Impairment

- No dose adjustment necessary for mild to moderate impairment
- Use in individuals with severe hepatic impairment has not been studied

Cardiac Impairment

- Use in patients with cardiac impairment has not been studied; however, the risk of orthostatic hypotension in pediatric patients is less than in adults, as children rely less on peripheral vasoconstriction to regulate blood pressure
- Use with caution if patient is taking concomitant antihypertensive or alpha 1 antagonist

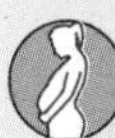

Pregnancy

- Controlled studies have not been conducted in pregnant women
- There is a risk of abnormal muscle movements and withdrawal symptoms in newborns whose mothers took an antipsychotic during the third trimester; symptoms may include agitation, abnormally increased or decreased muscle tone, tremor, sleepiness, severe difficulty breathing, and difficulty feeding
- Psychotic symptoms may worsen during pregnancy, and some form of treatment may be necessary

- Paliperidone may be preferable to anticonvulsant mood stabilizers if treatment is required during pregnancy
- Effects of hyperprolactinemia on the fetus are unknown
- National Pregnancy Registry for Atypical Antipsychotics: 1-866-961-2388 or http://womensmentalhealth.org/clinical-and-research-programs/pregnancyregistry/

Breast Feeding

- Some drug is found in breast milk
- Recommended either to discontinue drug or formula feed
- Infants of women who choose to breast feed while on paliperidone should be monitored for possible adverse effects; sedation, failure to thrive, jitteriness, tremor, and abnormal muscle movements have been reported

THE ART OF PSYCHOPHARMACOLOGY

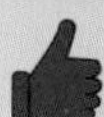

Potential Advantages

- In children:
  - May have a longer duration of action than risperidone in some patients
- In adolescents:
  - Approved for schizophrenia
- All ages:
  - Patients requiring rapid onset of antipsychotic action without dosage titration

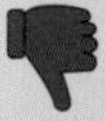

Potential Disadvantages

- In children:
  - Fewer studies and clinical experience than with the related compound risperidone
  - May be more susceptible to side effects than adults, particularly sedation, weight gain, drug-induced parkinsonism, and akathisia
- In adolescents:
  - May be more susceptible to side effects than adults
  - Pubescent girls with amenorrhea (because of prolactin elevation)
  - Boys who are sensitive to the effects of prolactin elevations and develop gynecomastia
- All ages:
  - Possible weight gain and dyslipidemia
  - Possible adverse reactions to prolactin elevation including sexual dysfunction and amenorrhea

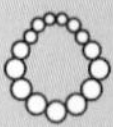

Pearls

- Use caution when converting from risperidone to paliperidone. In general, 1 mg of paliperidone might be considered equivalent to 2–3 mg of risperidone. However, this is a rough rule of thumb.
- Can cause a zombie-like syndrome of inattention, sedation and amotivation associated with reduced socialization and falling grades
- May cause less sedation than some other atypical antipsychotics, more than others
- May cause more motor side effects than some other atypical antipsychotics and motor side effects appear dose related in studies of adolescents
- Some patients may respond to paliperidone or tolerate paliperidone better than the parent drug risperidone
- Patients with inadequate responses to paliperidone may benefit either from switching to another atypical antipsychotic, or for experts, determination of plasma drug levels of paliperidone (i.e., 9-hydroxyrisperidone) to guide dosage increase even beyond the usual prescribing limits
- May cause more motor side effects than some other atypical antipsychotics
- Trilayer tablet consists of three compartments (two containing drug, one a "push" compartment) and an orifice at the head of the first drug compartment; water fills the push compartment and gradually pushes the drug up and out of the tablet through the orifice

SUGGESTED READING

Dunbar F, Kusumakar V, Daneman D, Schulz M. Growth and sexual maturation during long-term treatment with risperidone. Am J Psychiatry 2004;161(5):918–20.

Kloosterboer SM, de Winter BCM, Reichart CG et al. Risperidone plasma concentrations are associated with side effects and effectiveness in children and adolescents with autism spectrum disorder. Br J Clin Pharmacol 2021;87(3):1069–81.

Koch MT, Carlson HE, Kazimi MM, Correll CU. Antipsychotic-related prolactin levels and sexual dysfunction in mentally ill youth: a 3-month cohort-study. J Am Acad Child Adolesc Psychiatry 2023;62(9): 1021–50.

Lytle S, McVoy M, Sajatovic M. Long-acting injectable antipsychotics in children and adolescents. J Child Adolesc Psychopharmacol 2017;27(1):2–9.

Miklowitz DJ, Schneck CD, Walshaw PD et al. Effects of family-focused therapy vs enhanced usual care for symptomatic youths at high risk for bipolar disorder: a randomized clinical trial. JAMA Psychiatry 2020;77(5):455–63.

Pillay J, Boylan K, Carrey N et al. First- and Second-Generation Antipsychotics in Children and Young Adults: Systematic Review Update [Internet]. Rockville, MD: Agency for Healthcare Research and Quality (US); 2017 Mar. Report No.: 17-EHC001-EF. AHRQ Comparative Effectiveness Reviews.

Savitz A, Lane R, Nuamah I et al. Long-term safety of paliperidone extended release in adolescents with schizophrenia: an open-label, flexible dose study. J Child Adolesc Psychopharmacol 2015;25(7):548–57.

Savitz A, Lane R, Nuamah I, Gopal S, Hough D. Efficacy and safety of paliperidone extended release in adolescents with schizophrenia: a randomized, double-blind study. J Am Acad Child Adolesc Psychiatry 2015;54(2):126–37.

THERAPEUTICS

Brands
- Brisdelle
- Paxil
- Paxil CR

Generic
Yes

US FDA Approved for Pediatric Use
- None

Off-Label for Pediatric Use
- Approved in adults
  - Major depressive disorder (paroxetine and paroxetine CR)
  - Obsessive-compulsive disorder (OCD) (paroxetine)
  - Panic disorder (paroxetine and paroxetine CR)
  - Social anxiety disorder (paroxetine and paroxetine CR)
  - Posttraumatic stress disorder (PTSD) (paroxetine)
  - Generalized anxiety disorder (GAD) (paroxetine)
  - Premenstrual dysphoric disorder (PMDD) (paroxetine CR)
  - Vasomotor symptoms (Brisdelle)
- Other off-label uses
- Separation anxiety disorder

Class and Mechanism of Action
- Neuroscience-based Nomenclature: serotonin reuptake inhibitor (S-RI)
- SSRI (selective serotonin reuptake inhibitor); often classified as a drug for depression (i.e., antidepressant), but it is not just an antidepressant
- Paroxetine presumably increases serotonergic neurotransmission by blocking the serotonin reuptake pump (transporter, SERT), which results in the desensitization of serotonin receptors, especially serotonin 1A receptors
- Paroxetine also has mild anticholinergic actions
- Paroxetine may have mild norepinephrine reuptake blocking actions

SAFETY AND TOLERABILITY

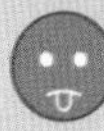

Notable Side Effects
- Mostly central nervous system side effects (insomnia but more so sedation, especially if not sleeping at night; agitation, tremors, headache, dizziness)
- Note: patients with diagnosed or undiagnosed bipolar or psychotic disorders may be more vulnerable to CNS-activating actions of SSRIs like paroxetine; pay particular attention to signs of activation in children with developmental disorders or autism spectrum disorders
- Treatment-emergent activation syndrome (TEAS) includes agitation, anxiety, panic attacks, irritability, aggression, impulsivity, and insomnia
- TEAS can represent side effects but should not be confused with bipolar mania or the onset of suicidality and should be monitored and investigated with consideration of discontinuing or decreasing the dose of paroxetine or addition of another agent or switching to another agent to reduce these symptoms
- Gastrointestinal (decreased appetite, nausea, diarrhea, constipation, dry mouth)
- Sexual dysfunction (boys: delayed ejaculation, erectile dysfunction; boys and girls: decreased sexual desire, anorgasmia)
- Autonomic (sweating)
- Bruising and rare bleeding
- Syndrome of inappropriate antidiuretic hormone secretion (SIADH)

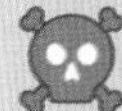

Life-Threatening or Dangerous Side Effects
- Rare seizures
- Rare induction of mania
- Rare suicidal ideation and behavior (suicidality) (short-term regulatory studies did not show any actual suicides in any age group and also did not show an increase in the risk of suicidality with antidepressants compared to placebo beyond age 24)

Growth and Maturation
- Decreased appetite and weight loss have been observed in patients taking SSRIs; however, paroxetine may be associated

with weight gain. In children treated with paroxetine, growth should be monitored.

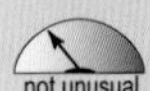

Weight Gain

- Not unusual

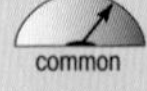

Sedation

- Many experience and/or can be significant in amount
- Generally transient; may be dose dependent

What to Do About Side Effects

- Wait, wait, wait: mild side effects are common, happen early, and usually improve with time, but treatment benefits can be delayed and often begin just as the side effects wear off. However, some side effects may emerge later, such as weight gain.
- Monitor side effects closely, especially when initiating treatment and following dose increases since the pharmacokinetics of paroxetine in children and adolescents are nonlinear
- May wish to give some drugs at night if not tolerated during the day, particularly if the medication is associated with sedation. However, with immediate-release forms of paroxetine, this may be difficult in youth as some studies suggest the need to administer paroxetine several times per day.
- For activation (jitteriness, anxiety, insomnia):
  - Consider a temporary dose reduction or a more gradual up-titration
  - Consider switching to another SSRI or potentially an SNRI (other than venlafaxine)
  - Optimize psychotherapeutic interventions
  - Activation and agitation may represent the induction of a bipolar state, especially a mixed dysphoric bipolar II condition sometimes associated with suicidal ideation, and may require the addition of lithium or an atypical antipsychotic, and/or discontinuation of paroxetine
- Often best to try another monotherapy prior to resorting to augmentation strategies to treat side effects
- For insomnia: consider adding melatonin
- For GI upset: try giving medication with a meal
- For sexual dysfunction:
  - Probably best to discontinue and try another agent. Dose reduction with paroxetine may not alleviate sexual dysfunction.
  - Consider adding daytime exercise, bupropion, or buspirone
- For emotional flattening, apathy: consider adding bupropion (with caution as little experience in children)

How Drug Causes Side Effects

- Theoretically due to increases in serotonin concentrations at serotonin receptors in parts of the brain and body other than those that cause therapeutic actions (e.g., unwanted actions of serotonin in sleep centers causing insomnia, unwanted actions of serotonin in the gut causing diarrhea)
- Increasing serotonin can cause diminished dopamine release and might contribute to emotional flattening, cognitive slowing, and apathy in some patients
- Paroxetine's weak antimuscarinic properties can cause constipation, dry mouth, sedation and weight gain

Warnings and Precautions

- Consider distributing the brochures provided by the FDA and the drug companies as well as the medication guides from the American Academy of Child & Adolescent Psychiatry (AACAP)
- Carefully consider monitoring patients regularly and within the practical limits, particularly during the first several weeks of treatment
- Warn patients and their caregivers when possible about the possibility of activating side effects and advise them to report such symptoms
- Carefully weigh the risks and benefits of pharmacological treatment against the risks and benefits of nontreatment with antidepressants and it is a good idea to document this in the patient's chart
- Add or initiate other antidepressants with caution for up to 2 weeks after discontinuing paroxetine
- As with any antidepressant, use with caution in patients with history of seizure

- As with any antidepressant, use with caution in patients with bipolar disorder unless treated with concomitant mood-stabilizing agent
- Monitor patients for activation and suicidal ideation and involve parents/guardians. Importantly, some studies suggest that the risk of suicidal thinking and behavior may be higher in youth treated with paroxetine compared to other antidepressant medications.

When Not to Prescribe

- If patient is taking an MAO inhibitor
- If patient is taking pimozide
- Not generally recommended in patients taking tricyclic antidepressants (see Drug Interactions)
- If there is a proven allergy to paroxetine

Long-Term Use

- Weight gain has been described in paroxetine-treated youth, so growth should be monitored; long-term effects are unknown

Habit Forming

- No

Overdose

- Rarely lethal in monotherapy overdose; vomiting, sedation, heart rhythm disturbances, dilated pupils, dry mouth

DOSING AND USE

Usual Dosage Range

- Depression: 20–60 mg/day (25–75 mg CR)
- Anxiety disorders and OCD: 10–60 mg/day (12.5–75 mg CR)

Dosage Forms

- Tablet 10 mg scored, 20 mg scored, 30 mg, 40 mg
- Capsule 7.5 mg
- Controlled-release tablets 12.5 mg, 25 mg, 37.5 mg
- Liquid 10 mg/5 mL

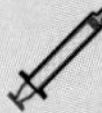

How to Dose

- In children:
  - Initial dose 10 mg/day (12.5–25 mg CR); usually wait a few weeks to assess drug effects; then can increase by 10 mg/day (12.5 mg CR) weekly; maximum dose generally 60 mg/day (75 mg CR) in a single dose
- In adolescents:
  - Depression: initial 20 mg (25 mg CR); usually wait a few weeks to assess drug effects before increasing dose, but can increase by 10 mg/day (12.5 mg/day CR) once a week; maximum generally 50 mg/day (62.5 mg/day CR); single dose
  - Panic disorder: initial 10 mg/day (12.5 mg/day CR); usually wait a few weeks to assess drug effects before increasing dose, but can increase by 10 mg/day (12.5 mg/ day CR) once a week; maximum generally 60 mg/day (75 mg/day CR); single dose
  - Social anxiety disorder: initial 10 mg/day (25 mg/day CR); usually wait a few weeks to assess drug effects before increasing dose, but can increase by 10 mg/day (12.5 mg/day CR) once a week; maximum 60 mg/day (75 mg/day CR); single dose
  - Other anxiety disorders and OCD: initial 10 mg/day (25 mg/day CR); usually wait a few weeks to assess drug effects before increasing dose, but can increase by 10 mg/day (12.5 mg/day CR) once a week; maximum 60 mg/day (75 mg/day CR); single dose
  - Premenstrual dysphoric disorder: initial dose 12.5 mg/day CR; should be administered as a single dose in the morning, with or without food; can be administered either daily or only during the luteal phase of the menstrual cycle

Options for Administration

- Liquid formulation can be beneficial for patients requiring very slow titration and in patients who cannot swallow pills or tablets

Tests

- None for healthy individuals

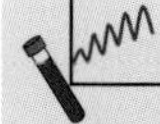

Pharmacokinetics

- Paroxetine is well absorbed from the gastrointestinal tract and is highly protein bound
- In adults, paroxetine reaches steady state within 7–14 days using daily doses of 20–30 mg; however, in youth, this is shorter. For a 10 mg dose of paroxetine, the

average half-life is 11 hours in children and adolescents, considerably shorter than the half-life reported in adults (21 hours) (Kaye et al., 1989).

- Importantly, just like in adults (Kaye et al., 1989), paroxetine exhibits nonlinear kinetics in youth (Findling et al., 1999, 2006) (Figure 1). At steady state, when the CYP2D6 pathway is essentially saturated, paroxetine clearance is governed by alternative P450 isozymes, which, unlike CYP2D6, show no evidence of saturation (Figure 2).

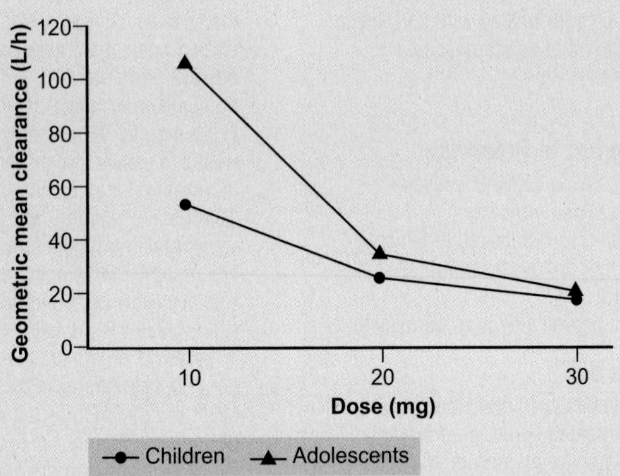

Figure 1 Relationship of paroxetine oral clearance and daily dose in pediatric patients. Reproduced from Findling et al., 2006.

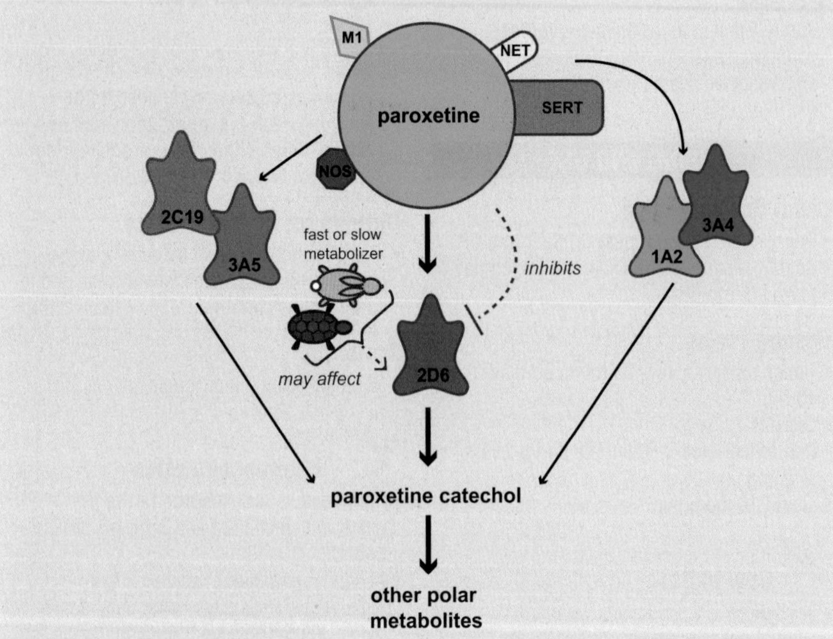

Figure 2 Paroxetine metabolism.

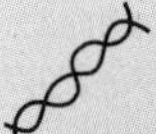

Pharmacogenetics

- Paroxetine undergoes first-pass metabolism in the liver through a high-affinity saturable process (related to CYP2D6 activity), although other enzymes may be involved in metabolism as follows: CYP2D6 ≫ CYP3A4 > CYP1A2 > CYP2C19 > CYP3A5 (Jornil et al., 2010)
- CYP3A4 and CYP1A2 are most likely to be involved in paroxetine metabolism in individuals with impaired CYP2D6 activity (Jornil et al., 2010)
- Because paroxetine is a strong CYP2D6 inhibitor, it influences its own metabolism leading to phenoconversion. In other words, a normal CYP2D6 metabolizer taking paroxetine is converted to an intermediate metabolizer and an intermediate metabolizer taking paroxetine is converted to a poor metabolizer, and so on.
- Current recommendations from the Clinical Pharmacogenetics Implementation Consortium (CPIC) include:
  - **CYP2D6 ultrarapid metabolizers:** CPIC recommends clinicians select alternative drug not predominantly metabolized by CYP2D6
  - **CYP2D6 normal metabolizers:** CPIC recommends that clinicians initiate therapy with recommended starting dose. If patient does not adequately respond to recommended maintenance dosing, consider titrating to a higher maintenance dose or switching to a clinically appropriate alternative antidepressant.
  - **CYP2D6 intermediate metabolizers:** CPIC recommends clinicians should consider a lower starting dose and slower titration schedule as compared to normal metabolizers
  - **CYP2D6 poor metabolizers:** CPIC recommends that clinicians consider a 50% reduction in recommended starting dose, slower titration schedule, and a 50% lower maintenance dose as compared to normal metabolizers

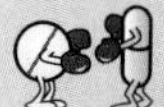

Drug Interactions

- Tramadol reported to increase the risk of seizures in adults taking an antidepressant
- Can increase tricyclic antidepressant (TCA) levels; use with caution with tricyclic antidepressants or when switching from a TCA to paroxetine
- Can cause a fatal "serotonin syndrome" when combined with MAO inhibitors, so do not use with MAO inhibitors or for at least 14 days after MAOIs are stopped
- Do not start an MAO inhibitor for at least 5 half-lives (5–7 days for most drugs)
- May displace highly protein-bound drugs (e.g., phenytoin, valproate)
- There are reports of elevated theophylline levels associated with paroxetine treatment, so it is recommended that theophylline levels be monitored when these drugs are administered together
- May increase anticholinergic effects of procyclidine and other drugs with anticholinergic properties
- Can theoretically cause weakness, hyperreflexia, and incoordination when combined with sumatriptan, or possibly with other triptans, requiring careful monitoring of patient
- Possible increased risk of bleeding
- Via CYP2D6 inhibition, could theoretically interfere with the analgesic actions of codeine, and increase the plasma levels of some beta blockers and of atomoxetine
- Via CYP2D6 inhibition, paroxetine could theoretically increase concentrations of thioridazine and cause dangerous cardiac arrhythmias

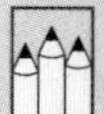

Dosing Tips

- Plasma levels are higher in lower-weight children; therefore, starting and target doses may be lower and longer intervals between dose increases may be needed (see How to Dose)
- Adolescents often need and receive adult doses
- Some pediatric pharmacokinetic studies suggest that paroxetine may need to be administered multiple times per day
- A dose of 20 mg/day (25 mg/day CR) is often sufficient for patients with social anxiety disorder and depression
- Other anxiety disorders, as well as difficult cases in general, may require higher dosing
- Occasional patients are dosed above 60 mg/day (75 mg/day CR), but this is for experts and requires caution
- Liquid formulation easiest for doses below 10 mg when used for cases that are very intolerant to paroxetine or especially for very slow down-titration during

discontinuation for patients with withdrawal symptoms

- Paroxetine CR tablets not scored; chewing or cutting in half can destroy controlled-release properties
- Unlike other SSRIs and antidepressants where dosage increments can be double and triple the starting dose, paroxetine's dosing increments are in 50% increments (i.e., 20, 30, 40; or 25, 37.5, 50 CR)
- Paroxetine inhibits its own metabolism and thus plasma concentrations can double when oral doses increase by 50%; plasma concentrations can increase 2–7-fold when oral doses are doubled
- For patients with severe problems discontinuing paroxetine, dosing may need to be tapered over many months (i.e., reduce dose by 1% every 3 days by crushing tablet and suspending or dissolving in 100 mL of fruit juice and then disposing of 1 mL while drinking the rest; 3–7 days later, dispose of 2 mL, and so on). This is both a form of very slow biological tapering and a form of behavioral desensitization (not for CR)
- For some patients with severe problems discontinuing paroxetine, it may be useful to add an SSRI with a long half-life, especially fluoxetine, prior to taper of paroxetine; while maintaining fluoxetine dosing, first slowly taper paroxetine and then taper fluoxetine
- Be sure to differentiate between the reemergence of symptoms requiring reinstitution of treatment and withdrawal symptoms
- The more anxious the patient, the lower the starting dose, the slower the titration
- If intolerable anxiety, insomnia, agitation, akathisia, or activation occurs either upon dosing initiation or discontinuation, consider an alternative SSRI. Importantly, the risk of activation with one SSRI does not predict the likelihood of activation with another SSRI.

How to Switch

- From another antidepressant to paroxetine:
  - When tapering a prior antidepressant, see its entry in this manual for how to stop and how to taper off that specific drug
  - In situations when there are antidepressant-related side effects, try to stop the first agent before starting paroxetine so that new side effects of paroxetine can be distinguished from withdrawal effects of the first agent
  - If urgent, cross taper
- Off paroxetine to another antidepressant:
  - Generally, try to stop paroxetine before starting another antidepressant
  - Taper to avoid withdrawal effects (dizziness, nausea, stomach cramps, sweating, tingling, dysesthesias)
  - Can reduce paroxetine dose by 50% every 3 to 7 days, or slower if this rate still causes withdrawal symptoms
  - If necessary, can cross taper off paroxetine this way while dosing up on another antidepressant simultaneously in urgent situations, being aware of all specific drug interactions to avoid

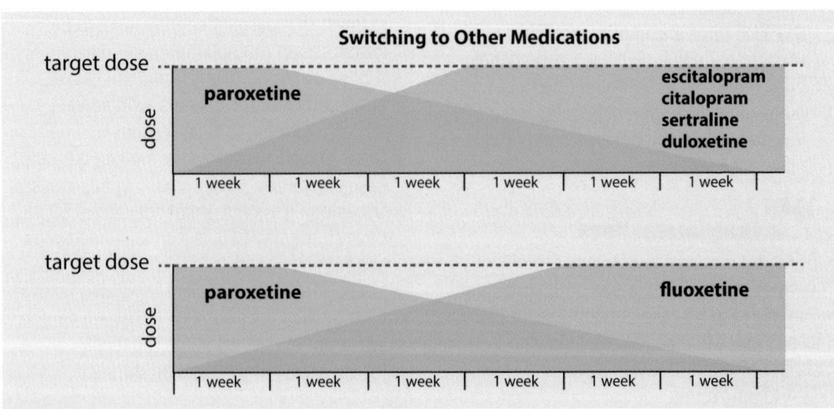

How to Stop

- Taper to avoid withdrawal effects (dizziness, nausea, stomach cramps, sweating, tingling, dysesthesias)
- Many patients tolerate 50% dose reduction for 5–7 days, then another 50% reduction for 5–7 days, then discontinuation. More recently however, hyperbolic discontinuation of SSRIs has been recommended in which the dose of the SSRI is halved every 4 weeks and this may be a preferable strategy in youth (Strawn et al., 2023). Also, when SSRIs are stopped, the risk of relapse is highest during the first 8 weeks after discontinuation.
- If withdrawal symptoms emerge during discontinuation, raise dose to stop symptoms and then restart withdrawal much more slowly
- Withdrawal effects can be more common or more severe with paroxetine than with some other SSRIs
- Paroxetine's withdrawal effects may be related in part to the fact that it inhibits its own metabolism
- Thus, when paroxetine is withdrawn, the rate of its decline can be faster as it stops inhibiting its metabolism (mechanism-based inhibition decreases)
- Controlled-release paroxetine may slow the rate of decline and thus reduce withdrawal reactions in some patients
- Readaptation of cholinergic receptors after prolonged blockade may contribute to withdrawal effects of paroxetine

WHAT TO EXPECT

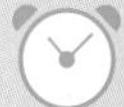

Onset of Action

- Some patients may experience increased energy or activation early after initiation of treatment
- Full onset of therapeutic actions is usually delayed by 2–4 weeks
- If it is not working within 6–8 weeks, it may require a dosage increase or it may not work at all

Duration of Action

- Effects are consistent over a 24-hour period
- May continue to work for many years to prevent relapse of symptoms

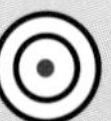

Primary Target Symptoms

- Depressed and/or irritable mood
- Obsessions, compulsions
- Anxiety (fear and worry are often target symptoms, but paroxetine can occasionally and transiently increase these symptoms short term before improving them)
- Sleep disturbances, especially insomnia
- Panic attacks, avoidant behavior, reexperiencing, hyperarousal
- Prior to initiation of treatment, it is helpful to develop a list of target symptoms of depression and/or anxiety to monitor during treatment to better assess treatment response

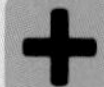

What Is Considered a Positive Result?

- The goal of treatment is complete remission of current symptoms as well as prevention of future relapses
- In practice, many patients have only a partial response where some symptoms are improved but others persist (especially insomnia, fatigue, and problems concentrating in depression), in which case higher doses of paroxetine, adding a second agent, or switching to an agent with a different mechanism of action can be considered
- If treatment works, it most often reduces or even eliminates symptoms, but is not a cure since symptoms can recur after medicine is stopped

How Long to Treat

- For adolescents with depression, generally, 9–12 months of antidepressant treatment is recommended (Hathaway et al., 2018)
- For anxiety disorders, 6–9 months of antidepressant treatment may be sufficient, though many clinicians extend treatment to 12 months based on extrapolation of data from adults with anxiety disorders (Hathaway et al., 2018; Strawn et al., 2023)
- Extended treatment periods may decrease the risk of long-term morbidity and recurrence; however, the goal of treatment is ultimately remission, rather than duration of antidepressant pharmacotherapy (Hathaway et al., 2018)
- In terms of the length of antidepressant treatment, evidence-based guidelines

represent a starting point; appropriate treatment duration varies, and patient-specific response, psychological factors, and timing of discontinuation must be considered for individual pediatric patients (Hathaway et al., 2018)

What If It Stops Working?

- Some patients who have an initial response may relapse even though they continue treatment, sometimes called "poop-out"
- Some patients may experience apparent lack of consistent efficacy due to activation syndrome or latent or underlying or newly evolved bipolar disorder, or major depressive episodes with mixed features, and require antidepressant discontinuation and a switch to a second generation antipsychotic

What If It Doesn't Work?

- Consider evaluation for another diagnosis (especially bipolar illness or depression with mixed features) or for a comorbid condition (e.g., medical illness, substance abuse)
- When treating youth with anxiety disorders, many patients will have had significant anxiety for years prior to beginning treatment. As such, when anxiety is treated with an SSRI, their symptoms may be improved, but the patient has likely missed important developmental milestones (e.g., spending the night with friends, being able to ask questions in class). Developing these skills will take time. Beyond this, the family may have lived with the anxious child for years and following treatment of the child, the family may need to readjust.
- Be mindful of family conflict contributing to the presentation; sometimes treating parental depression or anxiety disorders improves psychiatric and social function without any treatment of youth. Also, accommodation is common in families of youth with anxiety disorders and may need to be addressed specifically, as it can perpetuate symptoms.
- Consider factors associated with poor response to SSRIs in treatment-resistant depression or anxiety disorders, such as severe symptoms, long-lasting symptoms, poor treatment adherence, prior nonresponse to other treatments, and the presence of comorbid disorders
- Consider other important potential factors such as ongoing conflicts, family psychopathology, and an adverse environment (e.g., poverty, chaos, violence, prior and ongoing psychological trauma, abuse, neglect). Additionally, when symptoms are prominent at school, consider the presence of a learning disorder.
- Institute trauma-informed care for appropriate children and adolescents
- A 2007 meta-analysis of published and unpublished trials in pediatric patients found that antidepressants had a number needed to treat (NNT) of 10 for depression, 6 for OCD, and 3 for anxiety disorders; thus, paroxetine may not work in all children, so consider switching to another antidepressant (Bridge et al., 2007)
- Consider a dose adjustment
- Consider augmenting options:
    - Cognitive behavioral therapy (CBT), interpersonal psychotherapy for adolescents (IPT-A), light therapy, family therapy, and exercise especially in adolescents
    - For partial response (depression): use caution when adding medications to paroxetine, especially in children since there are not sufficient studies of augmentation in children or adolescents; however, for the expert, consider bupropion, aripiprazole, or other atypical antipsychotics such as quetiapine; use combinations of antidepressants with caution as this may activate bipolar disorder and suicidal ideation
    - For insomnia: sleep hygiene, CBT for insomnia, melatonin, or alpha 2 agonists
    - For anxiety: buspirone, antihistamines
    - Add lithium or atypical antipsychotics for bipolar depression, psychotic depression, treatment-resistant depression, or treatment-resistant anxiety disorders
    - TMS (transcranial magnetic stimulation) may have a role although pediatric trials of TMS have been hampered by high sham response rates (Croarkin et al., 2021)
    - ECT (case studies show effectiveness; cognitive side effects are similar to those in adults; reserve for treatment-resistant cases)

TALKING TO PATIENTS AND CAREGIVERS

What to Tell Parents About Efficacy

- Doesn't work right away; full therapeutic benefits may take up to 8 weeks, yet parents and teachers might see improvement before the patient does
- While the medicine helps by reducing symptoms and improving function, it is not a cure, and it is therefore necessary to keep taking the medication to sustain its therapeutic effects
- Since every treatment consideration depends on a risk/benefit analysis, parents should fully understand short- and long-term risks as well as benefits
- After successful treatment, continuation of paroxetine may be necessary to prevent relapse, especially in those who have had more than one episode or a very severe episode. In general, when treating depression in children and adolescents, medications are continued for 12 months after symptoms have resolved, while for anxiety disorders, clinicians have generally treated for 6–9 months (Hathaway et al., 2018).
- Often a good idea to tell parents whether the medication chosen is specifically approved for the disorder being treated, or whether it is being given for "unapproved" or "off-label" reasons based on good clinical practice, expert consensus, and/or prudent extrapolation of controlled data from adults

What to Tell Children and Adolescents About Efficacy

- We are trying to make you feel better
- It may be a good idea to give the medication a try; if it's not working very well, we can stop the medication and try something else
- A good try takes 2 to 3 months or even longer
- If it does make you feel better, you cannot stop it right away or you may feel sad or worried again
- Medications don't change who you are as a person; they give you the opportunity to be the best person you can be

What to Tell Parents About Side Effects

- Explain that side effects are expected in many when starting and are most common in the first 2–3 weeks of starting or increasing the dose
- Some SSRI side effects emerge early and resolve quickly (e.g., activation, gastrointestinal symptoms). In contrast, other side effects are late-emerging (e.g., weight gain) or persistent (e.g., sexual dysfunction). Discussing the temporal course of the side effects and distinguishing between persistent and transient side effects is critical. Ensuring that patients are aware not only of side effects but the tendency of some side effects to be transient is important and should be part of discussions with patients and their families. For many, knowing that a side effect is likely transient, as opposed to persistent, may significantly influence the patient and family's anxiety or fears related to medication (Strawn et al., 2023).
- Tell parents many side effects go away and do so about the same time that therapeutic effects start
- Predict side effects in advance (you will look clever and competent to the parents, unless you scare them with too much information and cause nocebo effects, in which case you won't look so clever when the patient develops lots of side effects and stops medication; use your judgment here); a balanced but honest presentation is an art rather than a science
- Ask them to help monitor for increased suicidality and if present, report any such symptoms immediately
- Ask parents to support the patient while side effects are occurring
- Parents should fully understand short- and long-term risks as well as benefits
- Explaining to the parents what to expect from medication treatment, and especially potential side effects, can help prevent early termination of medication

What to Tell Children and Adolescents About Side Effects

- Even if you get side effects, most of them get better or go away in a few days to a few weeks
- Consider having a conversation about sexual side effects in some adolescents who can find these side effects confusing and especially burdensome
- Explaining to child/adolescent what to expect from medication treatment, and

especially potential side effects, can help prevent early termination of medication
- Tell adolescents and children capable of understanding that some young patients, especially those who are depressed, may develop thoughts of hurting themselves, and if this happens, not to be alarmed but to tell their parents right away

What to Tell Teachers About the Medication (If Parents Consent)

- Paroxetine can make children/adolescents jittery or restless
- This medication may cause some tiredness
- It is not abusable
- Encourage dialogue with parents/guardians about any behavior or mood changes

SPECIAL POPULATIONS

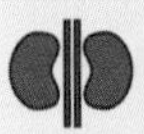

Renal Impairment

- Lower dose [initial 10 mg/day (12.5 mg CR), maximum 40 mg/day (50 mg/day CR)]

Hepatic Impairment

- Lower dose [initial 10 mg/day (12.5 mg CR), maximum 40 mg/day (50 mg/day CR)]

Cardiac Impairment

- Preliminary research suggests that paroxetine is safe in these patients
- In a study using US claims data, the crude incident rate of adverse cardiac events in pediatric patients taking paroxetine was 6.1/10,000 person-years (Czaja et al., 2013)

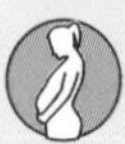

Pregnancy

- Not generally recommended for use during pregnancy, especially during first trimester
- Epidemiological data have shown an increased risk of cardiovascular malformations (primarily ventricular and atrial septal defects) in infants born to women who took paroxetine during the first trimester (absolute risk is small)
- Unless the benefits of paroxetine to the mother justify continuing treatment, consider discontinuing paroxetine or switching to another antidepressant
- Paroxetine use late in pregnancy may be associated with higher risk of neonatal complications, including respiratory distress
- At delivery there may be more bleeding in the mother and transient irritability or sedation in the newborn
- Must weigh the risk of treatment (first trimester fetal development, third trimester newborn delivery) to the child against the risk of no treatment (recurrence of depression, maternal health, infant bonding) to the mother and child
- For many patients this may mean continuing treatment during pregnancy
- SSRI use beyond the 20th week of pregnancy may be associated with increased risk of pulmonary hypertension in newborns, and this effect may be greater with paroxetine compared to other SSRIs
- Exposure to SSRIs late in pregnancy may be associated with increased risk of gestational hypertension and preeclampsia
- Neonates exposed to SSRIs or SNRIs late in the third trimester have developed complications requiring prolonged hospitalization, respiratory support, and tube feeding; reported symptoms are consistent with either a direct toxic effect of SSRIs and SNRIs or, possibly, a drug discontinuation syndrome, and include respiratory distress, cyanosis, apnea, seizures, temperature instability, feeding difficulty, vomiting, hypoglycemia, hypotonia, hypertonia, hyperreflexia, tremor, jitteriness, irritability, and constant crying. These effects may be greater with paroxetine compared to other SSRIs.

Breast Feeding

- Some drug is found in breast milk
- Trace amounts may be present in nursing children whose mothers are on paroxetine
- If child becomes irritable or sedated, breast feeding or drug may need to be discontinued
- Immediate postpartum period is a high-risk time for depression, especially in women who have had prior depressive episodes, so drug may need to be reinstituted late in the third trimester or shortly after childbirth to prevent a recurrence during the postpartum period

- Must weigh benefits of breast feeding with risks and benefits of antidepressant treatment versus nontreatment to both the infant and the mother
- For many patients, this may mean continuing treatment during breast feeding

THE ART OF PSYCHOPHARMACOLOGY

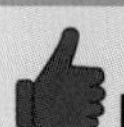

Potential Advantages

- In children:
  - Not specifically approved, but preliminary evidence suggests possible efficacy in children and adolescents with OCD or social anxiety disorder
- In adolescents:
  - Not specifically approved, but preliminary evidence suggests possible efficacy in children and adolescents with OCD or social anxiety disorder
- All ages:
  - Patients with anxiety disorders and insomnia

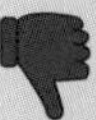

Potential Disadvantages

- In children:
  - Those who are already psychomotor agitated, angry, or irritable, and who do not have a psychiatric diagnosis
  - Results from three placebo-controlled trials in pediatric patients with depression were not sufficient to support approval in this population and data from these trials suggest that the risk of treatment-emergent suicidal ideation may be greater with paroxetine compared to other SSRIs in youth
- In adolescents:
  - Those who may possibly have a mood disorder with mixed or bipolar features, especially those with these features and a family history of bipolar disorder
  - Results from three placebo-controlled trials in pediatric patients with depression were not sufficient to support approval in this population and data from these trials suggest that the risk of treatment-emergent suicidal ideation may be greater with paroxetine compared to other SSRIs in youth
- All ages:
  - Patients with hypersomnia
  - Patients with psychomotor retardation, fatigue, and low energy

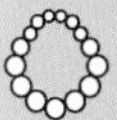

Pearls

- SSRIs show greater efficacy in pediatric anxiety disorders compared to depression; however, studies of paroxetine in youth with major depressive disorder have not consistently shown benefit. In youth with social anxiety disorder, one trial of paroxetine showed benefit compared to placebo.
- In anxious youth, SSRIs produce faster and greater improvement compared to SNRIs (Strawn et al., 2018)
- Withdrawal effects may be more likely for paroxetine than for some other SSRIs when discontinued (especially akathisia, restlessness, gastrointestinal symptoms, dizziness, tingling, dysesthesias, nausea, stomach cramps, restlessness). In fact, paroxetine is notorious for causing withdrawal reactions upon sudden discontinuation, especially when suddenly discontinued from long-term high-dose treatment. This is possibly due not only to SERT inhibition, since all SSRIs can cause discontinuation reactions, but also to anticholinergic rebound and potentially to mechanism-based inhibition. Importantly, youth may be more susceptible to these effects since the half-life of paroxetine is considerably shorter in youth compared to adults (Findling et al., 1999,).
- Paroxetine is a potent CYP2D6 inhibitor and inhibits its own metabolism, so change in blood levels with dose titration are not linear (see Figure 1). If combining with some second generation antipsychotics, such as aripiprazole, clinicians must consider that aripiprazole levels will be much greater than expected
- Paroxetine has mild anticholinergic actions that can enhance the rapid onset of anxiolytic and hypnotic efficacy but also cause mild anticholinergic side effects
- Combinations of CBT (cognitive behavioral therapy) and paroxetine may have better results than either treatment alone both for anxiety disorders and depression, especially for more severe cases

- Can cause cognitive and affective "flattening"
- Some reports suggest greater weight gain and sexual dysfunction than some other SSRIs. Paroxetine inhibits nitric oxide synthase, which theoretically contributes to sexual dysfunction, especially in men.

SUGGESTED READING

Bridge JA, Iyengar S, Salary CB et al. Clinical response and risk for reported suicidal ideation and suicide attempts in pediatric antidepressant treatment: a meta-analysis of randomized controlled trials. JAMA 2007;297(15):1683–96.

Croarkin PE, Elmaadawi AZ, Aaronson ST et al. Left prefrontal transcranial magnetic stimulation for treatment-resistant depression in adolescents: a double-blind, randomized, sham-controlled trial. Neuropsychopharmacology 2021;46(2):462–9.

Czaja AS, Valuck RJ, Anderson HD. Comparative safety of selective serotonin reuptake inhibitors among pediatric users with respect to adverse cardiac events. Pharmacoepidemiol Drug Saf 2013;22(6):607–14.

Findling RL, Reed MD, Myers C et al. Paroxetine pharmacokinetics in depressed children and adolescents. J Am Child Adolesc Psychiatry 1999;38(8):952–9.

Findling RL, Nucci G, Peirgies AA et al. Multiple dose pharmacokinetics of paroxetine in children and adolescents with major depressive disorder or obsessive-compulsive disorder. Neuropsychopharmacology 2006;31(6):1274–85.

Geller DA, Wagner KD, Emslie G et al. Paroxetine treatment in children and adolescents with obsessive-compulsive disorder: a randomized, multicenter, double-blind, placebo-controlled trial. J Am Acad Child Adolesc Psychiatry 2004;43(11):1387–96.

Hathaway EE, Walkup JT, Strawn JR. Antidepressant treatment duration in pediatric depressive and anxiety disorders: how long is long enough? Curr Probl Pediatr Adolesc Health Care 2018;48(2):31–9.

Jornil J, Jensen KG, Larsen F, Linnet K. Identification of cytochrome P450 isoforms involved in the metabolism of paroxetine and estimation of their importance for human paroxetine metabolism using a population-based simulator. Drug Metab Dispos 2010;38(3):376–85.

Kaye CM, Haddock RE, Langley PF et al. A review of the metabolism and pharmacokinetics of paroxetine in man. Acta Psychiatr Scand Suppl 1989;350:60–75.

Strawn JR, Mills JA, Sauley BA, Welge JA. The impact of antidepressant dose and class on treatment response in pediatric anxiety disorders: a meta-analysis. J Am Acad Child Adolesc Psychiatry 2018;57(4):235–244.e2.

Strawn JR, Mills JA, Poweleit EA, Ramsey LB, Croarkin PE. Adverse effects of antidepressant medications and their management in children and adolescents. Pharmacotherapy 2023;43(7):675–90.

Wagner KD, Berard R, Stein MB et al. A multicenter, randomized, double-blind, placebo-controlled trial of paroxetine in children and adolescents with social anxiety disorder. Arch Gen Psychiatry 2004;61(11):1153–62.

THERAPEUTICS

Brands

- Orap

Generic

Yes

US FDA Approved for Pediatric Use

- Suppression of motor and phonic tics in patients with Tourette syndrome who have failed to respond satisfactorily to standard treatment (ages 8 and older)

Off-Label for Pediatric Use

- Approved in adults
  - Used in adults for psychotic disorders in patients who have failed to respond satisfactorily to standard treatment; however, pimozide is not recommended for use in any childhood disorder other than Tourette syndrome

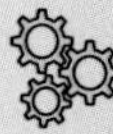

Class and Mechanism of Action

- Neuroscience-based Nomenclature: dopamine receptor antagonist (D-RAn)
- Tourette syndrome/tic suppressant; conventional antipsychotic (neuroleptic, dopamine 2 antagonist)
- Blocks dopamine 2 receptors in the nigrostriatal dopamine pathway, reducing tics in Tourette syndrome
- When used for psychosis, can block dopamine 2 receptors in the mesolimbic dopamine pathway, reducing positive symptoms of psychosis

SAFETY AND TOLERABILITY

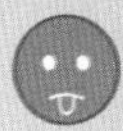

Notable Side Effects

- In adults:
  - Neuroleptic-induced deficit syndrome
  - Akathisia
  - Extrapyramidal symptoms (EPS, also called drug-induced parkinsonism)
  - Dizziness, sedation
  - Dry mouth, constipation, urinary retention, blurred vision
  - Decreased sweating
  - Hypotension, tachycardia, syncope
  - Weight gain
  - Galactorrhea, amenorrhea
  - Sexual dysfunction
  - Tardive dyskinesia (risk is higher in children than in adults)

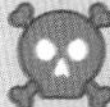

Life-Threatening or Dangerous Side Effects

- Possible lethal cardiac arrhythmias and sudden death when combined with drugs that raise pimozide levels such as macrolide antibiotics, azole antifungal agents, protease inhibitors, and certain antidepressants or that prolong QTc interval themselves (e.g., thioridazine, selected antiarrhythmics, moxifloxacin, sparfloxacin)
- Rare neuroleptic malignant syndrome
- Rare seizures
- Rare jaundice, agranulocytosis

Growth and Maturation

- Long-term effects are unknown

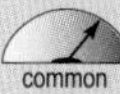

Weight Gain

- Many experience and/or can be significant in amount

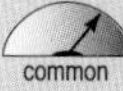

Sedation

- Many experience and/or can be significant in amount
- Sedation is usually transient

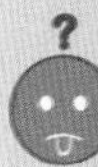

What to Do About Side Effects

- Wait, wait, wait: mild side effects are common, happen early, and usually improve with time, but treatment benefits can be delayed
- Monitor side effects closely, especially when initiating treatment
- May wish to give at night if not tolerated during the day and doesn't disrupt sleep
- Often best to try another monotherapy trial of a different antipsychotic prior to resorting to augmentation strategies to treat side effects
- Exercise and diet programs and medical management for high BMI percentiles, diabetes, dyslipidemia. Also, randomized controlled trials in youth suggest that omega-3 fatty acids can reduce SGA-related hypertriglyceridemia.

- Reduce the dose, particularly for drug-induced parkinsonism, akathisia, sedation, and tremor
- For drug-induced parkinsonism: consider reducing dose or switching to another agent. Augmenting with diphenhydramine or benztropine is less preferred in youth.
- For akathisia: reduce the dose or add a beta blocker. If these are ineffective, raising the dose of the beta blocker may be helpful.
- Using a 5HT2A antagonist such as mirtazapine or cyproheptadine to treat drug-induced akathisia is less common in children and adolescents compared to adults

How Drug Causes Side Effects

- By blocking dopamine 2 receptors in the striatum, it can cause motor side effects and akathisia
- By blocking dopamine 2 receptors in the pituitary, it can cause elevations in prolactin
- By blocking dopamine 2 receptors excessively in the mesocortical and mesolimbic dopamine pathways, especially at high doses, it can cause worsening of negative and cognitive symptoms (neuroleptic-induced deficit syndrome)
- Anticholinergic actions may cause sedation, blurred vision, constipation, dry mouth
- Antihistaminic actions may cause sedation, weight gain
- By blocking alpha 1 adrenergic receptors, it can cause dizziness, sedation, and hypotension
- Mechanism of any possible increased incidence of diabetes or dyslipidemia is unknown
- Mechanism of potentially dangerous QTc prolongation may be related to actions of pimozide on ion channels in the heart; mechanism is dose related so drug interactions that raise pimozide or overdose are more likely to cause potentially dangerous arrhythmias

Warnings and Precautions

- Carefully weigh the risks and benefits of pharmacological treatment against the risks and benefits of nontreatment with an antipsychotic and it is a good idea to document this in the patient's chart
- If signs of neuroleptic malignant syndrome develop, treatment should be immediately discontinued
- Use cautiously in patients with alcohol withdrawal or convulsive disorders because of possible lowering of seizure threshold
- Antiemetic effect can mask signs of other disorders or overdose
- Do not use epinephrine in event of overdose as interaction with some pressor agents may lower blood pressure
- Because pimozide may dose-dependently prolong QTc interval, use with caution in patients who have bradycardia or who are taking drugs that can induce bradycardia (e.g., beta blockers, calcium channel blockers, clonidine, digitalis)
- Because pimozide may dose-dependently prolong QTc interval, use with caution in patients who have hypokalemia and/or hypomagnesemia or who are taking drugs that can induce hypokalemia and/or hypomagnesemia (e.g., diuretics, stimulant laxatives, intravenous amphotericin B, glucocorticoids, tetracosactide)
- Pimozide can increase tumors in mice (dose-related effect)
- Pimozide can increase the QTc interval and potentially cause arrhythmia or sudden death, especially in combination with drugs that raise its levels

When Not to Prescribe

- If patient is taking an agent capable of significantly prolonging QTc interval (e.g., thioridazine, selected antiarrhythmics, moxifloxacin, and sparfloxacin)
- If patient is taking drugs that inhibit pimozide metabolism, such as macrolide antibiotics, azole antifungal agents (ketoconazole, itraconazole), protease inhibitors, nefazodone, fluvoxamine, fluoxetine, sertraline
- If there is a history of QTc prolongation or cardiac arrhythmia, recent acute myocardial infarction, uncompensated heart failure
- If patient is taking drugs that can cause tics
- If there is a proven allergy to pimozide
- If there is a known sensitivity to other antipsychotics
- Not recommended for use in any other childhood condition than Tourette syndrome
- If patient is in a comatose state or has CNS depression

Long-Term Use
- Some side effects may be irreversible (e.g., tardive dyskinesia)

Habit Forming
- No

Overdose
- Deaths have occurred; extrapyramidal symptoms, ECG changes, hypotension, respiratory depression, coma

DOSING AND USE

Usual Dosage Range
- 0.2 mg/kg/day (not to exceed 10 mg/day)

Dosage Forms
- Tablet 1 mg scored, 2 mg scored

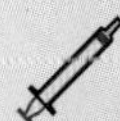

How to Dose
- Initial 0.05 mg/kg per day at night; can increase every 3 days; maximum 0.2 mg/kg/day (not to exceed 10 mg/day)
- CYP2D6 genotyping is recommended in the pimozide product label before exceeding 4 mg of pimozide daily in adults or 0.05 mg/kg/day in children
- Pimozide should not be titrated faster than 14 days in individuals who are identified as poor metabolizers of the CYP2D6

Options for Administration
- Oral dosage form is the only option

Tests
- Before starting pimozide:
  - Baseline ECG and serum potassium levels should be determined
  - Plan to monitor weight and metabolic parameters more closely than in adults since children and adolescents may be more prone to these side effects than adults
  - Weigh all patients and monitor weight gain against that expected for normal growth, using the pediatric height/weight chart to monitor
  - Get baseline personal and family history of diabetes, obesity, dyslipidemia, hypertension, and cardiovascular disease
  - Obtain blood pressure, fasting plasma glucose (or hemoglobin A1C), and a lipid profile
- After starting pimozide:
  - Periodic evaluation of ECG and serum potassium levels, especially during dose titration
  - Serum magnesium levels may also need to be monitored
  - Monitor weight and BMI percentile
  - Consider monitoring fasting triglycerides in patients at high risk for metabolic complications
  - Patients with low white blood cell count (WBC) or history of drug-induced leukopenia/neutropenia should have complete blood count (CBC) monitored frequently during the first few months and pimozide should be discontinued at the first sign of decline of WBC in the absence of other causative factors
  - Patients should be monitored periodically for the development of abnormal movements using neurological exam and the Abnormal Involuntary Movement Scale (AIMS)
  - Monitoring elevated prolactin levels is of dubious clinical benefit

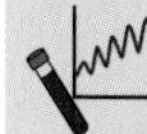

Pharmacokinetics
- Metabolized by CYP3A, CYP2D6, and to a lesser extent by CYP1A2 (Figure 1)
- In adults, pimozide has a half-life of approximately 60 hours in CYP2D6 poor metabolizers compared to approximately 30 hours in normal metabolizers. This doubling in half-life increases the time needed to achieve steady state in CYP2D6 poor metabolizers.
- Steady state occurs in 6 days in CYP2D6 normal metabolizers, but poor metabolizers require nearly 2 weeks to achieve steady state

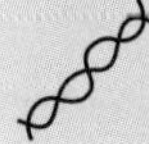

Pharmacogenetics
- CYP2D6 genotyping is recommended in the pimozide product label before exceeding 4 mg of pimozide daily in adults or 0.05 mg/kg/day in children
- In the past, it was advised to adjust the dose of pimozide every 3 days in order to attain the desired clinical response in all patients. However, the label has been updated to state that pimozide doses should not be increased sooner than 14 days

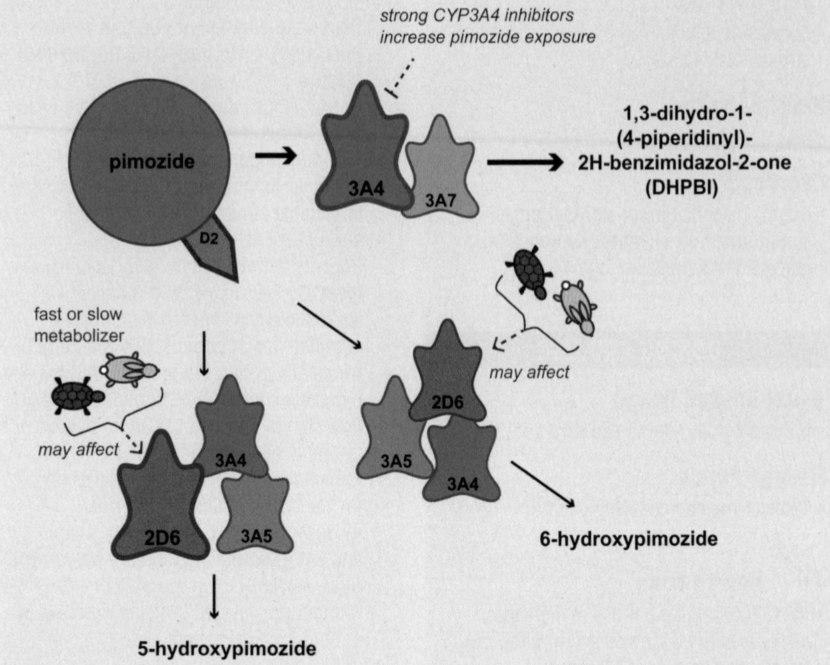

Figure 1 Metabolism of pimozide.

in individuals who are identified as poor metabolizers of the CYP2D6 enzyme.

- In a modeling study, 2 mg daily in CYP2D6 poor metabolizers produced higher blood levels and a longer time to steady-state concentrations (Figure 2)

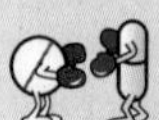

Drug Interactions

- May enhance QTc prolongation of other drugs capable of prolonging QT interval
- May increase the effects of antihypertensive drugs
- Use with CYP3A4 inhibitors (e.g., fluoxetine, sertraline, fluvoxamine, and nefazodone; foods such as grapefruit juice) can raise pimozide levels and increase the risks of dangerous arrhythmias
- Use with CYP2D6 inhibitors (e.g., fluoxetine, paroxetine, duloxetine and sertraline) can raise pimozide levels and increase the risks of dangerous arrhythmias
- Use with drugs capable of significantly prolonging QTc interval (e.g., thioridazine, selected antiarrhythmics, moxifloxacin, and sparfloxacin) can increase the risk of dangerous arrhythmias
- Additive effects may occur if used with CNS depressants

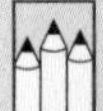

Dosing Tips

- In children and adolescents, CYP2D6 genotyping is recommended before exceeding 0.05 mg/kg/day
- The effects of pimozide on the QT interval are dose dependent, so start low and go slow while carefully monitoring QT interval
- Sudden, unexpected deaths have occurred in patients taking high doses of pimozide for conditions other than Tourette syndrome; therefore, patients should be instructed not to exceed the prescribed dose of pimozide
- Treatment should be suspended if absolute neutrophil count falls below 1,000/mm^3

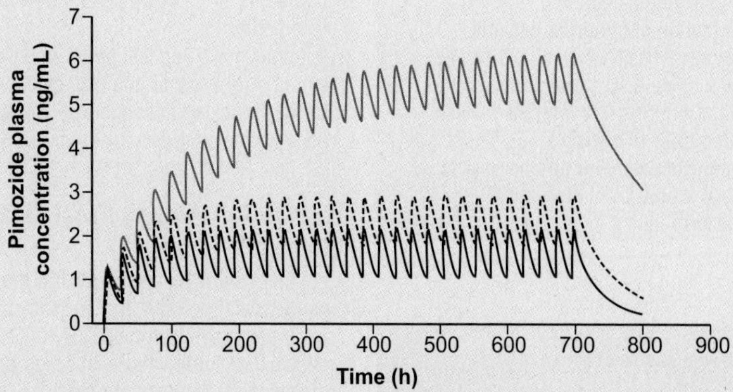

Figure 2 Concentration–time curves for pimozide in CYP2D6 poor metabolizers (light gray line) as well as normal (solid black line) and intermediate metabolizers (dotted line). Reproduced from Rogers et al., 2012.

How to Switch

- From another antipsychotic to pimozide:
  - When tapering a prior antipsychotic, see its entry in this manual for how to stop and how to taper off that specific drug. However, extreme caution should be used if cross-titrating to an antipsychotic that inhibits CYP2D6 or is associated with QTc prolongation.
  - Generally, stop the first agent before starting pimozide to decrease the chances of any adverse drug interaction and also so that new side effects of pimozide can be distinguished from withdrawal effects of the first agent
- Off pimozide to another antipsychotic:
  - Generally, stop pimozide before starting the new antipsychotic to decrease the chances of any adverse drug interaction and also so that new side effects of the next drug can be distinguished from any withdrawal effects from pimozide

How to Stop

- Slow down-titration of oral formulation (over 6–8 weeks), especially when simultaneously beginning a new antipsychotic while switching (i.e., cross-titration)
- Rapid discontinuation may lead to rebound worsening of tics

WHAT TO EXPECT

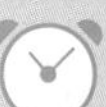

Onset of Action

- Relief from tics may occur rapidly

Duration of Action

- Effects are consistent over a 24-hour period

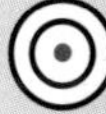

Primary Target Symptoms

- Vocal and motor tics in patients who fail to respond to treatment with other antipsychotics

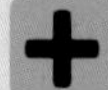

What Is Considered a Positive Result?

- Resolution of or reduction in vocal and motor tics

How Long to Treat

- Should continuously evaluate for switching to an antipsychotic with a better risk/benefit ratio

What If It Stops Working?

- Check for nonadherence and consider switching to another antipsychotic with fewer side effects

What If It Doesn't Work?

- Discontinue pimozide and try another drug for Tourette syndrome

- Consider trying haloperidol
- Augmentation of pimozide has not been systematically studied and can be dangerous, especially with drugs that can either prolong QTc interval or raise pimozide plasma levels
- Consider evaluation for another diagnosis including a possible neurological consultation

TALKING TO PATIENTS AND CAREGIVERS

What to Tell Parents About Efficacy

- Explain which use pimozide is being chosen for, how to tell if the drug is working by targeting specific symptoms, and why this is being done, especially since there are other options generally preferred for the treatment of Tourette syndrome because they are considered to be safer
- Specifically, tell parents pimozide is being chosen because of the failures of multiple first-line therapies and is justified despite its greater risks
- For acute symptoms, it can work right away
- Pimozide is usually given every day
- While the medicine helps by reducing symptoms and improving function, it is not a cure, and it therefore may be necessary to keep taking the medication long term to sustain its therapeutic effects
- Since every treatment consideration depends on a risk/benefit analysis, parents should fully understand short- and long-term risks as well as benefits
- Often a good idea to tell parents whether the medication chosen is specifically approved for the disorder being treated, or whether it is being given for "unapproved" or "off-label" reasons based on good clinical practice, expert consensus, and/or prudent extrapolation of controlled data from adults

What to Tell Children and Adolescents About Efficacy

- Be specific about the symptoms being targeted: we are trying to help you ...
- Give the medication a try; if it's not working very well, we can stop the medication and try something else
- A good try often takes several weeks with this medication
- If it does make you feel better, you cannot stop it right away or you may get sick again
- Medications don't change who you are as a person; they give you the opportunity to be the best person you can be

What to Tell Parents About Side Effects

- Let them know that pimozide is a more dangerous drug than first-line treatments for Tourette syndrome because of the effects that combinations of drugs with pimozide can have on the heart
- Tell them to let every doctor know the child is on pimozide, including emergency department physicians
- Let every physician the child is seeing know every drug the child is taking, and it is a good idea for you to become very familiar with every drug the child is taking
- Side effects (especially motor side effects) of pimozide are generally expected to be more severe than with second generation atypical antipsychotics
- Explain that side effects are expected in many when starting
- Tell parents many side effects go away and do so about the same time that therapeutic effects start
- Predict side effects in advance (you will look clever and competent to the parents, unless you scare them with too much information and cause nocebo effects, in which case you won't look so clever when the patient develops lots of side effects and stops medication; use your judgment here); a balanced but honest presentation is an art rather than a science
- Ask parents to support the patient while side effects are occurring
- Parents should fully understand short- and long-term risks as well as benefits
- Explaining to the parents what to expect from medication treatment, and especially what potential side effects to expect, can help prevent early termination of medication
- Specifically, it may be prudent to warn that tardive dyskinesia can be more common after treatment with haloperidol than with second generation atypical antipsychotics

What to Tell Children and Adolescents About Side Effects

- Even if you get side effects, most of them get better or go away in a few weeks
- If you have side effects that are bothering you, tell your parents and your parents should tell me
- Consider having a conversation about sexual side effects in some adolescents who can find these side effects confusing and especially burdensome
- Explaining to child/adolescent what to expect from medication treatment, and especially potential side effects, can help prevent early termination of medication

What to Tell Teachers About the Medication (If Parents Consent)

- Pimozide can make children/adolescents restless
- Pimozide can make children/adolescents sedated
- It is not abusable
- Encourage dialogue with parents/guardians about any behavior or mood changes
- Notify the clinician of increased restlessness or akathisia symptoms, which may be apparent in the school setting

SPECIAL POPULATIONS

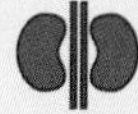

Renal Impairment

- Use with caution

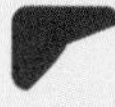

Hepatic Impairment

- Use with caution

Cardiac Impairment

- Pimozide produces a dose-dependent QT prolongation (Drolet et al., 2001), which may be enhanced by the existence of bradycardia, hypokalemia, congenital or acquired long QTc interval, which should be evaluated prior to administering pimozide
- Use with caution if treating concomitantly with a medication likely to produce prolonged bradycardia, hypokalemia, slowing of intracardiac conduction, or prolongation of the QTc interval
- Avoid pimozide in patients with a known history of QTc prolongation

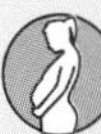

Pregnancy

- Controlled studies have not been conducted in pregnant women
- Renal papillary abnormalities have been seen in rats during pregnancy
- There is a risk of abnormal muscle movements and withdrawal symptoms in newborns whose mothers took an antipsychotic during the third trimester; symptoms may include agitation, abnormally increased or decreased muscle tone, tremor, sleepiness, severe difficulty breathing, and difficulty feeding
- Psychotic symptoms may worsen during pregnancy, and some form of treatment may be necessary
- Atypical antipsychotics may be preferable to conventional antipsychotics or anticonvulsant mood stabilizers if treatment is required during pregnancy
- Should evaluate for an antipsychotic with a better risk/benefit ratio if treatment required during pregnancy

Breast Feeding

- Unknown if pimozide is secreted in human breast milk, but all psychotropics assumed to be secreted in breast milk
- Not recommended for use because of potential for tumorigenicity or cardiovascular effects on infant
- Recommended either to discontinue drug or formula feed

THE ART OF PSYCHOPHARMACOLOGY

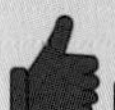

Potential Advantages

- In children and adolescents:
    - A 24-week open-label study of pimozide in 36 children ages 2 to 12 suggested a similar safety profile in this age group as in older patients
- All ages:
    - Only for patients who respond to this agent and not to other antipsychotics

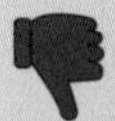

Potential Disadvantages

- In children and adolescents:
  - Limited data on the use and efficacy of pimozide in patients less than 12 years of age
- All ages:
  - Patients on other drugs

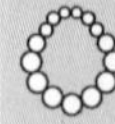

Pearls

- In the past, pimozide was a first-line choice for Tourette syndrome and for certain behavioral disorders, including monosymptomatic hypochondriasis; however, it is now recognized that the benefits of pimozide generally do not outweigh its risks in most patients
- Because of its effects on the QTc interval, pimozide is not intended for use unless other options for tic disorders (or psychotic disorders) have failed and is best prescribed by the expert
- CYP2D6 poor metabolizers are at an increased risk for QTc prolongation at standard doses of pimozide because of higher drug concentrations

SUGGESTED READING

Desta Z, Kerbusch T, Soukhova N et al. Identification and characterization of human cytochrome P450 isoforms interacting with pimozide. J Pharmacol Exp Ther 1998;285(2):428–37.

Drolet B, Rousseau G, Daleau P et al. Pimozide (Orap) prolongs cardiac repolarization by blocking the rapid component of the delayed rectifier potassium current in native cardiac myocytes. J Cardiovasc Pharmacol Ther 2001;6(3):255–60.

Pringsheim T, Marras C. Pimozide for tics in Tourette syndrome. Cochrane Database Syst Rev 2009;(2):CD006996.

Rogers HL, Bhattaram A, Zineh I et al. CYP2D6 genotype information to guide pimozide treatment in adult and pediatric patients: basis for the U.S. Food and Drug Administration's new dosing recommendations. J Clin Psychiatry 2012;73(9):1187–90.

Sallee FR, Nesbitt L, Jackson C et al. Relative efficacy of haloperidol and pimozide in children and adolescents with Tourette's disorder. Am J Psychiatry 1997;154(8):1057–62.

Shapiro AK, Shapiro E. Controlled study of pimozide vs placebo in Tourette's syndrome. J Am Acad Child Psychiatry 1984;23(2):161–73.

Shapiro E, Shapiro AK, Fulop G et al. Controlled study of haloperidol, pimozide and placebo for the treatment of Gilles de la Tourette's syndrome. Arch Gen Psychiatry 1989;46(8):722–30.

THERAPEUTICS

Brands
- Minipress

Generic
Yes

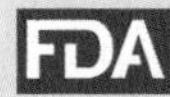

US FDA Approved for Pediatric Use
- None

Off-Label for Pediatric Use
- Approved in adults
  - Hypertension
- Other off-label uses
  - Nightmares associated with PTSD
  - Blood circulation disorders

Class and Mechanism of Action
- Blocks alpha 1 adrenergic receptors to reduce noradrenergic hyperactivation
- Stimulation of central noradrenergic receptors during sleep may activate traumatic memories, so blocking this activation may reduce nightmares

SAFETY AND TOLERABILITY

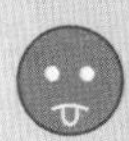

Notable Side Effects
- Dizziness, lightheadedness, headache, fatigue, blurred vision
- Nausea
- Orthostatic hypotension

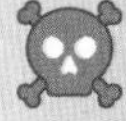

Life-Threatening or Dangerous Side Effects
- Syncope with sudden loss of consciousness

Growth and Maturation
- Not studied

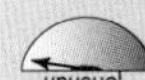

Weight Gain
- Reported but not expected

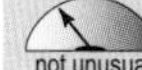

Sedation
- Occurs in significant minority

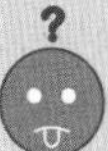

What to Do About Side Effects
- Lower the dose
- In a few weeks, switch to another agent

How Drug Causes Side Effects
- Excessive blockade of alpha 1 peripheral noradrenergic receptors

Warnings and Precautions
- Prazosin can cause syncope with sudden loss of consciousness, most often in association with rapid dose increases or the introduction of another antihypertensive drug
- Intraoperative floppy iris syndrome (IFIS) has been observed during cataract surgery in some patients treated with alpha 1 adrenergic blockers, which may require modifications to the surgical technique; however, there does not appear to be a benefit of stopping the alpha 1 adrenergic blocker prior to cataract surgery
- Avoid situations that can cause orthostatic hypotension, such as extensive periods of standing, prolonged or intense exercise, and exposure to heat

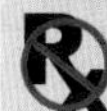

When Not to Prescribe
- If there is a proven allergy to quinazolines or prazosin

Long-Term Use
- Has not been evaluated in controlled studies
- Nightmares may return if prazosin is stopped

Habit Forming
- No

Overdose
- No fatalities have been reported; sedation, depressive reflexes, hypotension

DOSING AND USE

Usual Dosage Range

- 1–16 mg/day, generally in divided doses

Dosage Forms

- Capsule 1 mg, 2 mg, 5 mg

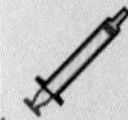

How to Dose

- Due to concern for first-dose hypotension, begin prazosin at 1 mg given 30 minutes before bedtime
- Titrate by 1 mg every 3 to 4 days for the first 2 weeks, with a clinical reevaluation once the patient is at 2 or 3 mg
- In children under 6 or in those with side effects (e.g., nausea, dizziness) start at 0.5 mg and titrate weekly, as more gradual titration minimizes orthostatic side effects. Increase the dose until nightmares and overall quality of sleep have significantly improved, which generally occurs at a dose between 2 and 5 mg, and then monitor.
- Monitor blood pressure and pulse (sitting and standing) at baseline and at each follow-up appointment. If morning dizziness or other orthostatic symptoms are present, administer the medication 30 to 60 minutes earlier in the evening. If symptoms persist, decrease the dose in 1 mg increments until tolerated.

Options for Administration

- Only available as a capsule

Tests

- Monitor blood pressure and pulse (sitting and standing) at baseline and at each follow-up appointment
- False-positive results may occur in screening tests for pheochromocytoma in patients who are being treated with prazosin; if an elevated urinary vanillylmandelic acid (VMA) is found, prazosin should be discontinued and the patient retested after a month

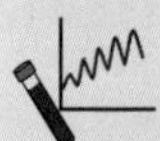

Pharmacokinetics

- Prazosin is well absorbed after oral administration in adults, and its peak plasma concentration (Cmax) is reached within 1 to 3 hours. However, data related to its pharmacokinetics in children and adolescents are extremely limited.
- Prazosin is highly bound to plasma proteins, particularly to albumin (97%–99%), meaning only a small fraction of the drug is in its unbound, active form and available to exert its pharmacological effect
- Prazosin has a moderate volume of distribution, indicating that it distributes relatively well throughout the body tissues
- Prazosin is primarily metabolized in the liver and involves conjugation with glucuronic acid to form inactive metabolites
- Prazosin and its metabolites are primarily renally excreted, and the elimination half-life (in adults) is approximately 2 to 3 hours

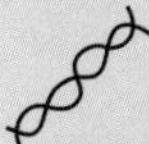

Pharmacogenetics

- No recommendations

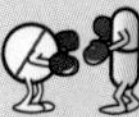

Drug Interactions

- Concomitant use with a phosphodiesterase-5 inhibitor (PDE-5) can have additive effects on blood pressure, potentially leading to hypotension; thus, a PDE-5 inhibitor should be initiated at the lowest possible dose
- Concomitant use with a beta blocker (e.g., propranolol) or other alpha blockers can have additive effects on blood pressure
- Concomitant use with other alpha 1 blockers, which include many psychotropic agents, can have additive effects leading to hypotension

Dosing Tips

- Dosing may be extremely individualized, with as little as 2 mg/day helpful for some patients
- Risk of syncope can be decreased by limiting the initial dose to 1 mg and using slow dose titration

How to Switch

- From another medication to prazosin:
  - Generally, try to stop the first agent before starting prazosin so that any side effects of prazosin can be distinguished from withdrawal effects of the first agent
- Off prazosin to another medication:
  - Generally, try to stop prazosin before starting the new medication, particularly if the new medication is also an alpha

1 blocker or has other alpha 1 blocking properties
  - Taper; may need to adjust dosage of concurrent medications as prazosin is being discontinued

How to Stop

- Taper to avoid the theoretical risk of rebound hypertension. However, this has not been well described in the literature.

WHAT TO EXPECT

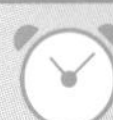

Onset of Action

- Within a few days; however, full effect may require appropriate dosing

Duration of Action

- Effects are consistent over an 8–10-hour period and the medication is primarily used for overnight symptoms (e.g., nightmares)
- May continue to work for many years to prevent relapse of symptoms

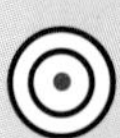

Primary Target Symptoms

- Nightmares

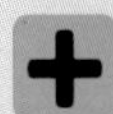

What Is Considered a Positive Result?

- Reduces the severity and frequency of nightmares associated with PTSD (consider assessing with structured scale)

How Long to Treat

- Continue treatment until all symptoms are gone or until improvement is stable. Encourage a trial off medication at regular intervals or at completion of an evidence-based trauma treatment to avoid unnecessary long-term treatment.

What If It Stops Working?

- Check for nonadherence and consider switching to another agent with fewer side effects
- Screen for the development of a new comorbid disorder, especially substance abuse
- Screen for adverse changes in the home or school environment that may increase trauma reminders

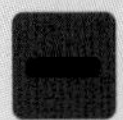

What If It Doesn't Work?

- Increase dose (see How to Dose)
- For individuals who do not respond to prazosin or cannot tolerate prazosin, may consider an alpha 2 adrenergic agonist (e.g., clonidine or guanfacine)
- Consider evaluation for another diagnosis or for a comorbid condition (e.g., medical illness, substance use)
- Consider other important potential factors such as ongoing conflicts, family psychopathology, and an adverse environment (e.g., poverty, chaos, violence, prior and ongoing psychological trauma, abuse, neglect)
- Institute trauma-focused psychotherapy

TALKING TO PATIENTS AND CAREGIVERS

What to Tell Parents About Efficacy

- It can work right away
- Explain which use prazosin is being chosen for, how to tell if the drug is working by targeting specific symptoms, and why this is being done
- Since every treatment consideration depends on a risk/benefit analysis, parents should fully understand short- and long-term risks as well as benefits
- Often a good idea to tell parents whether the medication chosen is specifically approved for the disorder being treated, or whether it is being given for "off-label" reasons based on good clinical practice, expert consensus, and/or prudent extrapolation of controlled data from adults

What to Tell Children and Adolescents About Efficacy

- Be specific about the symptoms being targeted: we are trying to help you …
- Give the medication a try; if it's not working very well, we can stop the medication and try something else
- Medications don't change who you are as a person; they give you the opportunity to be the best person you can be

What to Tell Parents About Side Effects

- Explain that side effects are expected in many when starting and that the most common side

effects may include lightheadedness in the morning
- Encourage their children to remain hydrated
- Predict side effects in advance (you will look clever and competent to the parents, unless you scare them with too much information and cause nocebo effects, in which case you won't look so clever when the patient develops lots of side effects and stops medication; use your judgment here); a balanced but honest presentation is an art rather than a science
- Ask parents to support the patient while side effects are occurring
- Parents should fully understand short- and long-term risks as well as benefits
- Explaining to the parents what to expect from medication treatment, and especially what potential side effects to expect, can help prevent early termination of medication

What to Tell Children and Adolescents About Side Effects

- Even if you get a side effect, we can usually reduce it over time and it is important to stay hydrated
- If you have side effects that are bothering you, tell your parents and your parents should tell me
- Explaining to child/adolescent what to expect from medication treatment, and especially potential side effects, can help prevent early termination of medication

What to Tell Teachers About the Medication (If Parents Consent)

- Prazosin can make children/adolescents sedated or may cause lightheadedness
- It is not abusable
- Encourage dialogue with parents/guardians about any behavior or mood changes

SPECIAL POPULATIONS

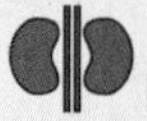

Renal Impairment

- Use with caution in patients with severe impairment
- May require lower dose

Hepatic Impairment

- Use with caution

Cardiac Impairment

- Use with caution in patients who are predisposed to hypotensive or syncopal episodes

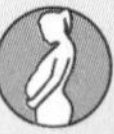

Pregnancy

- Controlled studies have not been conducted in pregnant women
- Prazosin has been used alone or in combination with other hypotensive agents in severe hypertension of pregnancy, with no fetal or neonatal abnormalities reported
- Prazosin should be used during pregnancy only if the potential benefits justify the potential risks to the mother and fetus

Breast Feeding

- Some drug is present in breast milk
- If child becomes irritable or sedated, breast feeding or drug may need to be discontinued
- Must weigh benefits of breast feeding with risks and benefits of treatment versus nontreatment to both the infant and the mother

THE ART OF PSYCHOPHARMACOLOGY

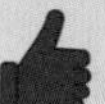

Potential Advantages

- Specifically for nightmares and other symptoms of autonomic arousal

Potential Disadvantages

- Patients with orthostatic symptoms and dysautonomia
- Patients taking concomitant psychotropic drugs with alpha 1 antagonist properties

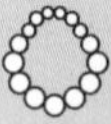

Pearls

- The evidence base for using prazosin to treat nightmares associated with PTSD is children and adolescents and draws largely from studies in adults and several retrospective trials in youth
- Given that studies of SSRIs have consistently failed to demonstrate benefits in pediatric patients with PTSD (Keeshin and Strawn, 2014), prazosin likely plays

an important role for PTSD symptoms in youth – particularly intrusive symptoms
- Monitor blood pressure and pulse (sitting and standing) at baseline and at follow-up visits. If morning dizziness or other orthostatic symptoms are present, administer the medication 30 to 60 minutes earlier in the evening.
- In youth with PTSD, trauma-focused CBT also improves reactive behaviors that may be driven by persistent hyperarousal and intrusive symptoms. Improving sleep can dramatically increase the patient's ability to cope with daytime trauma symptoms.
- Avoid multiple adrenergic modulator agents in the same patient
- Maximize the effectiveness of prazosin and ensure good and sustained engagement in trauma-focused cognitive behavioral therapy (TF-CBT). This may decrease the need for polypharmacy that often occurs in kids with PTSD.

SUGGESTED READING

Ferrafiat V, Soleimani M, Chaumette B, et al. Use of prazosin for pediatric post-traumatic stress disorder with nightmares and/or sleep disorder: case series of 18 patients prospectively assessed. Front Psychiatry 2020;11:724.

Hudson N, Burghart S, Reynoldson J, Grauer D. Evaluation of low dose prazosin for PTSD-associated nightmares in children and adolescents. Ment Health Clin 2021;11(2):45–9.

Keeshin BR, Strawn JR. Psychological and pharmacologic treatment of youth with posttraumatic stress disorder: an evidence-based review. Child Adolesc Psychiatr Clin N Am 2014;23(2):399–411.

Keeshin BR, Strawn JR, Out D, Granger DA, Putnam FW. Elevated salivary alpha amylase in adolescent sexual abuse survivors with posttraumatic stress disorder symptoms. J Child Adolesc Psychopharmacol 2015;25(4):344–50.

Keeshin BR, Ding Q, Presson AP, Berkowitz SJ, Strawn JR. Use of prazosin for pediatric PTSD-associated nightmares and sleep disturbances: a retrospective chart review. Neurol Ther 2017;6(2):247–57.

Strawn JR, Keeshin BR, Cohen JA. Posttraumatic stress disorder in children and adolescents: treatment and overview. UpToDate 2023. Last updated Sept. 6, 2023.

THERAPEUTICS

Brands

- Seroquel
- Seroquel XR

Generic

Yes

US FDA Approved for Pediatric Use

- Schizophrenia (quetiapine, ages 13 and older)
- Acute mania (quetiapine, ages 10 and older, monotherapy and adjunct)

Off-Label for Pediatric Use

- Approved in adults
  - Schizophrenia (quetiapine XR)
  - Maintaining response in schizophrenia (quetiapine XR)
  - Acute mania (quetiapine XR, monotherapy and adjunct)
  - Bipolar maintenance (quetiapine, quetiapine XR)
  - Bipolar depression (quetiapine, quetiapine XR)
  - Depression (quetiapine XR, adjunct)
- Other off-label uses
  - Other psychotic disorder
  - Mixed mania
  - Behavioral disturbances in children and adolescents
  - Disorders associated with problems with impulse control
  - Severe treatment-resistant anxiety
  - Posttraumatic stress disorder

Class and Mechanism of Action

- Neuroscience-based Nomenclature: dopamine, serotonin multimodal (DS-MM)
- Atypical antipsychotic (serotonin-dopamine antagonist; second generation antipsychotic; also a mood stabilizer)
- Blocks dopamine 2 receptors, reducing positive symptoms of psychosis and stabilizing affective symptoms
- Blockade of serotonin type 2A receptors may also contribute at clinical doses to the enhancement of dopamine release in certain brain regions, thus theoretically reducing motor side effects
- Interactions at a myriad of other neurotransmitter receptors may contribute to quetiapine's efficacy
- Specifically, antagonist actions at 5HT2C receptors may contribute to efficacy for cognitive and affective symptoms in some patients
- Specifically, actions at 5HT1A receptors may contribute to efficacy for cognitive and affective symptoms in some patients, especially at moderate to high doses

SAFETY AND TOLERABILITY

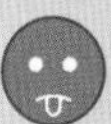

Notable Side Effects

- Probably increases risk for diabetes and dyslipidemia
- Weight gain, increased appetite
- Dizziness, sedation, fatigue
- Nausea, vomiting
- Dry mouth
- Tachycardia
- Hyperprolactinemia: in children and adolescents, quetiapine is associated with hyperprolactinemia; however, the incidence of this is lower than for some other second generation antipsychotics. In a prospective study of youth treated with quetiapine, the incidence of elevated prolactin was approximately 40% and was lower than risperidone and olanzapine but higher than aripiprazole (Koch et al., 2023)
- Orthostatic hypotension, usually during initial dose titration
- Risk of drug-induced parkinsonism and dystonic reactions may be higher in children than it is in adults
- Risk of withdrawal dyskinesias, although this is generally lower for quetiapine than for other antipsychotics

Life-Threatening or Dangerous Side Effects

- Hyperglycemia, in some cases extreme and associated with ketoacidosis or hyperosmolar coma or death, has been reported in patients taking atypical antipsychotics
- Rare neuroleptic malignant syndrome (NMS) may cause hyperpyrexia, muscle rigidity, delirium, and autonomic instability with elevated creatine phosphokinase,

myoglobinuria (rhabdomyolysis), and acute renal failure
- Rare seizures
- As a class, antidepressants have been reported to increase the risk of suicidal thoughts and behaviors in children and young adults

Growth and Maturation

- Long-term effects are unknown

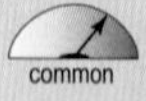

Weight Gain

- Many patients experience and/or can be significant in amount at effective antipsychotic doses
- Can become a health problem in some
- May be even more risk of weight gain and metabolic effects in children than in adults

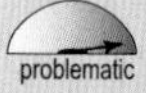

Sedation

- Frequent and can be significant in amount
- Some patients may not tolerate it
- Can wear off over time
- Can reemerge as dose increases and then wear off again over time
- Not necessarily increased as dose is raised
- May be more likely to be sedating in children than in adults

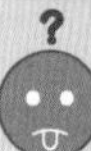

What to Do About Side Effects

- Wait, wait, wait: mild side effects are common, happen early, and usually improve with time, but treatment benefits can be delayed. However, weight gain and metabolic disturbance can emerge at any point (although they are more common earlier).
- Monitor side effects closely, especially when initiating treatment
- Usually dosed twice daily, so take more of the total daily dose at bedtime to help reduce daytime sedation
- Start dosing low and increase slowly as side effects wear off at each dosing increment
- Often best to try another monotherapy trial of a different antipsychotic prior to resorting to augmentation strategies to treat side effects
- Exercise and diet programs and medical management for high BMI percentiles, diabetes, dyslipidemia. Also, randomized controlled trials in youth suggest that omega-3 fatty acids can reduce SGA-related hypertriglyceridemia.
- Reduce the dose, particularly for drug-induced parkinsonism, akathisia, sedation, and tremor
- For drug-induced parkinsonism: consider reducing dose or switching to another agent. Augmenting with diphenhydramine or benztropine is less preferred in youth.
- For akathisia: reduce the dose or add a beta blocker. If these are ineffective, raising the dose of the beta blocker may be helpful.
- Using a 5HT2A antagonist such as mirtazapine or cyproheptadine to treat drug-induced akathisia is less common in children and adolescents compared to adults

How Drug Causes Side Effects

- By blocking histamine 1 receptors in the brain, it can cause sedation and possibly weight gain
- Blocking alpha 1 adrenergic receptors can cause dizziness, hypotension, and syncope
- Blocking muscarinic cholinergic receptors can cause dry mouth, blurred vision, urinary retention, constipation, and paralytic ileus
- By blocking dopamine 2 receptors in the striatum, it can cause drug-induced parkinsonism and akathisia
- Mechanism of any possible weight gain is unknown but may relate to effects at 5HT2C receptors
- Mechanism of any possible increased incidence of diabetes or dyslipidemia is unknown

Warnings and Precautions

- Consider distributing brochures provided by the FDA and the drug companies or have the pharmacy do this for the parents
- When quetiapine is used to treat depressive mood disorders off-label in children, either as a monotherapy or an augmenting agent to an SSRI/SNRI, it is a good idea to warn patients and their caregivers about the possibility of activating side effects and suicidality as for any antidepressant in this age group and advise them to report such symptoms immediately
- Carefully weigh the risks and benefits of pharmacological treatment against the risks and benefits of nontreatment with

an antipsychotic and it is a good idea to document this in the patient's chart
- Quetiapine should be used cautiously in patients at risk for aspiration pneumonia, as dysphagia has been reported
- Priapism has been reported
- Use with caution in patients with known cardiovascular disease, cerebrovascular disease
- Avoid use with drugs that increase the QTc interval and in patients with risk factors for prolonged QTc interval
- Atypical antipsychotics have the potential for cognitive and motor impairment, especially related to sedation
- Atypical antipsychotics can cause body temperature dysregulation; use caution in patients who may experience conditions that increase body temperature (e.g., strenuous exercise, saunas, extreme heat, dehydration, or concomitant anticholinergic medication)
- Dysphagia has been associated with antipsychotic use, and quetiapine should be used cautiously in patients at risk for aspiration pneumonia
- Antipsychotics may cause somnolence, postural hypotension, motor and sensory instability, which may lead to falls; for patients with diseases, conditions, or medications that could exacerbate these effects, complete fall risk assessments when initiating antipsychotic treatment and recurrently for patients on long-term antipsychotic therapy
- As with any antipsychotic, use with caution in patients with history of seizures

When Not to Prescribe
- If there is a proven allergy to quetiapine

Long-Term Use
- Approved in adults for long-term maintenance in bipolar disorder
- Approved in adults to maintain response in long-term treatment of schizophrenia
- Often used for long-term maintenance in various behavioral disorders

Habit Forming
- No

Overdose
- Rarely lethal in monotherapy overdose; sedation, slurred speech, hypotension

DOSING AND USE

Usual Dosage Range
- Schizophrenia: 400–800 mg/day
- Bipolar mania: 400–600 mg/day

Dosage Forms
- Tablet 25 mg, 50 mg, 100 mg, 150 mg, 200 mg, 300 mg, 400 mg
- Extended-release tablet 50 mg, 150 mg, 200 mg, 300 mg, 400 mg

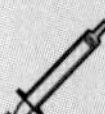

How to Dose
- Schizophrenia: day 1, initial 25 mg twice per day; day 2, twice-daily dosing totaling 100 mg; day 3, twice-daily dosing totaling 200 mg; day 4, twice-daily dosing totaling 300 mg; day 5, twice-daily dosing totaling 400 mg; further adjustments should be in increments no greater than 100 mg/day; recommended dose range 400–800 mg/day
- Bipolar mania: day 1, initial 25 mg twice per day; day 2, twice-daily dosing totaling 100 mg; day 3, twice-daily dosing totaling 200 mg; day 4, twice-daily dosing totaling 300 mg; day 5, twice-daily dosing totaling 400 mg; further adjustments should be in increments no greater than 100 mg/day; recommended dose range 400–600 mg/day

Options for Administration
- Oral tablet options only

Tests
- Before starting quetiapine:
  - Plan to monitor weight and metabolic parameters more closely than in adults since children and adolescents may be more prone to metabolic side effects than adults
  - Weigh all patients and monitor weight gain against that expected for normal growth, using the pediatric height/weight chart to monitor. In particular, monitor BMI percentiles.
  - Get baseline personal and family history of diabetes, obesity, dyslipidemia, hypertension, and cardiovascular disease
  - Obtain blood pressure, fasting plasma glucose (or hemoglobin A1C), and a lipid profile
- After starting quetiapine:
  - BMI percentile monthly for 3 months, then quarterly

- Consider monitoring fasting triglycerides monthly in patients at high risk for metabolic complications
- Blood pressure, fasting plasma glucose (or hemoglobin A1C), lipid profile within 3 months and then annually
- Treat or refer for treatment and consider switching to another atypical antipsychotic for patients who become overweight, obese, pre-diabetic, diabetic, or dyslipidemic while receiving an atypical antipsychotic
- Even in patients without known diabetes, be vigilant for the rare but life-threatening onset of diabetic ketoacidosis, which always requires immediate treatment, by monitoring for the rapid onset of polyuria, polydipsia, weight loss, nausea, vomiting, dehydration, rapid respiration, weakness, and clouding of sensorium, even coma
- Patients with low white blood cell count (WBC) or history of drug-induced leukopenia/neutropenia should have complete blood count (CBC) monitored frequently during the first few months and quetiapine should be discontinued at the first sign of decline of WBC in the absence of other causative factors
- Although U.S. manufacturer recommends 6-month eye checks for cataracts, clinical experience suggests this may be unnecessary
- Plasma drug levels of quetiapine are not reliable and thus monitoring is not recommended
- Patients should be monitored periodically for the development of abnormal movements using neurological exam and the Abnormal Involuntary Movement Scale (AIMS)

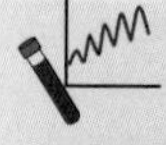

Pharmacokinetics

- Quetiapine is well absorbed after oral administration in pediatric patients. However, the absorption rate may vary among individuals and can be affected by factors such as food intake. Taking quetiapine with a meal delays its absorption but does not significantly alter the overall extent of absorption.
- In pharmacokinetic studies of children and adolescents, quetiapine pharmacokinetics are linear and the elimination half-life is 3–4 hours (in adults the half-life is 6–7 hours)
- Quetiapine is a substrate for CYP3A4 with minor contributions by CYP2D6 (Figure 1)

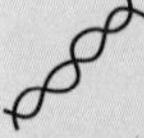

Pharmacogenetics

- No recommendations

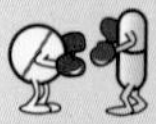

Drug Interactions

- CYP3A4 inhibitors and CYP2D6 inhibitors may reduce clearance of quetiapine and thus raise quetiapine plasma levels, but dosage reduction of quetiapine usually not necessary
- There are case reports in adults of increased international normalized ratio (INR) (used to monitor the degree of anticoagulation) when quetiapine is coadministered with warfarin, which is also a substrate of CYP3A4

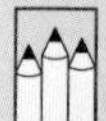

Dosing Tips

- Children and adolescents may tolerate lower doses better
- Clinical practice suggests that at low doses it may be a sedative-hypnotic, possibly due to potent H1 antihistamine actions, but this can risk numerous antipsychotic-related side effects and there are many other options
- Many patients do well with immediate-release form as a single daily oral dose, usually at bedtime
- Higher doses generally achieve greater response for manic or psychotic symptoms
- Dosing in major depression may be even lower than in bipolar depression, and dosing may be even lower still in generalized anxiety disorder
- Quetiapine XR is controlled-release and therefore should not be chewed or crushed but rather should be swallowed whole
- Treatment should be suspended if absolute neutrophil count falls below 1,000/mm^3

How to Switch

- From another antipsychotic to quetiapine:
  - When tapering a prior antipsychotic, see its entry in this manual for how to stop and how to taper off that specific drug
  - Generally, try to stop the first agent before starting quetiapine so that new side effects of quetiapine can be distinguished from withdrawal effects of the first agent

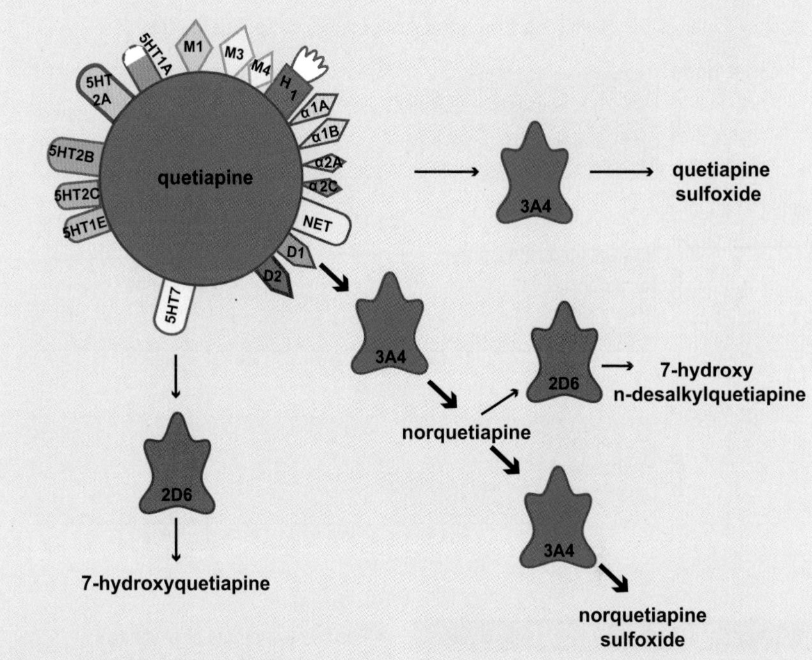

Figure 1 Quetiapine metabolism.

- If urgent, cross taper off the other antipsychotic while quetiapine is started at a low dose, with dose adjustments down of the other antipsychotic, and up for quetiapine every 3 to 7 days
- Off quetiapine to another antipsychotic:
  - Generally, try to stop quetiapine before starting the new antipsychotic so that new side effects of the next drug can be distinguished from any withdrawal effects from quetiapine
  - If urgent, cross taper off quetiapine by cutting the dose in half as the new antipsychotic is also started with dose adjustments down of quetiapine and up for the new antipsychotic

How to Stop

- Slow down-titration of oral formulation (over 6–8 weeks), especially when simultaneously beginning a new antipsychotic while switching (i.e., cross-titration)
- Make down-titration even slower if any signs of anticholinergic rebound such as tachycardia, tremor, gastrointestinal symptoms
- Rapid oral discontinuation may lead to rebound psychosis and worsening of symptoms
- Rapid oral discontinuation may lead to withdrawal dyskinesias, which are generally reversible in the pediatric population. Of note, withdrawal dyskinesias are more common in pediatric patients than in adults.
- If antiparkinsonian agents are being used, they should be continued for a few weeks after quetiapine is discontinued

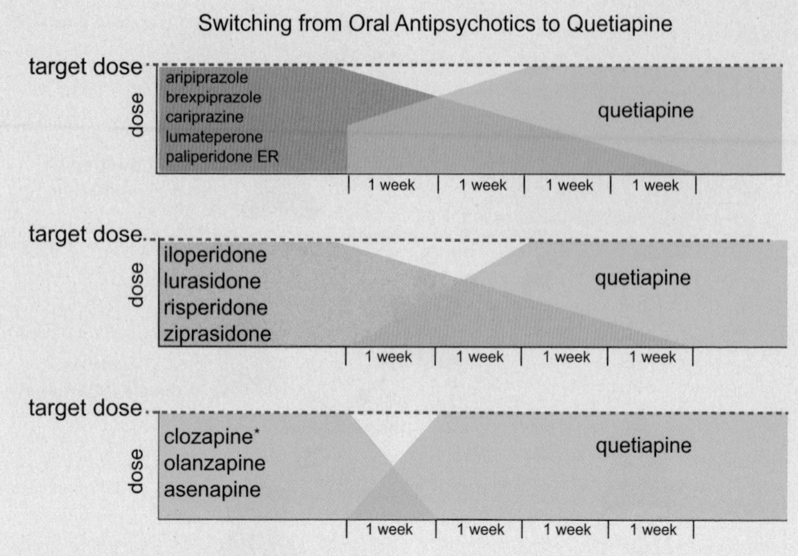

WHAT TO EXPECT

Onset of Action

- Psychotic and manic symptoms can improve within 1 week of oral dosing, but it may take several weeks for full effect on behavior as well as on cognition and affective stabilization
- Interestingly, in several randomized, prospective trials, quetiapine has been associated with greater and faster improvements in manic symptoms compared to both lithium and divalproex. In a head-to-head comparison of quetiapine and lithium in manic adolescents, 72% of youth were considered responders compared to 49% of patients receiving lithium (Patino et al., 2021).
- If it is not working within 6–8 weeks, it may require a dosage increase or it may not work at all

Duration of Action

- Effects of oral medication are consistent over a 24-hour period
- Oral medication may continue to work for many years to prevent relapse of symptoms

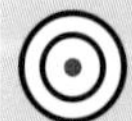

Primary Target Symptoms

- Mania
- Positive symptoms of psychosis
- Negative symptoms of psychosis
- Unstable mood (both depressed mood and mania)
- Aggressive symptoms
- Insomnia and anxiety

What Is Considered a Positive Result?

- In schizophrenia:
  - Most often reduces positive symptoms but does not eliminate them
  - Can improve negative symptoms, as well as aggressive, cognitive, and affective symptoms but less so than for positive symptoms
  - Can improve acute agitation
  - In children or adolescents with a first episode of psychosis, initial response may be greater than for recurrent episodes of psychosis in adults
- In bipolar disorder:
  - Many patients may experience a reduction of symptoms by half or more
  - Can improve agitation in bipolar mania
- In depression:
  - Full elimination of depressed mood, anxiety, and other symptoms of depression is the goal

How Long to Treat

- In schizophrenia and bipolar disorder:
  - Continue treatment until reaching a plateau of improvement
  - After reaching a satisfactory plateau, continue treatment for at least a year after first episode of psychosis or mania
  - For second and subsequent episodes of psychosis or mania, treatment may need to be indefinite
- In depression:
  - If it is the first episode, continue for 6–12 months after reaching full remission
  - If it is the second episode, continue for 12–24 months after reaching full remission
  - If it is the third or greater episode, continue treatment indefinitely

What If It Stops Working?

- Check for nonadherence and consider switching to another antipsychotic with fewer side effects
- Some patients who have an initial response may relapse even though they continue treatment, sometimes called "poop-out"
- Growth/developmental changes may contribute to apparent loss of efficacy as well as to new onset of side effects as metabolism slows and drug levels rise in transition from childhood to adolescence; dose adjustment (increase or decrease) should be considered
- Screen for the development of a new comorbid disorder, especially substance use
- Screen for adverse changes in the home or school environment

What If It Doesn't Work?

- Consider evaluation for another diagnosis (especially bipolar illness or depression with mixed features) or for a comorbid condition (e.g., medical illness, substance use)
- Consider other important potential factors such as ongoing conflicts, family psychopathology, and an adverse environment (e.g., poverty, chaos, violence, prior and ongoing psychological trauma, abuse, neglect)
- Institute trauma-informed care for appropriate children and adolescents
- For schizophrenia or bipolar disorder:
  - Try one of the other atypical antipsychotics
  - If no first-line atypical antipsychotic is effective, consider higher doses or augmentation with lithium or lamotrigine; however, in adolescents with mania, quetiapine produces faster and greater improvements compared to lithium (Patino et al., 2021)
  - Consider initiating psychotherapy. In adolescents with bipolar disorder (and those with affective symptoms who are at risk of developing bipolar disorder), family-focused psychotherapy can be particularly helpful (Miklowitz et al., 2020).
  - Consider presence of concomitant drug abuse

TALKING TO PATIENTS AND CAREGIVERS

What to Tell Parents About Efficacy

- For acute symptoms, it can work right away
- Oral quetiapine is usually given every day
- Explain which use quetiapine is being chosen for, how to tell if the drug is working by targeting specific symptoms, and why this is being done
- Once the child/adolescent calms down, at some point after one dose or after several days of dosing or after long-term dosing, we should all assess whether the medication should be continued
- While the medicine helps by reducing symptoms and improving function, it is not a cure, and it therefore may be necessary to keep taking the medication long term to sustain its therapeutic effects
- Since every treatment consideration depends on a risk/benefit analysis, parents should fully understand short- and long-term risks as well as benefits
- Often a good idea to tell parents whether the medication chosen is specifically approved for the disorder being treated, or whether it is being given for "unapproved" or "off-label" reasons based on good clinical practice, expert consensus, and/or prudent extrapolation of controlled data from adults

What to Tell Children and Adolescents About Efficacy

- Be specific about the symptoms being targeted: we are trying to help you …
- Give the medication a try; if it's not working very well, we can stop the medication and try something else
- A good try often takes several weeks
- If it does make you feel better, you cannot stop it right away or you may get sick again
- Medications don't change who you are as a person; they give you the opportunity to be the best person you can be

What to Tell Parents About Side Effects

- Explain that side effects are expected in many when starting
- Tell parents many side effects go away and do so about the same time that therapeutic effects start
- Predict side effects in advance (you will look clever and competent to the parents, unless you scare them with too much information and cause nocebo effects, in which case you won't look so clever when the patient develops lots of side effects and stops medication; use your judgment here); a balanced but honest presentation is an art rather than a science
- Ask parents to support the patient while side effects are occurring
- Parents should fully understand short- and long-term risks as well as benefits
- Explaining to the parents what to expect from medication treatment, and especially what potential side effects to expect, can help prevent early termination of medication

What to Tell Children and Adolescents About Side Effects

- Even if you get side effects, most of them get better or go away in a few weeks
- If you have side effects that are bothering you, tell your parents and your parents should tell me
- Consider having a conversation about sexual side effects in some adolescents who can find these side effects confusing and especially burdensome
- Explaining to child/adolescent what to expect from medication treatment, and especially potential side effects, can help prevent early termination of medication

What to Tell Teachers About the Medication (If Parents Consent)

- Quetiapine can make children/adolescents sedated
- It is not abusable
- Encourage dialogue with parents/guardians about any behavior or mood changes
- Notify the clinician of increased restlessness or akathisia symptoms, which may be apparent in the school setting

SPECIAL POPULATIONS

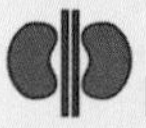

Renal Impairment

- No dose adjustment required

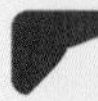

Hepatic Impairment

- Downward dose adjustment may be necessary

Cardiac Impairment

- Use in patients with cardiac impairment has not been studied; however, the risk of orthostatic hypotension in pediatric patients is less than in adults, as children rely less on peripheral vasoconstriction to regulate blood pressure
- Use with caution if patient is taking concomitant antihypertensive or alpha 1 antagonist

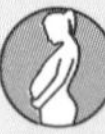

Pregnancy

- Controlled studies have not been conducted in pregnant women
- There is a risk of abnormal muscle movements and withdrawal symptoms in newborns whose mothers took an antipsychotic during the third trimester; symptoms may include agitation, abnormally increased or decreased muscle tone, tremor, sleepiness, severe difficulty breathing, and difficulty feeding
- When administered to pregnant rats and rabbits, embryo-fetal toxicity occurred at doses 1- and 2-times the maximum recommended human dose (MRHD), and maternal toxicity occurred at 2 times the MRHD in rats and 1–2 times the MRHD in rabbits

- Psychotic symptoms may worsen during pregnancy, and some form of treatment may be necessary
- National Pregnancy Registry for Atypical Antipsychotics: 1-866-961-2388 or http://womensmentalhealth.org/clinical-and-research-programs/pregnancyregistry/

Breast Feeding

- Unknown if quetiapine is secreted in human breast milk, but all psychotropics assumed to be secreted in breast milk
- Recommended either to discontinue drug or formula feed
- Infants of women who choose to breast feed while on quetiapine should be monitored for possible adverse effects; sedation, failure to thrive, jitteriness, tremor, and abnormal muscle movements have been reported

THE ART OF PSYCHOPHARMACOLOGY

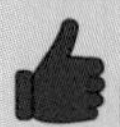

Potential Advantages

- In children:
  - Can provide more sedation than some other atypical antipsychotics if that is desired for symptom control
- In adolescents:
  - Approved for schizophrenia and manic episodes
- All ages:
  - Some cases of psychosis and bipolar disorder refractory to treatment with other antipsychotics
  - Often a preferred augmenting agent in bipolar depression or treatment-resistant unipolar depression

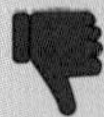

Potential Disadvantages

- In children and adolescents:
  - Can provide more sedation than some other atypical antipsychotics if that is NOT desired for symptom control
  - May be more susceptible to side effects, including sedation and weight gain
  - Efficacy was not demonstrated in a clinical study evaluating quetiapine for the treatment of bipolar depression in children ages 10–17
- All ages:
  - Patients concerned about gaining weight
  - Patients with diabetes mellitus, obesity, and/or dyslipidemia

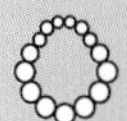

Pearls

- The active metabolite of quetiapine, norquetiapine, has the additional properties of norepinephrine reuptake inhibition and antagonism of 5HT2C receptors, which may contribute to therapeutic effects for mood and cognition
- Dosing differs depending on the indication, with high-dose mechanisms including robust blockade of D2 receptors above 60% occupancy and equal or greater 5HT2A blockade; medium-dose mechanisms including moderate amounts of NET inhibition combined with 5HT2C antagonism and 5HT1A partial agonism; and low-dose mechanisms including H1 antagonism and 5HT1A partial agonism and, to a lesser extent, NET inhibition and 5HT2C antagonism
- More sedation than some other antipsychotics, which may be of benefit in acutely manic or psychotic patients but not for stabilized patients in long-term maintenance
- Unlike in studies of adults, quetiapine has not demonstrated superiority to placebo in controlled trials of adolescents with bipolar I or bipolar II depression (DelBello et al., 2009; Findling et al., 2014)
- In prospective trials, quetiapine has been associated with the normalization of prefrontal functional activity in manic adolescents (Lei et al., 2023)
- Essentially no motor side effects

SUGGESTED READING

DelBello MP, Chang K, Welge JA et al. A double-blind, placebo-controlled pilot study of quetiapine for depressed adolescents with bipolar disorder. Bipolar Disord 2009;11(5):483–93.

Findling RL, McKenna K, Early WR et al. Efficacy and safety of quetiapine in adolescents with schizophrenia investigated in a 6-week, double-blind, placebo-controlled trial. J Child Adolesc Psychopharmacol 2012;22(5):327–42.

Findling RL, Pathak S, Earley WR et al. Efficacy and safety of extended-release quetiapine fumarate in youth with bipolar depression: an 8 week, double-blind, placebo-controlled trial. J Child Adolesc Psychopharmacol 2014;24(6):325–35.

Koch MT, Carlson HE, Kazimi MM, Correll CU. Antipsychotic-related prolactin levels and sexual dysfunction in mentally ill youth: a 3-month cohort-study. J Am Acad Child Adolesc Psychiatry 2023;62(9):1021–50.

Lei D, Li W, Qin K et al. Effects of short-term quetiapine and lithium therapy for acute manic or mixed episodes on the limbic system and emotion regulation circuitry in youth with bipolar disorder. Neuropsychopharmacology 2023;48(4):615–22.

Miklowitz DJ, Schneck CD, Walshaw PD et al. Effects of family-focused therapy vs enhanced usual care for symptomatic youths at high risk for bipolar disorder: a randomized clinical trial. JAMA Psychiatry 2020;77(5):455–63.

Pathak S, Findling RL, Earley WR et al. Efficacy and safety of quetiapine in children and adolescents with mania associated with bipolar I disorder: a 3-week, double-blind, placebo-controlled trial. J Clin Psychiatry 2013;74(1):e100–9.

Patino LR, Klein CC, Strawn JR et al. A randomized, double-blind, controlled trial of lithium versus quetiapine for the treatment of acute mania in youth with early course bipolar disorder. J Child Adolesc Psychopharmacol 2021;31(7):485–93.

Pillay J, Boylan K, Carrey N et al. First- and Second-Generation Antipsychotics in Children and Young Adults: Systematic Review Update [Internet]. Rockville, MD: Agency for Healthcare Research and Quality (US); 2017 Mar. Report No.: 17-EHC001-EF. AHRQ Comparative Effectiveness Reviews.

THERAPEUTICS

Brands
- CONSTA
- Perseris
- Risperdal
- Rykindo
- Uzedy

Generic
Yes

US FDA Approved for Pediatric Use
- Schizophrenia (Risperdal, ages 13 and older)
- Acute mania/mixed mania (Risperdal, ages 10 and older, monotherapy and adjunct)
- Autism-related irritability (Risperdal, ages 5–16)

Off-Label for Pediatric Use
- Approved in adults
  - Schizophrenia (CONSTA, Perseris, Rykindo, Uzedy)
  - Delaying relapse in schizophrenia (Risperdal)
  - Other psychotic disorder (Risperdal)
  - Bipolar maintenance [monotherapy and adjunct (CONSTA, Rykindo)]
- Other off-label uses
  - Bipolar depression
  - Behavioral disturbances in children and adolescents
  - Disorders associated with problems with impulse control
  - Posttraumatic stress disorder

Class and Mechanism of Action
- Neuroscience-based Nomenclature: dopamine, serotonin, norepinephrine receptor antagonist (DSN RAn)
- Atypical antipsychotic (serotonin-dopamine antagonist; second generation antipsychotic; also a mood stabilizer)
- Blocks dopamine 2 receptors, reducing positive symptoms of psychosis and stabilizing affective symptoms
- Blockade of serotonin type 2A receptors may also contribute at clinical doses to the enhancement of dopamine release in certain brain regions, thus theoretically reducing motor side effects
- Interactions at a myriad of other neurotransmitter receptors may contribute to risperidone's efficacy
- Specifically, 5HT7 antagonist properties may contribute to antidepressant actions

SAFETY AND TOLERABILITY

Notable Side Effects
- May increase risk for diabetes and dyslipidemia
- Dose-dependent extrapyramidal symptoms (EPS, also called drug-induced parkinsonism)
- Dose-dependent hyperprolactinemia (in children and adolescents, serum prolactin levels tend to rise and peak within the first 1 to 2 months and then steadily decline to values within or very close to the normal range within 6 months)
- Dose-dependent sedation, tremor, akathisia
- Nausea, vomiting, constipation, abdominal pain
- Weight gain, increased appetite
- Risk of drug-induced parkinsonism and dystonic reactions may be higher in children than it is in adults
- Risk of withdrawal dyskinesias
- Galactorrhea/amenorrhea (girls)
- Gynecomastia (boys)

Life-Threatening or Dangerous Side Effects
- Hyperglycemia, in some cases extreme and associated with ketoacidosis or hyperosmolar coma or death, has been reported in patients taking atypical antipsychotics
- Rare neuroleptic malignant syndrome (NMS) may cause hyperpyrexia, muscle rigidity, delirium, and autonomic instability with elevated creatine phosphokinase, myoglobinuria (rhabdomyolysis), and acute renal failure
- Rare seizures

Growth and Maturation
- Retrospective analyses have not shown a clinically significant growth failure or delay in pubertal onset or progression in children treated for up to 1 year with risperidone

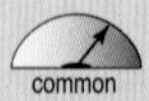

Weight Gain

- Many patients experience and/or can be significant in amount. In pediatric samples, higher plasma concentrations of risperidone are associated with more weight gain (Kloosterboer et al., 2021).
- May be more weight gain in children and adolescents than in adults. Current practice often includes adding metformin in pediatric patients who experience early weight gain (or are at high risk of antipsychotic weight gain, that is, greater than 85%ile for BMI).
- Can become a health problem in some

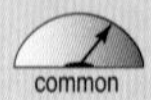

Sedation

- Many patients experience and/or can be significant. In pediatric samples, higher plasma concentrations are associated with more sedation (Kloosterboer et al., 2021).

What to Do About Side Effects

- Wait, wait, wait: mild side effects are common, happen early, and usually improve with time, but treatment benefits can be delayed
- Monitor side effects closely, especially when initiating treatment
- Children and adolescents with autism spectrum disorders may be particularly sensitive to side effects, so start with low doses and titrate slowly
- May wish to give at night if not tolerated during the day and doesn't disrupt sleep
- Often best to try another monotherapy trial of a different antipsychotic prior to resorting to augmentation strategies to treat side effects
- Exercise and diet programs and medical management for high BMI percentiles, diabetes, dyslipidemia. Also, randomized controlled trials in youth suggest that omega-3 fatty acids can reduce SGA-related hypertriglyceridemia.
- Reduce the dose, particularly for drug-induced parkinsonism, akathisia, sedation, and tremor
- For drug-induced parkinsonism: consider reducing dose or switching to another agent. Augmenting with diphenhydramine or benztropine is less preferred in youth.
- For akathisia: reduce the dose or add a beta blocker; if these are ineffective, raising the dose of the beta blocker may be helpful. Using a 5HT2A antagonist such as cyproheptadine to treat drug-induced akathisia is less common in children and adolescents compared to adults.

How Drug Causes Side Effects

- Blocking alpha 1 adrenergic receptors can cause dizziness, hypotension, and syncope. However, these effects may be less commonly seen as side effects in pediatric patients compared to adults.
- By blocking dopamine 2 receptors in the striatum, it can cause drug-induced parkinsonism, especially at high doses
- By blocking dopamine 2 receptors in the pituitary, it can cause elevations in prolactin
- Mechanism of any possible weight gain is unknown but may relate to effects at 5HT2C receptors
- Mechanism of any possible increased incidence of diabetes or dyslipidemia is unknown

Warnings and Precautions

- Carefully weigh the risks and benefits of pharmacological treatment against the risks and benefits of nontreatment with an antipsychotic and it is a good idea to document this in the patient's chart
- Use with caution in patients with conditions that predispose to hypotension (dehydration, overheating)
- Atypical antipsychotics have the potential for cognitive and motor impairment, especially related to sedation
- Atypical antipsychotics can cause body temperature dysregulation; use caution in patients who may experience conditions that increase body temperature (e.g., strenuous exercise, saunas, extreme heat, dehydration, or concomitant anticholinergic medication)
- Priapism has been reported
- As with any antipsychotic, use with caution in patients with history of seizures

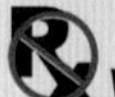

When Not to Prescribe

- If there is a proven allergy to risperidone and paliperidone

Long-Term Use

- In adults, oral risperidone is approved to delay relapse in long-term treatment of schizophrenia
- Often used for long-term maintenance in bipolar disorder and various behavioral disorders

Habit Forming

- No

Overdose

- Rarely lethal in monotherapy overdose; sedation, rapid heartbeat, convulsions, low blood pressure, difficulty breathing

DOSING AND USE

Usual Dosage Range

- 0.5–3 mg/day for aggression or irritability due to autism
- 1–2.5 mg/day for bipolar mania
- 3 mg/day (1 to 6 mg/day) for schizophrenia

Dosage Forms

- Tablet 0.25 mg, 0.5 mg, 1 mg, 2 mg, 3 mg, 4 mg, 6 mg
- Orally disintegrating tablet 0.5 mg, 1 mg, 2 mg, 3 mg, 4 mg
- Liquid 1 mg/mL
- CONSTA (risperidone microspheres) 12.5 mg, 25 mg, 37.5 mg, 50 mg
- Rykindo (risperidone microspheres) 12.5 mg, 25 mg, 37.5 mg, 50 mg
- Perseris (risperidone subcutaneous) 90 mg, 120 mg
- Uzedy (risperidone subcutaneous) 50 mg, 75 mg, 100 mg, 125 mg, 150 mg, 200 mg, 250 mg

How to Dose

- Can be dosed once or twice daily, usually starting at twice a day in divided doses, then when tolerated, full daily dose once a day, often at night
- If clinical effects wear off with once-daily administration, give as twice a day dosing
- Autism (patients weighing less than 20 kg): initial dose 0.25 mg/day; after at least 4 days can increase to target dose of 0.5 mg/day; this dose should be maintained for at least 14 days, after which, depending on response, dose can be increased at intervals of no less than 2 weeks in increments of 0.25 mg/day; effective dose range 0.5–3 mg/day
- Autism (patients weighing at least 20 kg): initial dose 0.5 mg/day; after at least 4 days can increase to target dose of 1 mg/day; this dose should be maintained for at least 14 days, after which, depending on response, dose can be increased at intervals of no less than 2 weeks in increments of 0.5 mg/day; effective dose range 0.5–3 mg/day
- Schizophrenia: initial dose 0.5 mg/day; can increase every 24 hours in increments of 0.5–1 mg/day; target dose 3 mg/day; effective dose range 1–6 mg/day
- Bipolar mania: initial dose 0.5 mg/day; can increase every 24 hours in increments of 0.5–1 mg/day; target dose 1–2.5 mg/day; effective dose range 1–6 mg/day

Options for Administration

- Multiple formulation alternatives for patients with difficulty swallowing pills, including oral solution and orally disintegrating tablet
- Long-acting injectable formulations not approved in children/adolescents and few studies; probably best not to use long-acting injectables in children at all, and only with caution off-label in adolescents who are older and have adult body weights

Tests

- Before starting risperidone:
  - Plan to monitor weight and metabolic parameters more closely than in adults since children and adolescents may be more prone to metabolic side effects than adults
  - Weigh all patients and monitor weight gain against that expected for normal growth, using the pediatric height/weight chart to monitor. In particular, monitor BMI percentiles.
  - Get baseline personal and family history of diabetes, obesity, dyslipidemia, hypertension, and cardiovascular disease
  - Obtain blood pressure, fasting plasma glucose (or hemoglobin A1C), and a lipid profile
- After starting risperidone:
  - BMI percentile monthly for 3 months, then quarterly

- Consider monitoring fasting triglycerides in patients at high risk for metabolic complications
- Blood pressure, fasting plasma glucose (or hemoglobin A1C), lipid profile within 3 months and then annually
- Treat or refer for treatment and consider switching to another atypical antipsychotic for patients who become overweight, obese, pre-diabetic, diabetic, or dyslipidemic while receiving an atypical antipsychotic
- Even in patients without known diabetes, be vigilant for the rare but life-threatening onset of diabetic ketoacidosis, which always requires immediate treatment, by monitoring for the rapid onset of polyuria, polydipsia, weight loss, nausea, vomiting, dehydration, rapid respiration, weakness, and clouding of sensorium, even coma
- Patients with low white blood cell count (WBC) or history of drug-induced leukopenia/neutropenia should have complete blood count (CBC) monitored frequently during the first few months and risperdone should be discontinued at the first sign of decline of WBC in the absence of other causative factors
- Monitoring elevated prolactin levels is of dubious clinical benefit, although risperidone is known to increase prolactin levels and cause galactorrhea and amenorrhea in girls and gynecomastia in boys. Prolactin levels should be obtained in female patients with secondary amenorrhea.
- Consider monitoring plasma levels of risperidone (i.e., 9-hydroxyrisperidone) if not responding, or questions about compliance or side effects
- Patients should be monitored periodically for the development of abnormal movements using neurological exam and the Abnormal Involuntary Movement Scale (AIMS)

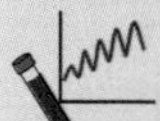

Pharmacokinetics

- Metabolized by CYP2D6 to the active metabolite 9-hydroxyrisperidone, also known as paliperidone (Figure 1)
- Metabolites are active
- Following oral administration, risperidone is rapidly absorbed (Tmax = 2 hours) in both children and adolescents (Figure 2)
- Parent drug of oral formulation has 20–24-hour half-life in adults; same for active metabolite 9-hydroxyrisperidone (paliperidone)
- In pediatric clinical trials, the body weight corrected pharmacokinetics of risperidone and 9-hydroxyrisperidone (paliperidone) were similar to those in adults
- Food does not affect absorption

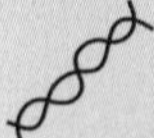

Pharmacogenetics

- In patients who are poor CYP2D6 metabolizers, concentrations of risperidone are increased compared to concentrations of 9-OH risperidone
- In ultrarapid CYP2D6 metabolizers, the ratio of 9-hydroxyrisperidone (paliperidone) to risperidone will be increased, which may produce more risk for hyperprolactinemia
- The dose of oral risperidone should be adjusted when used in combination with CYP2D6 inhibitors; however, there are no current Clinical Pharmacogenetics Implementation Consortium (CPIC) recommendations for risperidone dosing based on CYP2D6 phenotype

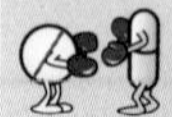

Drug Interactions

- Clearance of risperidone may be reduced and thus plasma levels increased by clozapine; dosing adjustment usually not necessary
- Coadministration with carbamazepine may decrease plasma levels of risperidone
- Coadministration with fluoxetine and paroxetine may increase plasma levels of risperidone
- Since risperidone is metabolized by CYP2D6, any agent that inhibits this enzyme could theoretically raise risperidone plasma levels and lower 9-hydroxyrisperidone levels

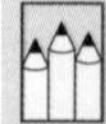

Dosing Tips

- In pediatric clinical trials, no additional benefit was observed above 2.5 mg per day (bipolar disorder) or 3 mg per day (schizophrenia); higher doses were associated with more adverse events, particularly weight gain
- Doses higher than 6 mg per day have not been studied in the pediatric population

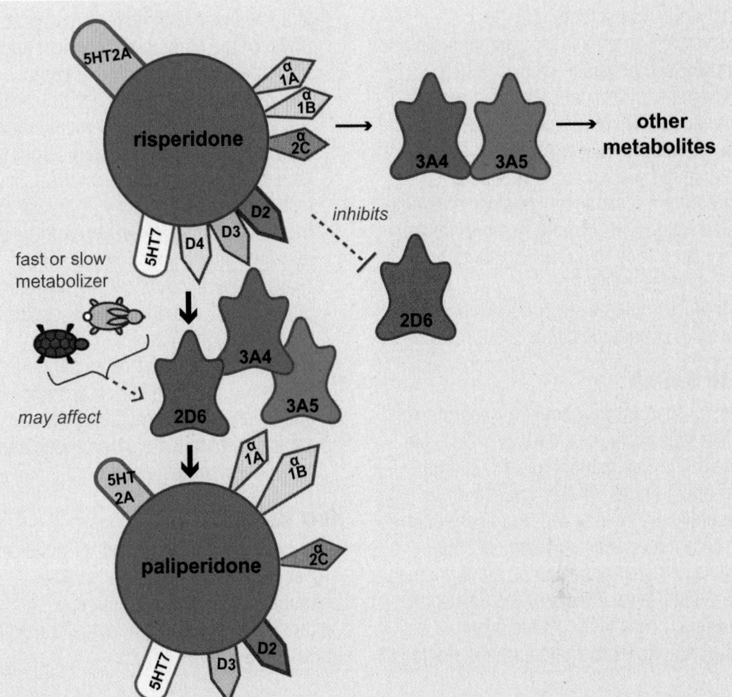

Figure 1 Risperidone metabolism. Risperidone is metabolized to 9-OH-risperidone (paliperidone) primarily by CYP2D6 and, in adults, variation in CYP2D6 produces differences in the ratio of risperidone to its metabolite, 9-OH-risperidone. Additionally, risperidone inhibits CYP2D6.

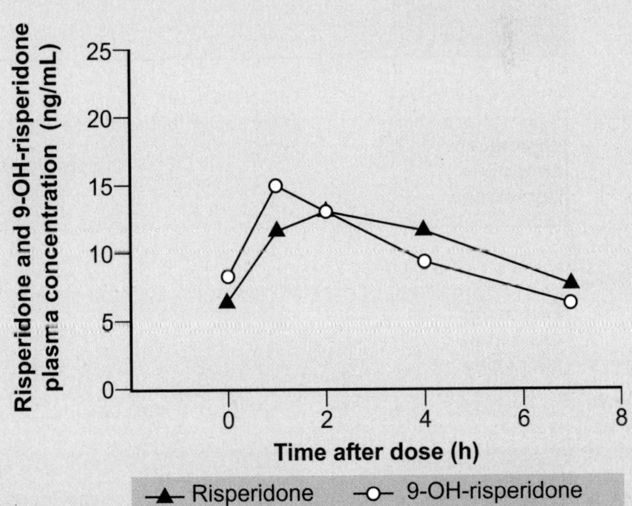

Figure 2 Risperidone plasma concentrations and 9-OH-risperidone concentrations following administration in youth.

- Risperidone oral solution can be administered directly from calibrated pipette or mixed with beverage (water, coffee, orange juice, or low-fat milk); it is not compatible with soft drinks or tea
- Orally disintegrating tablet can be administered with or without liquid
- For treatment resistance, consider obtaining plasma drug levels of both risperidone and 9-OH risperidone to guide dosing above recommended levels
- Treatment should be suspended if absolute neutrophil count falls below 1,000/mm^3

How to Switch

- From another antipsychotic to risperidone:
  - When tapering a prior antipsychotic, see its entry in this manual for how to stop and how to taper off that specific drug
  - Generally, try to stop the first agent before starting risperidone so that new side effects of risperidone can be distinguished from withdrawal effects of the first agent
  - If urgent, cross taper off the other antipsychotic while risperidone is started at a low dose, with dose adjustments down of the other antipsychotic, and up for risperidone, every 5 to 7 days
- Off risperidone to another antipsychotic:
  - Generally, try to stop risperidone before starting the new antipsychotic so that new side effects of the next drug can be distinguished from any withdrawal effects from risperidone. However, withdrawal dyskinesias are very common with risperidone discontinuation in pediatric patients and should not be mistaken for tardive dyskinesia.
  - If urgent, cross taper off risperidone by cutting the dose in half as the new antipsychotic is also started with dose adjustments down of risperidone and up for the new antipsychotic

How to Stop

- Slow down-titration of oral formulation (over 6–8 weeks), especially when simultaneously beginning a new antipsychotic while switching (i.e., cross-titration)

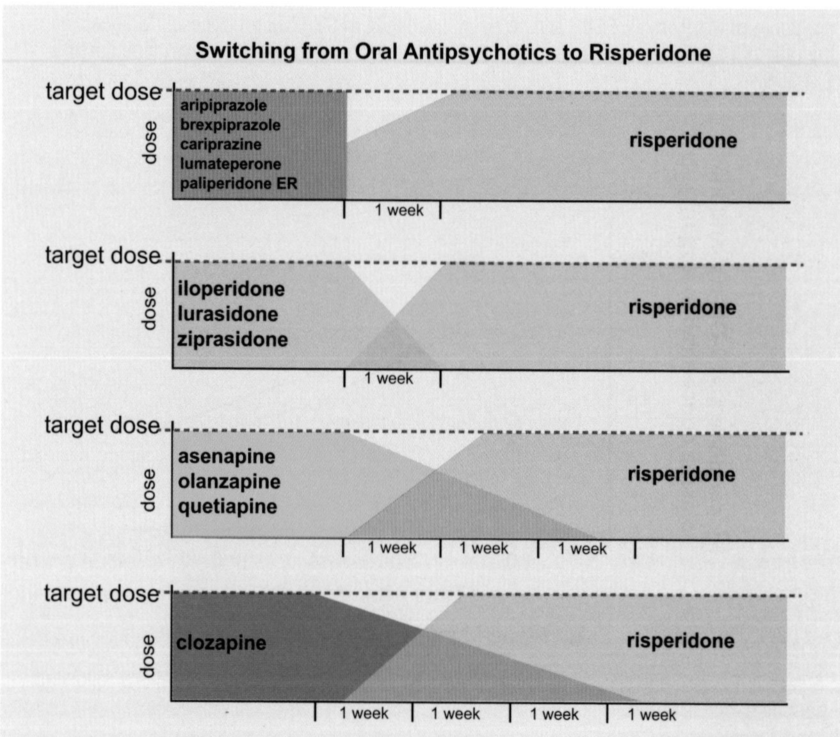

- Rapid oral discontinuation may lead to rebound psychosis and worsening of symptoms
- Rapid oral discontinuation may lead to withdrawal dyskinesias, which are generally reversible in the pediatric population. Of note, withdrawal dyskinesias are more common in pediatric patients than in adults.
- If antiparkinsonian agents are being used, they should be continued for a few weeks after risperidone is discontinued

WHAT TO EXPECT

Onset of Action

- Psychotic and manic symptoms can improve within 1 week of oral dosing, but it may take several weeks for full effect on behavior as well as on cognition and affective stabilization. In general, irritability in patients with autism spectrum disorders improves within the first week of treatment.
- If it is not working within 6–8 weeks, it may require a dosage increase or it may not work at all

Duration of Action

- Effects of oral medication are consistent over a 24-hour period
- However, in children with ultrarapid CYP2D6 metabolism, two divided doses may be necessary for consistent effects over 24 hours
- Some children may benefit from three divided doses in 24 hours
- Oral medication may continue to work for many years to prevent relapse of symptoms

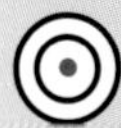

Primary Target Symptoms

- Positive symptoms of psychosis
- Negative symptoms of psychosis
- Cognitive symptoms
- Unstable mood and depression
- Aggressive symptoms
- Irritability and behavioral symptoms in autism

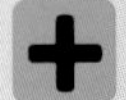

What Is Considered a Positive Result?

- In schizophrenia:
  - Most often reduces positive symptoms but does not eliminate them
  - Can improve negative symptoms, as well as aggressive, cognitive, and affective symptoms but less so than for positive symptoms
  - In children or adolescents with a first episode of psychosis, initial response may be greater than for recurrent episodes of psychosis in adults
- In bipolar disorder:
  - Many patients may experience a reduction of symptoms by half or more
- In autism:
  - Can decrease irritability, social withdrawal, stereotypy, and inappropriate speech

How Long to Treat

- In schizophrenia and bipolar disorder:
  - Continue treatment until reaching a plateau of improvement
  - After reaching a satisfactory plateau, continue treatment for at least a year after first episode of psychosis or mania
  - For second and subsequent episodes of psychosis or mania, treatment may need to be indefinite
- In autism:
  - Treat as long as risperidone improves irritability in autism; however, it may be prudent to periodically discontinue the medication if symptoms are well controlled to see if continued medication treatment is necessary as irritability can change as the patient with autism goes through neurodevelopmental changes and medication may become unnecessary

What If It Stops Working?

- Check for nonadherence, possibly by checking plasma drug level, and consider switching to another antipsychotic with fewer side effects
- Some patients who have an initial response may relapse even though they continue treatment, sometimes called "poop-out"
- Growth/developmental changes may contribute to apparent loss of efficacy as well as to new onset of side effects as metabolism slows and drug levels rise in transition from childhood to adolescence; dose adjustment (increase or decrease) should be considered
- Screen for the development of a new comorbid disorder, especially substance use

- Screen for adverse changes in the home or school environment

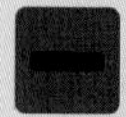

What If It Doesn't Work?

- Consider evaluation for another diagnosis (especially bipolar illness or depression with mixed features) or for a comorbid condition (e.g., medical illness, substance use)
- Consider other important potential factors such as ongoing conflicts, family psychopathology, and an adverse environment (e.g., inadequate school placement or educational services, bullying, poverty, chaos, violence, prior and ongoing psychological trauma, abuse, neglect)
- Institute trauma-informed care for appropriate children and adolescents
- For schizophrenia or bipolar disorder:
  - Try one of the other atypical antipsychotics
  - If no first-line atypical antipsychotic is effective, consider higher doses guided by plasma drug levels
  - If no first-line atypical antipsychotic is effective, consider augmentation with valproate, lithium, or lamotrigine
  - Consider initiating psychotherapy. In adolescents with bipolar disorder (and those with affective symptoms who are at risk of developing bipolar disorder), family-focused psychotherapy can be particularly helpful (Miklowitz et al., 2020).
  - Consider presence of concomitant drug abuse
- For autism spectrum disorders, consider aripiprazole

TALKING TO PATIENTS AND CAREGIVERS

What to Tell Parents About Efficacy

- For acute symptoms, it can work right away
- Oral risperidone is usually given every day
- Explain which use risperidone is being chosen for, how to tell if the drug is working by targeting specific symptoms, and why this is being done
- Once the child/adolescent calms down, at some point after one dose or after several days of dosing or after long-term dosing, we should all assess whether the medication should be continued
- While the medicine helps by reducing symptoms and improving function, it is not a cure, and it therefore may be necessary to keep taking the medication long term to sustain its therapeutic effects
- Since every treatment consideration depends on a risk/benefit analysis, parents should fully understand short- and long-term risks as well as benefits
- There are several studies and a lot of clinical experience giving risperidone to children and adolescents
- Often a good idea to tell parents whether the medication chosen is specifically approved for the disorder being treated, or whether it is being given for "unapproved" or "off-label" reasons based on good clinical practice, expert consensus, and/or prudent extrapolation of controlled data from adults

What to Tell Children and Adolescents About Efficacy

- Be specific about the symptoms being targeted: we are trying to help you ...
- Give the medication a try; if it's not working very well, we can stop the medication and try something else
- A good try often takes many months
- If it does make you feel better, you cannot stop it right away or you may get sick again
- Medications don't change who you are as a person; they give you the opportunity to be the best person you can be

What to Tell Parents About Side Effects

- Explain that side effects are expected in many when starting
- Tell parents many side effects go away and do so about the same time that therapeutic effects start
- Predict side effects in advance (you will look clever and competent to the parents, unless you scare them with too much information and cause nocebo effects, in which case you won't look so clever when the patient develops lots of side effects and stops medication; use your judgment here); a balanced but honest presentation is an art rather than a science
- Ask parents to support the patient while side effects are occurring
- Parents should fully understand short- and long-term risks as well as benefits

- Explaining to the parents what to expect from medication treatment, and especially what potential side effects to expect, can help prevent early termination of medication

What to Tell Children and Adolescents About Side Effects

- Even if you get side effects, most of them get better or go away in a few weeks
- If you have side effects that are bothering you, tell your parents and your parents should tell me
- Consider having a conversation about sexual side effects in some adolescents who can find these side effects confusing and especially burdensome
- Explaining to child/adolescent what to expect from medication treatment, and especially potential side effects, can help prevent early termination of medication

What to Tell Teachers About the Medication (If Parents Consent)

- Risperidone can make children/adolescents restless and have abnormal movements like tremor
- Risperidone can make children/adolescents sedated
- It is not abusable
- Encourage dialogue with parents/guardians about any behavior or mood changes
- Notify the clinician of increased restlessness or akathisia symptoms which may be apparent in the school setting

SPECIAL POPULATIONS

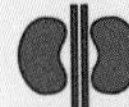

Renal Impairment

- In adults: initial 0.5 mg orally twice a day for first week; increase to 1 mg twice a day during second week; dosage increases above 1.5 mg twice a day should occur at least 1 week apart

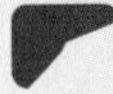

Hepatic Impairment

- In adults: initial 0.5 mg orally twice a day for first week; increase to 1 mg twice a day during second week

Cardiac Impairment

- Use in patients with cardiac impairment has not been studied; however, the risk of orthostatic hypotension in pediatric patients is less than in adults, as children rely less on peripheral vasoconstriction to regulate blood pressure

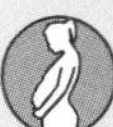

Pregnancy

- Controlled studies have not been conducted in pregnant women
- There is a risk of abnormal muscle movements and withdrawal symptoms in newborns whose mothers took an antipsychotic during the third trimester; symptoms may include agitation, abnormally increased or decreased muscle tone, tremor, sleepiness, severe difficulty breathing, and difficulty feeding
- Psychotic symptoms may worsen during pregnancy, and some form of treatment may be necessary
- Early findings of infants exposed to risperidone in utero do not show adverse consequences
- When administered to pregnant rats and rabbits, risperidone was not teratogenic at doses up to 6 times the maximum recommended human dose (MRHD); increased stillbirths and decreased birth weight occurred at 1.5 times the MRHD when administered to pregnant rats
- Risperidone may be preferable to anticonvulsant mood stabilizers if treatment is required during pregnancy
- Effects of hyperprolactinemia on the fetus are unknown
- National Pregnancy Registry for Psychiatric Medications: 1-866-961-2388 or https://womensmentalhealth.org/research/pregnancyregistry/

Breast Feeding

- Some drug is found in breast milk
- Recommended either to discontinue drug or formula feed
- Infants of women who choose to breast feed while on risperidone should be monitored for possible adverse effects; sedation, failure to thrive, jitteriness, tremor, and abnormal muscle movements have been reported

THE ART OF PSYCHOPHARMACOLOGY

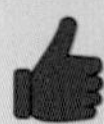

Potential Advantages

- In children:
  - Approved for manic/mixed episodes and irritability associated with autism
  - Often a preferred atypical antipsychotic for children with behavioral disturbances of multiple causations
  - Risperidone is the most frequently used atypical antipsychotic in children and adolescents
  - Well accepted for treatment of behavioral symptoms in children and adolescents
- In adolescents:
  - Approved for schizophrenia, manic/mixed episodes, and irritability associated with autism
  - Risperidone is the most frequently used atypical antipsychotic in children and adolescents
  - Well accepted for treatment of behavioral symptoms in children and adolescents

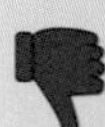

Potential Disadvantages

- In children:
  - May be more susceptible to side effects than adults, particularly sedation, weight gain, drug-induced parkinsonism, and akathisia
- In adolescents:
  - May be more susceptible to side effects than adults
  - Pubescent girls with amenorrhea (because of prolactin elevation)
  - Boys who are sensitive to the effects of prolactin elevations and develop gynecomastia
- All ages:
  - Possible weight gain and dyslipidemia
  - Possible adverse reactions to prolactin elevation including sexual dysfunction and amenorrhea

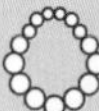

Pearls

- Can cause a zombie-like syndrome of inattention, sedation, and amotivation associated with reduced socialization and falling grades
- May cause less sedation than some other atypical antipsychotics, more than others
- May cause more motor side effects than some other atypical antipsychotics
- When discontinued, particularly if abrupt, risperidone may cause more withdrawal dyskinesias than some other atypical antipsychotics, which, in children and adolescents, generally reverse several weeks to months after discontinuation of risperidone
- Patients with inadequate responses to risperidone may benefit either from switching to another atypical antipsychotic, or for experts, determination of plasma drug levels of risperidone and its active metabolite 9-hydroxyrisperidone (paliperidone) to guide dosage increase even beyond the usual prescribing limits
- Meta-analysis suggests that short-term antipsychotic use can help reduce challenging behaviors in children with intellectual disabilities, but the quality of existing evidence is low and significant side effects also occurred
- Second generation antipsychotics (particularly risperidone) show moderate to large effects in decreasing irritability, disruptive behaviors, and aggression in children with and without autism spectrum disorders and developmental disabilities for short-term treatment
- Full symptomatic remission of mania may be more common than remission from schizophrenia, Tourette syndrome, or autism after treatment with risperidone, so augmenting options may often need to be considered for residual symptoms in these disorders, including CBT and additional medications

SUGGESTED READING

Dunbar F, Kusumakar V, Daneman D, Schulz M. Growth and sexual maturation during long-term treatment with risperidone. Am J Psychiatry 2004;161(5):918–20.

Earle JF. An introduction to the psychopharmacology of children and adolescents with autism spectrum disorder. J Child Adolesc Psychiatr Nurs 2016;29(2):62–71.

Fung LK, Mahajan R, Nozzolillo A et al. Pharmacologic treatment of severe irritability and problem behaviors in autism: a systematic review and meta-analysis. Pediatrics 2016;137(suppl 2):S124–35.

Haas M, Unis AS, Armenteros J et al. A 6-week, randomized, double-blind, placebo-controlled study of the efficacy and safety of risperidone in adolescents with schizophrenia. J Child Adolesc Psychopharmacol 2009;19(6):611–21.

Kloosterboer SM, de Winter BCM, Reichart CG et al. Risperidone plasma concentrations are associated with side effects and effectiveness in children and adolescents with autism spectrum disorder. Br J Clin Pharmacol 2021;87(3):1069–81.

Koch MT, Carlson HE, Kazimi MM, Correll CU. Antipsychotic-related prolactin levels and sexual dysfunction in mentally ill youth: a 3-month cohort-study. J Am Acad Child Adolesc Psychiatry 2023;62(9):1021–50.

Lytle S, McVoy M, Sajatovic M. Long-acting injectable antipsychotics in children and adolescents. J Child Adolesc Psychopharmacol 2017;27(1):2–9.

McQuire C, Hassiotis A, Harrison B, Pilling S. Pharmacological interventions for challenging behaviour in children with intellectual disabilities: a systematic review and meta-analysis. BMS Psychiatry 2015;15:303.

Miklowitz DJ, Schneck CD, Walshaw PD et al. Effects of family-focused therapy vs enhanced usual care for symptomatic youths at high risk for bipolar disorder: a randomized clinical trial. JAMA Psychiatry 2020;77(5):455–63.

Pillay J, Boylan K, Carrey N et al. First- and Second-Generation Antipsychotics in Children and Young Adults: Systematic Review Update [Internet]. Rockville, MD: Agency for Healthcare Research and Quality (US); 2017 Mar. Report No.: 17-EHC001-EF. AHRQ Comparative Effectiveness Reviews.

SERDEXMETHYLPHENIDATE

THERAPEUTICS

Brands

- AZSTARYS

Generic

No

US FDA Approved for Pediatric Use

- Attention deficit hyperactivity disorder (ADHD) (ages 6 and older)

Off-Label for Pediatric Use

- Approved in adults
  - None
- Other off-label uses
  - Narcolepsy
  - Treatment-resistant depression (rarely used for this in children)
  - Stimulants are sometimes used to augment antidepressants
  - Stimulants also sometimes used to treat amotivational or lethargic states in the elderly with dementia but rarely in children for these symptoms

Class and Mechanism of Action

- Neuroscience-based Nomenclature: dopamine, norepinephrine multimodal
- Stimulant
- AZSTARYS consists of serdexmethylphenidate, a prodrug of D-methylphenidate, co-formulated with immediate-release D-methylphenidate
- Serdexmethylphenidate is not active until after it has been absorbed by the lower intestinal tract and converted to D-methylphenidate (active component)
- D-Methylphenidate increases norepinephrine and especially dopamine actions by blocking their reuptake
- Enhancement of dopamine and norepinephrine actions in certain brain regions (e.g., dorsolateral prefrontal cortex) may improve attention, concentration, executive dysfunction, wakefulness, and cortical inhibitory control of striatum (i.e., theoretically "tunes" inefficient information processing in cortical–striatal pathways, improving "top-down" regulation of striatal and other subcortical drives)
- Enhancement of dopamine actions in other brain regions (e.g., basal ganglia) may decrease hyperactivity
- Enhancement of dopamine and norepinephrine in yet other brain regions (e.g., medial prefrontal cortex, hypothalamus) may improve depressive symptoms as well as nondepression-associated fatigue and sleepiness
- Hypothetically rebalances signal to noise ratios of cortical neurons: enhances focus on importance tasks (signal), theoretically due to norepinephrine, and reduces awareness of background activity (noise), theoretically due to dopamine

SAFETY AND TOLERABILITY

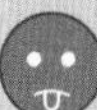

Notable Side Effects

- Anorexia and weight loss
- Nausea, abdominal pain
- Insomnia, headache, exacerbation of tics, tremor, dizziness, and possible irritability and anxiety. The risk of treatment-emergent irritability is lower with methylphenidate-based stimulants compared to amphetamine-based stimulants.
- Peripheral vasculopathy, including Raynaud's phenomenon

Life-Threatening or Dangerous Side Effects

- Psychosis
- Rare priapism
- Seizures
- Palpitations, tachycardia, hypertension
- Rare hypomania, mania, or suicidal ideation
- Cardiovascular adverse effects, death in patients with preexisting cardiac structural abnormalities often associated with a family history of cardiac disease

Growth and Maturation

- May temporarily slow normal growth in children (controversial): Multimodal Treatment of ADHD (MTA) study showed children/adolescents grew more slowly but eventually reached their expected adult height
- Controversy exists because theoretically stimulants might suppress appetite and reduce caloric intake, which could affect

potential growth; also, dopaminergic actions of stimulants might suppress growth hormone secretion and affect height development. However, expected adult height is likely attained with a delay if stimulants are continued, and slowing of growth is likely reversible with withdrawal of treatment.

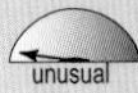

Weight Gain

- Patients may experience weight loss
- Weight gain is reported but not expected, rarely seen, controversial

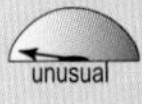

Sedation

- Activation much more common than sedation
- Sedation is reported but not expected, rarely seen, controversial

What to Do About Side Effects

- Wait, wait, wait: mild side effects are common, happen early, and usually improve with time, but treatment benefits can be delayed and often begin just as the side effects wear off
- Adjust dose
- Switch to a formulation of D,L-methylphenidate
- Switch to another agent
- For insomnia: avoid dosing in the midday, late afternoon, or evening
- However, insomnia is not always due to medication, but can be the result of relapse, rebound, and withdrawal effects from the daily dose, and in fact improves with additional late-day dosing of a short-acting stimulant
- Use beta blockers for peripheral autonomic side effects
- Often best to try another monotherapy prior to resorting to augmentation strategies to treat side effects, with the exception of an early-evening dose of a stimulant
- Monitor side effects closely, especially when initiating treatment
- For persistent insomnia: consider adding melatonin or an alpha 2 agonist
- For loss of appetite or loss of weight:
    - Give medication after breakfast
    - Switch to a nonstimulant
    - Eat a high-protein, high-carbohydrate breakfast prior to taking medication or within 10–15 minutes of ingesting medication; snack on high-protein, densely caloric foods throughout the school day and after school; eat dinner and then a second dinner or very heavy snack at bedtime
    - Add "liquid calories" (i.e., smoothies made with whole milk or ice cream, fruit, and protein powder; Boost or Ensure shakes)
    - Introduce "fourth meal" in the evening
    - Add cyproheptadine

How Drug Causes Side Effects

- Increases in norepinephrine peripherally can cause autonomic side effects, including tremor, tachycardia, hypertension, and cardiac arrhythmias
- Increases in norepinephrine and dopamine centrally can cause CNS side effects such as insomnia, agitation, psychosis (rarely)

Warnings and Precautions

- In children and adolescents:
    - Safety and efficacy not established in children under age 6
    - Use in young children should be reserved for the expert
    - Children who are not growing or gaining weight should stop treatment, at least temporarily
    - Usual dosing has been associated with sudden death in children with structural cardiac abnormalities
    - Consider distributing brochures provided by the FDA and the drug companies
- All ages:
    - Stimulants used to treat ADHD are associated with peripheral vasculopathy, including Raynaud's phenomenon; careful observation for digital changes is necessary during treatment with ADHD stimulants
    - Carefully weigh the risks and benefits of pharmacological treatment against the risks and benefits of nonpharmacological treatment and it is a good idea to document this in the patient's chart
    - Use with caution in patients with any degree of hypertension, hyperthyroidism, or history of drug abuse

- Many believe tics may be worsened by stimulants, but evidence does not support this association. A meta-analysis of 22 studies, including 2,385 individuals in treatment, found that the rate of new onset or worsening tics was 5.7% for those on stimulants versus 6.5% with placebo. In this analysis, there was no effect for type of stimulant, dose, duration of treatment, or age (Cohen et al., 2015). The presence of tics is not an absolute contraindication to use of stimulants.
- May worsen symptoms of thought disorder and behavioral disturbance in psychotic patients
- Stimulants have a high potential for abuse and must be used with caution in anyone with a current or past history of substance abuse or alcoholism, but stimulants for ADHD are less likely to be abused in terms of getting "high" and more likely to be used to stay awake, especially by college students. This misuse is the most common reason for diversion of prescription stimulants.
- Youth are neither more nor less likely to develop alcohol and substance use disorders as a result of being treated with stimulant medication. In fact, current data suggest that treating ADHD in children and adolescents decreases the likelihood of developing a substance use disorder.
- Adolescents and/or college students may divert/sell their medication to others for use in staying awake to study at the last minute, or to abuse; longer-acting preparations are harder to abuse than shorter-acting, immediate-release stimulants
- Particular attention should be paid to the possibility of adolescents you are seeing for the first time feigning ADHD in order to obtain stimulants for nontherapeutic use or distribution to others; the drugs should in general be prescribed sparingly with documentation of appropriate use, and if there is any doubt about the accuracy of their complaints, refer them for psychological-educational or neuropsychological testing
- Not an appropriate first-line treatment for depression or for normal fatigue
- May lower the seizure threshold; as long as seizures are well controlled, it is generally safe to use stimulants
- Emergence or worsening of activation and agitation may represent the induction of a bipolar state, especially a mixed dysphoric bipolar II condition sometimes associated with suicidal ideation, and may require the addition of lithium or an atypical antipsychotic, and/or discontinuation of D-methylphenidate

When Not to Prescribe

- Treating ADHD comorbid with tics or Tourette syndrome is not contraindicated, but may be for the expert
- Patients with ADHD who are comorbid for motor or vocal tics of Tourette syndrome, or even with just a family history of Tourette syndrome, may experience worsening/onset of tics with stimulant treatment (controversial). Decision to use stimulants in such cases should weigh the potential benefits for ADHD against the risks of worsening tics, and may require expert referral or consultation.
- Should generally not be administered with an MAOI, including within 14 days of MAOI use, except in heroic circumstances and by an expert
- If patient has glaucoma
- If patient has structural cardiac abnormalities
- If there is a proven allergy to methylphenidate
- If the patient has an eating disorder other than binge-eating disorder, be very cautious

Long-Term Use

- Methylphenidate is often used long-term for ADHD when ongoing monitoring documents continued efficacy
- Tolerance to therapeutic effects may develop in some patients
- Weight and height should be monitored during long-term treatment
- Periodic monitoring of blood pressure and heart rate

Habit Forming

- Paradoxically, stimulant abuse appears to be less likely in patients with ADHD than in those who do not have ADHD. In 2023, the FDA modified a boxed warning for stimulant medications, although they noted, "Our review found that nonmedical use has remained relatively stable over the past two decades,

despite the increasing number of prescription stimulants dispensed." The new warning notes that stimulants have a "high potential for abuse and misuse, which can lead to the development of a substance use disorder, including addiction." The new warning also notes that stimulant medications "can be diverted for non-medical use into illicit channels or distribution." They recommend:
  - Counsel patients not to give any of their medicine to anyone else
  - Monitor for signs and symptoms of diversion, such as requesting refills more frequently than needed
  - Regularly assess and monitor for signs and symptoms of nonmedical use and addiction
  - Keep careful records of prescribing information, including quantity, frequency, and renewal requests, as required by state and federal laws
- Stimulant abuse in ADHD patients more likely if there is a preexisting history of alcohol/drug abuse
- Tolerance to stimulants is surprisingly rare in ADHD; tolerance should not be confused with reduction of therapeutic effects over time due to growth: as youth grow, dose usually must be increased; otherwise, the appearance of tolerance occurs when this in reality is underdosing
- Misuse may be more likely with immediate-release stimulants than with controlled-release stimulants

Overdose

- Vomiting, tremor, coma, convulsion, hyperreflexia, euphoria, confusion, hallucination, tachycardia, flushing, palpitations, sweating, hyperpyrexia, hypertension, arrhythmia, mydriasis, agitation, delirium, headache

DOSING AND USE

Usual Dosage Range

- Ages 6–12: 26.1 mg/5.2 mg, 39.2 mg/7.8 mg, or 52.3 mg/10.4 mg
- Ages 13 and older: 39.2 mg/7.8 mg or 52.3 mg/10.4 mg

Dosage Forms

- Capsule (serdexmethylphenidate/dexmethylphenidate) 26.1 mg/5.2 mg, 39.2 mg/7.8 mg, 52.3 mg/10.4 mg

How to Dose

- Ages 6–12: initial dose 39.2 mg/7.8 mg orally once daily in the morning; can increase to 52.3 mg/10.4 mg daily or decrease to 26.1 mg/5.2 mg daily after 1 week; maximum recommended dose 52.3 mg/10.4 mg once daily
- Ages 13 and older: initial dose 39.2 mg/7.8 mg orally once daily in the morning; increase to 52.3 mg/10.4 mg daily after 1 week

Options for Administration

- Capsules can be opened and the contents sprinkled onto applesauce or dissolved in water for patients with difficulty swallowing pills
- Should have sufficient duration of action to eliminate the need for lunchtime dosing

Tests

- Before treatment, assess for presence of cardiac disease (history, family history, physical exam); consider whether electrocardiogram (ECG) is indicated
- Blood pressure and heart rate should be monitored regularly, sitting and standing
- Monitor weight and height
- Periodic complete blood cell and platelet counts may be considered during prolonged therapy (rare leukopenia and/or anemia)
- Current recommendations from the American Heart Association (AHA) are that it is reasonable but not mandatory to obtain an ECG prior to prescribing a stimulant to a child; the American Academy of Pediatrics (AAP) does not recommend an ECG prior to starting a stimulant for most children
- Document basic sleep patterns prior to starting a stimulant
- When necessary to rule out sleep apnea, nocturnal movements, or daytime sleepiness that may later be difficult to distinguish from side effects of stimulants, consider (rarely) a sleep study/polysomnogram (e.g., obese adolescents)

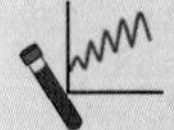

Pharmacokinetics

- Mean plasma elimination half-life approximately 5.7 hours

(serdexmethylphenidate) and 11.7 hours (D-methylphenidate) (Figure 1)
- Does not inhibit CYP450 enzymes

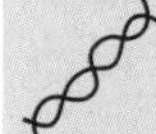

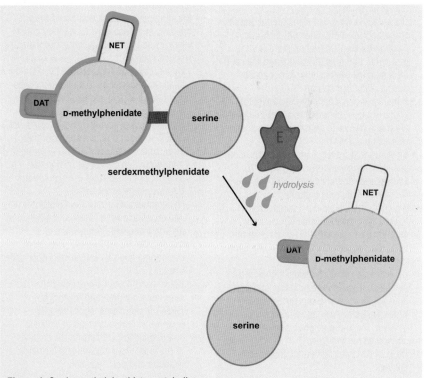

Pharmacogenetics

- Methylphenidate is not metabolized by CYP450 isoenzymes to a clinically relevant extent and therefore there are no pharmacogenetic recommendations related to methylphenidate based on pharmacokinetic genes. Additionally, there are no recommendations related to pharmacodynamic genes and stimulant selection.

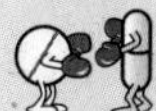

Drug Interactions

- May affect blood pressure and should be used cautiously with agents used to control blood pressure
- Methylphenidate is metabolized by carboxylesterase 1 and is not a substrate or inhibitor of the CYP450 drug-metabolizing system
- Most drug interactions are pharmacodynamic rather than pharmacokinetic
- CNS and cardiovascular actions of D-methylphenidate could theoretically be enhanced by combination with agents that block norepinephrine reuptake, such as the tricyclic antidepressants desipramine or protriptyline, venlafaxine, duloxetine, atomoxetine, milnacipran, and reboxetine
- Theoretically, D-methylphenidate could inhibit the antipsychotic actions of antipsychotics
- Theoretically, D-methylphenidate could inhibit the mood-stabilizing actions of atypical antipsychotics in some patients; however, stimulants can be safely combined with atypical antipsychotics by experts
- Combinations of D-methylphenidate with mood stabilizers (lithium, anticonvulsants,

Figure 1 Serdexmethylphenidate metabolism.

atypical antipsychotics) are generally something for experts only, when monitoring patients closely and when other options fail
- Antacids or acid suppressants could alter the release of extended-release formulation
- Use with MAOIs, including within 14 days of MAOI use, is not advised, but this can sometimes be considered by experts who monitor depressed patients closely when other treatment options for depression fail
- Use with halogenated anesthetics may increase the risk of sudden blood pressure and heart rate increase during surgery; avoid use of AZSTARYS (dexmethylphenidate and serdexmethylphenidate) in patients being treated with anesthetics on the day of surgery

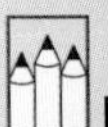

Dosing Tips

- Plasma levels are higher in lower-weight children; therefore, starting and target doses may be lower and longer intervals between dose increases may be needed (see How to Dose)
- Once-daily dosing can eliminate the hassle and pragmatic difficulties of lunchtime dosing at school, including storage problems, potential diversion, and the need for a medical professional to supervise dosing away from home
- If there are concerns about diversion or abuse, longer-acting stimulant preparations are much harder to abuse than immediate-release preparations
- Be aware that metabolism (and absorption) changes during puberty and entry into adolescence and becomes more like adults (i.e., slower than in children)
- If a child on a stable dose begins to lose tolerability with more side effects upon entering adolescence, this may signal the need for a dose reduction due to changing metabolism
- Capsules can either be taken whole or they can be opened and the contents sprinkled onto applesauce or dissolved in water
- When sprinkled over applesauce or taken in water, the entire solution should be consumed immediately
- Dose of a single capsule should not be divided
- Do not substitute methylphenidate products on a mg-per-mg basis due to differing methylphenidate base compositions and pharmacokinetic profiles (see Appendix)
- Avoid dosing late in the day because of the risk of insomnia
- Side effects are generally dose related
- Can be taken with or without food
-

Drug Holidays

- Drug holidays were originally done in an attempt to avoid the possibility that stimulants may blunt height
- May be able to give drug holidays over the summer in order to reassess therapeutic utility and effects on growth and theoretically to allow catch-up from any growth suppression and assess any other side effects and the need to reinstitute stimulant treatment for the next school term
- However, most studies show that parental height is what determines a patient's final height, and that most children/adolescents taking stimulants reach their expected height, just more slowly than children/adolescents not exposed to stimulants
- May be possible to give weekend drug holidays and dose only during the school week for some ADHD patients, but there are risks as well:
  - Hyperactivity and impulsivity increase the chances of accidents (i.e., broken bones and head injuries) and illicit alcohol and drug abuse
  - Studies have shown that adolescents with ADHD who drive vehicles without their stimulants are much more likely to get into motor vehicle accidents and that the severity of the accident is much greater than would be expected
  - Hyperactive and impulsive children/adolescents tend to have more difficulties getting along with family members and friends, increasing the chances of developing low self-esteem and poor self-image
  - Social benefits can be lost over the summer if children/adolescents are taken off stimulants; social rejection by other children can lead to isolation and depression, increasing the chances of bullying, victimization, and further isolation and peer rejection

- Inattention makes it harder for kids to learn the rules of life and pay attention to what is going on around them (e.g., noticing when a peer is not being a true friend, when someone is starting to get annoyed, when a car is coming toward you and you're in the middle of the street)

How to Switch

- When switching from one stimulant to another, the first one can be abruptly stopped and the new one started the next morning. Side effects from abrupt discontinuation are not expected; however, some patients may experience marked fatigue and sleepiness for several days.
- See Appendix for approximate dosing equivalents when switching

How to Stop

- Taper not necessary, especially for patients who have only had short-term treatment or intermittent treatment
- However, if withdrawal symptoms develop, resume dosing the medication and then taper slowly over several days
- Withdrawal following chronic therapeutic use may unmask symptoms of the underlying disorder and may require follow-up and reinstitution of treatment
- Usually symptoms after discontinuation are return of symptoms of the underlying disorder rather than symptoms due to drug withdrawal
- Supervision during withdrawal is always recommended for any psychotropic medication

WHAT TO EXPECT

Onset of Action

- Some immediate effects can be seen with first dosing
- Takes a few days to attain therapeutic benefit generally

Duration of Action

- Up to 10-hour duration

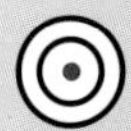

Primary Target Symptoms

- Concentration, attention span, distractibility
- Motor hyperactivity
- Impulsiveness
- Physical and mental fatigue
- Daytime sleepiness

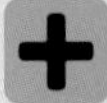

What Is Considered a Positive Result?

- The goal of treatment of ADHD is reduction of symptoms of inattentiveness, motor hyperactivity, and/or impulsiveness that disrupt social, school, and/or occupational functioning
- Can also improve oppositional and disruptive behaviors associated with ADHD
- The goal of treatment is complete remission of symptoms
- If treatment works, it most often reduces or even eliminates symptoms, but is not a cure since symptoms often recur after medicine is stopped

How Long to Treat

- ADHD is typically a lifelong illness; if any symptoms improve, hyperactivity is more likely to improve than inattention
- Can tell parents there is some chance that their child can grow out of this in adulthood, but many adults continue to have symptoms of ADHD throughout adolescence and adulthood
- Continue treatment until all symptoms are under control or improvement is stable and then continue treatment as long as improvement persists
- Reevaluate the need for treatment periodically; some clinicians advise to periodically stop stimulants in patients who are not severely symptomatic to observe how the patient responds, but not routinely done by most clinicians
- Treatment for ADHD begun in childhood may need to be continued into adolescence and adulthood if continued benefit is documented

What If It Stops Working?

- Some patients who have an initial response may relapse even though they continue treatment, sometimes called "poop-out"
- Growth/developmental changes may contribute to apparent loss of efficacy as well as to new onset of side effects as metabolism slows and drug levels rise in transition from childhood to adolescence; dose adjustment (increase or decrease) should be considered

- Some patients may experience apparent lack of consistent efficacy due to activation of latent or underlying or newly evolved bipolar disorder, major depressive episodes with mixed features of mania, new onset of major depression or an anxiety disorder (GAD, OCD, PD), and require stimulant discontinuation and a switch to the clinically appropriate medication(s)

What If It Doesn't Work?

- In practice, many patients have only a partial response where some symptoms are improved but others persist, in which case higher doses of serdexmethylphenidate, adding a second agent, or switching to an agent with a different mechanism of action can be considered
- Consider evaluation for another diagnosis or for a comorbid condition (e.g., medical illness, substance abuse). Also, when treating ADHD, consider the possibility of a learning disorder or learning weakness and consider school-based interventions.
- Consider adjusting dose or switching to another formulation of D-methylphenidate or to another agent
- Consider the presence of nonadherence and counsel patient and parents
- Some ADHD patients and some depressed patients may experience lack of consistent efficacy due to activation of latent or underlying bipolar disorder, and require either augmenting with a mood stabilizer or switching to a mood stabilizer
- Augmenting options:
  - Organizational skills training/executive function coaching
  - Exercise
  - Parent Management Training (PMT)
  - Coordinating with school for appropriate support
  - For the expert, can combine with modafinil, atomoxetine, or viloxazine for ADHD
  - For the expert, can occasionally combine with atypical antipsychotics in highly treatment-resistant cases of bipolar disorder or ADHD
  - For the expert, can combine with antidepressants to boost antidepressant efficacy in highly treatment-resistant cases of depression while carefully monitoring patient
  - Can combine with alpha 2 agonists such as guanfacine or clonidine
- Consider factors associated with poor response to any psychotropic medication in children and adolescents, such as severe symptoms, long-lasting symptoms, poor treatment adherence, prior nonresponse to other treatments, and the presence of comorbid psychiatric disorders or learning disorders
- Consider other important potential factors such as ongoing conflicts, family psychopathology, and an adverse environment (e.g., poverty, chaos, violence, prior and ongoing psychological trauma, abuse, bullying, less-than-ideal school placement, neglect)
- Institute trauma-informed care for appropriate children and adolescents

TALKING TO PATIENTS AND CAREGIVERS

What to Tell Parents About Efficacy

- Stimulant treatment for ADHD is one of the best studied of all medications in children and adolescents
- Often works right away once the dose is correct
- While the medicine helps ADHD by reducing symptoms and improving function, there are no cures for ADHD and it is therefore necessary to keep taking the medication to sustain its therapeutic effects
- It does not work that day if the child/adolescent has not taken their medication in the morning
- For longer-acting stimulants, be careful not to give too late (i.e., after 11 a.m.) because it can cause insomnia that night
- Does not stay in the body for a long time, so it stops working rapidly after you stop it
- Since every treatment consideration depends on a risk/benefit analysis, parents should fully understand short- and long-term risks as well as benefits compared to nontreatment of ADHD
- Although many stimulants are approved for ADHD, if using off-label, often a good idea to tell parents whether the medication chosen is specifically approved for the disorder being treated, or whether it is being given for "unapproved" or

"off-label" reasons based on good clinical practice, expert consensus, and/or prudent extrapolation of controlled data from adults
- Best results are often obtained when medications are combined with behavioral therapy
- Stimulants wear off after a number of hours and symptoms may return. Therefore, parents may complain that the medication isn't working if their child/adolescent is using a stimulant that lasts 8 hours, because it may have worn off after the patient has come home from school (and that is when the parents are seeing the child/adolescent) in comparison to a stimulant that lasts 10–12 hours and may keep working after the child/adolescent comes home from school.
- The American Academy of Child & Adolescent Psychiatry (AACAP) has helpful handouts for parents

What to Tell Children and Adolescents About Efficacy

- Be specific about the symptoms being targeted: we are trying to help you remember things better, do your best at school, follow the rules, get into less trouble (as applicable)
- It may be a good idea to give the medication a try; if it's not working very well, we can stop the medication and try something else
- You can be part of a special plan to help us figure out if the medicine is helpful for you. Would you like to do that? (for the parents and prescriber, can consider here a trial both on and then off medication, and then on again to see if the effects are clear and thus worth continuing the medication)
- The medication can work right away but a good try can take a few months to find the right dose
- Even if it does make you feel better, it will wear off and no longer work shortly after you stop it
- This medicine does not last very long in your body, so even if it does work, it won't work if you don't take it that day
- The medication can help you decide what you want to do, like making good choices versus bad choices; the medicine does not make you do something you don't want to do
- Medications don't change who you are as a person; they give you the opportunity to be the best person you can be

What to Tell Parents About Side Effects

- Explain that side effects are expected in many when starting
- Tell parents many side effects of stimulants often go away in a few days to weeks, especially nausea and insomnia, but if they don't we will change the treatment
- Predict side effects in advance (you will look clever and competent to the parents, unless you scare them with too much information and cause nocebo effects, in which case you won't look so clever when the patient develops lots of side effects and stops medication; use your judgment here); a balanced but honest presentation is an art rather than a science
- Sometimes a trial off medication and then on again can clarify what the true therapeutic effects of the medication are
- Ask parents to support the patient while side effects are occurring
- Parents should fully understand short- and long-term risks as well as benefits
- Explaining to the parents what to expect from medication treatment, and especially what potential side effects to expect, can help prevent early termination

What to Tell Children and Adolescents About Side Effects

- When a medicine starts to work, your body can first experience this by giving you unpleasant sensations – just like if you take a cough medicine it may taste bad – these body sensations include loss of appetite and problems sleeping. So, just like with a cough medicine, the bad taste will often go away before the medicine begins to stop the cough – many medicines work like that. It's important for you to pay attention to what your body is telling you, and we'll go over some of the ways that can happen.
- Even if you get a side effect, it's not permanent (it won't last forever)
- In a way, a side effect tells you the medication is working on your body and good effects should come soon
- Explaining to child/adolescent what to expect from medication treatment, and

especially potential side effects, can help prevent early termination

What to Tell Teachers About the Medication (If Parents Consent)

- Stimulants can be very helpful in improving the symptoms of ADHD: namely, inattention, impulsivity, and hyperactivity
- It does not work if the child/adolescent has not taken their medication that morning
- If the patient is sleepy, ask whether the medication is keeping them up at night or if they are eating enough food
- If the patient won't eat lunch or snacks, ask whether the medication is making them lose their appetite
- Medically speaking, methylphenidate is not a narcotic, because doctors define a narcotic as something that is sedating and sleep-inducing, like opioids such as heroin and Oxycontin and not stimulants like methylphenidate
- Methylphenidate should be kept in school under lock and key or at the nurse's office or not brought to school at all because it can be diverted and misused by those who do not have ADHD. Some schools will suspend students who are caught with medications on their person or in their backpacks; most schools know the misuse or even abuse potential of stimulants.

SPECIAL POPULATIONS

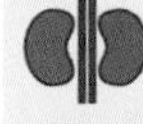

Renal Impairment

- No dose adjustment necessary

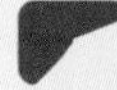

Hepatic Impairment

- No dose adjustment necessary

Cardiac Impairment

- Use with caution, particularly in patients with recent myocardial infarction or other conditions that could be negatively affected by increased blood pressure
- Do not use in patients with structural cardiac abnormalities without consultation with a cardiologist

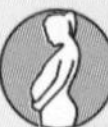

Pregnancy

- Controlled studies have not been conducted in pregnant women
- Infants whose mothers took methylphenidate during pregnancy may experience withdrawal symptoms
- In animal studies, D-methylphenidate caused delayed skeletal ossification and decreased postweaning weight gain in rats; no major malformations occurred in rat or rabbit studies
- Racemic methylphenidate has been shown to have teratogenic effects in rabbits when given in doses of 200 mg/kg/day throughout organogenesis
- No evidence of developmental effects were found in an embryo-fetal development study with oral administration of serdexmethylphenidate in rabbits during organogenesis at doses of up to 374 mg/kg/day
- Use in women of childbearing potential requires weighing potential benefits to the mother against potential risks to the fetus
- For ADHD patients, methylphenidate should generally be discontinued before anticipated pregnancies
- National Pregnancy Registry for Psychiatric Medications: 1-866-961-2388 or https://womensmentalhealth.org/research/pregnancyregistry/

Breast Feeding

- Unknown if methylphenidate is secreted in human breast milk, but all psychotropics assumed to be secreted in breast milk
- Recommended either to discontinue drug or formula feed
- If infant shows signs of irritability, drug may need to be discontinued

THE ART OF PSYCHOPHARMACOLOGY

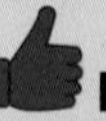

Potential Advantages

- In children:
  - Stimulants are probably the best studied psychotropic medications for use in children
  - Methylphenidate is one of the best studied stimulants in children
- In adolescents:

- Can improve school performance and grades, especially if ADHD has been unrecognized and untreated prior to adolescence
- Can improve performance in high school and college students whose ADHD is compromising academic performance due to the increased demands of higher levels of study
- All ages:
  - Methylphenidate has established long-term efficacy as a first-line treatment for ADHD
  - Combines an immediate-release dose of D-methylphenidate with the slower released dose of the prodrug serdexmethylphenidate

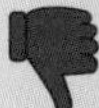

Potential Disadvantages

- Adolescents and especially college-age patients who divert their medication
- Patients with current substance abuse
- Patients with current manic or mixed symptoms associated with bipolar disorder or psychosis
- Patients with anorexia

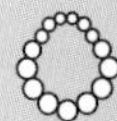

Pearls

- Half-life and duration of clinical action tend to be shorter in younger children than in adolescents and may require more frequent dosing or preferential use of long-acting preparations
- Drug abuse is no more likely and may even be lower (controversial) in ADHD adolescents treated with stimulants than in ADHD adolescents who are not treated with stimulants
- Stimulants have a moderate effect on decreasing ADHD symptoms and a moderate to large effect on decreasing aggression, oppositional behavior, and conduct problems in children with ADHD
- Meta-analyses suggest that when taking into account both efficacy and safety, methylphenidate is the best first-line stimulant in children and adolescents, whereas amphetamine is best in adults (Cortese et al., 2018)
- Stimulant dosing and titration are critical to optimizing response. Meta-analyses involving nearly 8,000 children/adolescents show that both methylphenidate and amphetamine salts have increased efficacy (but increased likelihood of discontinuation due to side effects) with higher doses (Farhat et al., 2022). In general, goal doses are often in the range of 0.8 mg/kg for methylphenidate and 0.5 mg/kg for amphetamine salts. However, these are rough guides that may not always be applicable depending on the formulation used and how completely (or incompletely) it's absorbed.
- Combinations of behavioral therapy or other nonmedication treatments along with stimulants may have better results than either treatment alone
- Capsule contents can be sprinkled over applesauce or dissolved in water for patients unable to swallow the capsule
- Rebound hyperactivity may occur in the afternoon and present with increased hyperactivity, restlessness, and irritability; if this occurs, can consider switching to a longer-acting agent or a nonstimulant or adding a short-acting stimulant
- On the other hand, too-high medication dosing may lead to cognitive rigidity, difficulty shifting attention, and seeming "spaced out" or "different"
- Many patients taking stimulants have early-morning ADHD symptoms and can be hard to get going, prepare for school, and be cooperative, especially for a few hours after awakening. In these patients delayed-release/extended-release formulations may be especially helpful.
- Stimulants are a classic augmentation strategy for treatment-refractory depression, although this is most established in adults
- Interestingly, in some studies combining stimulants with alpha 2 agonists, decreased side effects are seen with the combination compared to either medication as monotherapy. This is likely because of complementary side effects.

SUGGESTED READING

Biederman J, Spencer TJ, Monuteaux MC, Faraone SV. A naturalistic 10-year prospective study of height and weight in children with attention-deficit hyperactivity disorder grown up: sex and treatment effects. J Pediatr 2010 Oct;157(4):635–40.

Childress AC, Braeckman R, Guenther S et al. Safety and tolerability of KP415 (serdexmethylphenidate and d-methylphenidate) capsules in children with ADHD: a 12-month, open-label safety study. Poster presented at the American Professional Society of ADHD and Related Disorders (APSARD) 2021; January 15–17.

Cohen SC, Mulqueen JM, Ferracioli-Oda E et al. Meta-analysis: risk of tics associated with psychostimulant use in randomized, placebo-controlled trials. J Am Acad Child Adolesc Psychiatry 2015;54(9):728–36.

Cortese S, Adamo N, Del Giovane C et al. Comparative efficacy and tolerability of medications for attention-deficit hyperactivity disorder in children, adolescents, and adults: a systematic review and network meta-analysis. Lancet Psychiatry 2018;5(9):727–38.

Farhat LC, Flores JM, Behling E et al. The effects of stimulant dose and dosing strategy on treatment outcomes in attention-deficit/hyperactivity disorder in children and adolescents: a meta-analysis. Mol Psychiatry 2022;27(3):1562–72.

Jensen PS, Arnold LE, Swanson JM et al. 3-year follow-up of the NIMH MTA study. J Am Acad Child Adolesc Psychiatry 2007;46(8):989–1002.

Kollin SH, Braeckman R, Guenther S et al. Efficacy and safety of KP415 (serdexmethylphenidate and d-methylphenidate) capsules in children with ADHD: a randomized, double-blind, placebo-controlled laboratory classroom study. Poster presented at the American Professional Society of ADHD and Related Disorders (APSARD) 2021; January 15–17.

The MTA Cooperative Group. A 14-month randomized clinical trial of treatment strategies for attention-deficit/hyperactivity disorder. The MTA Cooperative Group. Multimodal Treatment Study of Children with ADHD. Arch Gen Psychiatry 1999;56(12):1073–86.

Po MD, Gomeni R, Incledon B. Quantitative characterization of the smoothness of extended-release methylphenidate pharmacokinetic profiles. Innov Clin Neurosci 2022;19(7–9):32–7.

Posner K, Melvin GA, Murray DW et al. Clinical presentation of attention-deficit/hyperactivity disorder in preschool children: the Preschoolers with Attention-Deficit/Hyperactivity Disorder Treatment Study (PATS). J Child Adolesc Psychopharmacol 2007;17(5):547–62.

Riddle MA, Yershova K, Lazzaretto D et al. The Preschool Attention-Deficit/Hyperactivity Disorder Treatment Study (PATS) 6-year follow-up. J Am Acad Child Adolesc Psychiatry 2013;52(3):264–78.

Swanson JM, Arnold LE, Molina BSG et al. Young adult outcomes in the follow-up of the multimodal treatment study of attention-deficit/hyperactivity disorder: symptom persistence, source discrepancy, and height suppression. J Child Psychol Psychiatry 2017;58(6):663–78.

Zhang L, Yao H, Li L, et al. Risk of cardiovascular diseases associated with medications used in attention-deficit/hyperactivity disorder: a systematic review and meta-analysis. JAMA Netw Open 2022;5(11):e2243597.

THERAPEUTICS

Brands

- Zoloft

Generic

Yes

US FDA Approved for Pediatric Use

- Obsessive-compulsive disorder (OCD) (ages 6 and older)

Off-Label for Pediatric Use

- Approved in adults
  - Major depressive disorder
  - Panic disorder
  - Posttraumatic stress disorder (PTSD)
  - Social anxiety disorder
  - Premenstrual dysphoric disorder (PMDD)
- Other off-label uses
  - Separation anxiety disorder

Class and Mechanism of Action

- Neuroscience-based Nomenclature: serotonin reuptake inhibitor (S-RI)
- SSRI (selective serotonin reuptake inhibitor); often classified as an antidepressant, but it is not just an antidepressant
- Sertraline presumably increases serotonergic neurotransmission by blocking the serotonin reuptake pump (transporter, SERT), which results in the desensitization of serotonin receptors, especially serotonin 1A receptors
- Sertraline also has some ability to block dopamine reuptake pump (dopamine transporter), which could increase dopamine neurotransmission and contribute to its therapeutic actions
- Sertraline also has moderate affinity for sigma 1 receptors

SAFETY AND TOLERABILITY

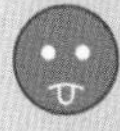

Notable Side Effects

- Gastrointestinal (decreased appetite, nausea, diarrhea, constipation, dry mouth)
- Several central nervous system side effects (insomnia but also sedation especially if not sleeping at night, agitation, tremors, headache, dizziness)
- Note: patients with diagnosed or undiagnosed bipolar or psychotic disorders may be more vulnerable to CNS-activating actions of SSRIs; pay particular attention to signs of activation in children with developmental disorders or autism spectrum disorders
- Treatment-emergent activation syndrome (TEAS) includes agitation, anxiety, panic attacks, irritability, aggression, impulsivity, and insomnia
- TEAS can represent side effects but should not be confused with bipolar mania or the onset of suicidality and should be monitored and investigated with consideration of discontinuing or decreasing the dose of sertraline or addition of another agent or switching to another agent to reduce these symptoms
- Sexual dysfunction (boys: delayed ejaculation, erectile dysfunction; boys and girls: decreased sexual desire, anorgasmia)
- Autonomic (sweating)
- Bruising and rare bleeding
- Syndrome of inappropriate antidiuretic hormone secretion (SIADH)
- Rare hyponatremia (mostly in elderly patients and generally reversible on discontinuation of sertraline)
- Rare hypotension

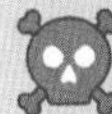

Life-Threatening or Dangerous Side Effects

- Rare seizures
- Rare induction of mania
- Rare suicidal ideation and behavior (suicidality) (short-term regulatory studies did not show any actual suicides in any age group and also did not show an increase in the risk of suicidality with antidepressants compared to placebo beyond age 24)

Growth and Maturation

- Long-term effects on growth were recently evaluated in a long-term study of children and adolescents ages 6–16 years over a 3-year period. No effects were observed for standardized height or Tanner stage based on sertraline exposure (Kolitsopoulos et al., 2023).

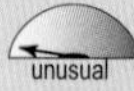

Weight Gain

- Weight gain was recently evaluated in a long-term study of children and adolescents ages 6–16 years over a 3-year period. Standardized weight over time was associated with cumulative sertraline exposure. In other words, being on higher doses of sertraline for longer periods was associated with more weight gain. But standardized body mass index was not affected by sertraline over the 3-year follow-up period (Kolitsopoulos et al., 2023).

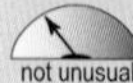

Sedation

- Reported but not expected
- Possibly activating in some patients

What to Do About Side Effects

- Wait, wait, wait: mild side effects are common, happen early, and usually improve with time, but treatment benefits can be delayed and often begin just as the side effects wear off. However, some side effects may emerge later such as weight gain.
- May wish to give some drugs at night if not tolerated during the day, particularly if the medication is associated with sedation
- Monitor side effects closely, especially when initiating treatment
- For activation (jitteriness, anxiety, insomnia):
  - Administer dose in the morning
  - Consider a more gradual up-titration
  - Consider a temporary dose reduction to 25 mg or even 12.5 mg until side effects abate, then increase dose as tolerated
  - Consider switching to another SSRI or potentially an SNRI (other than venlafaxine)
  - Optimize psychotherapeutic interventions
  - Activation and agitation may represent the induction of a bipolar state, especially a mixed dysphoric bipolar II condition sometimes associated with suicidal ideation, and may require the addition of lithium or an atypical antipsychotic, and/or discontinuation of sertraline
- Often best to try another monotherapy prior to resorting to augmentation strategies to treat side effects
- For insomnia: consider adding melatonin or an alpha 2 agonist
- For GI upset: try giving medication with a meal
- For sexual dysfunction:
  - Consider adding daytime exercise, bupropion, or buspirone
  - Probably best to reduce dose or discontinue and try another agent
- For emotional flattening, apathy: consider adding bupropion (with caution as little experience in children)

How Drug Causes Side Effects

- Theoretically due to increases in serotonin concentrations at serotonin receptors in parts of the brain and body other than those that cause therapeutic actions (e.g., unwanted actions of serotonin in sleep centers causing insomnia, unwanted actions of serotonin in the gut causing diarrhea)
- Increasing serotonin can cause diminished dopamine release and might contribute to emotional flattening, cognitive slowing, and apathy in some patients
- On the other hand, sertraline's possible dopamine reuptake blocking properties could contribute to agitation, anxiety, and undesirable activation, especially early in dosing

Warnings and Precautions

- Consider distributing brochures provided by the FDA and the drug companies as well as the medication guides from the American Academy of Child & Adolescent Psychiatry (AACAP)
- Carefully consider monitoring patients regularly within the practical limits, particularly during the first several weeks of treatment
- Warn patients and their caregivers when possible about the possibility of activating side effects and advise them to report such symptoms
- Carefully weigh the risks and benefits of pharmacological treatment against the risks and benefits of nontreatment with antidepressants and make sure to document this in the patient's chart
- As with any antidepressant, use with caution in patients with history of seizure
- As with any antidepressant, use with caution in patients with bipolar disorder unless treated with concomitant mood-stabilizing agent

- Monitor patients for activation and suicidal ideation and involve parents/guardians

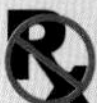

When Not to Prescribe

- If patient is taking an MAO inhibitor
- If patient is taking thioridazine
- If patient is taking pimozide
- Not generally recommended in patients taking tricyclic antidepressants (see Drug Interactions)
- Use of sertraline oral concentrate is contraindicated with disulfiram due to the alcohol content of the concentrate
- If there is a proven allergy to sertraline

Long-Term Use

- In adults, long-term use is safe

Habit Forming

- No

Overdose

- Rarely lethal in monotherapy overdose; symptoms can include vomiting, sedation, heart rhythm disturbances, dilated pupils, agitation; fatalities have been reported in sertraline overdose combined with other drugs or alcohol

DOSING AND USE

Usual Dosage Range

- In children for OCD and off-label uses: 25–200 mg/day
- In adolescents for OCD and most off-label uses: 50–200 mg/day

Dosage Forms

- Tablet 25 mg scored, 50 mg scored, 100 mg scored
- Oral solution 20 mg/mL

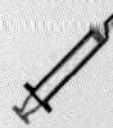

How to Dose

- In children:
  - OCD: initial 25 mg/day; usually wait a few weeks to assess drug effects before increasing dose, but can increase once a week by 25–50 mg/day; maximum dose generally 200 mg/day in a single dose
  - Dosing is generally the same for off-label uses
- In adolescents:
  - OCD: initial 50 mg/day; usually wait a few weeks to assess drug effects before increasing dose, but can increase once a week by 50 mg/day; maximum dose generally 200 mg/day in a single dose
  - Dosing is generally the same as adult dosing for off-label uses (i.e., anxiety, MDD)
  - Because sertraline concentrations vary so significantly in adolescents based on their CYP2C19 activity, clinicians could consider adjusting the dose based on CYP2C19 activity (Figure 1)

Options for Administration

- Scoring of tablets allows for initial dose of 12.5 mg for patients who require slower titration
- Oral solution can be beneficial for patients requiring very slow titration and in those who cannot swallow tablets; can be mixed with 4 oz of water, ginger ale, lemon/lime soda, lemonade, or orange juice only and must be consumed immediately after mixing

Tests

- None for healthy individuals

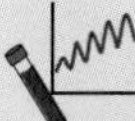

Pharmacokinetics

- Metabolized primarily by CYP2C19 and CYP2B6 and may weakly inhibit CYP2D6 and CYP3A4 at low doses. However, CYP2C19 is the primary pathway.
- Parent drug has 22–36-hour half-life (based on adult studies), and its metabolite has a 62–104-hour half-life (based on adult studies). In children and adolescents, the half-life of sertraline is related to CYP2C19. CYP2C19 poor metabolizers have a half-life of 62 hours compared to 37 hours in intermediate CYP2C19 metabolizers and 24 hours in other metabolizer groups.
- In pediatric patients – like in adults – sertraline metabolism is related to CYP2C19 variation
- Relative to the adults, both the 6- to 12-year-olds and the 13- to 17-year-olds showed about 22% lower concentrations over the course of the day. These data suggest that pediatric patients metabolize sertraline with slightly greater efficiency than adults.

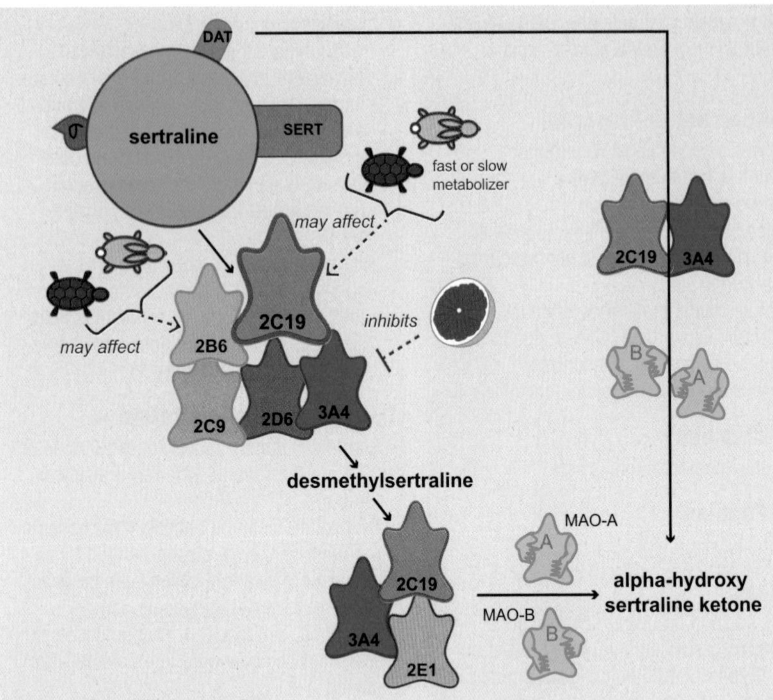

Figure 1 Sertraline metabolism.

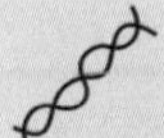

Pharmacogenetics

- Clearance of sertraline is reduced in children and adolescents who are slower CYP2C19 metabolizers (i.e., poor metabolizers and intermediate metabolizers) (Figure 2)
  - **CYP2C19 ultrarapid metabolizers:** The Clinical Pharmacogenetics Implementation Consortium (CPIC) recommends clinicians initiate therapy with recommended starting dose
  - **CYP2C19 rapid metabolizers:** CPIC recommends that clinicians initiate sertraline at the recommended starting dose
  - **CYP2C19 normal metabolizers:** CPIC recommends clinicians initiate sertraline at the recommended starting dose
  - **CYP2C19 intermediate metabolizers:** CPIC recommends clinicians initiate sertraline at the recommended starting dose. Consider a slower titration schedule and lower maintenance dose than normal metabolizers.
  - **CYP2C19 poor metabolizers:** CPIC recommends clinicians consider a lower starting dose, slower titration schedule, and 50% reduction of standard maintenance dose as compared to normal metabolizers or select an alternative

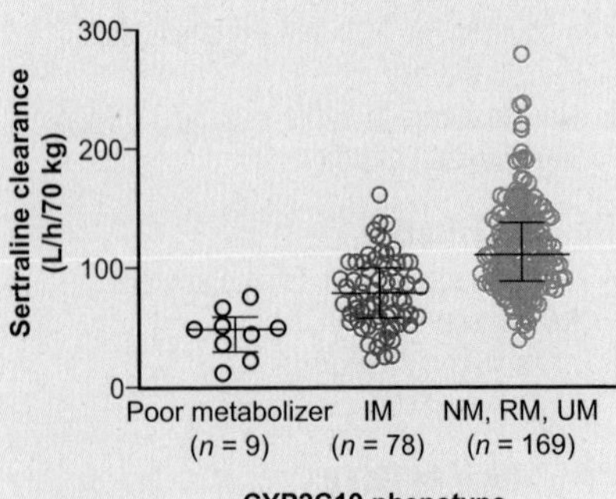

Figure 2 Sertraline clearance based on CYP2C19 phenotype. Children and adolescents who have reduced CYP2C19 activity have decreased sertraline clearance. IM, intermediate metabolzer; NM, normal metabolizer; RM, rapid metabolizer; UM, ultrarapid metabolizer. Reproduced from Poweleit et al, 2023.

antidepressant not predominantly metabolized by CYP2C19
  - CPIC also recommends that clinicians considering sertraline consider CYP2B6 status, drug–drug interactions, and other patient characteristics (e.g., age, renal function, liver function)

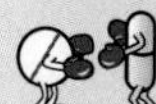

Drug Interactions

- Tramadol increases the risk of seizures in adults taking an antidepressant
- Can increase tricyclic antidepressant (TCA) levels; use with caution with TCAs or when switching from a TCA to sertraline
- Can cause a fatal "serotonin syndrome" when combined with MAOIs, so do not use with MAOIs or for at least 14 days after MAOIs are stopped
- Do not start an MAOI for at least 5 half-lives (5 to 7 days) after discontinuing sertraline
- May displace highly protein-bound drugs (e.g., phenytoin, valproate)
- Can theoretically cause weakness, hyperreflexia, and incoordination when combined with sumatriptan or possibly with other triptans, requiring careful monitoring of patient
- Possible increased risk of bleeding
- Via CYP2D6 inhibition, sertraline could theoretically interfere with the analgesic actions of codeine, and increase the plasma levels of some beta blockers and of atomoxetine
- Via CYP2D6 inhibition, sertraline could theoretically increase concentrations of thioridazine and cause dangerous cardiac arrhythmias
- Via CYP3A4 inhibition, sertraline may increase the levels of alprazolam, buspirone, and triazolam
- Via CYP3A4 inhibition, sertraline could theoretically increase the concentrations of pimozide, and cause QTc prolongation and dangerous cardiac arrhythmias
- False-positive urine immunoassay screening tests for benzodiazepine have been reported in patients taking sertraline due to a lack of specificity of the screening tests. False-positive results may be expected for several days following discontinuation of sertraline.
- Caution when used with drugs metabolized by CYP2D6 and 3A4, since plasma levels of those drugs may increase in patients also taking sertraline
- Cannabis and CBD increase sertraline concentrations in adolescents (Vaughn et al., 2021)

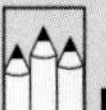

Dosing Tips

- If a child loses efficacy between daily doses, it may indicate rapid metabolism and the need to increase the dose or give twice daily. Also, some recent data suggest that dosing may need to be adjusted based on adolescent patients' CYP2C19 metabolism (Figure 3).
- Give once daily, often in the mornings to reduce chances of insomnia
- The more anxious and agitated the patient, the lower the starting dose, the slower the titration
- Utilize half a 25 mg tablet (12.5 mg) when initiating treatment in children, particularly those with anxiety
- If intolerable anxiety, insomnia, agitation, akathisia, or activation occurs either upon dosing initiation or discontinuation, consider an alternative SSRI. Importantly, for activation, the risk of activation with one SSRI does not predict the likelihood of activation with another SSRI.
- These symptoms may also indicate the need to evaluate for a mixed features episode and thus discontinuing sertraline and considering an atypical antipsychotic or a mood stabilizer or lithium

How to Switch

- From another antidepressant to sertraline:
  - When tapering a prior antidepressant, see its entry in this manual for how to stop and how to taper off that specific drug
  - In situations when there are antidepressant-related side effects, try to stop the first agent before starting sertraline so that new side effects of sertraline can be distinguished from withdrawal effects of the first agent
  - If necessary, can cross taper off the prior antidepressant and dose up on sertraline simultaneously in urgent situations, being aware of all specific drug interactions to avoid
- Off sertraline to another antidepressant:
  - Generally, try to stop sertraline before starting another antidepressant

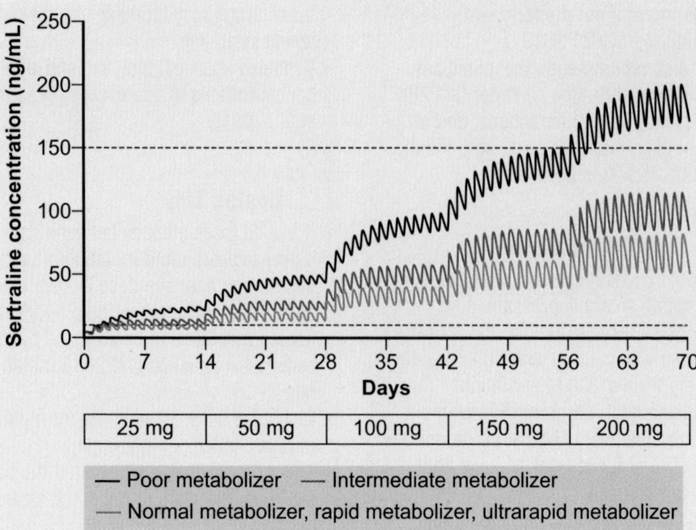

Figure 3 Sertraline concentration based on CYP2C19 phenotype. Sertraline exposure is influenced by CYP2C19 metabolizer status in children and adolescents. Reproduced from Poweleit et al., 2023.

- Stopping sertraline usually means tapering off since discontinuing many SSRIs can cause withdrawal symptoms
- If sertraline needs to be stopped quickly, one can reduce the sertraline dose by 50 mg every 3 to 7 days, or slower if this rate still causes withdrawal symptoms
- If necessary, can cross taper from sertraline to another antidepressant simultaneously in urgent situations, being aware of all specific drug interactions to avoid

How to Stop

- Taper to avoid withdrawal effects (dizziness, nausea, stomach cramps, sweating, tingling, dysesthesias)
- Many patients tolerate 50% dose reduction for 4–6 days, then another 50% reduction for 4–6 days, then discontinuation. More recently, however, hyperbolic discontinuation of SSRIs has been recommended in which the dose of the SSRI is halved every 4 weeks, and this may be a preferable strategy in

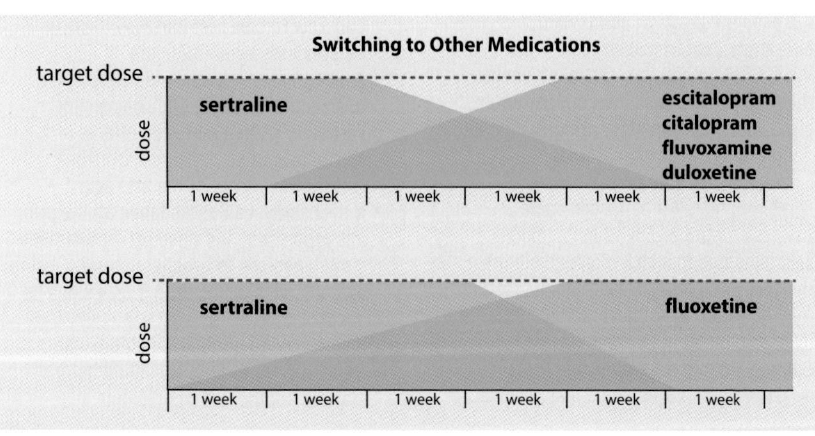

youth (Strawn et al., 2023). Also, when SSRIs are stopped, the risk of relapse is highest during the first 8 weeks after discontinuation.
- If withdrawal symptoms emerge during discontinuation, raise dose to stop symptoms and then restart withdrawal much more slowly

WHAT TO EXPECT

Onset of Action

- Some patients may experience increased energy or activation early after initiation of treatment
- Full onset of therapeutic actions is usually delayed by 2–4 weeks
- If it is not working within 6–8 weeks, it may require a dosage increase or it may not work at all

Duration of Action

- Effects are consistent over a 24-hour period
- May continue to work for many years to prevent relapse of symptoms

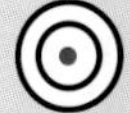

Primary Target Symptoms

- Obsessions, compulsions
- Depressed and/or irritable mood
- Anxiety (fear and worry are often target symptoms, but sertraline can occasionally and transiently increase these symptoms short term before improving them)
- Sleep disturbance, both hypersomnia and insomnia (eventually, but can actually cause insomnia, especially short term)
- Panic attacks, avoidant behavior, reexperiencing, hyperarousal
- Prior to initiation of treatment, it is helpful to develop a list of target symptoms of depression and/or anxiety to monitor during treatment to better assess treatment response

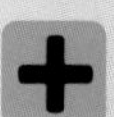

What Is Considered a Positive Result?

- The goal of treatment is complete remission of current symptoms as well as prevention of future relapses
- In practice, many patients have only a partial response where some symptoms are improved but others persist (especially insomnia, fatigue, and problems concentrating in depression), in which case higher doses of sertraline, adding a second agent, or switching to an agent with a different mechanism of action can be considered
- If treatment works, it most often reduces or even eliminates symptoms, but is not a cure since symptoms can recur after medicine is stopped

How Long to Treat

- For adolescents with depression, generally, 9–12 months of antidepressant treatment is recommended (Hathaway et al., 2018)
- For anxiety disorders, 6–9 months of antidepressant treatment may be sufficient, though many clinicians extend treatment to 12 months based on extrapolation of data from adults with anxiety disorders (Hathaway et al., 2018; Strawn et al., 2023)
- Extended treatment periods may decrease the risk of long-term morbidity and recurrence; however, the goal of treatment is ultimately remission, rather than duration of antidepressant pharmacotherapy (Hathaway et al., 2018)
- In terms of the length of antidepressant treatment, evidence-based guidelines represent a starting point; appropriate treatment duration varies, and patient-specific response, psychological factors, and timing of discontinuation must be considered for individual pediatric patients (Hathaway et al., 2018)

What If It Stops Working?

- Some patients who have an initial response may relapse even though they continue treatment, sometimes called "poop-out"
- Some patients may experience apparent lack of consistent efficacy due to activation syndrome or latent or underlying or newly evolved bipolar disorder, or major depressive episodes with mixed features, and require antidepressant discontinuation and a switch to a second generation antidepressant

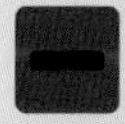

What If It Doesn't Work?

- Consider evaluation for another diagnosis (especially bipolar illness or depression with mixed features) or for a comorbid condition (e.g., medical illness, substance abuse)

- When treating youth with anxiety disorders, many patients will have had significant anxiety for years prior to beginning treatment. As such, when anxiety is treated with an SSRI, their symptoms may be improved, but the patient has likely missed important developmental milestones (e.g., spending the night with friends, being able to ask questions in class). Developing these skills will take time. Beyond this, the family may have lived with the anxious child for years and following treatment of the child, the family may need to readjust.
- Be mindful of family conflict contributing to the presentation; sometimes treating parental depression, if present, can improve psychiatric and social function without any treatment of youth. Also, accommodation is common in families of youth with anxiety disorders and may need to be addressed specifically, as it can perpetuate symptoms.
- Consider factors associated with poor response to SSRIs in treatment-resistant depression or anxiety disorders, such as severe symptoms, long-lasting symptoms, poor treatment adherence, prior nonresponse to other treatments, and the presence of comorbid disorders
- Consider other important potential factors such as ongoing conflicts, family psychopathology, and an adverse environment (e.g., poverty, chaos, violence, prior and ongoing psychological trauma, abuse, neglect). Additionally, when symptoms are prominent at school, consider the presence of a learning disorder.
- Institute trauma-informed care for appropriate children and adolescents
- A 2007 meta-analysis of published and unpublished trials in pediatric patients found that antidepressants had a number needed to treat (NNT) of 10 for depression, 6 for OCD, and 3 for anxiety disorders; thus, sertraline may not work in all children, so consider switching to another antidepressant (Bridge et al., 2007)
- Consider a dose adjustment in sertraline-treated patients, particularly if the patient is a CYP2C19 ultrarapid metabolizer
- Consider augmenting options:
  - Cognitive behavioral therapy (CBT), interpersonal psychotherapy for adolescents (IPT-A), light therapy, family therapy, and exercise especially in adolescents
  - For partial response (depression): use caution when adding medications to sertraline, especially in children since there are not sufficient studies of augmentation in children or adolescents; however, for the expert, consider bupropion, aripiprazole, or other atypical antipsychotics such as quetiapine; use combinations of antidepressants with caution as this may activate bipolar disorder and suicidal ideation
  - For insomnia: sleep hygiene, CBT for insomnia, melatonin, or alpha 2 agonists
  - For fatigue/sleepiness or lack of concentration: modafinil or armodafinil. However, first attempt to administer sertraline in the evening.
  - For anxiety: buspirone, antihistamines
  - Add lithium or atypical antipsychotics for bipolar depression, psychotic depression, treatment-resistant depression, or treatment-resistant anxiety disorders
  - TMS (transcranial magnetic stimulation) may have a role although pediatric trials of TMS have been hampered by high sham response rates (Croarkin et al., 2021)
  - ECT (case studies show effectiveness; cognitive side effects are similar to those in adults; reserve for treatment-resistant cases)

TALKING TO PATIENTS AND CAREGIVERS

What to Tell Parents About Efficacy

- Doesn't work right away; full therapeutic benefits may take 2–8 weeks, yet parents and teachers might see improvement before the patient does
- While the medicine helps by reducing symptoms and improving function, it is not a cure, and it is therefore necessary to keep taking the medication to sustain its therapeutic effects
- Since every treatment consideration depends on a risk/benefit analysis, parents should fully understand short- and long-term risks as well as benefits
- One of the SSRIs specifically approved for children and adolescents with OCD (obsessive-compulsive disorder)
- After successful treatment, continuation of sertraline may be necessary to prevent relapse. In general, when treating

depression in children and adolescents, medications are continued for 12 months after symptoms have resolved, while for anxiety disorders, clinicians have generally treated for 6–9 months (Hathaway et al., 2018).

- Often a good idea to tell parents whether the medication chosen is specifically approved for the disorder being treated, or if it is "unapproved" or "off-label" but nevertheless good clinical practice and based upon prudent extrapolation of controlled data from adults and from experience in children and adolescents instead of formal FDA approval

What to Tell Children and Adolescents About Efficacy

- We are trying to make you feel better
- It may be a good idea to give the medication a try; if it's not working very well, we can stop the medication and try something else
- A good try takes 2 to 3 months or even longer
- If it does make you feel better, you cannot stop it right away or you may feel sad or worried again
- Medications don't change who you are as a person; they give you the opportunity to be the best person you can be

What to Tell Parents About Side Effects

- Explain that side effects are expected in many when starting and are most common in the first 2–3 weeks of starting or increasing the dose
- Some SSRI side effects emerge early and resolve quickly (e.g., activation, gastrointestinal symptoms). In contrast, other side effects are late-emerging (e.g., weight gain) or persistent (e.g., sexual dysfunction). Discussing the temporal course of the side effects and distinguishing between persistent and transient side effects is critical. Ensuring that patients are aware not only of side effects but the tendency of some side effects to be transient is important and should be part of discussions with patients and their families. For many, knowing that a side effect is likely transient, as opposed to persistent, may significantly influence the patient and family's anxiety or fears related to medication (Strawn et al., 2023).
- Tell parents many side effects go away and do so about the same time that therapeutic effects start
- Predict side effects in advance (you will look clever and competent to the parents, unless you scare them with too much information and cause nocebo effects, in which case you won't look so clever when the patient develops lots of side effects and stops medication; use your judgment here); a balanced but honest presentation is an art rather than a science
- Ask them to help monitor for increased suicidality and if present, report any such symptoms immediately
- Ask parents to support the patient while side effects are occurring
- Parents should fully understand short- and long-term risks as well as benefits
- Explaining to the parents what to expect from medication treatment, and especially potential side effects, can help prevent early termination

What to Tell Children and Adolescents About Side Effects

- Even if you get side effects, most of them get better or go away in a few days to a few weeks
- Consider having a conversation about sexual side effects in some adolescents who can find these side effects confusing and especially burdensome
- Explaining to child/adolescent what to expect from medication treatment, and especially potential side effects, can help prevent early termination of medication
- Tell adolescents and children capable of understanding that some young patients, especially those who are depressed, may develop thoughts of hurting themselves, and if this happens, not to be alarmed but to tell their parents right away

What to Tell Teachers About the Medication (If Parents Consent)

- It is not abusable
- Encourage dialogue with parents/guardians about any behavior or mood changes

SPECIAL POPULATIONS

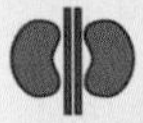

Renal Impairment

- No dose adjustment
- Not removed by hemodialysis

Hepatic Impairment

- Lower dose or give less frequently, perhaps by half

Cardiac Impairment

- Proven cardiovascular safety in adult depressed patients with recent myocardial infarction or angina
- Treating depression with SSRIs in patients with acute angina or following myocardial infarction may reduce cardiac events and improve survival as well as mood
- A study of US claims data found that the risk of adverse cardiac events for sertraline users was low (incidence rate was 10.3 per 10,000 person-years) (Czaja et al., 2013)

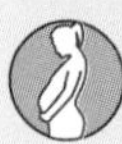

Pregnancy

- Controlled studies have not been conducted in pregnant women
- Not generally recommended for use during pregnancy, especially during first trimester
- Nonetheless, continuous treatment during pregnancy may be necessary and has not been proven to be harmful to the fetus
- At delivery there may be more bleeding in the mother and transient irritability or sedation in the newborn
- Must weigh the risk of treatment (first trimester fetal development, third trimester newborn delivery) to the child against the risk of no treatment (recurrence of depression, maternal health, infant bonding) to the mother and child
- For many patients, this may mean continuing treatment during pregnancy
- Exposure to serotonin reuptake inhibitors early in pregnancy may be associated with increased risk of septal heart defects (absolute risk is small)
- Use of serotonin reuptake inhibitors beyond the 20th week of pregnancy may be associated with increased risk of pulmonary hypertension in newborns, although this is not proven
- Exposure to serotonin reuptake inhibitors late in pregnancy may be associated with increased risk of gestational hypertension and preeclampsia
- Neonates exposed to SSRIs or SNRIs late in the third trimester have developed complications requiring prolonged hospitalization, respiratory support, and tube feeding; reported symptoms are consistent with either a direct toxic effect of SSRIs and SNRIs or, possibly, a drug discontinuation syndrome, and include respiratory distress, cyanosis, apnea, seizures, temperature instability, feeding difficulty, vomiting, hypoglycemia, hypotonia, hypertonia, hyperreflexia, tremor, jitteriness, irritability, and constant crying

Breast Feeding

- Some drug is found in breast milk
- Trace amounts may be present in nursing children whose mothers are on sertraline
- Sertraline has shown efficacy in treating postpartum depression
- If child becomes irritable or sedated, breast feeding or drug may need to be discontinued
- Immediate postpartum period is a high-risk time for depression, especially in women who have had prior depressive episodes, so drug may need to be reinstituted late in the third trimester or shortly after childbirth to prevent a recurrence during the postpartum period
- Must weigh benefits of breast feeding with risks and benefits of antidepressant treatment versus non-treatment to both the infant and the mother
- For many patients, this may mean continuing treatment during breast feeding

THE ART OF PSYCHOPHARMACOLOGY

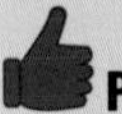

Potential Advantages

- In children:
  - One of only four agents specifically approved for OCD in children (also fluvoxamine, fluoxetine, and clomipramine)
- In adolescents:
  - One of only four agents specifically approved for OCD in adolescents

(also fluvoxamine, fluoxetine, and clomipramine)
- All ages:
  - Patients with atypical depression (hypersomnia, increased appetite)
  - Patients with fatigue and low energy
  - Patients who are sensitive to the prolactin-elevating properties of other SSRIs, girls and women with galactorrhea or unexplained amenorrhea, boys and men with gynecomastia

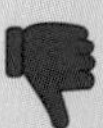

Potential Disadvantages

- In children:
  - Two placebo-controlled trials were conducted in pediatric patients with MDD, but the data were not sufficient to support an indication for use in pediatric patients
  - Does not mean sertraline doesn't work, but that clinical trials have not proven that despite clinical experience that sertraline does work in pediatric MDD
  - Those who are already psychomotor agitated, angry, or irritable, and who do not have a psychiatric diagnosis
- In adolescents:
  - Those who may possibly have a mood disorder with mixed or bipolar features, especially those with these features and a family history of bipolar disorder
- All ages:
  - Initiating treatment in anxious, agitated patients
  - Initiating treatment in patients with insomnia
  - Patients with comorbid irritable bowel syndrome
  - Can require dose titration

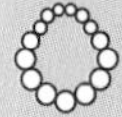

Pearls

- SSRIs show greater efficacy in pediatric anxiety disorders compared to depression
- In anxious youth, SSRIs produce faster and greater improvement compared to SNRIs (Strawn et al., 2018)
- In adolescents with anxiety disorders, SSRIs may improve emotional processing within 2 weeks and enhance the connection between the prefrontal cortex and the amygdala (Lu et al., 2022)
- Some SSRIs can cause cognitive and affective "flattening"; however, this may be theoretically diminished in some patients by sertraline's dopamine reuptake blocking properties
- Binding at sigma 1 receptors may enhance sertraline's anxiolytic actions
- Cannabis and CBD may increase sertraline concentrations in adolescents through effects at CYP2C19 (Vaughn et al., 2021)
- Can have more gastrointestinal effects, particularly diarrhea, than some other antidepressants; however, in the largest trial of youth with anxiety disorders, sertraline produced improvement in some gastrointestinal symptoms, including abdominal pain and nausea (Strawn et al., 2023)
- In meta-analyses examining the risk of insomnia for specific SSRIs in youth with anxiety and obsessive-compulsive disorders, sertraline was associated with twice the likelihood of insomnia compared to placebo (relative risk: 1.94)
- In the largest trial of sertraline in pediatric patients, patients who did not have improvement by the eighth week of treatment had a 3:1 odds against improvement with continued treatment. Therefore, it may make sense to switch from sertraline if a patient has had no response by week 8 (Strawn et al., 2018)
- Finally, some data suggest that adolescents who are ultrarapid and rapid CYP2C19 metabolizers may require bid dosing to produce similar pharmacokinetic profiles to normal metabolizers (Strawn et al., 2018)

SUGGESTED READING

Bridge JA, Iyengar S, Salary CB et al. Clinical response and risk for reported suicidal ideation and suicide attempts in pediatric antidepressant treatment: a meta-analysis of randomized controlled trials. JAMA 2007;297(15):1683–96.

Croarkin PE, Elmaadawi AZ, Aaronson ST et al. Left prefrontal transcranial magnetic stimulation for treatment-resistant depression in adolescents: a double-blind, randomized, sham-controlled trial. Neuropsychopharmacology 2021;46(2):462–9.

Czaja AS, Valuck RJ, Anderson HD. Comparative safety of selective serotonin reuptake inhibitors among pediatric users with respect to adverse cardiac events. Pharmacoepidemiol Drug Saf 2013;22(6):607–14.

Hathaway EE, Walkup JT, Strawn JR. Antidepressant treatment duration in pediatric depressive and anxiety disorders: how long is long enough? Curr Probl Pediatr Adolesc Health Care 2018 Feb;48(2):31–9.

Hicks JK, Bishop JR, Sangkuhl K et al. Clinical Pharmacogenetics Implementation Consortium (CPIC) guideline for CYP2D6 and CYP2C19 genotypes and dosing of selective serotonin reuptake inhibitors. Clin Pharmacol Ther 2015;98(2):127–34.

Kolitsopoulos F, Ramaker S, Compton SN et al. Effects of long-term sertraline use on pediatric growth and development: the sertraline pediatric registry for the evaluation of safety (SPRITES). J Child Adolesc Psychopharmacol 2023;33(1):2–13.

Lu L, Li H, Baumel WT et al. Acute neurofunctional effects of escitalopram during emotional processing in pediatric anxiety: a double-blind, placebo-controlled trial. Neuropsychopharmacology 2022;47(5):1081–7.

Pediatric OCD Treatment Study Team (POTS). Cognitive-behavior therapy, sertraline, and their combination for children and adolescents with obsessive-compulsive disorder: the Pediatric OCD Treatment Study (POTS) randomized controlled trial. JAMA 2004;292:1969–76.

Strawn JR, Mills JA, Sauley BA, Welge JA. The impact of antidepressant dose and class on treatment response in pediatric anxiety disorders: a meta-analysis. J Am Acad Child Adolesc Psychiatry 2018;57(4):235–244.e2.

Strawn JR, Poweleit EA, Ramsey LB. CYP2C19-guided escitalopram and sertraline dosing in pediatric patients: a pharmacokinetic modeling study. J Child Adolesc Psychopharmacol 2019;29(5):340–7.

Strawn JR, Lu L, Peris TS, Levine A, Walkup JT. Research review: pediatric anxiety disorders – what have we learnt in the last 10 years? J Child Psychol Psychiatry 2021;62(2):114–39.

Strawn JR, Mills JA, Poweleit EA, Ramsey LB, Croarkin PE. Adverse effects of antidepressant medications and their management in children and adolescents. Pharmacotherapy 2023;43(7):675–90.

Vaughn SE, Strawn JR, Poweleit EA, Sarangdhar M, Ramsey LB. The impact of marijuana on antidepressant treatment in adolescents: clinical and pharmacologic considerations. J Pers Med 2021;11(7):615.

Walkup JT, Albano AM, Piacentini J et al. Cognitive behavioral therapy, sertraline, or a combination in childhood anxiety. N Engl J Med 2008;359:2753–66.

THERAPEUTICS

Brands

- Epitomax
- Topamac
- Topamax
- Topimax
- Trokendi XR
- Qsymia
- Qudexy XR

Generic

Yes

US FDA Approved for Pediatric Use

- Partial onset seizures (for immediate-release: adjunct for adults and pediatric patients 2–16 years of age; for extended-release: monotherapy or adjunct for patients 2 years and older)
- Primary generalized tonic-clonic seizures (adjunct and monotherapy for patients 2 years of age and older)
- Seizures associated with Lennox–Gastaut syndrome (adjunct; 2 years of age and older)
- Migraine prophylaxis (ages 12 and older)
- Chronic weight management (adjunct to reduced-calorie diet and increased physical activity) in pediatric patients aged 12 years and older with BMI in the 95th percentile or greater standardized for age and sex [in combination with phentermine (Qsymia)]

Off-Label for Pediatric Use

- Approved in adults
  - Chronic weight management (adjunct to reduced-calorie diet and increased physical activity) in adults with an initial body mass index (BMI) of at least 30 kg/m^2 (obese) or at least 27 kg/m^2 (overweight) in the presence of at least one weight-related comorbid condition [in combination with phentermine (Qsymia)]
- Other off label uses
  - Bipolar disorder (adjunctive; no longer in development)
  - Psychotropic drug-induced weight gain
  - Binge-eating disorder

Class and Mechanism of Action

- Anticonvulsant, voltage-sensitive sodium channel modulator

SAFETY AND TOLERABILITY

Notable Side Effects

- Sedation, asthenia, dose-dependent dizziness, ataxia, dose-dependent paresthesia, nystagmus, nervousness, tremor
- Dose-dependent nausea, appetite loss, weight loss
- Visual field defects
- Problems concentrating, confusion, memory problems, psychomotor retardation, language problems, speech problems
- Mood problems, dose-dependent fatigue, taste perversion

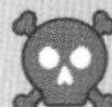

Life-Threatening or Dangerous Side Effects

- Metabolic acidosis (bicarbonate decrements are usually mild–moderate (average decrease of 4 mEq/L at daily doses of 400 mg in adults and at approximately 6 mg/kg/day in pediatric patients)
- Kidney stones
- Hyperammonemia with or without encephalopathy has been reported (may be dose related; may be more likely with concomitant valproate use)
- Secondary angle-closure glaucoma
- Rare severe dermatological reactions (purpura, Stevens–Johnson syndrome)
- Oligohidrosis and hyperthermia (more common in children)
- Sudden unexplained deaths have occurred in epilepsy (unknown if related to topiramate use)
- Rare activation of suicidal ideation and behavior (suicidality)

Growth and Maturation

- Although topiramate can cause weight loss, the existing limited literature does not show a negative effect on height growth in pediatric patients

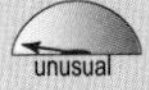

Weight Gain

- Patients may experience weight loss

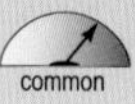

Sedation

- Many experience and/or can be significant in amount
- May be dose dependent

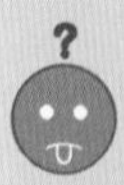

What to Do About Side Effects

- Wait
- Wait
- Wait
- Take at night to reduce daytime sedation
- Increase fluid intake to reduce the risk of kidney stones
- Switch to another agent

How Drug Causes Side Effects

- CNS side effects theoretically due to excessive actions at voltage-sensitive sodium channels
- Weak inhibition of carbonic anhydrase may lead to kidney stones and paresthesia
- Inhibition of carbonic anhydrase may also lead to metabolic acidosis

Warnings and Precautions

- A syndrome consisting of acute myopia associated with secondary angle-closure glaucoma has been reported in adult and pediatric patients taking topiramate; if secondary angle-closure glaucoma occurs, topiramate should be discontinued
- If symptoms of metabolic acidosis develop and persist (hyperventilation, fatigue, anorexia, cardiac arrhythmias, stupor), then dose may need to be reduced or treatment may need to be discontinued
- Depressive effects may be increased by other CNS depressants (alcohol, MAOIs, other anticonvulsants, etc.)
- Use with caution when combining with other drugs that predispose patients to heat-related disorders, including carbonic anhydrase inhibitors and anticholinergics
- Warn patients and their caregivers about the possibility of activation of suicidal ideation and advise them to report such side effects immediately

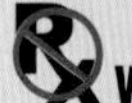

When Not to Prescribe

- Within 6 hours prior to and 6 hours after alcohol use (extended release)
- In patients with metabolic acidosis who are taking metformin (extended-release)
- If there is a proven allergy to topiramate

Long-Term Use

- Probably safe
- Periodic monitoring of serum bicarbonate levels may be required

Habit Forming

- No

Overdose

- No fatalities have been reported in monotherapy; convulsions, sedation, speech disturbance, blurred or double vision, metabolic acidosis, impaired coordination, hypotension, abdominal pain, agitation, dizziness

DOSING AND USE

Usual Dosage Range

- Seizures (patients 10 years of age and younger): 6–9 mg/kg/day
- Migraine (ages 10 and older): 100 mg/day in two divided doses

Dosage Forms

- Tablet 25 mg, 50 mg, 100 mg, 200 mg
- Sprinkle capsule 15 mg, 25 mg
- Extended-release capsule 25 mg, 50 mg, 100 mg, 150 mg, 200 mg
- Oral solution 25 mg/mL

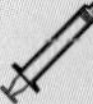

How to Dose

- Migraine (ages 10 and older): initial 25 mg/night for the first week; increase weekly in 25 mg increments; approved dose 100 mg/day in two divided doses
- Seizures (monotherapy, patients' ages 10 and older): initial 50 mg once daily; increase by 50 mg weekly for 4 weeks, increase by 100 mg weekly for weeks 5 and 6; recommended dose 400 mg/day
- Seizures (immediate-release, ages 2–16): initial 1–3 mg/kg per day at night; after 1 week increase by 1–3 mg/kg per day every 1–2 weeks with total daily dose administered in 2 divided doses; recommended dose generally 5–9 mg/kg per day in 2 divided doses

- Seizures (extended release, adjunct): initial 25 mg once nightly (1–3 mg/kg/night) for first week; increase at 1- or 2-week intervals by increments of 1–3 mg/kg/night; recommended dose 5–9 mg/kg/night
- Seizures (extended release, monotherapy, ages 2 through 9): initial 25 mg once at night for the first week; titrate over 5 to 7 weeks; recommended dose is based on weight
- See accompanying table

Weight (kg)	Total daily dose (mg/day)*
Up to 11	150–250
12–22	200–300
23–31	200–350
32–38	250–350
Greater than 38	250–400

* Administered in two equally divided doses

Options for Administration

- Available as a sprinkle capsule and as an oral liquid formulation

Tests

- Baseline and periodic serum bicarbonate levels to monitor for hyperchloremic, nonanion gap metabolic acidosis (i.e., decreased serum bicarbonate below the normal reference range in the absence of chronic respiratory alkalosis)
- Monitor height and weight

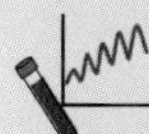

Pharmacokinetics

- Topiramate is well absorbed orally and reaches peak plasma concentrations within 2 to 4 hours after administration
- Food can slightly delay its absorption, but it does not significantly affect the overall bioavailability
- Topiramate has a relatively high volume of distribution, indicating that it distributes extensively into body tissues. It binds moderately (approximately 13–17%) to plasma proteins, such as albumin.
- Topiramate undergoes minimal metabolism in the liver but enzyme-inducing comedication (i.e., carbamazepine) decreases serum topiramate concentration by approximately one-half and one-third in children and adults, respectively
- Inhibits CYP2C19 and induces CYP3A4
- Topiramate clearance is highest in young children and decreases progressively with age until puberty, presumably due to age-dependent changes in the rate of drug metabolism
- Younger patients require higher dosages to achieve serum topiramate concentrations comparable with those found in older children and adults

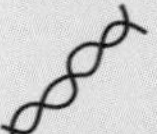

Pharmacogenetics

- No recommendations

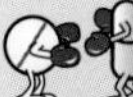

Drug Interactions

- Carbamazepine, phenytoin, and valproate may increase the clearance of topiramate, and thus decrease topiramate levels, possibly requiring a higher dose of topiramate
- Topiramate may increase the clearance of phenytoin and thus decrease phenytoin levels, possibly requiring a higher dose of phenytoin
- Topiramate may increase the clearance of valproate and thus decrease valproate levels, possibly requiring a higher dose of valproate
- Topiramate may increase plasma levels of metformin; also, metformin may reduce clearance of topiramate and increase topiramate levels
- Topiramate may interact with carbonic anhydrase inhibitors to increase the risk of kidney stones
- Topiramate may reduce the effectiveness of oral contraceptives; though only a mild enzyme-inducing antiepileptic drug, concomitant topiramate use led to inferior serum etonogestrel concentrations among implant users, with a significant proportion reaching etonogestrel concentrations below the threshold for ovulatory suppression when taking antiepileptic dosages of topiramate
- Topiramate levels may increase in the presence of hydrochlorothiazide (HCTZ), possibly requiring a dose decrease of topiramate
- Topiramate may decrease the exposure of pioglitazone and its active metabolites; patients taking both medications should be carefully monitored for adequate control of their diabetic disease state

- At high doses, topiramate may increase systemic exposure of lithium by increasing the excretion of sodium
- Reports of hypothermia and hyperammonemia with or without encephalopathy in patients taking topiramate combined with valproate, though this is not due to a pharmacokinetic interaction; in patients who develop unexplained lethargy, vomiting, or change in mental status, an ammonia level should be measured

Dosing Tips

- For migraine, the individual dose may vary widely. Some patients benefit from doses as low as 25 mg/day, but others may require much higher doses than the 100 mg/day approved for migraine prophylaxis.
- Headaches may return within days to months of stopping, but patients often continue to do well for 6 or more months after stopping
- Adverse effects may increase as dose increases
- Topiramate is available in a sprinkle capsule formulation, which can be swallowed whole or sprinkled over approximately a teaspoon of soft food (e.g., applesauce); the mixture should be consumed immediately
- Slow upward titration from doses as low as 25 mg/day can reduce the incidence of unacceptable sedation
- Weight loss is dose related but most patients treated for weight gain receive doses at the lower end of the dosing range
- Effectiveness was not demonstrated in infants/toddlers 1 to 24 months of age with refractory partial onset seizures; some adverse effects/toxicities not observed in older patients did occur

How to Switch

- From another medication to topiramate:
  - When tapering a prior medication, see its entry in this manual for how to stop and how to taper off that specific drug
  - Generally, try to stop the first agent before starting topiramate so that new side effects of topiramate can be distinguished from withdrawal effects of the first agent
  - If urgent, cross taper
- Off topiramate to another medication:
  - Generally, try to stop topiramate before starting the new medication so that new side effects of the next drug can be distinguished from any withdrawal effects from topiramate
  - Taper; may need to adjust dosage of concurrent medications as topiramate is being discontinued
  - If urgent, cross taper

How to Stop

- Taper
- Epilepsy patients may seize upon withdrawal, especially if withdrawal is abrupt
- Rapid discontinuation may increase the risk of relapse in bipolar patients
- Discontinuation symptoms uncommon

WHAT TO EXPECT

Onset of Action

- Should reduce seizures by 2 weeks
- Not clear that it has mood-stabilizing properties, but some bipolar patients may respond and if so, it may take several weeks to months to optimize an effect on mood stabilization

Duration of Action

- Effects are consistent over a 24-hour period
- May continue to work for many years to prevent relapse of symptoms

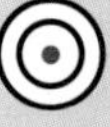

Primary Target Symptoms

- Increased appetite/obesity
- Incidence of seizures
- Migraine prophylaxis
- Unstable mood

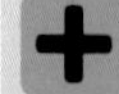

What Is Considered a Positive Result?

- The goal of treatment is complete remission of symptoms (e.g., seizures, migraine)

How Long to Treat

- Continue treatment until all symptoms are gone or until improvement is stable and then continue treating indefinitely as long as improvement persists
- Continue treatment indefinitely to avoid recurrence of seizures, and headaches

What If It Stops Working?

- Check for nonadherence, possibly by checking plasma drug level, and consider switching to another agent with fewer side effects
- Screen for the development of a new comorbid disorder, especially substance abuse
- Screen for adverse changes in the home or school environment

What If It Doesn't Work?

- Consider evaluation for another diagnosis or for a comorbid condition (e.g., medical illness, substance abuse)
- Consider other important potential factors such as ongoing conflicts, family psychopathology, and an adverse environment (e.g., poverty, chaos, violence, prior and ongoing psychological trauma, abuse, neglect)
- Institute trauma-informed care for appropriate children and adolescents
- May be effective only in a subset of bipolar patients, in some patients who fail to respond to other mood stabilizers, or it may not work at all
- Consider increasing dose or switching to another agent with better demonstrated efficacy in bipolar disorder (one of the atypical antipsychotics or lithium)
- Consider initiating rehabilitation and psychotherapy such as cognitive remediation, although these may be less well standardized for children/adolescents than for adults
- Consider presence of concomitant drug abuse
- Consider augmentation with lithium, an atypical antipsychotic, or an antidepressant (with caution because antidepressants can destabilize mood in some patients, including induction of rapid cycling or suicidal ideation; in particular, consider bupropion; also SSRIs, SNRIs, others; generally, avoid TCAs, MAOIs)

TALKING TO PATIENTS AND CAREGIVERS

What to Tell Parents About Efficacy

- For appetite suppression, it can work right away
- Explain which use topiramate is being chosen for, how to tell if the drug is working by targeting specific symptoms, and why this is being done
- Since every treatment consideration depends on a risk/benefit analysis, parents should fully understand short- and long-term risks as well as benefits
- Often a good idea to tell parents whether the medication chosen is specifically approved for the disorder being treated, or whether it is being given for "unapproved" or "off-label" reasons based on good clinical practice, expert consensus, and/or prudent extrapolation of controlled data from adults

What to Tell Children and Adolescents About Efficacy

- Be specific about the symptoms being targeted: we are trying to help you …
- Give the medication a try; if it's not working very well, we can stop the medication and try something else
- A good try often takes 2 to 3 months
- If it does make you feel better, you cannot stop it right away or you may get sick again
- Medications don't change who you are as a person; they give you the opportunity to be the best person you can be

What to Tell Parents About Side Effects

- Explain that side effects are expected in many when starting
- Tell parents many side effects go away and do so about the same time that therapeutic effects start
- Predict side effects in advance (you will look clever and competent to the parents, unless you scare them with too much information and cause nocebo effects, in which case you won't look so clever when the patient develops lots of side effects and stops medication; use your judgment here); a balanced but honest presentation is an art rather than a science
- Ask parents to support the patient while side effects are occurring

- Parents should fully understand short- and long-term risks as well as benefits
- Explaining to the parents what to expect from medication treatment, and especially what potential side effects to expect, can help prevent early termination of medication

What to Tell Children and Adolescents About Side Effects

- Even if you get a side effect, we can usually reduce it over time
- If you have side effects that are bothering you, tell your parents and your parents should tell me
- Explaining to child/adolescent what to expect from medication treatment, and especially potential side effects, can help prevent early termination of medication

What to Tell Teachers About the Medication (If Parents Consent)

- Topiramate can make children/adolescents tired
- It is not abusable
- Encourage dialogue with parents/guardians about any behavior or mood changes

SPECIAL POPULATIONS

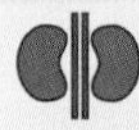

Renal Impairment

- Topiramate is renally excreted, so the dose should be lowered by half
- Can be removed by hemodialysis; patients receiving hemodialysis may require supplemental doses of topiramate

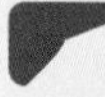

Hepatic Impairment

- Reduce dose and increase intervals between dosing

Cardiac Impairment

- Drug should be used with caution

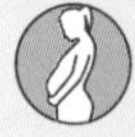

Pregnancy

- Increased risk of cleft lip/palate
- Increased risk of being small for gestational age
- Use in women of childbearing potential requires weighing potential benefits to the mother against the risks to the fetus
- Hypospadias has occurred in some male infants whose mothers took topiramate during pregnancy
- Lack of convincing efficacy for treatment of bipolar disorder suggests risk/benefit ratio is in favor of discontinuing topiramate in bipolar patients during pregnancy
- For bipolar patients, topiramate should generally be discontinued before anticipated pregnancies
- Antiepileptic Drug Pregnancy Registry: (888) 233-2334 or www.aedpregnancyregistry.org
- Taper drug if discontinuing
- For bipolar patients, given the risk of relapse in the postpartum period, mood stabilizer treatment, especially with agents with better evidence of efficacy than topiramate, should generally be restarted immediately after delivery if patient is unmedicated during pregnancy
- Atypical antipsychotics may be preferable to topiramate if treatment of bipolar disorder is required during pregnancy
- Bipolar symptoms may recur or worsen during pregnancy, and some form of treatment may be necessary
- Seizures, even mild seizures, may cause harm to the embryo/fetus

Breast Feeding

- Some drug is found in breast milk
- Recommended either to discontinue drug or formula feed
- If drug is continued while breast feeding, infant should be monitored for possible adverse effects
- If infant shows signs of irritability or sedation, drug may need to be discontinued

THE ART OF PSYCHOPHARMACOLOGY

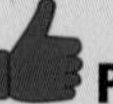

Potential Advantages

- Patients who wish to avoid weight gain

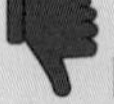

Potential Disadvantages

- Efficacy in pediatric patients with bipolar disorder unlikely
- Patients with a history of kidney stones or risks for metabolic acidosis

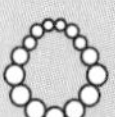

Pearls

- Topiramate treatment produced a dose-related increased shift in serum creatinine from normal at baseline to an increased value at the end of 4 months' treatment in adolescent patients (ages 12–16 years) who were treated for migraine prophylaxis in a double-blind, placebo-controlled study
- Topiramate may significantly affect word finding and working memory. Interestingly, in one study, each 1 µg/mL of topiramate plasma concentration was associated with nearly a 4% decrease in accuracy for working memory (Callisto et al., 2020).
- In double-blind, placebo-controlled trials of adolescents treated with second generation antipsychotics, adjunctive topiramate decreases weight gain (Wozniak et al., 2009; DelBello et al., 2023), although in adolescents with acute mania, adding topiramate to second generation antipsychotics does not appear to improve symptoms of mania (Woznick et al., 2009)
- Side effects may occur less often in pediatric patients, although nephrolithiasis occurs at similar rates in children and adults. In topiramate-treated youth, risk factors for nephrolithiasis in spot urine include hypocitraturia and hypercalciuria, and these are independent of topiramate dose and duration. High urine pH is found in nearly 70% of youth taking topiramate and correlates with dose (Corbin Bush et al., 2013).
- Has been studied in a wide range of psychiatric disorders, including bipolar disorder, posttraumatic stress disorder, binge-eating disorder, obesity, and others
- Randomized clinical trials do not suggest efficacy in bipolar disorder
- Misperceptions about topiramate's efficacy in bipolar disorder have led to its use in more patients than other agents with proven efficacy, such as lamotrigine
- Migraines may decrease in as little as 2 weeks, but can take up to 3 months on a stable dose to see full effect
- The goal when using topiramate for migraine prophylaxis is a 50% or greater reduction in migraine frequency or severity; consider tapering or stopping if headaches remit for more than 6 months or if considering pregnancy
- Augmenting options for migraine include beta blockers, antidepressants, natural products, other anticonvulsants, and nonmedication treatments such as biofeedback to improve headache control
- Due to reported weight loss in some patients in trials with epilepsy, topiramate is commonly used to treat weight gain, especially in patients with psychotropic drug-induced weight gain
- Weight loss in epilepsy patients is dose related with more weight loss at high doses (mean 6.5 kg or 7.3% decline) and less weight loss at lower doses (mean 1.6 kg or 2.2% decline)
- Changes in weight were greatest in epilepsy patients who weighed the most at baseline (>100 kg), with mean loss of 9.6 kg or 8.4% decline, while those weighing <60 kg had only a mean loss of 1.3 kg or 2.5% decline
- Long-term studies demonstrate that weight losses in epilepsy patients were seen within the first 3 months of treatment and peaked at a mean of 6 kg after 12–18 months of treatment; however, weight tended to return to pretreatment levels after 18 months
- Some patients with psychotropic drug-induced weight gain may experience significant weight loss (>7% of body weight) with topiramate up to 200 mg/day for 3 months, but this is not typical, is not often sustained, and has not been systemically studied

SUGGESTED READING

Alrifai MT, Alsubaie NA, Abodarahem AB et al. What is the effect of topiramate use on growth in children with epilepsy? Cureus 2022;14(8):e28503.

Battino D, Croci D, Rossini A et al. Topiramate pharmacokinetics in children and adults with epilepsy: a case-matched comparison based on therapeutic drug monitoring data. Clin Pharmacokinet 2005;44(4):407–16.

Callisto SP, Illamola SM, Birnbaum AK et al. Severity of topiramate-related working memory impairment is modulated by plasma concentration and working memory capacity. J Clin Pharmacol 2020;60(9):1166–76.

Corbin Bush N, Twombley K, Ahn J et al. Prevalence and spot urine risk factors for renal stones in children taking topiramate. J Pediatr Urol 2013;9(6 Pt A):884–9.

DelBello MP, Bruns KM, Bloom T et al. A double-blind placebo-controlled pilot study of topiramate in manic adolescents treated with olanzapine. J Child Adolesc Psychopharmacol 2023;33(4):12633.

Dhillon S. Phentermine/topiramate: pediatric first approval. Paediatr Drugs 2022;24(6):715–20.

Girgis IG, Nandy P, Nye JS et al. Pharmacokinetic-pharmacodynamic assessment of topiramate dosing regimens for children with epilepsy 2 to <10 years of age. Epilepsia 2010;51(10):1954–62.

Lazorwitz A, Pena M, Sheeder J, Teal S. Effect of topiramate on serum etonogestrel concentrations among contraceptive implant users. Obstet Gynecol 2022;139(4):579–87.

Wozniak J, Mick E, Waxmonsky J, et al. Comparison of open-label, 8-week trials of olanzapine monotherapy and topiramate augmentation of olanzapine for the treatment of pediatric bipolar disorder. J Child Adolesc Psychopharmacol 2009;19(5):539–45.

THERAPEUTICS

Brands

- Desyrel
- Oleptro

Generic

Yes

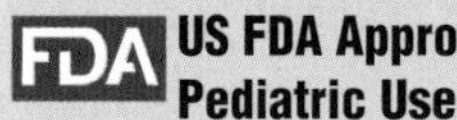

US FDA Approved for Pediatric Use

- None

Off-Label for Pediatric Use

- Approved in adults
  - Depression
- Other off-label uses
  - Insomnia (primary and secondary)
  - Anxiety

Class and Mechanism of Action

- Neuroscience-based Nomenclature: serotonin receptor antagonist (S-MM)
- SARI (serotonin 2 antagonist/reuptake inhibitor); antidepressant; hypnotic
- Blocks serotonin 2A receptors potently
- Trazodone presumably increases serotonergic neurotransmission by blocking the serotonin reuptake pump (transporter, SERT), which results in the desensitization of serotonin receptors, especially serotonin 1A receptors

SAFETY AND TOLERABILITY

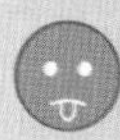

Notable Side Effects

- Nausea, vomiting, constipation, dry mouth, blurred vision
- Dizziness, sedation, fatigue, headache
- Sinus bradycardia (long term)
- Hypotension, syncope
- Incoordination, tremor
- Rare rash
- Bruising and rare bleeding

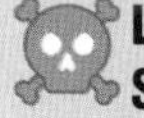

Life-Threatening or Dangerous Side Effects

- Rare priapism
- Rare seizures
- Rare induction of mania
- Rare suicidal ideation and behavior (suicidality) (short-term regulatory studies did not show any actual suicides in any age group and also did not show an increase in the risk of suicidality with antidepressants compared to placebo beyond age 24)

Growth and Maturation

- Growth should be monitored; long-term effects are unknown

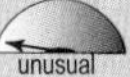

Weight Gain

- Reported but not expected

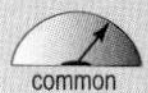

Sedation

- Many experience and/or can be significant in amount

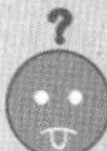

What to Do About Side Effects

- Wait, wait, wait: mild side effects are common, happen early, and usually improve with time
- Monitor side effects closely, especially when initiating treatment

How Drug Causes Side Effects

- Sedative effects may be due to antihistamine properties
- Blockade of alpha adrenergic 1 receptors may explain dizziness, sedation, and hypotension

Warnings and Precautions

- Consider distributing brochures provided by the FDA and the drug companies as well as the medication guides from the American Academy of Child & Adolescent Psychiatry (AACAP)
- Carefully consider monitoring patients regularly within the practical limits, particularly during the first several weeks of treatment
- Warn patients and their caregivers when possible about the possibility of activating side effects and advise them to report such symptoms
- Carefully weigh the risks and benefits of pharmacological treatment against the risks and benefits of nontreatment with antidepressants and it is a good idea to document this in the patient's chart

- Possibility of additive effects if trazodone is used with other CNS depressants
- Treatment should be discontinued if prolonged penile erection occurs because of the risk of permanent erectile dysfunction
- Advise patients to seek medical attention immediately if painful erections occur lasting more than 1 hour
- Generally, priapism reverses spontaneously, while penile blood flow and other signs being monitored, but in urgent cases, local phenylephrine injections or even surgery may be indicated
- As with any antidepressant, use with caution in patients with history of seizure
- As with any antidepressant, use with caution in patients with bipolar disorder unless treated with concomitant mood-stabilizing agent
- Monitor patients for activation and suicidal ideation and involve parents/guardians

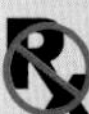

When Not to Prescribe

- If patient is taking an MAO inhibitor
- If there is a proven allergy to trazodone

Long-Term Use

- Growth should be monitored; long-term effects are unknown

Habit Forming

- No

Overdose

- Rarely lethal; sedation, vomiting, priapism, respiratory arrest, seizure, ECG changes

DOSING AND USE

Usual Dosage Range

- In children:
  - Insomnia: as low as 1.25–100 mg/night (generally 0.8–1 mg/kg)
- In adolescents:
  - Insomnia: 50–150 mg/night (generally 1 mg/kg)

Dosage Forms

- Tablet 50 mg scored, 100 mg scored, 150 mg, 150 mg with povidone scored, 300 mg with povidone scored

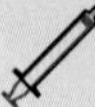

How to Dose

- Insomnia: initial 25–50 mg at bedtime; increase as tolerated, usually to 50–100 mg/day, but some patients may require up to full antidepressant dose range

Options for Administration

- Tablets are scored

Tests

- None for healthy individuals

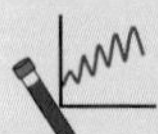

Pharmacokinetics

- Trazodone is metabolized by CYP3A4 to the active metabolite m-chlorophenylpiperazine (mCPP), which in turn is metabolized by CYP2D6 (Figure 1)
- Half-life is biphasic; in adults first phase is approximately 3–6 hours and second phase is approximately 5–9 hours

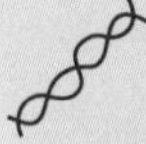

Pharmacogenetics

- The Clinical Pharmacogenetics Implementation Consortium does not provide dosing recommendations for trazodone

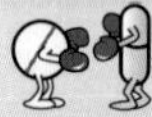

Drug Interactions

- Tramadol reported to increase the risk of seizures in adults taking an antidepressant
- Antidepressants that inhibit CYP2D6 may increase levels of the trazodone metabolite mCPP. In several studies of adolescents with depression who were treated with antidepressants that inhibited CYP2D6, those who received trazodone failed to improve in terms of their depression. This was attributed to increases in mCPP (Figure 1). Interestingly, mCPP, when administered experimentally, can produce irritability, malaise, fatigue.
- Trazodone may increase phenytoin concentrations
- Generally, do not use with MAO inhibitors, including 14 days after MAOIs are stopped

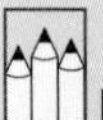

Dosing Tips

- In general, trazodone is primarily used for sleep in children and adolescents, when it is used

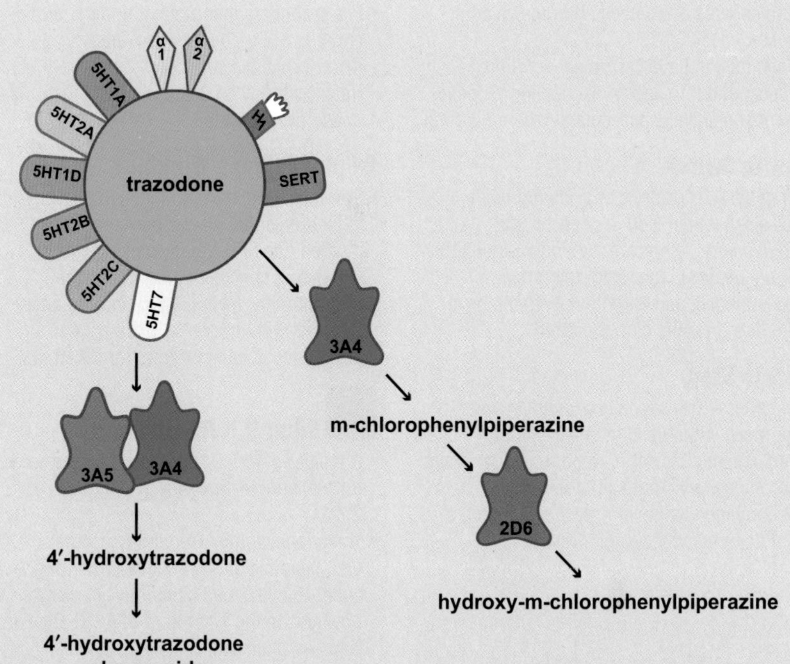

Figure 1 Trazodone metabolism.

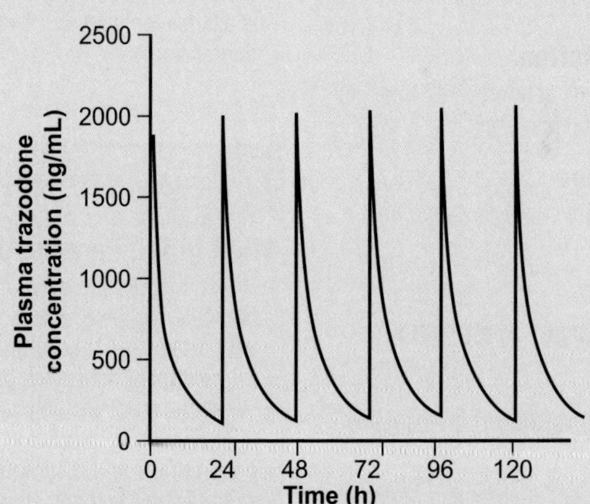

Figure 2 Nightly trazodone concentration over five days.

- Adolescents often need and receive adult doses
- Patients can have carryover sedation, ataxia, and intoxicated-like feeling if dosed too aggressively, particularly when initiating

How to Switch

- In general, trazodone is primarily used for sleep when used in children and adolescents; therefore, tapering is generally not necessary. That said, tolerance, dependence, and withdrawal effects have not been reliably demonstrated.

How to Stop

- In general, trazodone is primarily used for sleep when used in children and adolescents; therefore, tapering is generally not necessary. That said, tolerance, dependence, and withdrawal effects have not been reliably demonstrated.

WHAT TO EXPECT

Onset of Action

- Onset of therapeutic actions in insomnia is immediate if dosing is correct

Duration of Action

- Sedating effects are consistent over an 8–12-hour period

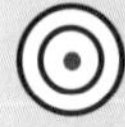

Primary Target Symptoms

- Insomnia

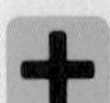

What Is Considered a Positive Result?

- The goal of treatment is complete remission of current symptoms as well as prevention of future relapses

How Long to Treat

- For insomnia, use possibly can be indefinite as there is no reliable evidence of tolerance, dependence, or withdrawal, but few long-term studies
- For secondary insomnia, if underlying condition (e.g., depression, anxiety disorder) is in remission, trazodone treatment may be discontinued if insomnia does not reemerge

What If It Stops Working?

- Some patients have an initial improvement in insomnia that wanes over time; this is often due to tachyphylaxis. In these situations, consider using trazodone intermittently, switching to another agent to assist with insomnia, or re-trying psychosocial interventions for insomnia.

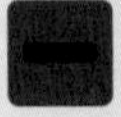

What If It Doesn't Work?

- Consider other evidence-based treatments for pediatric insomnia (e.g., Hamill et al., 2022)
- Trazodone is most frequently used in depression in adults as an augmenting agent to numerous psychotropic drugs; however, in the Treatment of SSRI-Resistant Depression in Adolescents (TORDIA) study, combination of trazodone with antidepressants that inhibit CYP2D6 did not lead to improvement of depressive symptoms (Brent et al., 20080). This may be due to increases in the trazodone metabolite m-chlorophenylpiperazine, which is associated with dysphoria, irritability, and depression.

TALKING TO PATIENTS AND CAREGIVERS

What to Tell Parents About Efficacy

- Doesn't work right away; full therapeutic benefits may take up to 8 weeks, yet parents and teachers might see improvement before the patient does
- While the medicine helps by reducing symptoms and improving function, it is not a cure, and it is therefore necessary to keep taking the medication to sustain its therapeutic effects
- Since every treatment consideration depends on a risk/benefit analysis, parents should fully understand short- and long-term risks as well as benefits
- After successful treatment, continuation of trazodone may be necessary to prevent relapse, especially in those who have had

more than one episode or a very severe episode. In general, when treating depression in children and adolescents, medications are continued for 12 months after symptoms have resolved, while for anxiety disorders, clinicians have generally treated for 6–9 months (Hathaway et al., 2018).
- Often a good idea to tell parents whether the medication chosen is specifically approved for the disorder being treated, or whether it is being given for "unapproved" or "off-label" reasons based on good clinical practice, expert consensus, and/or prudent extrapolation of controlled data from adults

What to Tell Children and Adolescents About Efficacy

- We are trying to make you feel better
- It may be a good idea to give the medication a try; if it's not working very well, we can stop the medication and try something else
- A good try takes 2 to 3 months or even longer
- If it does make you feel better, you cannot stop it right away or you may feel sad or worried again
- Medications don't change who you are as a person; they give you the opportunity to be the best person you can be

What to Tell Parents About Side Effects

- Explain that side effects are expected in many when starting and are most common in the first 2–3 weeks of starting or increasing the dose
- Tell parents many side effects go away and do so about the same time that therapeutic effects start
- Predict side effects in advance (you will look clever and competent to the parents, unless you scare them with too much information and cause nocebo effects, in which case you won't look so clever when the patient develops lots of side effects and stops medication; use your judgment here); a balanced but honest presentation is an art rather than a science
- Ask them to help monitor for increased suicidality and if present, report any such symptoms immediately
- Ask parents to support the patient while side effects are occurring
- Parents should fully understand short- and long-term risks as well as benefits
- Explaining to the parents what to expect from medication treatment, and especially potential side effects, can help prevent early termination of medication

What to Tell Children and Adolescents About Side Effects

- Even if you get side effects, most of them get better or go away in a few days to a few weeks
- Explaining to child/adolescent what to expect from medication treatment, and especially potential side effects, can help prevent early termination of medication
- Tell adolescents and children capable of understanding that some young patients, especially those who are depressed, may develop thoughts of hurting themselves, and if this happens, not to be alarmed but to tell their parents right away

What to Tell Teachers About the Medication (If Parents Consent)

- Trazodone can make children/adolescents sleepy
- It is not abusable
- Encourage dialogue with parents/guardians about any behavior or mood changes

SPECIAL POPULATIONS

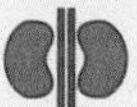

Renal Impairment

- No dose adjustment

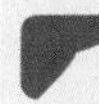

Hepatic Impairment

- Drug should be used with caution

Cardiac Impairment

- Trazodone may be arrhythmogenic and, in adults, has a modest, dose-dependent effect on cardiac repolarization and dose-dependent QTc prolongation (Tellone et al., 2020)
- Monitor patients closely

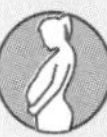

Pregnancy

- Controlled studies have not been conducted in pregnant women
- Case report documents that trazodone and its active metabolite were transferred into the placenta and breast milk (Saito et al., 2021)

- Avoid use during first trimester
- Must weigh the risk of treatment (first trimester fetal development, third trimester newborn delivery) to the child against the risk of no treatment (recurrence of depression, maternal health, infant bonding) to the mother and child
- For many patients this may mean continuing treatment during pregnancy
- National Pregnancy Registry for Psychiatric Medications: 1-866-961-2388 or https://womensmentalhealth.org/research/pregnancyregistry/

Breast Feeding

- Trazodone and its metabolites are found in breast milk
- If child becomes irritable or sedated, breast feeding or drug may need to be discontinued
- Immediate postpartum period is a high-risk time for depression, especially in women who have had prior depressive episodes, so drug may need to be reinstituted late in the third trimester or shortly after childbirth to prevent a recurrence during the postpartum period
- Must weigh benefits of breast feeding with risks and benefits of antidepressant treatment versus nontreatment to both the infant and the mother
- For many patients this may mean continuing treatment during breast feeding

THE ART OF PSYCHOPHARMACOLOGY

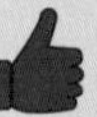

Potential Advantages

- In children and adolescents:
  - For patients who need a hypnotic but wish to avoid benzodiazepines and Z-drug hypnotics
- All ages:
  - For insomnia when it is preferred to avoid the use of dependence-forming agents
  - As an adjunct to the treatment of residual anxiety and insomnia with other antidepressants
  - Depressed patients with anxiety
  - For patients who wish to avoid sexual dysfunction and weight gain

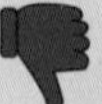

Potential Disadvantages

- In children and adolescents:
  - Boys may be even more sensitive to having prolonged erections than adult men
- All ages:
  - For patients with fatigue, hypersomnia
  - For patients who cannot tolerate sedation

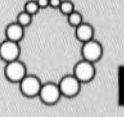

Pearls

- Open-label studies of children and toddlers suggest that trazodone may be well-tolerated and improve sleep
- Sleep studies suggest that while trazodone (median dosage 50 mg/day, range 25–200 mg/day) may be commonly used for insomnia, it is associated with more increased periodic limb movements and increased muscle tone in all sleep stages
- Pharmacokinetic modeling studies suggest that to achieve similar pharmacokinetics to an adult treated with 75 mg qHS, children ages 2–6 years require 0.8 mg/kg, children ages 7–12 require 1 mg/kg, and patients ages 13–17 require 1.1 mg/kg
- Some studies in adolescents with depression suggest that caution should be used when combining trazodone with medications that inhibit CYP2D6. In the Treatment of SSRI-Resistant Depression in Adolescents study, none of the patients who were treated with trazodone (vs. other soporifics) improved. This may relate to CYP2D6 interactions and accumulation of m-chlorophenylpiperazine (mCPP), a trazodone metabolite associated with dysphoria, irritability, and depression (Shamseddeen et al., 2012). This finding has been replicated in a separate cohort of depressed adolescents (Sultan et al., 2017).
- Can cause carryover sedation, sometimes severe, if dosed too high
- Priapism may occur in 1 in 8,000 men
- Early indications of impending priapism may be slow penile detumescence when awakening from REM sleep
- When using to treat insomnia, remember that insomnia may be a symptom of some other primary disorder, and not a primary disorder itself, and thus warrant evaluation for comorbid psychiatric and/or medical conditions
- Rarely, patients may complain of visual “trails” or after-images on trazodone

SUGGESTED READING

Brent D, Emslie G, Clarke G et al. Switching to another SSRI or to venlafaxine with or without cognitive behavioral therapy for adolescents with SSRI-resistant depression: the TORDIA randomized controlled trial. JAMA 2008;299(8):901–13.

Bridge JA, Iyengar S, Salary CB et al. Clinical response and risk for reported suicidal ideation and suicide attempts in pediatric antidepressant treatment: a meta-analysis of randomized controlled trials. JAMA 2007;297(15):1683–96.

DelRosso LM, Mogavero MP, Bruni O et al. Trazodone affects periodic leg movements and chin muscle tone during sleep less than selective serotonin reuptake inhibitor antidepressants in children. J Clin Sleep Med 2022;18(12):2829–36.

Hamill S, Koch SK, Stimpfl J, Strawn JR. Pediatric insomnia: treatment. Curr Psychiatry 2022;21(1):15–21.

Hathaway EE, Walkup JT, Strawn JR. Antidepressant treatment duration in pediatric depressive and anxiety disorders: how long is long enough? Curr Probl Pediatr Adolesc Health Care 2018;48(2):31–9.

Oggianu L, Ke AB, Chetty M et al. Estimation of an appropriate dose of trazodone for pediatric insomnia and the potential for a trazodone-atomoxetine interaction. CPT Pharmacometrics Syst Pharmacol 2020;9(2):77–86.

Saito J, Ishii M, Mito A et al. Trazodone levels in maternal serum, cord blood, breast milk, and neonatal serum. Breastfeed Med 2021;16(11):922–5.

Shamseddeen W, Clarke G, Keller MB et al. Adjunctive sleep medications and depression outcome in the treatment of serotonin-selective reuptake inhibitor resistant depression in adolescents study. J Child Adolesc Psychopharmacol 2012;22(1):29–36.

Strawn JR, Mills JA, Poweleit EA, Ramsey LB, Croarkin PE. Adverse effects of antidepressant medications and their management in children and adolescents. Pharmacotherapy 2023;43(7):675–90.

Sultan MA, Courtney DB. Adjunctive trazodone and depression outcome in adolescents treated with serotonin re-uptake inhibitors. J Can Acad Child Adolesc Psychiatry 2017;26(3):233–40.

Tellone V, Rosignoli MT, Picollo R et al. Effect of 3 single doses of trazodone on QTc interval in healthy subjects. J Clin Pharmacol 2020;60(11):1483–95.

THERAPEUTICS

Brands

- Depacon
- Depakene
- Depakote
- Depakote ER
- Stavzor

Generic

Yes

US FDA Approved for Pediatric Use

- Complex partial seizures that occur either in isolation or in association with other types of seizures (monotherapy and adjunctive) (ages 10 and older)

Off-Label for Pediatric Use

- Approved in adults
  - Acute mania (divalproex) and mixed episodes (divalproex, divalproex ER, valproic acid delayed-release)
  - Simple and complex absence seizures (monotherapy and adjunctive)
  - Multiple seizure types, which include absence seizures (adjunctive)
  - Migraine prophylaxis (divalproex, divalproex ER, valproic acid delayed-release)
  - Maintenance treatment of bipolar disorder
- Other off-label uses
  - Bipolar depression
  - Psychosis, schizophrenia (adjunctive)

Class and Mechanism of Action

- Neuroscience-based Nomenclature: glutamate (Glu); yet to be determined
- Anticonvulsant, mood stabilizer, migraine prophylaxis, voltage-sensitive sodium channel modulator
- Blocks voltage-sensitive sodium channels by an unknown mechanism
- Increases brain concentrations of gamma-aminobutyric acid (GABA) by an unknown mechanism

SAFETY AND TOLERABILITY

Notable Side Effects

- Sedation, dose-dependent tremor, dizziness
- Abdominal pain, nausea, vomiting, diarrhea, reduced appetite, constipation, dyspepsia, weight gain
- Ataxia, asthenia, headache
- Alopecia (unusual)
- Polycystic ovaries (controversial)
- Hyperandrogenism, hyperinsulinemia, lipid dysregulation (controversial)
- Decreased bone mineral density (controversial)

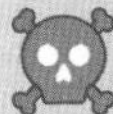

Life-Threatening or Dangerous Side Effects

- Can cause tachycardia or bradycardia
- Rare hepatotoxicity with liver failure sometimes severe and fatal, particularly in children under 2 years
- Rare pancreatitis, sometimes fatal
- Rare but serious skin condition known as Drug Reaction with Eosinophilia and Systemic Symptoms (DRESS)
- Rare activation of suicidal ideation and behavior (suicidality)

Growth and Maturation

- Long-term effects are unknown

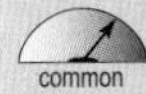

Weight Gain

- Many experience and/or can be significant in amount
- Can become a health problem in some

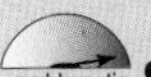

Sedation

- Frequent and can be significant in amount
- Some patients may not tolerate it
- Can wear off over time
- Can reemerge as dose increases and then wear off again over time

What to Do About Side Effects

- Wait, wait, wait: mild side effects are common, happen early (often before therapeutic effects), and usually improve with time
- Monitor side effects closely, especially when initiating treatment

- Take at night to reduce daytime sedation, especially with divalproex ER
- Consider adjusting dose
- For tremor, avoid caffeine; propranolol 20–30 mg 2–3 times/day may also reduce tremor
- Exercise and diet programs and medical management for high BMIs, diabetes, dyslipidemia
- Multivitamins fortified with zinc and selenium may help reduce alopecia
- Often best to try another monotherapy prior to resorting to augmentation strategies to treat side effects

How Drug Causes Side Effects

- CNS side effects theoretically due to excessive actions at voltage-sensitive sodium channels

Warnings and Precautions

- Consider distributing brochures provided by the FDA and the drug companies or have the pharmacy do this for the parents
- Carefully weigh the risks and benefits of pharmacological treatment against the risks and benefits of nontreatment and it is a good idea to document this in the patient's chart
- Be alert to the following symptoms of hepatotoxicity that require immediate attention: malaise, weakness, lethargy, facial edema, anorexia, vomiting, yellowing of the skin and eyes
- Be alert to the possibility of hyperammonemia, which may not correlate with changes in transaminases
- Be alert to the following symptoms of pancreatitis that require immediate attention: abdominal pain, nausea, vomiting, anorexia
- Teratogenic effects in developing fetuses, such as neural tube defects, may occur with valproate use
- Somnolence may be more common in the elderly and may be associated with dehydration, reduced nutritional intake, and weight loss, requiring slower dosage increases, lower doses, and monitoring of fluid and nutritional intake
- Use in patients with thrombocytopenia is not recommended; patients should report easy bruising or bleeding
- Evaluate for urea cycle disorders, as hyperammonemic encephalopathy, sometimes fatal, has been associated with valproate administration in these uncommon disorders; urea cycle disorders, such as ornithine transcarbamylase deficiency, are associated with unexplained encephalopathy, intellectual disability, elevated plasma ammonia, cyclical vomiting, and lethargy
- Valproate is associated with a rare but serious skin condition known as Drug Reaction with Eosinophilia and Systemic Symptoms (DRESS). DRESS may begin as a rash but can progress to other parts of the body and can include symptoms such as fever, swollen lymph nodes, inflammation of organs, and an increase in white blood cells known as eosinophilia. In some cases, DRESS can lead to death.
- Warn patients and their caregivers about the possibility of activation of suicidal ideation and advise them to report such side effects immediately

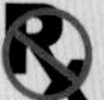

When Not to Prescribe

- If patient has pancreatitis
- If patient has serious liver disease
- If patient has urea cycle disorder
- If there is a proven allergy to valproic acid, valproate, or divalproex

Long-Term Use

- Requires regular liver function tests and platelet counts

Habit Forming

- No

Overdose

- Fatalities have been reported; coma, restlessness, hallucinations, sedation, heart block

DOSING AND USE

Usual Dosage Range

- Generally dosed the same as in adults
- Mania: 1,200–1,500 mg/day
- Migraine: 500–1,000 mg/day
- Epilepsy: 10–60 mg/kg per day

Dosage Forms

- Tablet [delayed-release, as divalproex sodium (Depakote)] 125 mg, 250 mg, 500 mg

- Tablet [extended-release, as divalproex sodium (Depakote ER)] 250 mg, 500 mg
- Capsule [sprinkle, as divalproex sodium (Depakote Sprinkle)] 125 mg
- Capsule [as valproic acid (Depakene)] 250 mg
- Injection [as sodium valproate (Depacon)] 100 mg/mL (5 mL)

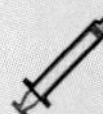

How to Dose

- Younger children, especially those receiving enzyme-inducing drugs, will require larger maintenance doses to attain targeted total and unbound valproate concentrations
- Over the age of 10 years, children have pharmacokinetic parameters that approximate those of adults
- In pediatric trials of youth with mania, divalproex was titrated up to 15 mg/kg/day over the first 3 days of treatment; serum level may be obtained after 5 days and targeted to 80–120 µg/mL trough
- In adults:
  - Usual starting dose for mania or epilepsy is 15 mg/kg in 2 divided doses (once daily for extended-release valproate)
  - Acute mania: initial 1,000 mg/day; increase dose rapidly; maximum dose generally 60 mg/kg per day
  - For less acute mania, may begin at 250–500 mg the first day, and then titrate upward as tolerated
  - Migraine: initial 500 mg/day in two doses; maximum recommended dose 1,000 mg/day
  - Epilepsy: initial 10–15 mg/kg per day; increase by 5–10 mg/kg per week; maximum dose generally 60 mg/kg per day

Options for Administration

- Oral solution can be beneficial for patients with difficulty swallowing pills

Tests

- Before starting treatment, complete blood counts, coagulation tests, and liver function tests
- Consider coagulation tests prior to planned surgery or if there is a history of bleeding
- During the first few months of treatment, regular liver function tests and platelet counts; this can be shifted to once or twice a year for the remainder of treatment
- Plasma drug levels can assist monitoring of efficacy, side effects, and adherence
- Since valproate is frequently associated with weight gain, before starting treatment, weigh all patients and determine whether the patient is already overweight (BMI 25.0–29.9) or obese (BMI ≥ 30)
- Before giving a drug that can cause weight gain to an overweight or obese patient, consider determining whether the patient already has pre-diabetes (fasting plasma glucose 100–125 mg/dL), diabetes (fasting plasma glucose > 126 mg/dL), or dyslipidemia (increased total cholesterol, LDL cholesterol, and triglycerides; decreased HDL cholesterol), and treat or refer such patients for treatment, including nutrition and weight management, physical activity counseling, smoking cessation, and medical management
- Monitor weight and BMI during treatment
- While giving a drug to a patient who has gained >5% of initial weight, consider evaluating for the presence of pre-diabetes, diabetes, or dyslipidemia, or consider switching to a different agent

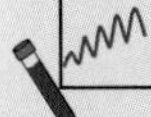

Pharmacokinetics

- Valproic acid is rapidly distributed; distribution appears to be restricted to plasma and rapidly exchangeable extracellular water.
- Plasma protein binding of valproic acid is concentration dependent; the free fraction of drug increases from 10% at a concentration of 40 mcg/mL to 18.5% at a concentration of 130 mcg/mL. When increasing the dose, an unbound concentration of valproate increases because protein-binding sites become saturated.
- Theoretically, because serum albumin concentration increases with age in children and the unbound concentration of valproate correlates with albumin concentrations, free valproate concentrations could vary according to age, although studies have not consistently observed this (Tauzin et al., 2019)
- Pediatric patients (i.e., age range 3 months to 10 years) have 50% higher clearance of the drug expressed by weight (i.e., mL/minute per kg); over the age of 10 years,

pharmacokinetic parameters of valproic acid approximate those in adults
- Metabolized primarily by the liver, approximately 25% dependent upon CYP2C9 and 2C19; also inhibits CYP2C9 (Figure 1)
- In pediatric patients, there is a nonlinear relationship between dose and clearance: clearance increases with increasing doses, so that concentrations do not rise proportionally with the dose
- Food slows rate but not extent of absorption

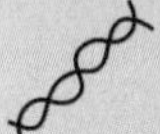

Pharmacogenetics

- No recommendations

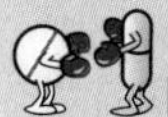

Drug Interactions

- Carbamazepine, phenytoin, and phenobarbital interact with valproate by inducing the metabolism of CYP3A4, CYP2C19, CYP2C9, UGT1A6, UGT1A9, and UGT2B7; this leads to a reduction in plasma valproate levels
- Lamotrigine dose should be reduced by perhaps 50% if used with valproate, as valproate inhibits metabolism of lamotrigine and raises lamotrigine plasma levels, theoretically increasing the risk of rash
- Plasma levels of valproate may be lowered by rifampin
- Aspirin may inhibit metabolism of valproate and increase valproate plasma levels
- Plasma levels of valproate may also be increased by felbamate, chlorpromazine, fluoxetine, fluvoxamine, topiramate, cimetidine, erythromycin, and ibuprofen
- Valproate inhibits metabolism of ethosuximide, phenobarbital, and phenytoin, and can thus increase their plasma levels
- No likely pharmacokinetic interactions of valproate with lithium or atypical antipsychotics
- Reports of hypothermia and hyperammonemia with or without encephalopathy in patients taking topiramate combined with valproate, though this is not due to a pharmacokinetic

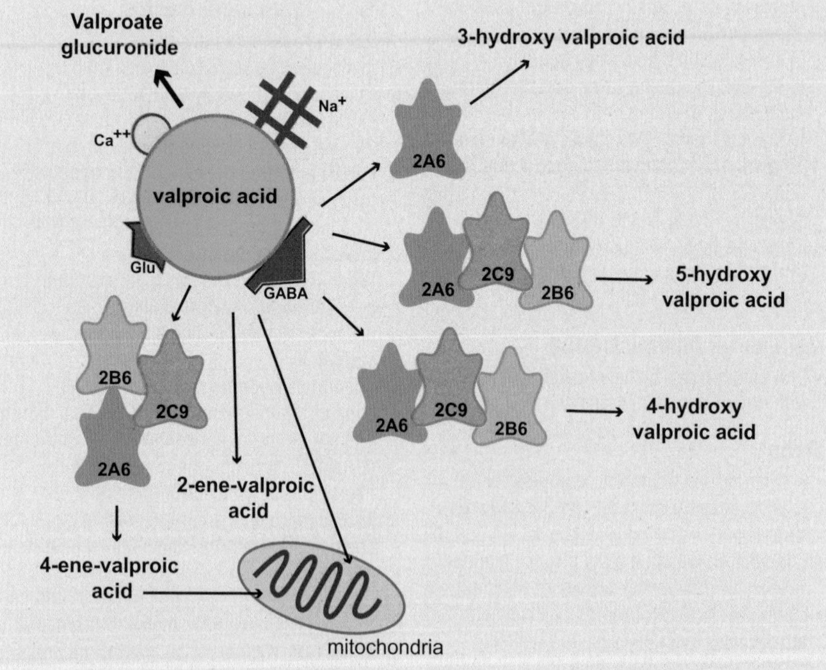

Figure 1 Valproic acid metabolism.

interaction; in patients who develop unexplained lethargy, vomiting, or change in mental status, an ammonia level should be measured

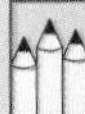

Dosing Tips

- Dosing can be guided by plasma drug levels (usual range approximately 45–125 mcg/mL)
- In adults, oral loading with 20–30 mg/kg per day may reduce onset of action to 5 days or less and may be especially useful for treatment of acute mania in inpatient settings
- Given the half-life of immediate-release valproate (e.g., Depakene, Depakote),twice-daily dosing is probably ideal
- Extended-release valproate (e.g., Depakote ER) can be given once daily
- However, extended-release valproate is only about 80% as bioavailable as immediate-release valproate, producing plasma drug levels 10–20% lower than with immediate-release valproate
- Thus, extended-release valproate is dosed approximately 8–20% higher when converting patients to the ER formulation
- Depakote (divalproex sodium) is an enteric-coated stable compound containing both valproic acid and sodium valproate
- Divalproex immediate-release formulation reduces gastrointestinal side effects compared to generic valproate
- Divalproex ER improves gastrointestinal side effects and alopecia compared to immediate-release divalproex or generic valproate
- The amide of valproic acid is available in Europe [valpromide (Depamide)]
- Trough plasma drug levels > 45 μg/ml may be required for either antimanic effects or anticonvulsant actions
- Trough plasma drug levels up to 100 μg/mL are generally well tolerated
- Trough plasma drug levels up to 125 μg/mL may be required in some acutely manic patients
- Dosages to achieve therapeutic plasma levels vary widely, often between 750 and 3,000 mg/day

How to Switch

- From another medication to valproate:
  - When tapering a prior medication, see its entry in this manual for how to stop and how to taper off that specific drug
  - Generally, try to stop the first agent before starting valproate so that new side effects of valproate can be distinguished from withdrawal effects of the first agent
  - If urgent, cross taper
- Off valproate to another medication:
  - Generally, try to stop valproate before starting the new medication so that new side effects of the next drug can be distinguished from any withdrawal effects from valproate
  - Taper; may need to adjust dosage of concurrent medications as valproate is being discontinued
  - If urgent, cross taper

How to Stop

- Taper; may need to adjust dosage of concurrent medications as valproate is being discontinued
- Patients may seize upon withdrawal, especially if withdrawal is abrupt
- Rapid discontinuation increases the risk of relapse in bipolar disorder
- Discontinuation symptoms uncommon

WHAT TO EXPECT

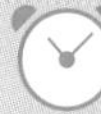

Onset of Action

- For acute mania, effects should occur within a few days depending on the formulation of the drug
- May take several weeks to months to optimize an effect on mood stabilization
- Should also reduce seizures and improve migraine within a few weeks

Duration of Action

- Effects are consistent over a 24-hour period
- May continue to work for many years to prevent relapse of symptoms

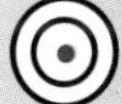

Primary Target Symptoms

- Unstable mood
- Incidence of migraine
- Incidence of partial complex seizures

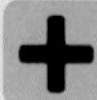

What Is Considered a Positive Result?

- Many patients may experience a reduction of symptoms by half or more

How Long to Treat

- Continue treatment until all symptoms are gone or until improvement is stable and then continue treating indefinitely as long as improvement persists
- Continue treatment indefinitely to avoid recurrence of mania, depression, seizures, and headaches

What If It Stops Working?

- Check for nonadherence, possibly by checking plasma drug level, and consider switching to another agent with fewer side effects
- Some patients who have an initial response may relapse even though they continue treatment, sometimes called "poop-out"
- Growth/developmental changes may contribute to apparent loss of efficacy as well as to new onset of side effects as metabolism slows and drug levels rise in transition from childhood to adolescence; dose adjustment (increase or decrease) should be considered
- Screen for the development of a new comorbid disorder, especially substance abuse
- Screen for adverse changes in the home or school environment

What If It Doesn't Work?

- Consider evaluation for another diagnosis or for a comorbid condition (e.g., medical illness, substance abuse)
- Consider other important potential factors such as ongoing conflicts, family psychopathology, and an adverse environment (e.g., poverty, chaos, violence, prior and ongoing psychological trauma, abuse, neglect)
- Institute trauma-informed care for appropriate children and adolescents
- Try one of the atypical antipsychotics or lithium
- Consider initiating rehabilitation and psychotherapy such as cognitive remediation, although these may be less well standardized for children/adolescents than for adults
- Consider presence of concomitant drug abuse
- Consider augmentation with lithium, an atypical antipsychotic, or an antidepressant (with caution because antidepressants can destabilize mood in some patients, including induction of rapid cycling or suicidal ideation; in particular, consider bupropion; also SSRIs, SNRIs, others; generally, avoid TCAs, MAOIs)
- Consider augmentation with lamotrigine (with caution and at half the dose in the presence of valproate because valproate can double lamotrigine levels)

TALKING TO PATIENTS AND CAREGIVERS

What to Tell Parents About Efficacy

- For acute symptoms, it can work right away
- Explain which use valproate is being chosen for, how to tell if the drug is working by targeting specific symptoms, and why this is being done
- Once the child/adolescent calms down, at some point after one dose or after several days of dosing or after long-term dosing, we should all assess whether the medication should be continued
- While the medicine helps by reducing symptoms and improving function, it is not a cure, and it therefore may be necessary to keep taking the medication long term to sustain its therapeutic effects
- Since every treatment consideration depends on a risk/benefit analysis, parents should fully understand short- and long-term risks as well as benefits
- Often a good idea to tell parents whether the medication chosen is specifically approved for the disorder being treated, or whether it is being given for "unapproved" or "off-label" reasons based on good clinical practice, expert consensus, and/or prudent extrapolation of controlled data from adults

What to Tell Children and Adolescents About Efficacy

- Be specific about the symptoms being targeted: we are trying to help you …
- Give the medication a try; if it's not working very well, we can stop the medication and try something else

- A good try often takes 2 to 3 months
- If it does make you feel better, you cannot stop it right away or you may get sick again
- Medications don't change who you are as a person; they give you the opportunity to be the best person you can be

What to Tell Parents About Side Effects

- Explain that side effects are expected in many when starting
- Tell parents many side effects go away and do so about the same time that therapeutic effects start
- Predict side effects in advance (you will look clever and competent to the parents, unless you scare them with too much information and cause nocebo effects, in which case you won't look so clever when the patient develops lots of side effects and stops medication; use your judgment here); a balanced but honest presentation is an art rather than a science
- Ask parents to support the patient while side effects are occurring
- Parents should fully understand short- and long-term risks as well as benefits
- Explaining to the parents what to expect from medication treatment, and especially what potential side effects to expect, can help prevent early termination of medication

What to Tell Children and Adolescents About Side Effects

- Even if you get a side effect, we can usually reduce it over time
- If you have side effects that are bothering you, tell your parents and your parents should tell me
- Consider having a conversation about sexual side effects in some adolescents who can find these side effects confusing and especially burdensome
- Explaining to child/adolescent what to expect from medication treatment, and especially potential side effects, can help prevent early termination of medication

What to Tell Teachers About the Medication (If Parents Consent)

- Valproate can make children/adolescents sedated
- It is not abusable
- Encourage dialogue with parents/guardians about any behavior or mood changes

SPECIAL POPULATIONS

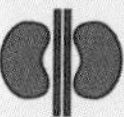

Renal Impairment

- No dose adjustment necessary

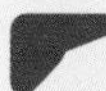

Hepatic Impairment

- Contraindicated

Cardiac Impairment

- No dose adjustment necessary

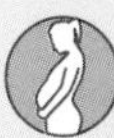

Pregnancy

- Use during first trimester may raise risk of neural tube defects (e.g., spina bifida) or other congenital anomalies
- Cases of developmental delay in the absence of teratogenicity associated with fetal exposure have been identified
- Increased risk of lower cognitive test scores in children whose mothers took valproate during pregnancy
- Use in women of childbearing potential requires weighing potential benefits to the mother against the risks to the fetus
- If drug is continued, monitor clotting parameters and perform tests to detect birth defects
- If drug is continued, start on folate 1 mg/day early in pregnancy to reduce risk of neural tube defects
- If drug is continued, consider vitamin K during the last 6 weeks of pregnancy to reduce risks of bleeding
- Antiepileptic Drug Pregnancy Registry: (888) 233-2334 or www.aedpregnancyregistry.org
- Taper drug if discontinuing
- Seizures, even mild seizures, may cause harm to the embryo/fetus
- For bipolar patients, valproate should generally be discontinued before anticipated pregnancies
- Recurrent bipolar illness during pregnancy can be quite disruptive
- For bipolar patients, given the risk of relapse in the postpartum period, mood stabilizer treatment such as valproate should generally be restarted immediately after delivery if patient is unmedicated during pregnancy
- Atypical antipsychotics may be preferable to lithium or anticonvulsants such as valproate

if treatment of bipolar disorder is required during pregnancy
- Bipolar symptoms may recur or worsen during pregnancy, and some form of treatment may be necessary

Breast Feeding

- Some drug is found in breast milk
- Generally considered safe to breast feed while taking valproate
- If drug is continued while breast feeding, infant should be monitored for possible adverse effects
- If infant shows signs of irritability or sedation, drug may need to be discontinued
- Bipolar disorder may recur during the postpartum period, particularly if there is a history of prior postpartum episodes of either depression or psychosis
- Relapse rates may be lower in women who receive prophylactic treatment for postpartum episodes of bipolar disorder
- Atypical antipsychotics and anticonvulsants such as valproate may be safer than lithium during the postpartum period when breast feeding

THE ART OF PSYCHOPHARMACOLOGY

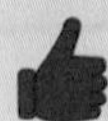

Potential Advantages

- Manic phase of bipolar disorder
- Works well in combination with lithium and/or atypical antipsychotics
- Patients for whom therapeutic drug monitoring is desirable

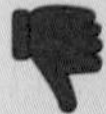

Potential Disadvantages

- In children and adolescents:
  - Not generally recommended for use in children under age 10 for bipolar disorder except by experts and when other options have been considered
  - Children under age 2 have significantly increased risk of hepatotoxicity, as they have a markedly decreased ability to eliminate valproate compared to older children and adults
  - Use requires close medical supervision
- All ages:
  - Depressed phase of bipolar disorder
  - Patients unable to tolerate sedation or weight gain
  - Multiple drug interactions
  - Multiple side-effect risks
  - Pregnant patients

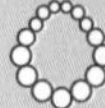

Pearls

- A ketone metabolite in the urine of patients receiving valproic acid may produce false-positive results for urine ketones
- Combining antipsychotics with mood stabilizers seems to lead to greater weight gain than treatment with one or two mood stabilizers in children and adolescents (Correll, 2007)
- Meta-analyses of traditional mood stabilizers like divalproex suggest that they are less effective than SGAs in children and adolescents with manic or mixed episodes (effect size for SGAs 0.65 vs. 0.24). However, SGAs caused more weight gain than mood stabilizers in youth (ES = 0.53 vs. 0.10) (Correll et al., 2010).
- Valproate is a first-line treatment option in adults that may be best for patients with mixed states of bipolar disorder or for patients with rapid-cycling bipolar disorder
- Seems to be more effective in treating manic episodes than depressive episodes in bipolar disorder (treats from above better than it treats from below)
- May also be more effective in preventing manic relapses than in preventing depressive episodes (stabilizes from above better than it stabilizes from below)
- Only a third of bipolar patients experience adequate relief with a monotherapy, so most patients need multiple medications for best control
- Useful in combination with atypical antipsychotics and/or lithium for acute mania
- May also be useful for bipolar disorder in combination with lamotrigine, but must reduce lamotrigine dose by half when combined with valproate
- Usefulness for bipolar disorder in combination with anticonvulsants other than lamotrigine is not well demonstrated; such combinations can be expensive and are possibly ineffective or even irrational
- May be useful as an adjunct to atypical antipsychotics for rapid onset of action in schizophrenia
- Used to treat aggression, agitation, and impulsivity not only in bipolar disorder

and schizophrenia but also in many other disorders, including dementia, personality disorders, and brain injury
- Patients with acute mania tend to tolerate side effects better than patients with hypomania or depression
- Multivitamins fortified with zinc and selenium may help reduce alopecia
- Association of valproate with polycystic ovaries is controversial and may be related to weight gain, obesity, or epilepsy
- Nevertheless, may wish to be cautious in administering valproate to women of childbearing potential, especially adolescent female bipolar patients, and carefully monitor weight, endocrine status, and ovarian size and function
- In women of childbearing potential who are or are likely to become sexually active, should inform about risk of harm to the fetus and monitor contraceptive status
- Association of valproate with decreased bone mass is controversial and may be related to activity levels, exposure to sunlight, and epilepsy, and might be prevented by supplemental vitamin D 2,000 IU/day and calcium 600–1,000 mg/day
- Delayed-release capsule of valproic acid (Stavzor) may be easier to swallow than other formulations
- A prodrug of valproic acid, valpromide, is available in several European countries
- Although valpromide is rapidly transformed to valproic acid, it has some unique characteristics that can affect drug interactions
- In particular, valpromide is a potent inhibitor of liver microsomal epoxide hydrolase and thus causes clinically significant increases in the plasma levels of carbamazepine-10,11-epoxide (the active metabolite of carbamazepine)

SUGGESTED READING

Correll CU. Weight gain and metabolic effects of mood stabilizers and antipsychotics in pediatric bipolar disorder: a systematic review and pooled analysis of short-term trials. J Am Acad Child Adolesc Psychiatry 2007;46(6):687–700.

Correll CU, Sheridan EM, DelBello MP. Antipsychotic and mood stabilizer efficacy and tolerability in pediatric and adult patients with bipolar I mania: a comparative analysis of acute, randomized, placebo-controlled trials. Bipolar Disord 2010;12(2):116–41.

Delbello MP, Kowatch RA, Adler CM et al. A double-blind randomized pilot study comparing quetiapine and divalproex for adolescent mania. J Am Acad Child Adolesc Psychiatry 2006;45(3):305–13.

Findling RL, McNamara NK, Youngstrom EA et al. Double-blind 18-month trial of lithium versus divalproex maintenance treatment in pediatric bipolar disorder. J Am Acad Child Adolesc Psychiatry 2005;44(5):409–17.

Geller B, Luby JL, Joshi P et al. A randomized controlled trial of risperidone, lithium, or divalproex sodium for initial treatment of bipolar I disorder, manic or mixed phase, in children and adolescents. Arch Gen Psychiatry 2012;69(5):515–28.

Pavuluri MN, Henry DB, Findling RL et al. Double-blind randomized trial of risperidone versus divalproex in pediatric bipolar disorder. Bipolar Disord 2010;12(6):593–605.

Tauzin M, Tréluyer JM, Nabbout R et al. Simulations of valproate doses based on an external evaluation of pediatric population pharmacokinetic models. J Clin Pharmacol 2019;59(3):406–17.

Teixeira-da-Silva P, Pérez-Blanco JS, Santos-Buelga D, Otero MJ, García MJ. Population pharmacokinetics of valproic acid in pediatric and adult Caucasian patients. Pharmaceutics 2022;14(4):811.

VENLAFAXINE

THERAPEUTICS

Brands

- Effexor
- Effexor XR

Generic

Yes

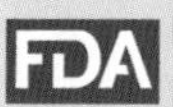

US FDA Approved for Pediatric Use

- None

Off-Label for Pediatric Use

- Approved in adults
  - Depression
  - Generalized anxiety disorder (GAD)
  - Social anxiety disorder
  - Panic disorder
- Other off-label uses
  - Separation anxiety disorder
  - Premenstrual dysphoric disorder (PMDD)
  - Posttraumatic stress disorder (PTSD)

Class and Mechanism of Action

- Neuroscience-based Nomenclature: serotonin norepinephrine reuptake inhibitor (SN-RI)
- SNRI (dual serotonin and norepinephrine reuptake inhibitor); often classified as a drug for depression (i.e., antidepressant), but it is not just an antidepressant
- Venlafaxine presumably increases serotonergic neurotransmission by blocking the serotonin reuptake pump (transporter, SERT), which results in the desensitization of serotonin receptors, especially serotonin 1A receptors
- Venlafaxine presumably increases noradrenergic neurotransmission by blocking the norepinephrine reuptake pump (transporter, NET), which results in the desensitization of beta adrenergic receptors
- Since dopamine is inactivated by norepinephrine reuptake in the frontal cortex, which largely lacks dopamine transporters, venlafaxine can increase dopamine neurotransmission in this part of the brain
- Venlafaxine weakly blocks the dopamine reuptake pump (dopamine transporter), and may increase dopamine neurotransmission

SAFETY AND TOLERABILITY

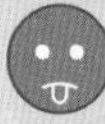

Notable Side Effects

- Most side effects increase with higher doses, at least transiently
- Mostly central nervous system side effects (insomnia but also sedation especially if not sleeping at night; agitation, tremors, headache, dizziness)
- Note: patients with diagnosed or undiagnosed bipolar or psychotic disorders may be more vulnerable to CNS-activating actions of antidepressants like venlafaxine; pay particular attention to signs of activation in children with developmental disorders or autism spectrum disorders
- Treatment-emergent activation syndrome (TEAS) includes agitation, anxiety, panic attacks, irritability, aggression, impulsivity, and insomnia; however, in pediatric patients, this is less with SNRIs compared to SSRIs (Mills and Strawn, 2020)
- TEAS can represent side effects but should not be confused with bipolar mania or the onset of suicidality and should be monitored and investigated with consideration of discontinuing or decreasing the dose of venlafaxine or addition of another agent or switching to another agent to reduce these symptoms
- Gastrointestinal (decreased appetite, nausea, diarrhea, constipation, dry mouth)
- Sexual dysfunction (boys: delayed ejaculation, erectile dysfunction; boys and girls: decreased sexual desire, anorgasmia)
- Autonomic (sweating)
- Dose-dependent increase in blood pressure and in patients who are faster CYP2D6 metabolizers (see Pharmacogenetics)
- Syndrome of inappropriate antidiuretic hormone secretion (SIADH)

Life-Threatening or Dangerous Side Effects

- Rare seizures
- Rare hyponatremia
- Rare induction of mania
- Rare suicidal ideation and behavior (suicidality) (short-term regulatory studies did not show any actual suicides in any age group and also did not show an increase in the risk of suicidality with antidepressants compared to placebo beyond age 24)

Growth and Maturation

- Limited data suggest less than expected weight gain and less than expected height increases in children and adolescents taking venlafaxine; the differences between observed and expected growth rates were greater for children than for adolescents

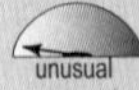

Weight Gain

- Limited data suggest weight loss in children and adolescents taking venlafaxine

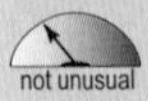

Sedation

- Occurs in significant minority

What to Do About Side Effects

- Wait, wait, wait: mild side effects are common, happen early, and usually improve with time, but treatment benefits can be delayed and often begin just as the side effects wear off
- Monitor side effects closely, especially when initiating treatment
- For activation (jitteriness, anxiety, insomnia):
  - Administer dose in the morning
  - Consider a temporary dose reduction or a more gradual up-titration
  - Consider switching to another antidepressant
  - Optimize psychotherapeutic interventions
  - Activation and agitation may represent the induction of a bipolar state, especially a mixed dysphoric bipolar II condition sometimes associated with suicidal ideation, and may require the addition of lithium or an atypical antipsychotic, and/ or discontinuation of venlafaxine
- Often best to try another monotherapy prior to resorting to augmentation strategies to treat side effects
- For insomnia: consider adding melatonin
- For GI upset: try giving medication with a meal
- For sexual dysfunction:
  - Probably best to reduce dose or discontinue and try another agent
  - Consider adding daytime exercise, bupropion, or buspirone
- For emotional flattening, apathy: consider adding bupropion (with caution as little experience in children)

How Drug Causes Side Effects

- Theoretically due to increases in serotonin and norepinephrine concentrations at receptors in parts of the brain and body other than those that cause therapeutic actions (e.g., unwanted actions of serotonin in sleep centers causing insomnia, unwanted actions of norepinephrine on acetylcholine release causing constipation and dry mouth)

Warnings and Precautions

- Consider distributing the brochures provided by the FDA and the drug companies as well as the medication guides from the American Academy of Child & Adolescent Psychiatry (AACAP)
- Carefully consider monitoring patients regularly and within the practical limits, particularly during the first several weeks of treatment
- Warn patients and their caregivers when possible about the possibility of activating side effects and advise them to report such symptoms immediately
- Carefully weigh the risks and benefits of pharmacological treatment against the risks and benefits of nontreatment with antidepressants and it is a good idea to document this in the patient's chart
- Use with caution in patients with heart disease
- As with any antidepressant, use with caution in patients with history of seizure
- As with any antidepressant, use with caution in patients with bipolar disorder unless treated with concomitant mood-stabilizing agent
- Monitor patients for activation and suicidal ideation and involve parents/guardians

When Not to Prescribe

- If patient is taking an MAO inhibitor
- If patient has uncontrolled angle-closure glaucoma
- If there is a proven allergy to venlafaxine

Long-Term Use

- Growth should be monitored; long-term effects are unknown
- Regularly monitor blood pressure, especially at doses >225 mg/day

Habit Forming

- No

Overdose

- Can be lethal; may cause no symptoms; possible symptoms include sedation, convulsions, rapid heartbeat
- Fatal toxicity index data from the UK suggest a higher rate of deaths from overdose with venlafaxine than with SSRIs
- Unknown whether this is related to differences in patients who receive venlafaxine or to potential cardiovascular toxicity of venlafaxine

DOSING AND USE

Usual Dosage Range

- 37.5–225 mg/day

Dosage Forms

- Capsule (extended-release) 37.5 mg, 75 mg, 150 mg
- Tablet (extended-release) 37.5 mg, 75 mg, 150 mg, 225 mg
- Tablet 25 mg scored, 37.5 mg scored, 50 mg scored, 75 mg scored, 100 mg scored

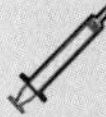

How to Dose

- In children: initial 37.5 mg once daily (extended-release); usually avoid immediate-release formulation; caution for doses above 150 mg/day
- In adolescents: initial 37.5 mg/day extended-release for 1 week; if tolerated increase daily dose generally no faster than 37.5 mg every week until desired efficacy is reached; maximum dose generally 225 mg/day

Options for Administration

- Do not cut or crush extended-release capsules

Tests

- Check blood pressure before initiating treatment and regularly during treatment
- Monitor weight and height against that expected for normal growth

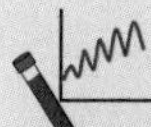

Pharmacokinetics

- Compared to other antidepressants, venlafaxine has low protein binding (27% for venlafaxine and 30% for its metabolite, desvenlafaxine)
- Venlafaxine is metabolized via CYP2D6 to its active metabolite, O-desmethylvenlafaxine; other metabolites include *N*-desmethylvenlafaxine and *N*,O-didesmethylvenlafaxine (Figure 1)
- In adults, the bioavailability of venlafaxine is approximately 45%. However, venlafaxine absorption from the gastrointestinal tract is lower in children and adolescents than in adults.
- In adults treated with immediate-release formulations, peak venlafaxine concentrations generally occur 2 hours after administration (Tmax) while peak concentrations of O-desmethylvenlafaxine occur at approximately 3 hours. In adults treated with extended-release formulations, peak concentrations are observed at approximately 6 hours for venlafaxine and 11½ hours for O-desmethylvenlafaxine.
- In pediatric patients, the pharmacokinetics vary by age group: in children ages 6–11 years of age, venlafaxine reaches peak concentrations in 4–5 hours, whereas in adolescents ages 12–17 years, peak concentrations are reached in approximately 6½ hours
- In pediatric patients, the half-life of venlafaxine also varies by age: half-life is approximately 8–10 hours in youth ages 6–11 years and 11–14 hours in adolescents
- Venlafaxine exposure (blood levels over time) is slightly lower in adolescents compared to adults when dosed at the same mg/kg dose. Some data suggest that with the XR formulation, children may need, on average, a 2- to 4-fold higher mg/kg dose as compared to adults and that adolescents may need a 1.75-fold higher mg/kg dose.

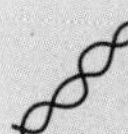

Pharmacogenetics

- CYP2D6 converts venlafaxine to the active metabolite O-desmethylvenlafaxine
- In adults, venlafaxine concentrations over time (i.e., area under the curve) are approximately 3–11 times higher in CYP2D6 poor metabolizers compared to normal metabolizers

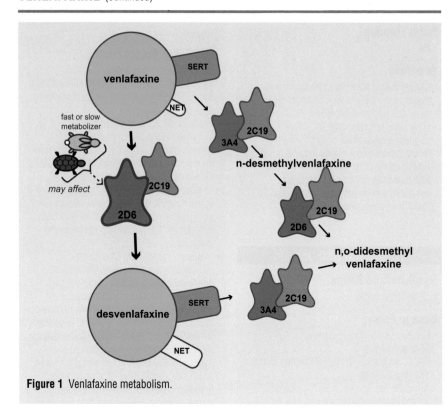

Figure 1 Venlafaxine metabolism.

- Peak concentrations of venlafaxine are approximately doubled in CYP2D6 poor metabolizers compared to normal metabolizers, while the peak concentration is approximately doubled in intermediate CYP2D6 metabolizers
- Importantly, faster CYP2D6 metabolizers have a lower concentration of venlafaxine compared to desvenlafaxine
- The Clinical Pharmacogenetics Implementation Consortium (CPIC) recommends that clinicians "consider a clinically appropriate alternative antidepressant not predominantly metabolized by CYP2D6" in CYP2D6 poor metabolizers
- The Dutch Pharmacogenetics Working Group (DPWG) recommends that for CYP2D6 poor metabolizers or intermediate metabolizers, venlafaxine should be avoided when possible and "if avoidance is not possible and side effects occur, reduce the dose and closely monitor clinical response and serum concentrations of venlafaxine and its O-desmethyl metabolite"

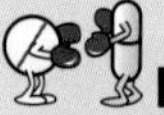

Drug Interactions

- Tramadol reported to increase the risk of seizures in adults taking an antidepressant
- Can cause a fatal "serotonin syndrome" when combined with MAO inhibitors, so do not use with MAO inhibitors or for at least 14 days after MAOIs are stopped
- Do not start an MAO inhibitor for at least 5 half-lives (5 to 7 days for most drugs) after discontinuing venlafaxine
- Possible increased risk of bleeding
- Concomitant use with cimetidine may reduce clearance of venlafaxine and raise venlafaxine levels
- Could theoretically interfere with the analgesic actions of codeine or possibly with other triptans
- Few known adverse drug interactions

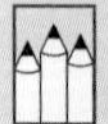

Dosing Tips

- Based on pharmacokinetic considerations, venlafaxine treatment has generally involved initial doses of 1.5 mg/kg/day and may be titrated upward to 3.0 to 5.0 mg/kg/day. However, it is important to remember that venlafaxine is cleared more quickly in pediatric patients compared to adults and is not as well absorbed in youth compared to adults. Further, because its half-life is shorter in youth, it may need to be dosed multiple times per day, even with extended-release formulations.

- At all doses, potent serotonin reuptake blockade; however, at higher doses, more noradrenergic effects may be observed:
  - 75–225 mg/day may be predominantly serotonergic in some patients, and dual serotonin and norepinephrine acting in other patients
  - 225–375 mg/day is dual serotonin and norepinephrine acting in most patients
- Recently, we have understood that slower CYP2D6 metabolizers will have greater ratios of venlafaxine to O-desmethylvenlafaxine (more serotonergic effect), whereas faster metabolizers will have greater concentrations of O-desmethylvenlafaxine compared to venlafaxine (more noradrenergic effects)
- CYP2D6 inhibition reduces the formation of O-desmethylvenlafaxine, but this is of uncertain clinical significance
- Do not break or chew venlafaxine XR capsules, as this will alter controlled-release properties
- The more anxious and agitated the patient, the lower the starting dose, the slower the titration
- If intolerable anxiety, insomnia, agitation, akathisia, or activation occurs either upon dosing initiation or discontinuation, consider the possibility of activated bipolar disorder and switch to an atypical antipsychotic or a mood stabilizer
- These symptoms may also indicate the need to evaluate for a mixed features episode and thus discontinuing venlafaxine and considering an atypical antipsychotic or a mood stabilizer or lithium

How to Switch

- From another antidepressant to venlafaxine:
  - When tapering a prior antidepressant, see its entry in this manual for how to stop and how to taper off that specific drug
  - In situations when there are antidepressant-related side effects, try to stop the first agent before starting venlafaxine so that new side effects of venlafaxine can be distinguished from withdrawal effects of the first agent
  - If urgent, cross taper
- Off venlafaxine to another antidepressant:
  - Generally, try to stop venlafaxine before starting another antidepressant
  - Taper to avoid withdrawal effects (dizziness, nausea, stomach cramps, sweating, tingling, dysesthesias)
  - Many patients tolerate 50% dose reduction for 5–7 days, then another 50% reduction for 5–7 days, then discontinuation
  - If necessary, can cross taper off venlafaxine this way while dosing up on another antidepressant simultaneously in urgent situations, being aware of all specific drug interactions to avoid

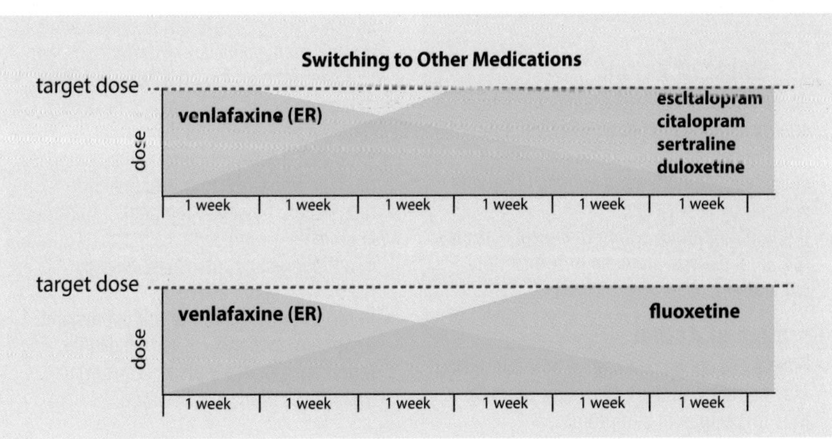

How to Stop

- Withdrawal effects can be more common or more severe with venlafaxine than with some other antidepressants
- Taper to avoid withdrawal effects (dizziness, nausea, stomach cramps, sweating, tingling, dysesthesias)
- Many patients tolerate 50% dose reduction for 5–7 days, then another 50% reduction for 5–7 days, then discontinuation
- If withdrawal symptoms emerge during discontinuation, raise dose to stop symptoms and then restart withdrawal much more slowly
- For patients with severe problems discontinuing venlafaxine, dosing may need to be tapered over many months (i.e., reduce dose by 1% every 3 days by crushing tablet and suspending or dissolving in 100 mL of fruit juice, and then disposing of 1 mL while drinking the rest; 3–7 days later, dispose of 2 mL, and so on). This is both a form of very slow biological tapering and a form of behavioral desensitization (not for XR).
- For some patients with severe problems discontinuing venlafaxine, it may be useful to add an SSRI with a long half-life, especially fluoxetine, prior to taper of venlafaxine; while maintaining fluoxetine dosing, first slowly taper venlafaxine and then taper fluoxetine
- Be sure to differentiate between reemergence of symptoms requiring reinstitution of treatment and withdrawal symptoms

WHAT TO EXPECT

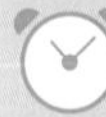

Onset of Action

- Some patients may experience increased energy or activation early after initiation of treatment
- Full onset of therapeutic actions is usually delayed by 2–4 weeks
- If it is not working within 6–8 weeks, it may require a dosage increase or it may not work at all

Duration of Action

- Effects are consistent over a 24-hour period
- May continue to work for many years to prevent relapse of symptoms

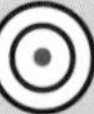

Primary Target Symptoms

- Depressed and/or irritable mood
- Energy, motivation, and interest
- Sleep disturbance
- Anxiety (fear and worry are often target symptoms, but venlafaxine can occasionally and transiently increase these symptoms short term before improving them)
- Prior to initiation of treatment, it is helpful to develop a list of target symptoms of depression and/or anxiety to monitor during treatment to better assess treatment response

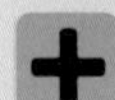

What Is Considered a Positive Result?

- The goal of treatment is complete remission of current symptoms as well as prevention of future relapses
- In practice, many patients have only a partial response where some symptoms are improved but others persist (especially insomnia, fatigue, and problems concentrating in depression), in which case higher doses of venlafaxine, adding a second agent, or switching to an agent with a different mechanism of action can be considered
- If treatment works, it most often reduces or even eliminates symptoms, but is not a cure since symptoms can recur after medicine is stopped

How Long to Treat

- For adolescents with depression, generally, 9–12 months of antidepressant treatment is recommended (Hathaway et al., 2018)
- For anxiety disorders, 6–9 months of antidepressant treatment may be sufficient, though many clinicians extend treatment to 12 months based on extrapolation of data from adults with anxiety disorders (Hathaway et al., 2018; Strawn et al., 2023)
- Extended treatment periods may decrease the risk of long-term morbidity and recurrence; however, the goal of treatment is ultimately remission, rather than duration of antidepressant pharmacotherapy (Hathaway et al., 2018)
- In terms of the length of antidepressant treatment, evidence-based guidelines represent a starting point; appropriate treatment duration varies, and

patient-specific response, psychological factors, and timing of discontinuation must be considered for individual pediatric patients (Hathaway et al., 2018)

What If It Stops Working?

- Some patients who have an initial response may relapse even though they continue treatment, sometimes called "poop-out"
- Some patients may experience apparent lack of consistent efficacy due to activation syndrome or latent or underlying or newly evolved bipolar disorder, or major depressive episodes with mixed features of mania, and require antidepressant discontinuation and a switch to a second generation antipsychotic

What If It Doesn't Work?

- Consider evaluation for another diagnosis (especially bipolar illness or depression with mixed features) or for a comorbid condition (e.g., medical illness, substance abuse)
- Be mindful of family conflict contributing to the presentation; sometimes treating parental depression or anxiety disorders improves psychiatric and social function without any treatment of youth. Also, accommodation is common in families of youth with anxiety disorders and may need to be addressed specifically, as it can perpetuate symptoms.
- Consider factors associated with poor response to antidepressants in treatment-resistant depression (Dwyer et al., 2020) or anxiety disorders (Strawn et al., 2023), such as severe symptoms, long-lasting symptoms, poor treatment adherence, prior nonresponse to other treatments, and the presence of comorbid disorders
- Consider other important potential factors such as ongoing conflicts, family psychopathology, and an adverse environment (e.g., poverty, chaos, violence, prior and ongoing psychological trauma, abuse, neglect). Additionally, when symptoms are prominent at school, consider the presence of a learning disorder.
- Institute trauma-informed care for appropriate children and adolescents
- A 2007 meta-analysis of published and unpublished trials in pediatric patients found that antidepressants had a number needed to treat (NNT) of 10 for depression, 6 for OCD, and 3 for anxiety disorders; thus, venlafaxine may not work in all children, so consider switching to another antidepressant (Bridge et al., 2007)
- Consider a dose adjustment
- Consider augmenting options:
  - Cognitive behavioral therapy (CBT), interpersonal psychotherapy for adolescents (IPT-A), light therapy, family therapy, and exercise, especially in adolescents
  - For partial response (depression): use caution when adding medications to venlafaxine, especially in children since there are not sufficient studies of augmentation in children or adolescents; however, for the expert, consider bupropion, aripiprazole, or other atypical antipsychotics such as quetiapine; use combinations of antidepressants with caution as this may activate bipolar disorder and suicidal ideation
  - For insomnia: sleep hygiene, CBT for insomnia, melatonin, or alpha 2 agonists
  - For anxiety: buspirone, antihistamines
  - Add lithium or atypical antipsychotics for bipolar depression, psychotic depression, treatment-resistant depression, or treatment-resistant anxiety disorders
  - TMS (transcranial magnetic stimulation) may have a role although pediatric trials of TMS have been hampered by high sham response rates (Croarkin et al., 2021)
  - ECT (case studies show effectiveness; cognitive side effects are similar to those in adults; reserve for treatment-resistant cases)

TALKING TO PATIENTS AND CAREGIVERS

What to Tell Parents About Efficacy

- Doesn't work right away; full therapeutic benefits may take up to 8 weeks, yet parents and teachers might see improvement before the patient does
- While the medicine helps by reducing symptoms and improving function, it is not a cure, and it is therefore necessary to keep taking the medication to sustain its therapeutic effects

- Since every treatment consideration depends on a risk/benefit analysis, parents should fully understand short- and long-term risks as well as benefits
- After successful treatment, continuation of venlafaxine may be necessary to prevent relapse, especially in those who have had more than one episode or a very severe episode. In general, when treating depression in children and adolescents, medications are continued for 12 months after symptoms have resolved, while for anxiety disorders, clinicians have generally treated for 6–9 months (Hathaway et al., 2018).
- Often a good idea to tell parents whether the medication chosen is specifically approved for the disorder being treated, or whether it is being given for "unapproved" or "off-label" reasons based on good clinical practice, expert consensus, and/or prudent extrapolation of controlled data from adults

What to Tell Children and Adolescents About Efficacy

- We are trying to make you feel better
- It may be a good idea to give the medication a try; if it's not working very well, we can stop the medication and try something else
- A good try takes 2 to 3 months or even longer
- If it does make you feel better, you cannot stop it right away or you may feel sad or worried again
- Medications don't change who you are as a person; they give you the opportunity to be the best person you can be

What to Tell Parents About Side Effects

- Explain that side effects are expected in many when starting and are most common in the first 2–3 weeks of starting or increasing the dose
- Tell parents many side effects go away and do so about the same time that therapeutic effects start
- Predict side effects in advance (you will look clever and competent to the parents, unless you scare them with too much information and cause nocebo effects, in which case you won't look so clever when the patient develops lots of side effects and stops medication; use your judgment here); a balanced but honest presentation is an art rather than a science
- Ask them to help monitor for increased suicidality and if present, report any such symptoms immediately
- Ask parents to support the patient while side effects are occurring
- Parents should fully understand short- and long-term risks as well as benefits
- Explaining to the parents what to expect from medication treatment, and especially potential side effects, can help prevent early termination of medication

What to Tell Children and Adolescents About Side Effects

- Even if you get side effects, most of them get better or go away in a few days to a few weeks
- Consider having a conversation about sexual side effects in some adolescents who can find these side effects confusing and especially burdensome
- Explaining to child/adolescent what to expect from medication treatment, and especially potential side effects, can help prevent early termination of medication
- Tell adolescents and children capable of understanding that some young patients, especially those who are depressed, may develop thoughts of hurting themselves, and if this happens, not to be alarmed but to tell their parents right away

What to Tell Teachers About the Medication (If Parents Consent)

- Venlafaxine can make children/adolescents jittery or restless
- If the patient is sleepy, ask whether the medication is keeping them up at night
- It is not abusable
- Encourage dialogue with parents/guardians about any behavior or mood changes

SPECIAL POPULATIONS

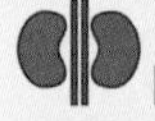

Renal Impairment

- Lower dose by 25–50%
- Patients on dialysis should not receive subsequent dose until dialysis is completed

Hepatic Impairment

- Lower dose by 50%

Cardiac Impairment

- Drug should be used with caution
- Hypertension should be controlled prior to initiation of venlafaxine and should be monitored regularly during treatment
- Venlafaxine has a dose-dependent effect on increasing blood pressure and, in adolescents, higher blood levels are associated with more cardiovascular adverse events (Sakolsky et al., 2011)
- Venlafaxine is contraindicated in patients with heart disease in the UK
- Venlafaxine can block cardiac ion channels in vitro

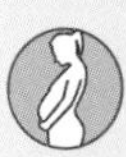

Pregnancy

- Controlled studies have not been conducted in pregnant women
- Not generally recommended for use during pregnancy, especially during first trimester
- Nonetheless, continuous treatment during pregnancy may be necessary and has not been proven to be harmful to the fetus
- Must weigh the risk of treatment (first trimester fetal development, third trimester newborn delivery) to the child against the risk of no treatment (recurrence of depression, maternal health, infant bonding) to the mother and child
- For many patients this may mean continuing treatment during pregnancy
- Neonates exposed to SSRIs or SNRIs late in the third trimester have developed complications requiring prolonged hospitalization, respiratory support, and tube feeding; reported symptoms are consistent with either a direct toxic effect of SSRIs and SNRIs or, possibly, a drug discontinuation syndrome, and include respiratory distress, cyanosis, apnea, seizures, temperature instability, feeding difficulty, vomiting, hypoglycemia, hypotonia, hypertonia, hyperreflexia, tremor, jitteriness, irritability, and constant crying

Breast Feeding

- Some drug is found in breast milk
- Trace amounts may be present in nursing children whose mothers are on venlafaxine
- If child becomes irritable or sedated, breast feeding or drug may need to be discontinued
- Immediate postpartum period is a high-risk time for depression, especially in women who have had prior depressive episodes, so drug may need to be reinstituted late in the third trimester or shortly after childbirth to prevent a recurrence during the postpartum period
- Must weigh benefits of breast feeding with risks and benefits of antidepressant treatment versus nontreatment to both the infant and the mother
- For many patients, this may mean continuing treatment during breast feeding

THE ART OF PSYCHOPHARMACOLOGY

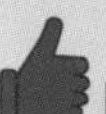

Potential Advantages

- In children and adolescents:
  - May be helpful in treatment-resistant depression or anxiety disorders; however, it should be used cautiously in patients who have higher suicidality prior to treatment as these patients are at greater risk for suicide attempts when treated with venlafaxine (Brent et al., 2009)
- All ages:
  - Patients with atypical depression (hypersomnia, increased appetite)
  - Depressed patients with somatic symptoms, fatigue, and pain
  - Patients who do not respond or remit on treatment with SSRIs; however, data from the Treatment of SSRI-Resistant Depression in Adolescents (TORDIA) Study (Brent et al., 2008) suggest that patients who have not responded to an initial SSRI should receive a trial of a second SSRI before pursuing a trial of an SNRI (Suresh et al., 2020)

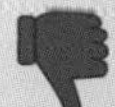

Potential Disadvantages

- In children:
  - Those who are already psychomotor agitated, angry, or irritable, and who do not have a psychiatric diagnosis
  - Results from two placebo-controlled trials in pediatric patients with depression were not sufficient to support approval in this population

- Results from two placebo-controlled trials in pediatric patients with GAD were not sufficient to support approval in this population
- In adolescents:
  - Those who may possibly have a mood disorder with mixed or bipolar features, especially those with these features and a family history of bipolar disorder
  - Results from two placebo-controlled trials in pediatric patients with depression were not sufficient to support approval in this population
  - Results from two placebo-controlled trials in pediatric patients with GAD were not sufficient to support approval in this population
- All ages:
  - Patients sensitive to nausea
  - Patients with borderline or uncontrolled hypertension
  - Patients with cardiac disease

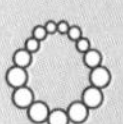

Pearls

- SNRIs appear less effective than SSRIs in reducing depressive and anxiety symptoms in youth (Strawn et al., 2018; Suresh et al., 2020)
- Many SSRIs and SNRIs have an even smaller effect and sometimes no effect in controlled clinical trials of child and adolescent depression
- Venlafaxine has been associated with more treatment-emergent suicidality in adolescents compared to other SNRIs or SSRIs in multiple studies and meta-analyses (Brent et al., 2009; Dobson et al., 2019)
- XR formulation improves tolerability, reduces nausea, and requires only once-daily dosing
- Has greater potency for serotonin reuptake blockade than for norepinephrine reuptake blockade, but this is of unclear clinical significance as a differentiating feature from other SNRIs
- In vitro binding studies tend to underestimate in vivo potency for reuptake blockade, as they do not factor in the presence of high concentrations of an active metabolite, higher oral mg dosing, or the lower protein binding, which can increase functional drug levels at receptor sites
- Efficacy as well as side effects (especially nausea and increased blood pressure) are dose dependent
- Blood pressure increases and heart rate increases have been observed in pediatric populations and may be more common in patients treated with higher doses
- More withdrawal reactions reported upon discontinuation than for some other antidepressants
- Because of recent studies from the UK that suggest a higher rate of deaths from overdose with venlafaxine than with SSRIs, and because of its potential to affect heart function, venlafaxine can only be prescribed in the UK by specialist doctors and is contraindicated there in patients with heart disease
- Venlafaxine's toxicity in overdose is less than that for tricyclic antidepressants

SUGGESTED READING

Bousman CA, Stevenson JM, Ramsey LB et al. Clinical Pharmacogenetics Implementation Consortium (CPIC) guideline for CYP2D6, CYP2C19, CYP2B6, SLC6A4, and HTR2A genotypes and serotonin reuptake inhibitor antidepressants. Clin Pharmacol Ther 2023;114(1):51–68.

Brent D, Emslie G, Clarke G et al. Switching to another SSRI or to venlafaxine with or without cognitive behavioral therapy for adolescents with SSRI-resistant depression: the TORDIA randomized controlled trial. JAMA 2008;299(8):901–13.

Brent DA, Emslie GJ, Clarke GN et al. Predictors of spontaneous and systematically assessed suicidal adverse events in the Treatment of SSRI-Resistant Depression in Adolescents (TORDIA) study. Am J Psychiatry 2009;166(4):418–26.

Bridge JA, Iyengar S, Salary CB et al. Clinical response and risk for reported suicidal ideation and suicide attempts in pediatric antidepressant treatment: a meta-analysis of randomized controlled trials. JAMA 2007;297(15):1683–96.

Croarkin PE, Elmaadawi AZ, Aaronson ST et al. Left prefrontal transcranial magnetic stimulation for treatment-resistant depression in adolescents: a double-blind, randomized, sham-controlled trial. Neuropsychopharmacology 2021;46(2):462–9.

Dobson ET, Bloch MH, Strawn JR. Efficacy and tolerability of pharmacotherapy for pediatric anxiety disorders: a network meta-analysis. J Clin Psychiatry 2019;80(1):17r12064.

Doroudgar S, Perry PJ, Lackey GD et al. An 11-year retrospective review of venlafaxine ingestion in children from the California Poison Control System. Hum Exp Toxicol 2016;35(7):767–74.

Dwyer JB, Stringaris A, Brent DA, Bloch MH. Annual Research Review: Defining and treating pediatric treatment-resistant depression. J Child Psychol Psychiatry 2020;61(3):312–32.

Emslie GJ, Findling RL, Yeung PP, Kunz NR, Li Y. Venlafaxine ER for the treatment of pediatric subjects with depression: results of two placebo-controlled trials. J Am Acad Child Adolesc Psychiatry 2007;46(4):479–88.

Hathaway EE, Walkup JT, Strawn JR. Antidepressant treatment duration in pediatric depressive and anxiety disorders: how long is long enough? Curr Probl Pediatr Adolesc Health Care 2018;48(2):31–9.

Mills JA, Strawn JR. Antidepressant tolerability in pediatric anxiety and obsessive-compulsive disorders: a Bayesian hierarchical modeling meta-analysis. J Am Acad Child Adolesc Psychiatry 2020;59(11):1240–51.

Rynn MA, Riddle MA, Yeung PP, Kunz NR. Efficacy and safety of extended-release venlafaxine in the treatment of generalized anxiety disorder in children and adolescents: two placebo-controlled trials. Am J Psychiatry 2007;164(2):290–300.

Sakolsky DJ, Perel JM, Emslie GJ et al. Antidepressant exposure as a predictor of clinical outcomes in the Treatment of Resistant Depression in Adolescents (TORDIA) study. J Clin Psychopharmacol 2011;31(1):92–7.

Sangkuhl K, Stingl JC, Turpeinen M, Altman RB, Klein TE. PharmGKB summary: venlafaxine pathway. Pharmacogenet Genomics 2014;24(1):62–72.

Strawn JR, Mills JA, Sauley BA, Welge JA. The impact of antidepressant dose and class on treatment response in pediatric anxiety disorders: a meta-analysis. J Am Acad Child Adolesc Psychiatry 2018;57(4):235–244.e2.

Strawn JR, Mills JA, Poweleit EA, Ramsey LB, Croarkin PE. Adverse effects of antidepressant medications and their management in children and adolescents. Pharmacotherapy 2023;43(7):675–90.

Suresh V, Mills JA, Croarkin PE, Strawn JR. What next? A Bayesian hierarchical modeling re-examination of treatments for adolescents with selective serotonin reuptake inhibitor-resistant depression. Depress Anxiety 2020;37(9):926–34.

THERAPEUTICS

Brands

- Viibryd

Generic

Yes

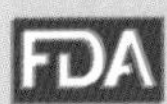

US FDA Approved for Pediatric Use

- None

Off-Label for Pediatric Use

- Approved in adults
  - Major depressive disorder
- Other off-label uses
  - Anxiety
  - Obsessive-compulsive disorder (OCD)

Class and Mechanism of Action

- Neuroscience-based Nomenclature: serotonin multimodal (S-MM)
- SPARI (serotonin partial agonist reuptake inhibitor)
- Dual-acting serotonin reuptake inhibitor plus 5HT1A partial agonist
- Vilazodone presumably increases serotonergic neurotransmission by blocking the serotonin reuptake pump (transporter, SERT), which results in the desensitization of serotonin receptors, especially serotonin 1A receptors
- Partial agonist actions at presynaptic somatodendritic serotonin 1A autoreceptors may theoretically enhance serotonergic activity and contribute to antidepressant actions
- Partial agonist actions at postsynaptic serotonin 1A receptors may theoretically diminish sexual dysfunction caused by serotonin reuptake inhibition

SAFETY AND TOLERABILITY

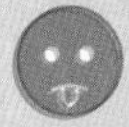

Notable Side Effects

- Several central nervous system side effects (insomnia but also sedation, especially if not sleeping at night, agitation, headache, dizziness). Rates of these symptoms in vilazodone-treated youth are similar to other antidepressant-treated children and adolescents in clinical trials.
- Note: patients with diagnosed or undiagnosed bipolar or psychotic disorders may be more vulnerable to CNS-activating actions of SSRIs like vilazodone; pay particular attention to signs of activation in children with developmental disorders or autism spectrum disorders
- Treatment-emergent activation syndrome (TEAS) includes agitation, anxiety, panic attacks, irritability, aggression, impulsivity, and insomnia
- TEAS can represent side effects but should not be confused with bipolar mania or the onset of suicidality and should be monitored and investigated with consideration of discontinuing or decreasing the dose of vilazodone or addition of another agent or switching to another agent to reduce these symptoms
- Gastrointestinal (nausea, vomiting, diarrhea). In some pediatric trials of vilazodone, which include fluoxetine as a reference treatment, rates of nausea (21%), vomiting (13%), diarrhea (9%), and abdominal pain (7%) are higher than for fluoxetine or placebo (Findling et al., 2020).
- Sexual dysfunction (boys: delayed ejaculation, erectile dysfunction; boys and girls: decreased sexual desire, anorgasmia); in adult studies sexual dysfunction is slightly greater than placebo and generally less than for SSRIs/SNRIs, but no head-to-head studies
- Bruising and rare bleeding
- Syndrome of inappropriate antidiuretic hormone secretion (SIADH)

Life-Threatening or Dangerous Side Effects

- Rare seizures
- Rare induction of mania
- Rare suicidal ideation and behavior (suicidality) (short-term regulatory studies did not show any actual suicides in any age group and also did not show an increase in the risk of suicidality with antidepressants compared to placebo beyond age 24)

Growth and Maturation

- Growth should be monitored; long-term effects are unknown

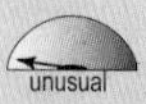

Weight Gain

- Reported but not common. In short-term trials of vilazodone in children and adolescents, weight increases were similar to placebo (Findling et al., 2020).

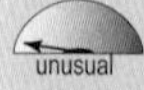

Sedation

- Reported but not common; may be slightly higher than for some other SSRIs (e.g., fluoxetine) (Findling et al., 2020)

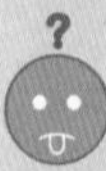

What to Do About Side Effects

- Wait, wait, wait: mild side effects are common, happen early, and usually improve with time, but treatment benefits can be delayed and often begin just as the side effects wear off. However, some side effects may emerge later such as weight gain.
- Monitor side effects closely, especially when initiating treatment
- May wish to give in the evening or at bedtime, particularly if the medication is associated with sedation
- For activation (jitteriness, anxiety, insomnia):
  - Consider a temporary dose reduction or a more gradual up-titration
  - Administer dose in the morning
  - Consider switching to an SSRI or potentially an SNRI (other than venlafaxine)
  - Optimize psychotherapeutic interventions
  - Activation and agitation may represent the induction of a bipolar state, especially a mixed dysphoric bipolar II condition sometimes associated with suicidal ideation, and may require the addition of lithium, or an atypical antipsychotic, and/or discontinuation of vilazodone
- Often best to try another monotherapy prior to resorting to augmentation strategies to treat side effects
- For insomnia: consider adding melatonin
- For GI upset: try giving medication with a meal
- For sexual dysfunction:
  - Probably best to reduce dose or discontinue and try another agent
  - Consider adding daytime exercise, bupropion. Importantly, adding buspirone may not have a significant effect in vilazodone-treated patients, given that vilazodone has serotonin 1A partial agonist effects.

How Drug Causes Side Effects

- Theoretically due to increases in serotonin concentrations at serotonin receptors in parts of the brain and body other than those that cause therapeutic actions (e.g., unwanted actions of serotonin in sleep centers causing insomnia, unwanted actions of serotonin in the gut causing diarrhea)
- Increasing serotonin can cause diminished dopamine release and might contribute to emotional flattening, cognitive slowing, and apathy in some patients

Warnings and Precautions

- Consider distributing the brochures provided by the FDA and the drug companies as well as the medication guides from the American Academy of Child & Adolescent Psychiatry (AACAP)
- Carefully consider monitoring patients regularly and within the practical limits, particularly during the first several weeks of treatment
- Warn patients and their caregivers when possible about the possibility of activating side effects and advise them to report such symptoms
- Carefully weigh the risks and benefits of pharmacological treatment against the risks and benefits of nontreatment with antidepressants and make sure to document this in the patient's chart
- As with any antidepressant, use with caution in patients with history of seizure
- As with any antidepressant, use with caution in patients with bipolar disorder unless treated with concomitant mood-stabilizing agent
- Monitor patients for activation and suicidal ideation and involve parents/guardians

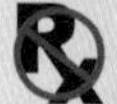

When Not to Prescribe

- If patient is taking an MAO inhibitor
- If there is a proven allergy to vilazodone

Long-Term Use

- Growth should be monitored; long-term effects are unknown

Habit Forming

- No

Overdose

- Few reports of vilazodone overdose
- No fatalities; serotonin syndrome, lethargy, restlessness, hallucinations, disorientation

DOSING AND USE

Usual Dosage Range

- In children (depression): 15–30 mg/day
- In adolescents (depression): 15–40 mg/day

Dosage Forms

- Tablet 10 mg, 20 mg, 40 mg

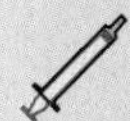

How to Dose

- In children (depression and anxiety disorders): initial dose 5–10 mg/day; after 4 weeks can increase to 20 mg/day
- In adolescents (depression): initial dose 10 mg/day; after 2 weeks can increase to 15 mg/day; after another 2–4 weeks can titrate to 30 mg/day; after another 2–4 weeks can titrate to 40 mg. However, in anxious youth, may consider starting at 5 mg/day for 2 days and then increasing to 10 mg/day.

Options for Administration

- Only available as a tablet

Tests

- None for healthy individuals

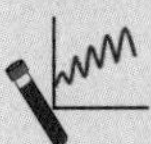

Pharmacokinetics

- Metabolized primarily by CYP3A4 with minor contributions from CYP2C19 and CYP2D6. Vilazodone concentrations are not impacted by CYP2D6 and/or CYP2C19 metabolism (Figure 1).
- Absorption and bioavailability are reduced by half when taken on an empty stomach
- Mean terminal half-life is 25 hours in adults

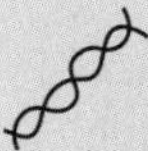

Pharmacogenetics

- The Clinical Pharmacogenetics Implementation Consortium does not provide dosing recommendations for vilazodone based on pharmacokinetic genes

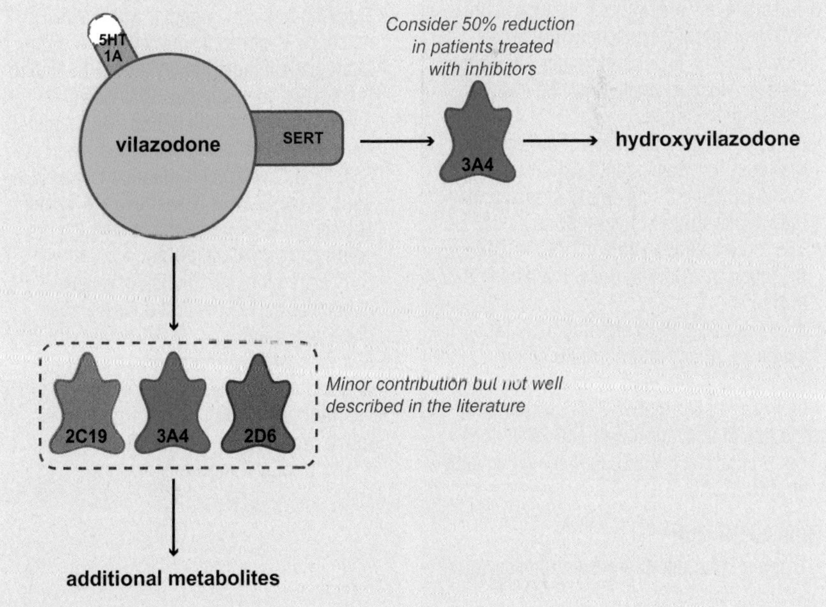

Figure 1 Vilazodone metabolism.

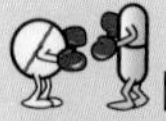

Drug Interactions

- Tramadol increases the risk of seizures in adults taking an antidepressant
- Can cause a fatal "serotonin syndrome" when combined with MAO inhibitors, so do not use with MAO inhibitors or for at least 14 days after MAOIs are stopped
- Do not start an MAO inhibitor for at least 5 half-lives (5 to 7 days for most drugs) after discontinuing vilazodone
- Inhibitors of CYP3A4, such as nefazodone, fluoxetine, and fluvoxamine, may decrease the clearance of vilazodone and thereby raise its plasma levels, so dose should be reduced by 50% when co-administered with strong CYP3A4 inhibitors
- Inducers of CYP3A4, such as carbamazepine, may increase clearance of vilazodone and thus lower its plasma levels and possibly reduce therapeutic effects
- Can theoretically cause weakness, hyperreflexia, and incoordination when combined with sumatriptan, or possibly with other triptans, requiring careful monitoring of patient
- Possible increased risk of bleeding

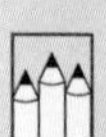

Dosing Tips

- Plasma levels are higher in lower-weight children; therefore, starting and target doses may be lower and longer intervals between dose increases may be needed (see How to Dose)
- Given once daily, any time of day tolerated but must be administered with food, because taking on an empty stomach may reduce absorption of vilazodone by 50%
- The more anxious and agitated the patient, the lower the starting dose, the slower the titration
- If intolerable anxiety, insomnia, agitation, akathisia, or activation occurs either upon dosing initiation or discontinuation, consider an alternative SSRI. Importantly, the risk of activation with one SSRI does not predict the likelihood of activation with another SSRI.

How to Switch

- From another antidepressant to vilazodone:
  - When tapering a prior antidepressant, see its entry in this manual for how to stop and how to taper off that specific drug
  - In situations when there are antidepressant-related side effects, try to stop the first agent before starting vilazodone so that new side effects of vilazodone can be distinguished from withdrawal effects of the first agent
  - If necessary, can cross taper off the prior antidepressant and dose up on vilazodone simultaneously in urgent situations, being aware of all specific drug interactions to avoid
- Off vilazodone to another antidepressant:
  - Generally, try to stop vilazodone before starting another antidepressant
  - Stopping vilazodone often means tapering off since discontinuing many SSRIs can cause withdrawal symptoms
  - If vilazodone needs to be stopped quickly, one can reduce vilazodone by 5 mg every 5–7 days, or slower if this rate still causes withdrawal symptoms
  - If necessary, can cross taper off vilazodone this way while dosing up on another antidepressant simultaneously in urgent situations, being aware of all specific drug interactions to avoid

How to Stop

- Tapering to avoid potential withdrawal reactions is generally prudent
- Many patients tolerate 50% dose reduction for 1 week, then another 50% reduction for 1 week, then discontinuation. More recently however, hyperbolic discontinuation of SSRIs has been recommended in which the dose of the SSRI is halved every 4 weeks and this may be a preferable strategy in youth (Strawn et al., 2023). Also, when SSRIs are stopped, the risk of relapse is highest during the first 8 weeks after discontinuation.
- If withdrawal symptoms emerge during discontinuation, raise dose to stop symptoms and then restart withdrawal much more slowly such as reducing vilazodone by 5 mg every 10 days

WHAT TO EXPECT

Onset of Action

- Some patients may experience increased energy or activation early after initiation of treatment
- Full onset of therapeutic actions is usually delayed by 2–4 weeks
- If it is not working within 6–8 weeks, it may require a dosage increase or it may not work at all

Duration of Action

- Effects are consistent over a 24-hour period
- May continue to work for many years to prevent relapse of symptoms

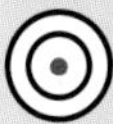

Primary Target Symptoms

- Depressed and/or irritable mood
- Anxiety (fear and worry are often target symptoms, but vilazodone can occasionally and transiently increase these symptoms short term before improving them)
- Sleep disturbance, both hypersomnia and insomnia (eventually, but can actually cause insomnia, especially short term)
- Prior to initiation of treatment, it is helpful to develop a list of target symptoms of depression and/or anxiety to monitor during treatment to better assess treatment response

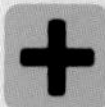

What Is Considered a Positive Result?

- The goal of treatment is complete remission of current symptoms as well as prevention of future relapses
- In practice, many patients have only a partial response where some symptoms are improved but others persist (especially insomnia, fatigue, and problems concentrating in depression), in which case higher doses of vilazodone, adding a second agent, or switching to an agent with a different mechanism of action can be considered
- If treatment works, it most often reduces or even eliminates symptoms, but is not a cure since symptoms can recur after medicine is stopped

How Long to Treat

- For adolescents with depression, generally, 9–12 months of antidepressant treatment is recommended (Hathaway et al., 2018)
- For anxiety disorders, 6–9 months of antidepressant treatment may be sufficient, though many clinicians extend treatment to 12 months based on extrapolation of data from adults with anxiety disorders (Hathaway et al., 2018; Strawn et al., 2021)
- Extended treatment periods may decrease the risk of long-term morbidity and recurrence; however, the goal of treatment is ultimately remission, rather than duration of antidepressant pharmacotherapy (Hathaway et al., 2018)
- In terms of the length of antidepressant treatment, evidence-based guidelines represent a starting point; appropriate treatment duration varies, and patient-specific response, psychological factors, and timing of discontinuation must be considered for individual pediatric patients (Hathaway et al., 2018)

What If It Stops Working?

- Some patients who have an initial response may relapse even though they continue treatment, sometimes called "poop-out"
- Some patients may experience apparent lack of consistent efficacy due to activation syndrome or latent or underlying or newly evolved bipolar disorder, or major depressive episodes with mixed features, and require antidepressant discontinuation and a switch to a second generation antipsychotic

What If It Doesn't Work?

- Consider evaluation for another diagnosis (especially bipolar illness or depression with mixed features) or for a comorbid condition (e.g., medical illness, substance abuse)
- When treating youth with anxiety disorders, many patients will have had significant anxiety for years prior to beginning treatment. As such, when anxiety is treated with an SSRI, their symptoms may be improved, but the patient has likely missed important developmental milestones (e.g., spending the night with friends, being able to ask questions in class). Developing these skills will take time. Beyond this, the family

may have lived with the anxious child for years and following treatment of the child, the family may need to readjust.

- Be mindful of family conflict contributing to the presentation; sometimes treating parental depression or anxiety disorders improves psychiatric and social function without any treatment of youth. Also, accommodation is common in families of youth with anxiety disorders and may need to be addressed specifically, as it can perpetuate symptoms.
- Consider factors associated with poor response to SSRIs in treatment-resistant depression or anxiety disorders, such as severe symptoms, long-lasting symptoms, poor treatment adherence, prior nonresponse to other treatments, and the presence of comorbid disorders
- Consider other important potential factors such as ongoing conflicts, family psychopathology, and an adverse environment (e.g., poverty, chaos, violence, prior and ongoing psychological trauma, abuse, neglect). Additionally, when symptoms are prominent at school, consider the presence of a learning disorder.
- Institute trauma-informed care for appropriate children and adolescents
- A 2007 meta-analysis of published and unpublished trials in pediatric patients found that antidepressants had a number needed to treat (NNT) of 10 for depression, 6 for OCD, and 3 for anxiety disorders; thus, vilazodone may not work in all children, so consider switching to another antidepressant (Bridge et al., 2007)
- Consider a dose adjustment
- Consider augmenting options:
  - Cognitive behavioral therapy (CBT), interpersonal psychotherapy for adolescents (IPT-A), light therapy, family therapy, and exercise especially in adolescents
  - For partial response (depression): use caution when adding medications to vilazodone, especially in children, since there are not sufficient studies of augmentation in children or adolescents; however, for the expert, consider bupropion, aripiprazole, or other atypical antipsychotics such as quetiapine; use combinations of antidepressants with caution as this may activate bipolar disorder and suicidal ideation
  - For insomnia: sleep hygiene, CBT for insomnia, melatonin, or alpha 2 agonists
  - For anxiety: buspirone, antihistamines
  - Add lithium or atypical antipsychotics for bipolar depression, psychotic depression, treatment-resistant depression, or treatment-resistant anxiety disorders
  - TMS (transcranial magnetic stimulation) may have a role although pediatric trials of TMS have been hampered by high sham response rates (Croarkin et al., 2021)
  - ECT (case studies show effectiveness; cognitive side effects are similar to those in adults; reserve for treatment-resistant cases)

TALKING TO PATIENTS AND CAREGIVERS

What to Tell Parents About Efficacy

- Doesn't work right away; full therapeutic benefits may take up to 8 weeks, yet parents and teachers might see improvement before the patient does
- While the medicine helps by reducing symptoms and improving function, it is not a cure, and it is therefore necessary to keep taking the medication to sustain its therapeutic effects
- Since every treatment consideration depends on a risk/benefit analysis, parents should fully understand short- and long-term risks as well as benefits
- After successful treatment, continuation of vilazodone may be necessary to prevent relapse, especially in those who have had more than one episode or a very severe episode. In general, when treating depression in children and adolescents, medications are continued for 12 months after symptoms have resolved, while for anxiety disorders, clinicians have generally treated for 6–9 months (Hathaway et al., 2018).
- Often a good idea to tell parents whether the medication chosen is specifically approved for the disorder being treated, or if it is "unapproved" or "off-label" but nevertheless good clinical practice and based upon prudent extrapolation of controlled data from adults and from

experience in children and adolescents instead of formal FDA approval

What to Tell Children and Adolescents About Efficacy

- We are trying to make you feel better
- It may be a good idea to give the medication a try; if it's not working very well, we can stop the medication and try something else
- A good try takes 2 to 3 months or even longer
- If it does make you feel better, you cannot stop it right away or you may feel sad or worried again
- Medications don't change who you are as a person; they give you the opportunity to be the best person you can be

What to Tell Parents About Side Effects

- Explain that side effects are expected in many when starting and are most common in the first 2–3 weeks of starting or increasing the dose
- Some SSRI side effects emerge early and resolve quickly (e.g., activation, gastrointestinal symptoms). In contrast, other side effects are late-emerging (e.g., weight gain) or persistent (e.g., sexual dysfunction). Discussing the temporal course of the side effects and distinguishing between persistent and transient side effects is critical. Ensuring that patients are aware not only of side effects but the tendency of some side effects to be transient is important and should be part of discussions with patients and their families. For many, knowing that a side effect is likely transient, as opposed to persistent, may significantly influence the patient and family's anxiety or fears related to medication (Strawn et al., 2023).
- Tell parents many side effects go away and do so about the same time that therapeutic effects start
- Predict side effects in advance (you will look clever and competent to the parents, unless you scare them with too much information and cause nocebo effects, in which case you won't look so clever when the patient develops lots of side effects and stops medication; use your judgment here); a balanced but honest presentation is an art rather than a science
- Ask them to help monitor for increased suicidality and if present, report any such symptoms immediately
- Ask parents to support the patient while side effects are occurring
- Parents should fully understand short- and long-term risks as well as benefits
- Explaining to the parents what to expect from medication treatment, and especially potential side effects, can help prevent early termination of medication

What to Tell Children and Adolescents About Side Effects

- Even if you get side effects, most of them get better or go away in a few days to a few weeks
- Consider having a conversation about sexual side effects in some adolescents who can find these side effects confusing and especially burdensome
- Explaining to child/adolescent what to expect from medication treatment, and especially potential side effects, can help prevent early termination of medication
- Tell adolescents and children capable of understanding that some young patients, especially those who are depressed, may develop thoughts of hurting themselves, and if this happens, not to be alarmed but to tell their parents right away

What to Tell Teachers About the Medication (If Parents Consent)

- It is not abusable
- Encourage dialogue with parents/guardians about any behavior or mood changes

SPECIAL POPULATIONS

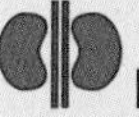

Renal Impairment

- No dose adjustment necessary

Hepatic Impairment

- No dose adjustment necessary for mild to moderate impairment
- Has not been studied in patients with severe hepatic impairment

Cardiac Impairment

- Not systematically evaluated in patients with cardiac impairment
- Vilazodone has not shown any significant effect on blood pressure, heart rate, or QTc interval in placebo-controlled trials in adults

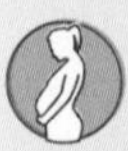

Pregnancy

- Controlled studies have not been conducted in pregnant women
- Not generally recommended for use during pregnancy, especially during first trimester
- Nonetheless, continuous treatment during pregnancy may be necessary and has not been proven to be harmful to the fetus
- At delivery there may be more bleeding in the mother and transient irritability or sedation in the newborn
- Must weigh the risk of treatment (first trimester fetal development, third trimester newborn delivery) to the child against the risk of no treatment (recurrence of depression, maternal health, infant bonding) to the mother and child
- For many patients, this may mean continuing treatment during pregnancy
- Exposure to SSRIs early in pregnancy may be associated with increased risk of septal heart defects (absolute risk is small)
- SSRI use beyond the 20th week of pregnancy may be associated with increased risk of pulmonary hypertension in newborns, although this is not proven
- Exposure to SSRIs late in pregnancy may be associated with increased risk of gestational hypertension and preeclampsia
- Neonates exposed to SSRIs or SNRIs late in the third trimester have developed complications requiring prolonged hospitalization, respiratory support, and tube feeding; reported symptoms are consistent with either a direct toxic effect of SSRIs and SNRIs or, possibly, a drug discontinuation syndrome, and include respiratory distress, cyanosis, apnea, seizures, temperature instability, feeding difficulty, vomiting, hypoglycemia, hypotonia, hypertonia, hyperreflexia, tremor, jitteriness, irritability, and constant crying
- National Pregnancy Registry for Psychiatric Medications: 1-866-961-2388 or https://womensmentalhealth.org/research/pregnancyregistry/

Breast Feeding

- Unknown if vilazodone is secreted in human breast milk, but all psychotropics assumed to be secreted in breast milk
- Trace amounts may be present in nursing children whose mothers are on vilazodone
- If child becomes irritable or sedated, breast feeding or drug may need to be discontinued
- Immediate postpartum period is a high-risk time for depression, especially in women who have had prior depressive episodes, so drug may need to be reinstituted late in the third trimester or shortly after childbirth to prevent a recurrence during the postpartum period
- Must weigh benefits of breast feeding with risks and benefits of antidepressant treatment versus nontreatment to both the infant and the mother
- For many patients, this may mean continuing treatment during breast feeding

THE ART OF PSYCHOPHARMACOLOGY

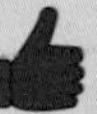

Potential Advantages

- Patients who wish to avoid sexual dysfunction and weight gain

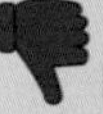

Potential Disadvantages

- Double-blind, randomized, placebo-controlled trial did not demonstrate efficacy of vilazodone in adolescents with major depressive disorder
- Patients who cannot take medication reliably with food
- Patients sensitive to gastrointestinal side effects such as diarrhea and nausea

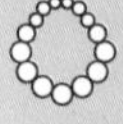

Pearls

- First member of a new antidepressant class, SPARIs, or serotonin partial agonist reuptake inhibitors
- Relative lack of sexual dysfunction and weight gain compared to many other antidepressants that block serotonin reuptake may be due to the serotonin 1A partial agonist properties of vilazodone

- High doses would theoretically raise brain serotonin levels more robustly than the standard dose, and may improve efficacy in some patients but reduce tolerability in some patients
- Regarding tolerability, the randomized controlled trials of vilazodone in adolescents with major depressive disorder suggested higher rates of treatment-emergent adverse events (67%) compared to both placebo and fluoxetine (both 50%) (Findling et al., 2020)

SUGGESTED READING

Bridge JA, Iyengar S, Salary CB et al. Clinical response and risk for reported suicidal ideation and suicide attempts in pediatric antidepressant treatment: a meta-analysis of randomized controlled trials. JAMA 2007;297(15):1683–96.

Croarkin PE, Elmaadawi AZ, Aaronson ST et al. Left prefrontal transcranial magnetic stimulation for treatment-resistant depression in adolescents: a double-blind, randomized, sham-controlled trial. *Neuropsychopharmacology* 2021;46(2):462–9.

Durgam S, Chen C, Migliore R et al. A phase 3, double-blind, randomized, placebo-controlled study of vilazodone in adolescents with major depressive disorder. Paediatr Drugs 2018;20(4):353–63.

Findling RL, McCusker E, Strawn JR. A randomized, double-blind, placebo-controlled trial of vilazodone in children and adolescents with major depressive disorder with twenty-six-week open-label follow-up. J Child Adolesc Psychopharmacol 2020;30(6):355–65.

Hathaway EE, Walkup JT, Strawn JR. Antidepressant treatment duration in pediatric depressive and anxiety disorders: how long is long enough? Curr Probl Pediatr Adolesc Health Care 2018;48(2):31–9.

Strawn JR, Lu L, Peris TS, Levine A, Walkup JT. Research review: pediatric anxiety disorders – what have we learnt in the last 10 years? J Child Psychol Psychiatry 2021 Feb;62(2):114–39.

Strawn JR, Mills JA, Poweleit EA, Ramsey LB, Croarkin PE. Adverse effects of antidepressant medications and their management in children and adolescents. Pharmacotherapy 2023;43(7):675–90.

THERAPEUTICS

Brands
- Qelbree

Generic
No

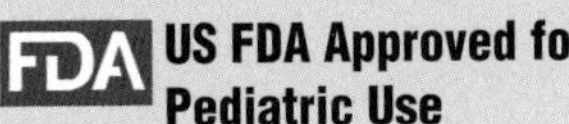

US FDA Approved for Pediatric Use
- Attention deficit hyperactivity disorder (ages 6 and older)

Off-Label for Pediatric Use
- Approved in adults
  - None
- Other off-label uses
  - Major depressive disorder

Class and Mechanism of Action
- Neuroscience-based Nomenclature: norepinephrine reuptake inhibitor (N-RI)
- Selective norepinephrine reuptake inhibitor (NRI)
- Boosts neurotransmitter norepinephrine/noradrenaline and may also increase dopamine in the prefrontal cortex
- Blocks norepinephrine reuptake pumps, also known as norepinephrine transporters
- Presumably this increases noradrenergic neurotransmission
- Since dopamine is inactivated by norepinephrine reuptake in the frontal cortex, which largely lacks dopamine transporters, viloxazine can also increase dopamine neurotransmission in this part of the brain
- Has antagonist actions at 5HT2B receptors and agonist actions at 5HT2C receptors and has been shown to increase serotonin levels

SAFETY AND TOLERABILITY

Notable Side Effects
- Fatigue, sleepiness, insomnia, irritability
- Decreased appetite, nausea, vomiting
- Increased heart rate
- Increased blood pressure

Life-Threatening or Dangerous Side Effects
- Rare hypomania, mania, or suicidal ideation

Growth and Maturation
- Changes not reported

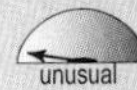

Weight Gain
- Patients may experience weight loss, but typically less than with stimulants because there is generally less appetite suppression
- Weight gain is not expected

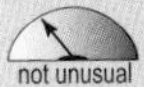

Sedation
- Occurs in significant minority
- Insomnia may occur

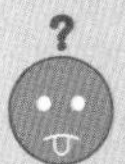

What to Do About Side Effects
- Wait, wait, wait: mild side effects are common, happen early, and usually improve with time, but treatment benefits can be delayed and often begin just as the side effects wear off
- Monitor side effects closely, especially when initiating treatment
- Lower the dose
- If viloxazine is sedating, take at night to reduce daytime drowsiness
- Often best to try another monotherapy prior to resorting to augmentation strategies to treat side effects
- Activation and agitation may represent the induction of a bipolar state, especially a mixed dysphoric bipolar II condition sometimes associated with suicidal ideation, and may require the addition of lithium or an atypical antipsychotic, and/or discontinuation of viloxazine

How Drug Causes Side Effects
- Norepinephrine increases in parts of the brain and body and at receptors other than those that cause therapeutic actions (e.g., unwanted actions of norepinephrine on acetylcholine release causing decreased appetite, increased heart rate and blood pressure, dry mouth, urinary retention)
- Lack of enhancing dopamine activity in limbic areas theoretically explains viloxazine's lack of abuse potential

Warnings and Precautions
- In children and adolescents:
  - Safety and efficacy not established in children under age 6

- Use in young children should be reserved for the expert
- Children who are not growing or gaining weight should stop treatment, at least temporarily
- Consider distributing brochures provided by the FDA and the drug companies
- Warn patients and their caregivers about the possibility of activating side effects and advise them to report such symptoms immediately

• All ages:

- Carefully weigh the risks and benefits of pharmacological treatment against the risks and benefits of nonpharmacological treatment and it is a good idea to document this in the patient's chart
- Use with caution if at all in patients with bipolar disorder
- Monitor patients for activation of suicidal ideation
- Emergence or worsening of activation and agitation may represent the induction of a bipolar state, especially a mixed dysphoric bipolar II condition sometimes associated with suicidal ideation, and may require the addition of lithium or an atypical antipsychotic, and/or discontinuation of viloxazine

When Not to Prescribe

- If patient is taking an MAO inhibitor (except as noted under Drug Interactions)
- If patient is taking a sensitive CYP1A2 substrate or CYP1A2 substrates with a narrow therapeutic range
- If there is a proven allergy to viloxazine

Long-Term Use

- Long-term data are not available

Habit Forming

- No

Overdose

- Limited experience; drowsiness, impaired consciousness, diminished reflexes, and increased heart rate have been reported with overdose of immediate-release viloxazine

DOSING AND USE

Usual Dosage Range

- Ages 6 to 11: 100–400 mg once daily
- Ages 12 to 17: 200–400 mg once daily

Dosage Forms

- Extended-release capsule 100 mg, 150 mg, 200 mg

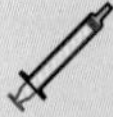

How to Dose

- Ages 6 to 11: initial dose 100 mg once daily; can increase by 100 mg each week; maximum recommended dose 400 mg once daily
- Ages 12 to 17: initial dose 200 mg once daily; can increase by 100 mg each week; maximum recommended dose 400 mg once daily

Options for Administration

- Capsule can be opened and the contents sprinkled over applesauce

Tests

- Blood pressure (sitting and standing) and pulse should be measured at baseline and monitored following dose increases and periodically during treatment
- Monitor weight and height

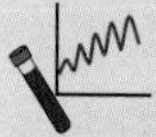

Pharmacokinetics

- Bioavailability of viloxazine extended-release relative to an immediate-release formulation is about 88%
- Linear kinetics over a dosage range from 100 mg to 600 mg once daily
- Steady-state reached after 2 days of once-daily administration
- Time to peak plasma concentration of viloxazine (Tmax) is 5 hours (range: 3 to 9 hours)
- Food decreases viloxazine Cmax and AUC by about 10% and slows absorption by 2 hours
- Viloxazine is 76–82% bound to plasma proteins
- Half-life is about 7 hours and the medication reaches steady state quickly; however, just one or two missed doses can drop blood levels to nearly zero (Figure 1)
- Metabolized primarily by CYP2D6, UGT1A9, and UGT2B15 (Figure 2)

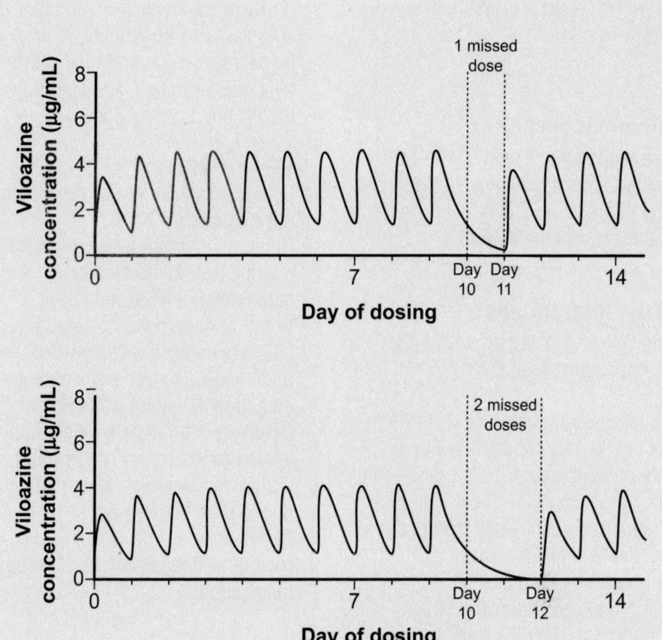

Figure 1 Concentration–time curves for viloxazine demonstrating the impact of 1 (top) or 2 (bottom) missed doses. From Nasser et al., 2021.

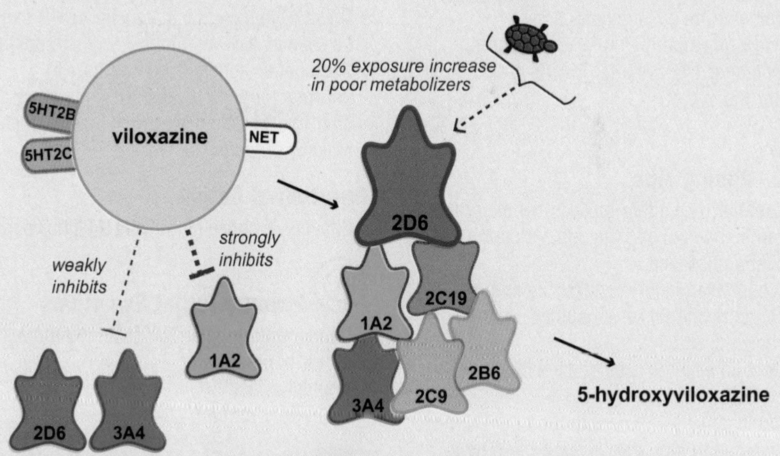

Figure 2 Viloxazine metabolism.

- Inhibits CYP1A2 (strong), CYP2D6 (weak), and CYP3A4 (weak)

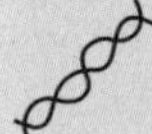

Pharmacogenetics

- No recommendations; however, CYP2D6 poor metabolizers have increased Cmax and AUC_{0-24} by about 20 and 25%, respectively, compared to normal metabolizers

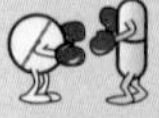

Drug Interactions

- Via strong CYP1A2 inhibition, viloxazine may increase exposure of CYP1A2 substrates
- Use of viloxazine with sensitive CYP1A2 substrate or CYP1A2 substrates with a narrow therapeutic range is contraindicated
- Viloxazine administered with caffeine (a CYP1A2 substrate) can cause jitteriness and excessive stimulation due to a 6-fold increase in caffeine exposure
- Via CYP2D6 inhibition, viloxazine may reduce clearance of CYP2D6 substrates (e.g., atomoxetine, venlafaxine, risperidone), and thus require dosage reduction
- Via CYP3A4 inhibition, viloxazine may reduce clearance of CYP3A4 substrates (e.g., avanafil, buspirone, triazolam), and thus require dosage reduction
- Use with caution with MAO inhibitors, including 14 days after MAOIs are stopped (for the expert)

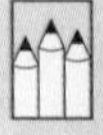

Dosing Tips

- Capsules can either be taken whole or they can be opened and the contents sprinkled over applesauce
- When taken in applesauce, the entire contents should be consumed, without chewing, within 2 hours
- Dose of a single capsule should not be divided
- Can be given with or without food. However, giving with food delays absorption by 2 hours.

How to Switch

- Generally, try to stop the first agent before starting a new drug so that side effects from the new medication can be distinguished from withdrawal effects of the first agent
- Side effects from abrupt discontinuation are not expected
- If urgent, can usually cross taper from a stimulant to a nonstimulant, or vice versa, by decreasing the first medication perhaps by a quarter to half, and starting the new medication at a low dose

How to Stop

- Side effects from abrupt discontinuation are not expected
- However, if withdrawal symptoms develop, resume dosing the medication and then taper slowly over several days
- Withdrawal following chronic therapeutic use may unmask symptoms of the underlying disorder and may require follow-up and reinstitution of treatment
- Usually symptoms after discontinuation of viloxazine are return of symptoms of the underlying disorder rather than symptoms due to drug withdrawal
- Supervision during withdrawal is always recommended for any psychotropic medication

WHAT TO EXPECT

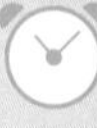

Onset of Action

- Onset of therapeutic actions in ADHD can be seen as early as the first week of dosing
- Therapeutic actions may continue to improve for 8–12 weeks; early response after two weeks of treatment may predict efficacy outcomes at week 6

Duration of Action

- Effects are consistent over a 24-hour period

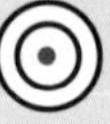

Primary Target Symptoms

- Concentration, attention span, distractibility
- Motor hyperactivity
- Impulsiveness
- Depressed mood

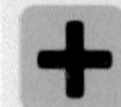

What Is Considered a Positive Result?

- The goal of treatment of ADHD is reduction of symptoms of inattentiveness, motor hyperactivity, and/or impulsiveness that disrupt social, school, and/or occupational functioning
- The goal of treatment is complete remission of symptoms

- If treatment works, it most often reduces or even eliminates symptoms, but is not a cure since symptoms often recur after medicine is stopped

How Long to Treat

- ADHD is typically a lifelong illness; if any symptoms improve, hyperactivity is more likely to improve than inattention
- Can tell parents there is some chance that their child can grow out of this in adulthood, but many adults continue to have symptoms of ADHD throughout adolescence and adulthood
- Continue treatment until all symptoms are under control or improvement is stable and then continue treatment as long as improvement persists
- Reevaluate the need for treatment periodically; some clinicians advise to periodically taper ADHD medication in patients who are not severely symptomatic to observe how the patient responds, but not routinely done by most clinicians
- Treatment for ADHD begun in childhood may need to be continued into adolescence and adulthood if continued benefit is documented

What If It Stops Working?

- Some patients may experience apparent lack of consistent efficacy due to activation of latent or underlying or newly evolved bipolar disorder, major depressive episodes with mixed features of mania, new onset of major depression or an anxiety disorder (GAD, OCD, PD), and require medication discontinuation and a switch to the clinically appropriate medication(s)

What If It Doesn't Work?

- In practice, many patients have only a partial response where some symptoms are improved but others persist, in which case higher doses of viloxazine, adding a second agent, or switching to an agent with a different mechanism of action can be considered
- Consider evaluation for another diagnosis or for a comorbid condition (e.g., medical illness, substance abuse). Also, when treating ADHD, consider the possibility of a learning disorder or learning weakness and consider school-based interventions.
- Consider the presence of nonadherence and counsel patient and parents
- Some ADHD patients and some depressed patients may experience lack of consistent efficacy due to activation of latent or underlying bipolar disorder, and require either augmenting with a mood stabilizer or switching to a mood stabilizer
- Augmenting options:
  - Cognitive behavioral therapy (CBT)
  - Parent Management Training (PMT)
  - Behavioral modification
  - Coordinating with school for appropriate support
  - Best to attempt other monotherapies prior to augmenting
  - Augmentation with a stimulant is commonly used for treatment-resistant ADHD symptoms, especially inattention and hyperactivity
  - Augmentation with an alpha 2 agonist can be used for treatment-resistant ADHD symptoms, especially oppositional and aggressive/impulsive behaviors
  - Triple therapy with a stimulant, alpha 2 agonist, and viloxazine for especially treatment-resistant cases is for the expert
  - Can combine with modafinil, methylphenidate, or amphetamine for ADHD. Methylphenidate and lisdexamfetamine do not affect concentrations of viloxazine.
  - For the expert, can occasionally combine with mood stabilizers or atypical antipsychotics in highly treatment-resistant cases of bipolar disorder including bipolar disorder comorbid with ADHD
- Consider factors associated with poor response to any psychotropic medication in children and adolescents, such as severe symptoms, long-lasting symptoms, poor treatment adherence, prior nonresponse to other treatments, and the presence of comorbid psychiatric disorders or learning disorders
- Consider other important potential factors such as ongoing conflicts, family psychopathology, and an adverse environment (e.g., poverty, chaos, violence, prior and ongoing psychological trauma, abuse, bullying, less than ideal school placement, neglect)
- Institute trauma-informed care for appropriate children and adolescents

TALKING TO PATIENTS AND CAREGIVERS

What to Tell Parents About Efficacy

- Doesn't work right away; full therapeutic benefits may take 2–6 weeks
- This medicine generally takes longer to start working than stimulants for ADHD
- It is not a stimulant
- While the medicine helps ADHD by reducing symptoms and improving function, there are no cures for ADHD and it is therefore necessary to keep taking the medication to sustain its therapeutic effects
- Since every treatment consideration depends on a risk/benefit analysis, parents should fully understand short- and long-term risks as well as benefits compared to nontreatment of ADHD
- Often a good idea to tell parents whether the medication chosen is specifically approved for the disorder being treated, or whether it is being given for "unapproved" or "off-label" reasons based on good clinical practice, expert consensus, and/or prudent extrapolation of controlled data from adults
- Best results are often obtained when medications are combined with behavioral therapy
- The American Academy of Child & Adolescent Psychiatry (AACAP) has helpful handouts for parents

What to Tell Children and Adolescents About Efficacy

- Be specific about the symptoms being targeted: we are trying to help you remember things better, do your best at school, follow the rules, get into less trouble (as applicable)
- It may be a good idea to give the medication a try; if it's not working very well, we can stop the medication and try something else
- You can be part of a special plan to help us figure out if the medicine is helpful for you. Would you like to do that? (for the parents and prescriber, can consider here a trial both on and then off medication, and then on again to see if the effects are clear and thus worth continuing the medication)
- A good try takes about 2 months
- Even if it does make you feel better, it will wear off and no longer work shortly after you stop it
- The medication can help you decide what you want to do, like making good choices versus bad choices; the medicine does not make you do something you don't want to do
- Medications don't change who you are as a person; they give you the opportunity to be the best person you can be

What to Tell Parents About Side Effects

- Explain that side effects are expected in many when starting
- Tell parents many side effects go away and do so about the same time that therapeutic effects start
- Predict side effects in advance (you will look clever and competent to the parents, unless you scare them with too much information and cause nocebo effects, in which case you won't look so clever when the patient develops lots of side effects and stops medication; use your judgment here); a balanced but honest presentation is an art rather than a science
- Tell them this medication works like some antidepressants, and all antidepressants have a warning in children and adolescents for increased suicidality (i.e., suicidal thoughts and behavior), but the FDA studies did not show any actual suicides in any age group nor risk beyond age 24 and this was observed in children and adolescents with depression, not ADHD
- Ask them to help monitor for these symptoms and if present, report any such symptoms immediately
- Ask parents to support the patient while side effects are occurring
- Parents should fully understand short- and long-term risks as well as benefits
- Explaining to the parents what to expect from medication treatment, and especially what potential side effects to expect, can help prevent early termination

What to Tell Children and Adolescents About Side Effects

- When a medicine starts to work, your body can first experience this by giving you unpleasant sensations – just like if you take a cough medicine it may taste bad – these body sensations include loss of appetite and feeling tired or sleepy. So, just like with a cough medicine, the bad taste will often

go away before the medicine begins to stop the cough – many medicines work like that. It's important for you to pay attention to what your body is telling you, and we'll go over some of the ways that can happen.
- Even if you get a side effect, it's not permanent (it won't last forever)
- Explaining to child/adolescent what to expect from medication treatment, and especially potential side effects, can help prevent early termination
- Tell adolescents and children capable of understanding that some young patients, especially those who are depressed, may develop thoughts of hurting themselves, and if this happens, not to be alarmed but to tell their parents right away

What to Tell Teachers About the Medication (If Parents Consent)

- Viloxazine can be helpful in improving the symptoms of ADHD: namely, inattention, impulsivity, and hyperactivity
- Some students will experience side effects from the medications that you may notice in or outside the classroom; many of these side effects can be modified
- If the patient is sleepy, ask whether the medication is keeping them up at night or if they are eating enough food

SPECIAL POPULATIONS

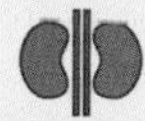

Renal Impairment

- Severe impairment [estimated glomerular filtration rate (eGFR) < 30 mL/min/1.73 m^2]: initial dose 100 mg once daily; can increase by 50–100 mg each week; maximum recommended dose 200 mg once daily
- Mild to moderate impairment (eGFR 30 to 89 mL/min/1.73 m^2): dose adjustment not necessary

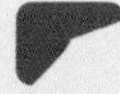

Hepatic Impairment

- Not recommended

Cardiac Impairment

- Use with caution because viloxazine can increase heart rate and blood pressure
- At a dose 3 times the maximum recommended dose, viloxazine does not prolong the QTc interval
- No effect on the PR interval or QRS duration; however, nonclinical studies suggest the potential to inhibit cardiac sodium channels

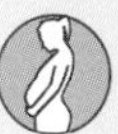

Pregnancy

- Controlled studies have not been conducted in pregnant women
- In rats, administration of viloxazine during organogenesis did not result in significant maternal toxicity but did cause fetal toxicities and delayed fetal development at doses 2 times the maximum recommended human dose (MRHD)
- In rabbits, administration of viloxazine during organogenesis caused maternal toxicity without significant fetal toxicity at doses ≥7 times the MRHD
- The no observed adverse effect levels (NOAELs) for fetal toxicity are approximately equal to 11 times the MRHD, based on mg/m^2 in rats and rabbits
- In rats and mice, administration of viloxazine during pregnancy and lactation caused maternal toxicities and deaths at doses approximately 2 and 1 times the MRHD, based on mg/m^2, respectively; at these maternally toxic doses, viloxazine caused offspring toxicities
- The NOAEL for maternal and developmental toxicity is approximately equal to or less than the MRHD, based on mg/m^2, in the rat and mouse, respectively
- Use in women of childbearing potential requires weighing potential risks and benefits to the mother against potential risks to the fetus
- For women of childbearing potential, viloxazine should generally be discontinued before anticipated pregnancies
- National Pregnancy Registry for Psychiatric Medications: 1-866-961-2388 or http://womensmentalhealth.org/clinical-and-research-programs/pregnancyregistry/

Breast Feeding

- Unknown if viloxazine is secreted in human breast milk, but all psychotropics assumed to be secreted in breast milk
- Recommend either to discontinue drug or formula feed

THE ART OF PSYCHOPHARMACOLOGY

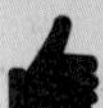

Potential Advantages

- In children:
  - For patients whose parents do not want them to take a stimulant or who cannot tolerate or do not respond to stimulants
- In adolescents:
  - For patients who have a history of diverting or abusing stimulants
  - Can improve school performance and grades, especially if ADHD has been unrecognized and untreated prior to adolescence
  - Can improve performance in high school and college students whose ADHD is compromising academic performance due to the increased demands of higher levels of study
- All ages:
  - No known abuse potential; not a controlled substance
  - No withdrawal reactions
  - Only nonstimulant with the option to open the capsule and sprinkle contents on applesauce for patients who cannot/won't swallow pills

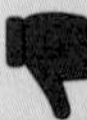

Potential Disadvantages

- In children:
  - Those who are psychomotor agitated, angry, or irritable, and who do not have a psychiatric diagnosis
  - Possible activation of suicidality/bipolar disorder
- In adolescents:
  - Those who may possibly have an untreated mood or anxiety disorder or who refuse treatment for them
  - Possible activation of suicidality/bipolar disorder
- All ages:
  - May not act as rapidly as stimulants when initiating treatment in some patients
  - May not act as robustly as stimulants in some patients
  - Those who need to take drugs that are CYP1A2 substrates

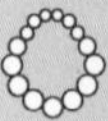

Pearls

- Can be a first-line treatment for children or adolescents who wish to avoid a trial of a stimulant and may produce faster response compared to atomoxetine
- Unlike stimulants, viloxazine is not abusable and has little or no value to friends of adolescent patients who may otherwise divert stimulant medications, especially when responsible for self-administration of medication in college settings
- Despite its name as a selective norepinephrine reuptake inhibitor, viloxazine also increases serotonin, presumably through its agonist actions at 5HT2B and 5HT2C receptors, which may contribute to its efficacy in depression and also suggests efficacy in anxiety disorders
- Viloxazine enhances both dopamine and norepinephrine in the frontal cortex, presumably accounting for its therapeutic actions on attention and concentration
- Since dopamine is inactivated by norepinephrine reuptake in the frontal cortex, which largely lacks dopamine transporters, viloxazine can increase dopamine as well as norepinephrine in this part of the brain, presumably causing therapeutic actions in ADHD
- Since dopamine is inactivated by dopamine reuptake in the nucleus accumbens, which largely lacks norepinephrine transporters, viloxazine does not increase dopamine in this part of the brain, presumably explaining why viloxazine lacks abuse potential
- Viloxazine has proven efficacy as an antidepressant and has been approved for depression in Europe for over 20 years
- Unlike stimulants, viloxazine may not exacerbate tics in Tourette syndrome patients with comorbid ADHD
- Does not improve tics in Tourette syndrome patients

SUGGESTED READING

Faraone SV, Gomeni R, Hull JT et al. Early response to SPN-812 (viloxazine extended-release) can predict efficacy outcome in pediatric subjects with ADHD: a machine learning post-hoc analysis of four randomized clinical trials. Psychiatry Res 2021;296:113664. doi: 10.1016/j.psychres.2020.113664.

Nasser A, Liranso T, Adewole T et al. Once-daily SPN-812 200 and 400 mg in the treatment of ADHD in school-aged children: a phase III randomized, controlled trial. Clin Ther 2021;43(4):684–700.

Nasser A, Gomeni R, Wang Z et al. Population pharmacokinetics of viloxazine extended-release capsules in pediatric subjects with attention deficit/hyperactivity disorder. J Clin Pharmacol 2021;61(12):1626–37.

Nasser A, Liranso T, Adewole T et al. A phase 3, placebo-controlled trial of once-daily viloxazine extended-release capsules in adolescents with attention-deficit/hyperactivity disorder. J Clin Psychopharmacol 2021;41(4):370–80.

Pliszka S ; AACAP Work Group on Quality Issues. Practice parameter for the assessment and treatment of children and adolescents with attention-deficit/hyperactivity disorder. J Am Acad Child Adolesc Psychiatry 2007;46(7):894–921.

THERAPEUTICS

Brands

- Trintellix

Generic

No

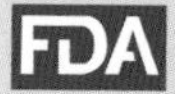

US FDA Approved for Pediatric Use

- None

Off-Label for Pediatric Use

- Approved in adults
  - Major depressive disorder
  - Other off-label uses
  - Anxiety

Class and Mechanism of Action

- Neuroscience-based Nomenclature: serotonin multimodal (S-MM)
- Increases release of several different neurotransmitters (serotonin, norepinephrine, dopamine, glutamate, acetylcholine, and histamine) and reduces the release of GABA through 3 different modes of action:
  - Mode 1: blocks serotonin reuptake pump (serotonin transporter)
  - Mode 2: binds to G protein-linked receptors (full agonist at serotonin 1A receptors; partial agonist at serotonin 1B receptors, antagonist at serotonin 1D and serotonin 7 receptors)
  - Mode 3: binds to ion channel-linked receptors (antagonist at serotonin 3 receptors)
- Full agonist actions at presynaptic somatodendritic serotonin 1A autoreceptors may theoretically enhance serotonergic activity and contribute to antidepressant actions
- Full agonist actions at postsynaptic serotonin 1A receptors may theoretically diminish sexual dysfunction caused by serotonin reuptake inhibition
- Antagonist actions at serotonin 3 receptors may theoretically enhance noradrenergic, acetylcholinergic, and glutamatergic activity and contribute to antidepressant and procognitive actions
- Antagonist actions at serotonin 3 receptors may theoretically reduce nausea and vomiting caused by serotonin reuptake inhibition
- Antagonist actions at serotonin 7 receptors may theoretically contribute to antidepressant and pro-cognitive actions as well as reduce insomnia caused by serotonin reuptake inhibition
- Partial agonist actions at serotonin 1B receptors may enhance not only serotonin release, but also acetylcholine and histamine release
- Antagonist actions at serotonin 1D receptors may enhance serotonin release

SAFETY AND TOLERABILITY

Notable Side Effects

- Several central nervous system side effects (insomnia but also sedation, especially if not sleeping at night, agitation, headache, dizziness)
- Note: patients with diagnosed or undiagnosed bipolar or psychotic disorders may be more vulnerable to CNS-activating actions of serotonergic agents like vortioxetine; pay particular attention to signs of activation in children with developmental disorders or autism spectrum disorders
- Treatment-emergent activation syndrome (TEAS) includes agitation, anxiety, panic attacks, irritability, aggression, impulsivity, and insomnia
- TEAS can represent side effects but should not be confused with bipolar mania or the onset of suicidality and should be monitored and investigated with consideration of discontinuing or decreasing the dose of vortioxetine or addition of another agent or switching to another agent to reduce these symptoms
- Gastrointestinal (nausea, diarrhea, constipation, dry mouth)
- Sexual dysfunction (boys: delayed ejaculation, erectile dysfunction; boys and girls: decreased sexual desire, anorgasmia)
- Bruising and rare bleeding
- Syndrome of inappropriate antidiuretic hormone secretion (SIADH)

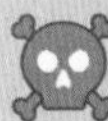

Life-Threatening or Dangerous Side Effects

- Rare seizures
- Rare induction of mania
- Rare suicidal ideation and behavior (suicidality) (short-term regulatory studies did not show any actual suicides in any age group and also did not show an increase in the risk of suicidality with antidepressants compared to placebo beyond age 24)

Growth and Maturation

- Growth should be monitored; long-term effects are unknown

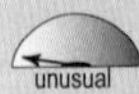

Weight Gain

- Reported but not common

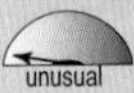

Sedation

- Reported but not common

What to Do About Side Effects

- Wait, wait, wait: mild side effects are common, happen early, and usually improve with time, but treatment benefits can be delayed and often begin just as the side effects wear off. However, some side effects may emerge later such as weight gain.
- Monitor side effects closely, especially when initiating treatment
- May wish to give in the evening or at bedtime, particularly if the medication is associated with sedation
- For activation (jitteriness, anxiety, insomnia):
  - Consider a temporary dose reduction or a more gradual up-titration
  - Administer dose in the morning
  - Consider switching to an SSRI or potentially an SNRI (other than venlafaxine)
  - Optimize psychotherapeutic interventions
  - Activation and agitation may represent the induction of a bipolar state, especially a mixed dysphoric bipolar II condition sometimes associated with suicidal ideation, and may require the addition of lithium, or an atypical antipsychotic, and/or discontinuation of vortioxetine
- Often best to try another monotherapy prior to resorting to augmentation strategies to treat side effects
- For insomnia: consider adding melatonin
- For GI upset: try giving medication with a meal
- For sexual dysfunction:
  - Probably best to reduce dose or discontinue and try another agent
  - Consider adding daytime exercise, bupropion, or buspirone
- For emotional flattening, apathy: consider adding bupropion (with caution as little experience in children)

How Drug Causes Side Effects

- Theoretically due to increases in serotonin concentrations at serotonin receptors in parts of the brain and body other than those that cause therapeutic actions (e.g., unwanted actions of serotonin in sleep centers causing insomnia, unwanted actions of serotonin in the gut causing diarrhea)
- Increasing serotonin can cause diminished dopamine release and might contribute to emotional flattening, cognitive slowing, and apathy in some patients

Warnings and Precautions

- Consider distributing the brochures provided by the FDA and the drug companies as well as the medication guides from the American Academy of Child & Adolescent Psychiatry (AACAP)
- Carefully consider monitoring patients regularly and within the practical limits, particularly during the first several weeks of treatment
- Warn patients and their caregivers when possible about the possibility of activating side effects and advise them to report such symptoms
- Carefully weigh the risks and benefits of pharmacological treatment against the risks and benefits of nontreatment with antidepressants and make sure to document this in the patient's chart
- As with any antidepressant, use with caution in patients with history of seizure
- As with any antidepressant, use with caution in patients with bipolar disorder unless treated with concomitant mood-stabilizing agent
- Monitor patients for activation and suicidal ideation and involve parents/guardians

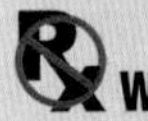

When Not to Prescribe

- If patient is taking an MAO inhibitor
- If there is a proven allergy to vortioxetine

Long-Term Use

- Growth should be monitored; long-term effects are unknown

Habit Forming

- No

Overdose

- No fatalities have been reported; nausea, dizziness, diarrhea, abdominal discomfort, generalized pruritus, somnolence, flushing

DOSING AND USE

Usual Dosage Range

- 10–20 mg/day

Dosage Forms

- Tablet 5 mg, 10 mg, 20 mg

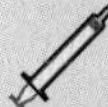

How to Dose

- In children, initiate at 5 mg daily for 2 weeks and then increase to 10 mg. May increase to 20 mg following 4 weeks of treatment at 10 mg.
- In adolescents, 10 mg daily for 1 month and then increase to 20 mg

Options for Administration

- Only available as a tablet

Tests

- None for healthy individuals

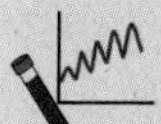

Pharmacokinetics

- Metabolized by CYP2D6, CYP3A4/5, CYP2C19, CYP2C9, CYP2A6, CYP2C8, and CYP2B6 (Figure 1). The main metabolites formed are pharmacologically inactive
- Vortioxetine is readily absorbed after ingestion and reaches peak plasma concentrations (Cmax) within 5–6.5 hours in children and between 4–8 hours in adolescents (Figure 2) (Findling et al., 2017)
- The bioavailability of vortioxetine is approximately 75% and it is highly protein-bound (greater than 98%) to human plasma proteins, primarily albumin
- In adults, the elimination half-life of vortioxetine is about 66 hours, meaning it takes several days for the drug to be eliminated from the body. However, in children,

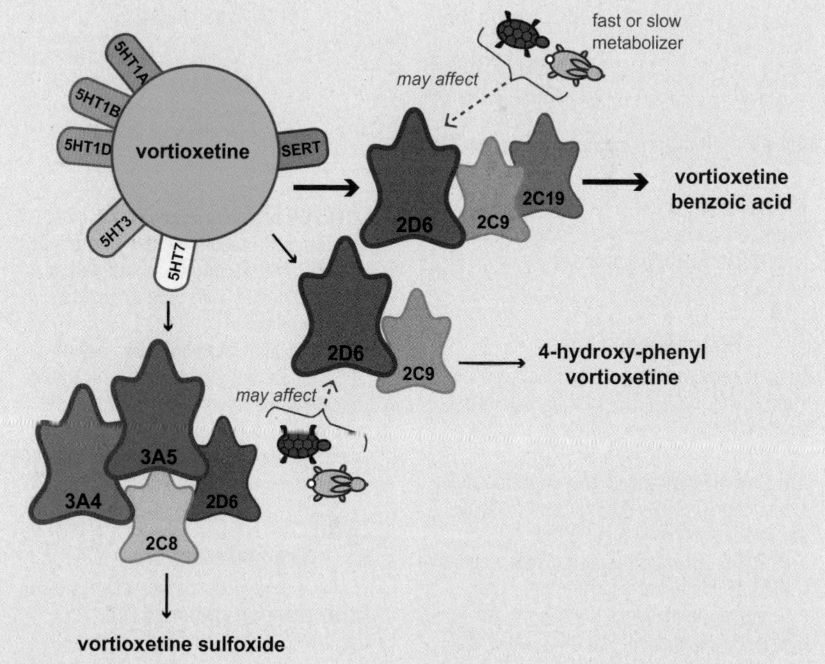

Figure 1 Vortioxetine metabolism.

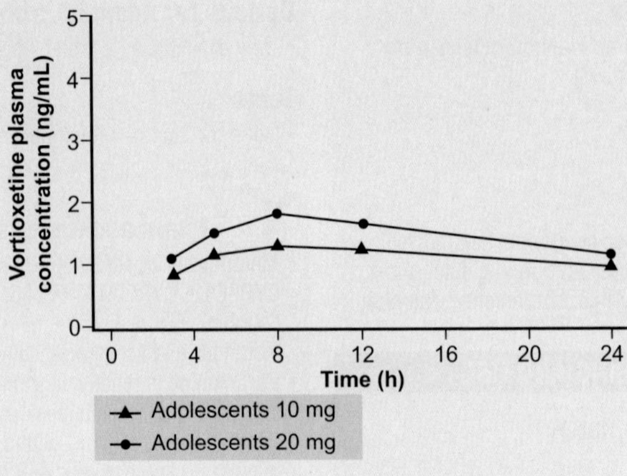

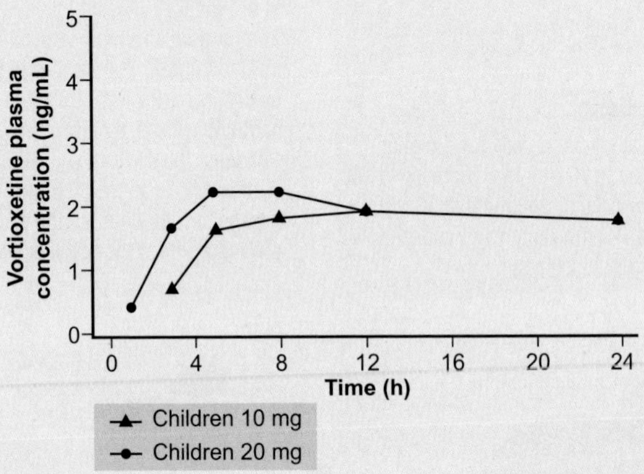

Figure 2 Vortioxetine concentration over 24 hours.

its elimination half-life is between 45 and 70 hours, while in adolescents it is between 40 and 56 hours (Findling et al., 2017).

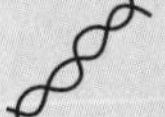

Pharmacogenetics

- In one small pediatric study, clearance was slower in CYP2D6 poor metabolizers than in CYP2D6 intermediate or normal metabolizers (Findling et al., 2017)
- The Clinical Pharmacogenetics Implementation Consortium provides dosing recommendations for vortioxetine based on CYP2D6:
  - **CYP2D6 ultrarapid metabolizers:** Initiate therapy at standard starting dose and titrate to maintenance dose based on efficacy and side effects. Increasing the target maintenance dose by 50% or more may be needed for efficacy.
  - **CYP2D6 normal metabolizers:** Initiate therapy with recommended starting dose
  - **CYP2D6 intermediate metabolizers:** Initiate therapy with recommended starting dose
  - **CYP2D6 poor metabolizers:** Initiate 50% of starting dose (e.g., 5 mg) and titrate to the maximum recommended dose of 10 mg, or consider a clinically appropriate alternative antidepressant not predominantly metabolized by CYP2D6

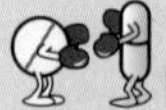

Drug Interactions

- Tramadol increases the risk of seizures in adults taking an antidepressant
- Can cause a fatal "serotonin syndrome" when combined with MAO inhibitors, so do

not use with MAO inhibitors or for at least 14 days after MAOIs are stopped
- Do not start an MAO inhibitor for at least 5 half-lives (5 to 7 days for most drugs) after discontinuing vortioxetine
- Strong CYP2D6 inhibitors can increase plasma levels of vortioxetine, possibly requiring its dose to be decreased
- Broad CYP2D6 inducers can decrease plasma levels of vortioxetine, possibly requiring its dose to be increased
- Possible increased risk of bleeding

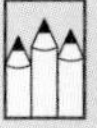

Dosing Tips

- Can be taken with or without food
- Tablet should not be divided, crushed, or dissolved
- The more anxious and agitated the patient, the lower the starting dose, the slower the titration
- If intolerable anxiety, insomnia, agitation, akathisia, or activation occurs either upon dosing initiation or discontinuation, consider an alternative SRI. Importantly, the risk of activation with one SRI does not predict the likelihood of activation with another SRI.

How to Switch

- From another antidepressant to vortioxetine:
  - When tapering a prior antidepressant, see its entry in this manual for how to stop and how to taper off that specific drug
  - In situations when there are antidepressant-related side effects, try to stop the first agent before starting vortioxetine so that new side effects of vortioxetine can be distinguished from withdrawal effects of the first agent
  - If necessary, can cross taper off the prior antidepressant and dose up on vortioxetine simultaneously in urgent situations, being aware of all specific drug interactions to avoid
- From vortioxetine to another antidepressant
  - Generally, try to stop vortioxetine before starting another antidepressant
  - Stopping vortioxetine often means tapering off since discontinuing many antidepressants can cause withdrawal symptoms; however, tapering may not be necessary with recommended doses

How to Stop

- Tapering may not be necessary with recommended doses

WHAT TO EXPECT

Onset of Action

- Some patients may experience increased energy or activation early after initiation of treatment
- Full onset of therapeutic actions is usually delayed by 2–4 weeks
- If it is not working within 6–8 weeks, it may require a dosage increase or it may not work at all

Duration of Action

- Effects are consistent over a 24-hour period
- May continue to work for many years to prevent relapse of symptoms

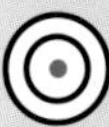

Primary Target Symptoms

- Depressed and/or irritable mood
- Anxiety (fear and worry are often target symptoms, but vortioxetine can occasionally and transiently increase these symptoms short term before improving them)
- Sleep disturbance, both hypersomnia and insomnia (eventually, but can actually cause insomnia, especially short term)
- Prior to initiation of treatment, it is helpful to develop a list of target symptoms of depression and/or anxiety to monitor during treatment to better assess treatment response

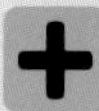

What Is Considered a Positive Result?

- The goal of treatment is complete remission of current symptoms as well as prevention of future relapses
- In practice, many patients have only a partial response where some symptoms are improved but others persist (especially insomnia, fatigue, and problems concentrating in depression), in which case higher doses of vortioxetine, adding a second agent, or switching to an agent with a different mechanism of action can be considered
- If treatment works, it most often reduces or even eliminates symptoms, but is not a cure since symptoms can recur after medicine is stopped

How Long to Treat

- For adolescents with depression, generally, 9–12 months of antidepressant treatment is recommended (Hathaway et al., 2018)
- For anxiety disorders, 6–9 months of antidepressant treatment may be sufficient, though many clinicians extend treatment to 12 months based on extrapolation of data from adults with anxiety disorders (Hathaway et al., 2018; Strawn et al., 2023)
- Extended treatment periods may decrease the risk of long-term morbidity and recurrence; however, the goal of treatment is ultimately remission, rather than duration of antidepressant pharmacotherapy (Hathaway et al., 2018)
- In terms of the length of antidepressant treatment, evidence-based guidelines represent a starting point; appropriate treatment duration varies, and patient-specific response, psychological factors, and timing of discontinuation must be considered for individual pediatric patients (Hathaway et al., 2018)

What If It Stops Working?

- Some patients who have an initial response may relapse even though they continue treatment, sometimes called "poop-out"
- Some patients may experience apparent lack of consistent efficacy due to activation syndrome or latent or underlying or newly evolved bipolar disorder, or major depressive episodes with mixed features, and require antidepressant discontinuation and a switch to a second generation antipsychotic

What If It Doesn't Work?

- Consider evaluation for another diagnosis (especially bipolar illness or depression with mixed features) or for a comorbid condition (e.g., medical illness, substance abuse)
- When treating youth with anxiety disorders, many patients will have had significant anxiety for years prior to beginning treatment. As such, when anxiety is treated with an SRI, their symptoms may be improved, but the patient has likely missed important developmental milestones (e.g., spending the night with friends, being able to ask questions in class). Developing these skills will take time. Beyond this, the family may have lived with the anxious child for years and following treatment of the child, the family may need to readjust.
- Be mindful of family conflict contributing to the presentation; sometimes treating parental depression or anxiety disorders improves psychiatric and social function without any treatment of youth. Also, accommodation is common in families of youth with anxiety disorders and may need to be addressed specifically, as it can perpetuate symptoms.
- Consider factors associated with poor response to SRIs in treatment-resistant depression or anxiety disorders, such as severe symptoms, long-lasting symptoms, poor treatment adherence, prior nonresponse to other treatments, and the presence of comorbid disorders
- Consider other important potential factors such as ongoing conflicts, family psychopathology, and an adverse environment (e.g., poverty, chaos, violence, prior and ongoing psychological trauma, abuse, neglect). Additionally, when symptoms are prominent at school, consider the presence of a learning disorder.
- Institute trauma-informed care for appropriate children and adolescents
- A 2007 meta-analysis of published and unpublished trials in pediatric patients found that antidepressants had a number needed to treat (NNT) of 10 for depression, 6 for OCD, and 3 for anxiety disorders; thus, vortioxetine may not work in all children, so consider switching to another antidepressant (Bridge et al., 2007)
- Consider a dose adjustment
- Consider augmenting options:
  - Cognitive behavioral therapy (CBT), interpersonal psychotherapy for adolescents (IPT-A), light therapy, family therapy, and exercise especially in adolescents
  - For partial response (depression): use caution when adding medications to vortioxetine, especially in children, since there are not sufficient studies of augmentation in children or adolescents; however, for the expert, consider bupropion, aripiprazole, or other atypical antipsychotics such as quetiapine; use combinations of antidepressants with

caution as this may activate bipolar disorder and suicidal ideation
- For insomnia: sleep hygiene, CBT for insomnia, melatonin, or alpha 2 agonists
- For anxiety: buspirone, antihistamines
- Add lithium or atypical antipsychotics for bipolar depression, psychotic depression, treatment-resistant depression, or treatment-resistant anxiety disorders
- TMS (transcranial magnetic stimulation) may have a role although pediatric trials of TMS have been hampered by high sham response rates (Croarkin et al., 2021)
- ECT (case studies show effectiveness; cognitive side effects are similar to those in adults; reserve for treatment-resistant cases)

TALKING TO PATIENTS AND CAREGIVERS

What to Tell Parents About Efficacy

- Doesn't work right away; full therapeutic benefits may take up to 8 weeks, yet parents and teachers might see improvement before the patient does
- While the medicine helps by reducing symptoms and improving function, it is not a cure, and it is therefore necessary to keep taking the medication to sustain its therapeutic effects
- Since every treatment consideration depends on a risk/benefit analysis, parents should fully understand short- and long-term risks as well as benefits
- After successful treatment, continuation of vortioxetine may be necessary to prevent relapse, especially in those who have had more than one episode or a very severe episode. In general, when treating depression in children and adolescents, medications are continued for 12 months after symptoms have resolved, while for anxiety disorders, clinicians have generally treated for 6–9 months (Hathaway et al., 2018).
- Often a good idea to tell parents whether the medication chosen is specifically approved for the disorder being treated, or if it is "unapproved" or "off-label" but nevertheless good clinical practice and based upon prudent extrapolation of controlled data from adults and from experience in children and adolescents instead of formal FDA approval

What to Tell Children and Adolescents About Efficacy

- We are trying to make you feel better
- It may be a good idea to give the medication a try; if it's not working very well, we can stop the medication and try something else
- A good try takes 2 to 3 months or even longer
- If it does make you feel better, you cannot stop it right away or you may feel sad or worried again
- Medications don't change who you are as a person; they give you the opportunity to be the best person you can be

What to Tell Parents About Side Effects

- Explain that side effects are expected in many when starting and are most common in the first 2–3 weeks of starting or increasing the dose
- Some antidepressant side effects emerge early and resolve quickly (e.g., activation, gastrointestinal symptoms). In contrast, other side effects are late-emerging (e.g., weight gain) or persistent (e.g., sexual dysfunction). Discussing the temporal course of the side effects and distinguishing between persistent and transient side effects is critical. Ensuring that patients are aware not only of side effects but the tendency of some side effects to be transient is important and should be part of discussions with patients and their families. For many, knowing that a side effect is likely transient, as opposed to persistent, may significantly influence the patient and family's anxiety or fears related to medication (Strawn et al., 2023).
- Tell parents many side effects go away and do so about the same time that therapeutic effects start
- Predict side effects in advance (you will look clever and competent to the parents, unless you scare them with too much information and cause nocebo effects, in which case you won't look so clever when the patient develops lots of side effects and stops medication; use your judgment here); a balanced but honest presentation is an art rather than a science
- Ask them to help monitor for increased suicidality and if present, report any such symptoms immediately
- Ask parents to support the patient while side effects are occurring

- Parents should fully understand short- and long-term risks as well as benefits
- Explaining to the parents what to expect from medication treatment, and especially potential side effects, can help prevent early termination of medication

What to Tell Children and Adolescents About Side Effects

- Even if you get side effects, most of them get better or go away in a few days to a few weeks
- Consider having a conversation about sexual side effects in some adolescents who can find these side effects confusing and especially burdensome
- Explaining to child/adolescent what to expect from medication treatment, and especially potential side effects, can help prevent early termination of medication
- Tell adolescents and children capable of understanding that some young patients, especially those who are depressed, may develop thoughts of hurting themselves, and if this happens, not to be alarmed but to tell their parents right away

What to Tell Teachers About the Medication (If Parents Consent)

- It is not abusable
- Encourage dialogue with parents/guardians about any behavior or mood changes

SPECIAL POPULATIONS

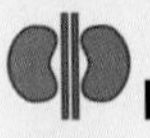

Renal Impairment

- No dose adjustment necessary

Hepatic Impairment

- No dose adjustment necessary for mild to moderate impairment
- Has not been studied in patients with severe hepatic impairment

Cardiac Impairment

- Not systematically evaluated in patients with cardiac impairment

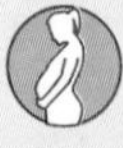

Pregnancy

- Controlled studies have not been conducted in pregnant women
- Not generally recommended for use during pregnancy, especially during first trimester
- Nonetheless, continuous treatment during pregnancy may be necessary and has not been proven to be harmful to the fetus
- At delivery there may be more bleeding in the mother and transient irritability or sedation in the newborn
- Must weigh the risk of treatment (first trimester fetal development, third trimester newborn delivery) to the child against the risk of no treatment (recurrence of depression, maternal health, infant bonding) to the mother and child
- For many patients, this may mean continuing treatment during pregnancy
- Exposure to SSRIs early in pregnancy may be associated with increased risk of septal heart defects (absolute risk is small)
- SSRI use beyond the 20th week of pregnancy may be associated with increased risk of pulmonary hypertension in newborns, although this is not proven
- Exposure to SSRIs late in pregnancy may be associated with increased risk of gestational hypertension and preeclampsia
- Neonates exposed to SSRIs or SNRIs late in the third trimester have developed complications requiring prolonged hospitalization, respiratory support, and tube feeding; reported symptoms are consistent with either a direct toxic effect of SSRIs and SNRIs or, possibly, a drug discontinuation syndrome, and include respiratory distress, cyanosis, apnea, seizures, temperature instability, feeding difficulty, vomiting, hypoglycemia, hypotonia, hypertonia, hyperreflexia, tremor, jitteriness, irritability, and constant crying
- National Pregnancy Registry for Psychiatric Medications: 1-866-961-2388 or https://womensmentalhealth.org/research/pregnancyregistry/

Breast Feeding

- Unknown if vortioxetine is secreted in human breast milk, but all psychotropics assumed to be secreted in breast milk
- Trace amounts may be present in nursing children whose mothers are on vortioxetine
- If child becomes irritable or sedated, breast feeding or drug may need to be discontinued

- Immediate postpartum period is a high-risk time for depression, especially in women who have had prior depressive episodes, so drug may need to be reinstituted late in the third trimester or shortly after childbirth to prevent a recurrence during the postpartum period
- Must weigh benefits of breast feeding with risks and benefits of antidepressant treatment versus nontreatment to both the infant and the mother
- For many patients, this may mean continuing treatment during breast feeding

THE ART OF PSYCHOPHARMACOLOGY

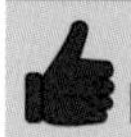

Potential Advantages

- Patients who wish to avoid sexual dysfunction

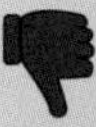

Potential Disadvantages

- Double-blind, randomized, placebo-controlled trial did not demonstrate efficacy of vortioxetine in adolescents with major depressive disorder, but this trial was complicated by a very high placebo response rate

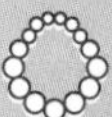

Pearls

- May have less sexual dysfunction than SSRIs
- Multiple studies show pro-cognitive effects greater than a comparator antidepressant in adult patients with major depressive episodes; however, this has not been explored in youth
- Patients who do not respond to antidepressants with other mechanisms of action may respond to vortioxetine

SUGGESTED READING

Bousman CA, Stevenson JM, Ramsey LB et al. Clinical Pharmacogenetics Implementation Consortium (CPIC) Guideline for CYP2D6, CYP2C19, CYP2B6, SLC6A4, and HTR2A genotypes and serotonin reuptake inhibitor antidepressants. Clin Pharmacol Ther 2023;114(1):51–68.

Bridge JA, Iyengar S, Salary CB et al. Clinical response and risk for reported suicidal ideation and suicide attempts in pediatric antidepressant treatment: a meta-analysis of randomized controlled trials. JAMA 2007;297(15):1683–96.

Croarkin PE, Elmaadawi AZ, Aaronson ST et al. Left prefrontal transcranial magnetic stimulation for treatment-resistant depression in adolescents: a double-blind, randomized, sham-controlled trial. Neuropsychopharmacology 2021;46(2):462–9.

Findling RL, Robb AS, DelBello M et al. Pharmacokinetics and safety of vortioxetine in pediatric patients. J Child Adolesc Psychopharmacol 2017;27(6):526–34.

Findling RL, DelBello MP, Zuddas A et al. Vortioxetine for major depressive disorder in adolescents: 12-week randomized, placebo-controlled, fluoxetine-referenced, fixed-dose study. J Am Acad Child Adolesc Psychiatry 2022;61(9):1106–18.e2.

Hathaway EE, Walkup JT, Strawn JR. Antidepressant treatment duration in pediatric depressive and anxiety disorders: how long is long enough? Curr Probl Pediatr Adolesc Health Care 2018;48(2):31–9.

Strawn JR, Mills JA, Poweleit EA, Ramsey LB, Croarkin PE. Adverse effects of antidepressant medications and their management in children and adolescents. Pharmacotherapy 2023;43(7):675–90.

THERAPEUTICS

Brands
- Ambien
- Ambien CR
- Intermezzo, other

Generic
Yes

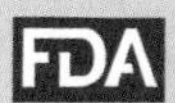

US FDA Approved for Pediatric Use
- None

Off-Label for Pediatric Use
- Approved in adults
  - Short-term treatment of insomnia (controlled-release indication is not restricted to short term)
  - As needed for the treatment of insomnia when a middle-of-the-night awakening is followed by difficulty returning to sleep and there are at least 4 hours of bedtime remaining before the planned time of wakening (Intermezzo)

Class and Mechanism of Action
- Neuroscience-based Nomenclature: GABA positive allosteric modulator (GABA-PAM)
- Nonbenzodiazepine hypnotic; alpha 1 isoform selective agonist of GABA-A/ benzodiazepine receptors

SAFETY AND TOLERABILITY

Notable Side Effects
- Sedation
- Dizziness, ataxia
- Dose-dependent amnesia
- Hyperexcitability, nervousness
- Diarrhea, nausea
- Headache
- Rare hallucinations

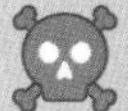

Life-Threatening or Dangerous Side Effects
- Respiratory depression, especially when taken with other CNS depressants in overdose
- Rare angioedema

Growth and Maturation
- Not studied

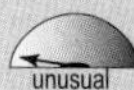

Weight Gain
- Reported but not expected

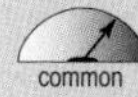

Sedation
- Many experience and/or can be significant in amount

What to Do About Side Effects
- Wait
- To avoid problems with memory, only take zolpidem or zolpidem CR if planning to have a full night's sleep
- Lower the dose
- Switch to a shorter-acting sedative-hypnotic or melatonin

How Drug Causes Side Effects
- Actions at benzodiazepine receptors that carry over to the next day can cause daytime sedation, amnesia, and ataxia
- Long-term adaptations of zolpidem immediate-release not well studied, but chronic studies of zolpidem CR and other alpha 1 selective nonbenzodiazepine hypnotics suggest lack of notable tolerance or dependence developing over time

Warnings and Precautions
- Insomnia may be a symptom of a primary disorder, rather than a primary disorder itself
- Some patients may exhibit abnormal thinking or behavioral changes similar to those caused by other CNS depressants (i.e., either depressant actions or disinhibiting actions)
- Some depressed patients may experience worsening of suicidal ideation
- Use only with extreme caution in patients with impaired respiratory function or obstructive sleep apnea
- Zolpidem and zolpidem CR should only be administered at bedtime
- Temporary memory loss may occur at doses above 10 mg/night in adults
- Rare angioedema has occurred with sedative-hypnotic use and could potentially cause fatal airway obstruction if it involves

the throat, glottis, or larynx; thus if angioedema occurs, treatment should be discontinued
- Sleep driving and other complex behaviors, such as eating and preparing food and making phone calls, have been reported in patients taking sedative-hypnotics; in some cases, these behaviors have resulted in serious injury or death, prompting the FDA to require a boxed warning

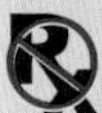

When Not to Prescribe
- If the patient has experienced an episode of complex sleep behaviors after taking a sleep medication
- If there is a proven allergy to zolpidem
- For Intermezzo, if the patient has fewer than 4 hours of bedtime remaining before the planned time of waking

Long-Term Use
- Increased wakefulness during the latter part of the night (wearing off) or an increase in daytime anxiety (rebound) may occur

Habit Forming
- Zolpidem is a Schedule IV drug
- Some patients may develop dependence and/or tolerance; risk may be greater with higher doses
- History of drug addiction may increase risk of dependence

Overdose
- No fatalities reported with zolpidem monotherapy; sedation, ataxia, confusion, hypotension, respiratory depression, coma

DOSING AND USE

Usual Dosage Range
- 0.25 mg/kg up to a dose of 10 mg at bedtime (immediate-release)
- 6.25–12.5 mg/day at bedtime (controlled-release)

Dosage Forms
- Immediate-release tablet 5 mg, 10 mg
- Immediate-release capsule 7.5 mg
- Extended-release tablet 6.25 mg, 12.5 mg
- Sublingual tablet 1.75 mg, 3.5 mg, 5 mg, 10 mg

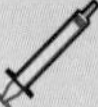

How to Dose
- In children, 2.5 mg to 5 mg initially or 6.25 mg initially if using the controlled-release formulation
- In adolescents, 5 mg initially or 6.25 mg initially if using the controlled-release formulation
- Post-pubertally, based on recommendations for adults, adolescent girls may begin lower doses compared to adolescent boys
- Adult men: 10 mg at bedtime for 7–10 days (immediate-release); 12.5 mg at bedtime for 7–10 days (controlled-release); 3.5 mg sublingually in the middle of the night if more than 4 hours of bedtime remain (Intermezzo)
- Adult women: 5 mg at bedtime for 7–10 days (immediate-release); 6.25 mg at bedtime for 7–10 days (controlled-release); 1.75 mg sublingually in the middle of the night if more than 4 hours of bedtime remain (Intermezzo)
- Intermezzo formulation is administered sublingually in the middle of the night; it should be placed under the tongue and allowed to dissolve completely before swallowing
- Intermezzo formulation should not be taken more than once per night

Options for Administration
- Low-dose sublingual tablet for middle-of-the-night administration

Tests
- None for healthy individuals

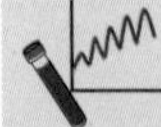

Pharmacokinetics
- Rapidly and well absorbed after oral administration
- Reaches peak plasma concentrations within 1 to 2 hours after ingestion in adults, 55 minutes after ingestion in children up to age 6, 60 minutes after ingestion in children between 7 and 12 years, and 80 minutes after administration in adolescents between 13 and 17 years (Blumer et al., 2008) (Figure 1)
- Food slightly delays absorption, but it does not significantly affect the overall extent of absorption

- Moderate volume of distribution, which means it is distributed throughout the body's tissues. It readily crosses the blood–brain barrier, leading to its rapid onset of action in inducing sleep.
- Undergoes extensive metabolism in the liver, via CYP3A4 and multiple other cytochromes (Figure 2). It is metabolized into several inactive metabolites, the main one being zolpidem carboxylic acid. Some of the metabolites may still have some activity at the GABA-A receptors, but their contribution to the overall pharmacological effects is minimal.
- Elimination half-life of zolpidem varies among individuals but is typically around 2.3 hours in children and adolescents (Blumer et al., 2008)

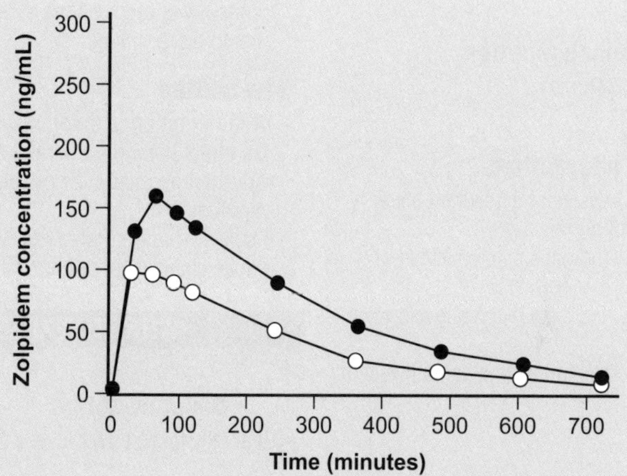

Figure 1 Concentration–time curves for immediate-release zolpidem in children and adolescents. Open circles represent 0.125 mg/kg and closed circles represent 0.5 mg/kg. Adapted from Blumer et al., 2008.

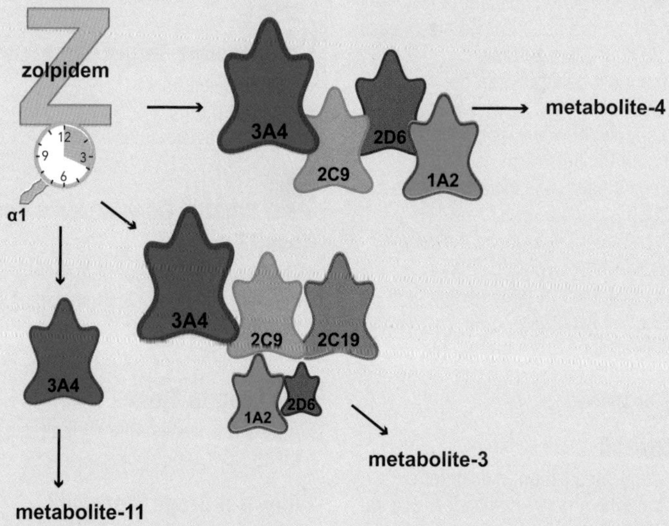

Figure 2 Zolpidem metabolism.

- Clearance decreases with age in pediatric patients, with children younger than 6 having a clearance of 12 mL/min/kg compared to about 10 mL/min/kg in children ages 7–12 and 5 mL/min/kg in adolescents 13–17 (Blumer et al., 2008)
- The majority of zolpidem and its metabolites are excreted in the urine, primarily as metabolites. Only a small amount is excreted unchanged in the urine.

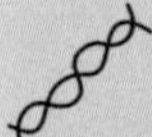

Pharmacogenetics

- No recommendations

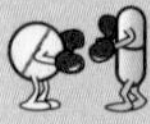

Drug Interactions

- Increased depressive effects when taken with other CNS depressants
- Sertraline may increase plasma levels of zolpidem
- Rifampin may decrease plasma levels of zolpidem
- Ketoconazole may increase plasma levels of zolpidem

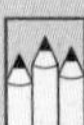

Dosing Tips

- Zolpidem is not absorbed as quickly if taken with food, which could reduce onset of action
- Patients with lower body weights may require only a 5 mg dose immediate-release or 6.25 mg controlled-release
- Zolpidem should generally not be prescribed in quantities greater than a 1-month supply; however, zolpidem CR is not restricted to short-term use
- Risk of dependence may increase with dose and duration of treatment
- However, treatment with alpha 1 selective nonbenzodiazepine hypnotics may cause less tolerance or dependence than benzodiazepine hypnotics
- Controlled-release tablets should be swallowed whole and should not be divided, crushed, or chewed

How to Switch

- From another medication to zolpidem:
  - When tapering a prior medication, see its entry in this manual for how to stop and how to taper off that specific drug
  - Generally, try to stop the first agent before starting zolpidem so that new side effects of zolpidem can be distinguished from withdrawal effects of the first agent
- From zolpidem to another medication:
  - Generally, try to stop zolpidem before starting the new medication so that new side effects of the next drug can be distinguished from any withdrawal effects from zolpidem
  - Taper; may need to adjust dosage of concurrent medications as zolpidem is being discontinued

How to Stop

- Although rebound insomnia could occur, this effect has not generally been seen with therapeutic doses of zolpidem or zolpidem CR
- If taken for more than a few weeks, taper to reduce chances of withdrawal effects

WHAT TO EXPECT

Onset of Action

- Generally takes effect in less than an hour

Duration of Action

- Duration of action is generally 2–4 hours for immediate-release and 6–8 hours for controlled-release

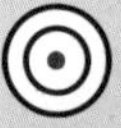

Primary Target Symptoms

- Time to sleep onset
- Total sleep time
- Nighttime awakenings

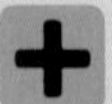

What Is Considered a Positive Result?

- The goal of treatment of insomnia is to improve quality of sleep, including effects on total wake time and number of nighttime awakenings

How Long to Treat

- After a few weeks, discontinue use or use on an "as-needed" basis

What If It Stops Working?

- Consider an alternative medication or melatonin and re-trying CBT-I

What If It Doesn't Work?

- If insomnia does not improve, it may be a manifestation of a primary psychiatric or physical illness, which requires independent evaluation. Also, re-trying other interventions for insomnia may be helpful.

TALKING TO PATIENTS AND CAREGIVERS

What to Tell Parents About Efficacy

- While the medicine helps by reducing symptoms and improving function, it is not a cure, and it is therefore necessary to keep taking the medication to sustain its therapeutic effects
- Since every treatment consideration depends on a risk/benefit analysis, parents should fully understand short- and long-term risks as well as benefits
- Often a good idea to tell parents whether the medication chosen is specifically approved for the disorder being treated, or whether it is being given for "unapproved" or "off-label" reasons based on good clinical practice, expert consensus, and/or prudent extrapolation of controlled data from adults

What to Tell Children and Adolescents About Efficacy

- We are trying to make you feel better
- It may be a good idea to give the medication a try; if it's not working very well, we can stop the medication and try something else

What to Tell Parents About Side Effects

- Explain that mild side effects are expected at initiation or when increasing the dose and are usually transitory
- Predict side effects in advance (you will look clever and competent to the parents, unless you scare them with too much information and cause nocebo effects, in which case you won't look so clever when the patient develops lots of side effects and stops medication; use your judgment here); a balanced but honest presentation is an art rather than a science
- Ask parents to support the patient while side effects are occurring
- Parents should fully understand short- and long-term risks as well as benefits
- Explaining to the parents what to expect from medication treatment, and especially potential side effects, can help prevent early termination of medication

What to Tell Children and Adolescents About Side Effects

- Even if you get side effects, most of them get better or go away in a few days to a few weeks; however, we will likely not use this medication for a long time
- Explaining to child/adolescent what to expect from medication treatment, and especially potential side effects, can help prevent early termination of medication

What to Tell Teachers About the Medication (If Parents Consent)

- Zolpidem can make children/adolescents sleepy
- Encourage dialogue with parents/guardians about any behavior or mood changes

SPECIAL POPULATIONS

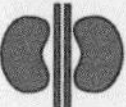

Renal Impairment

- No dose adjustment necessary
- Patients should be monitored

Hepatic Impairment

- Recommended dose 5 mg (immediate-release), 6.25 mg (controlled-release), 1.75 mg (Intermezzo)
- Patients should be monitored

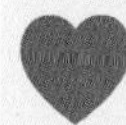

Cardiac Impairment

- No available data

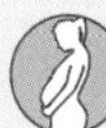

Pregnancy

- Controlled studies have not been conducted in pregnant women
- In animal studies, oral administration of zolpidem did not indicate a risk for adverse effects on fetal development at clinically relevant doses

- Infants whose mothers took sedative hypnotics during pregnancy may experience some withdrawal symptoms
- Neonatal flaccidity has been reported in infants whose mothers took sedative hypnotics during pregnancy

Breast Feeding

- Some drug is found in breast milk
- Recommended either to discontinue drug or formula feed

THE ART OF PSYCHOPHARMACOLOGY

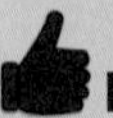

Potential Advantages

- May be helpful for initial insomnia in adolescents who have not responded to first- and second-line interventions for insomnia

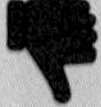

Potential Disadvantages

- Can have carryover effects
- Lack of controlled data in pediatric patients

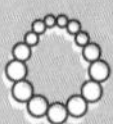

Pearls

- In a controlled study assessing zolpidem for the treatment of insomnia in children and adolescents with ADHD, zolpidem (0.25 mg/kg per day to a maximum of 10 mg) failed to reduce the latency to persistent sleep on polysomnographic recordings after 4 weeks of treatment (Blumer et al., 2009)
  - However, zolpidem was thought to be effective in adolescents – but not in children – with separation from placebo seen at weeks 4 and 8 (Blumer et al., 2009)
  - Despite data from adults, the pediatric trials did not observe next-day residual effects or rebound phenomena after discontinuation (Blumer et al., 2009)
- In some patients, zolpidem blood levels may be high enough the morning after use to impair activities that require alertness, including driving; this prompted the FDA to issue revised dosing requirements for adults
- Specifically, because clearance of zolpidem is slightly slower in adult women than in adult men, the FDA has required that the recommended dose be lowered for women
- A low-dose zolpidem product is approved in adults for middle-of-the-night awakenings by sublingual administration
- Not a benzodiazepine itself, but binds to benzodiazepine receptors
- May have fewer carryover side effects than some other sedative hypnotics

SUGGESTED READING

Blumer JL, Reed MD, Steinberg F et al.; NICHD PPRU Network. Potential pharmacokinetic basis for zolpidem dosing in children with sleep difficulties. Clin Pharmacol Ther 2008;83(4):551–8.

Blumer JL, Findling RL, Shih WJ, Soubrane C, Reed MD. Controlled clinical trial of zolpidem for the treatment of insomnia associated with attention-deficit/ hyperactivity disorder in children 6 to 17 years of age. Pediatrics 2009;123(5):e770–6.

Appendix

Anxiety

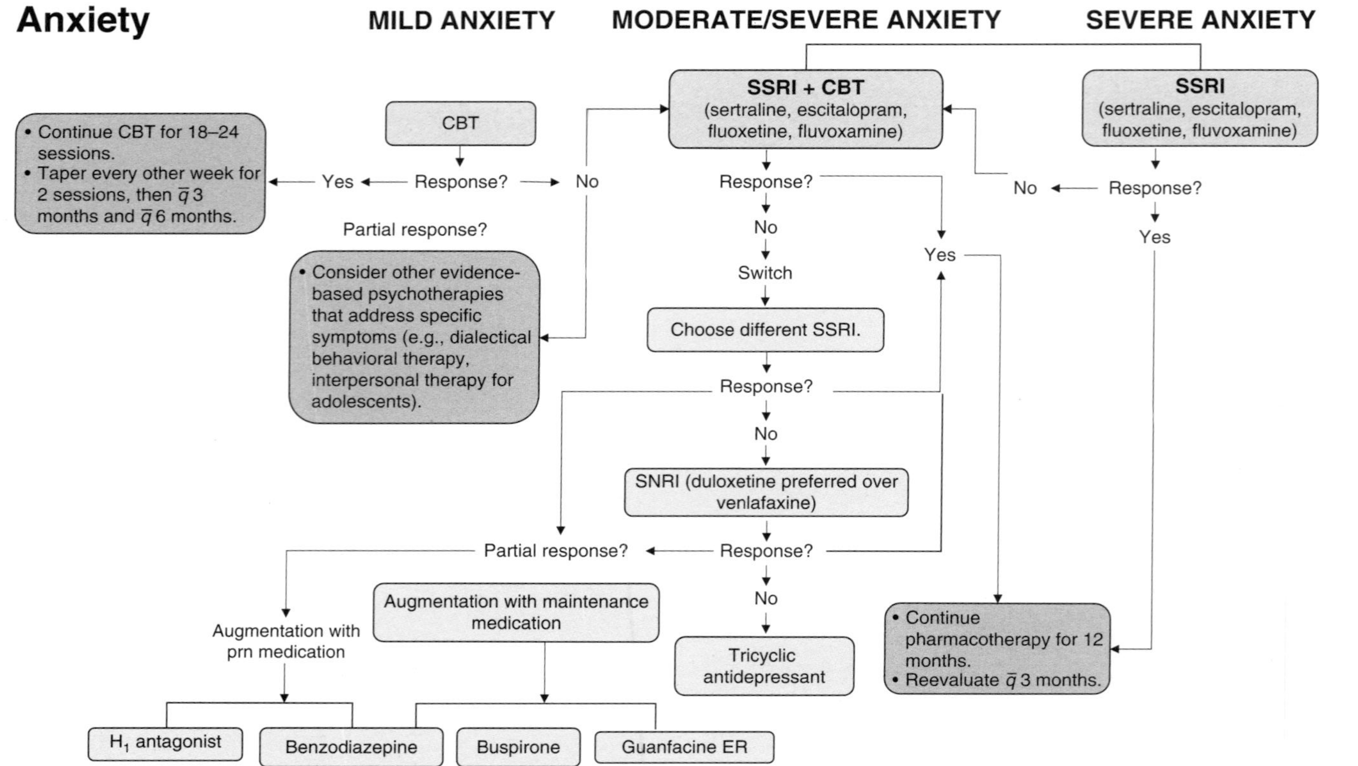

MILD ANXIETY
MODERATE/SEVERE ANXIETY
SEVERE ANXIETY
CBT
Response?
Yes
No
Partial response?
• Continue CBT for 18–24 sessions.
• Taper every other week for 2 sessions, then q̄ 3 months and q̄ 6 months.
• Consider other evidence-based psychotherapies that address specific symptoms (e.g., dialectical behavioral therapy, interpersonal therapy for adolescents).
SSRI + CBT
(sertraline, escitalopram, fluoxetine, fluvoxamine)
Response?
No
Switch
Choose different SSRI.
Response?
No
SNRI (duloxetine preferred over venlafaxine)
Response?
No
Tricyclic antidepressant
Yes
Partial response?
Augmentation with prn medication
Augmentation with maintenance medication
H1 antagonist
Benzodiazepine
Buspirone
Guanfacine ER
SSRI
(sertraline, escitalopram, fluoxetine, fluvoxamine)
Response?
No
Yes
• Continue pharmacotherapy for 12 months.
• Reevaluate q̄ 3 months.

ADHD

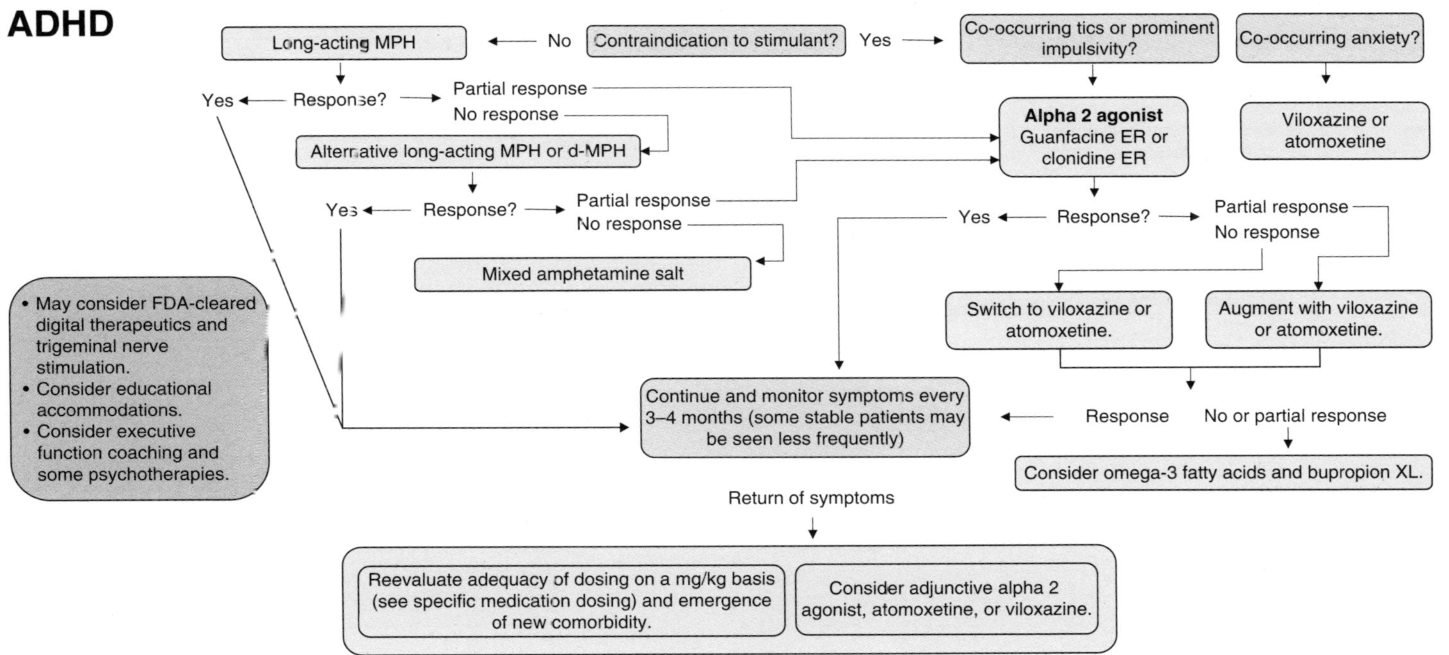

Long-acting MPH
No
Contraindication to stimulant?
Yes
Co-occurring tics or prominent impulsivity?
Co-occurring anxiety?
Yes
Response?
Partial response
No response
Alpha 2 agonist
Guanfacine ER or clonidine ER
Viloxazine or atomoxetine
Alternative long-acting MPH or d-MPH
Yes
Response?
Partial response
No response
Yes
Response?
Partial response
No response
Mixed amphetamine salt
Switch to viloxazine or atomoxetine.
Augment with viloxazine or atomoxetine.
• May consider FDA-cleared digital therapeutics and trigeminal nerve stimulation.
• Consider educational accommodations.
• Consider executive function coaching and some psychotherapies.
Continue and monitor symptoms every 3–4 months (some stable patients may be seen less frequently)
Response
No or partial response
Consider omega-3 fatty acids and bupropion XL.
Return of symptoms
Reevaluate adequacy of dosing on a mg/kg basis (see specific medication dosing) and emergence of new comorbidity.
Consider adjunctive alpha 2 agonist, atomoxetine, or viloxazine.

Bipolar Disorder

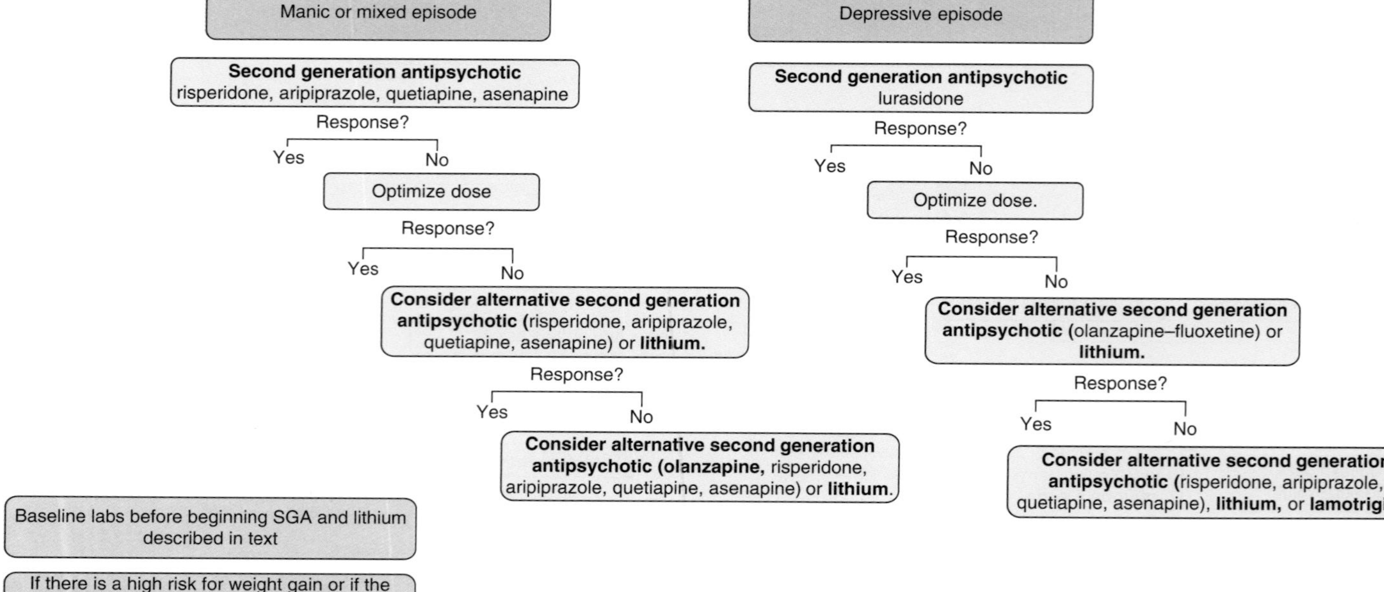

Insomnia

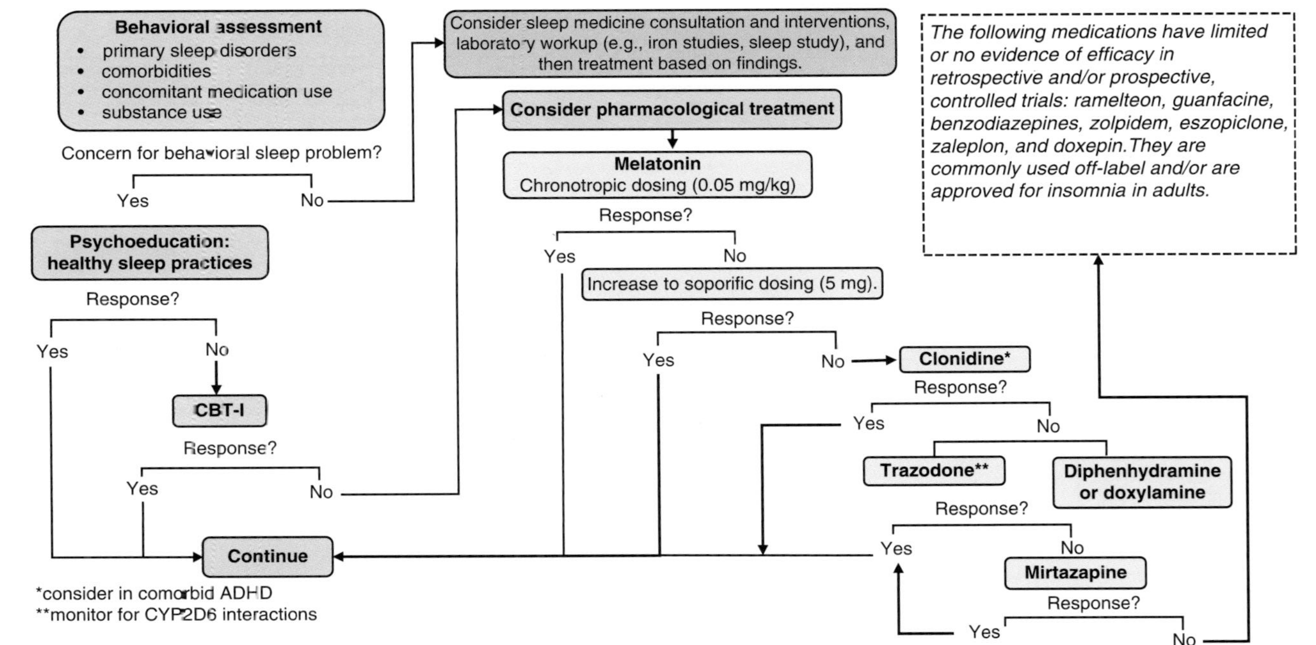
Behavioral assessment
primary sleep disorders
comorbidities
concomitant medication use
substance use
Concern for behavioral sleep problem?
Yes
No
Consider sleep medicine consultation and interventions, laboratory workup (e.g., iron studies, sleep study), and then treatment based on findings.
Psychoeducation: healthy sleep practices
Response?
Yes
No
CBT-I
Response?
Yes
No
Consider pharmacological treatment
Melatonin
Chronotropic dosing (0.05 mg/kg)
Response?
Yes
No
Increase to soporific dosing (5 mg).
Response?
Yes
No
Clonidine*
Response?
Yes
No
Trazodone**
Diphenhydramine or doxylamine
Response?
Yes
No
Mirtazapine
Response?
Yes
No
Continue
The following medications have limited or no evidence of efficacy in retrospective and/or prospective, controlled trials: ramelteon, guanfacine, benzodiazepines, zolpidem, eszopiclone, zaleplon, and doxepin. They are commonly used off-label and/or are approved for insomnia in adults.
*consider in comorbid ADHD
**monitor for CYP2D6 interactions

MDD

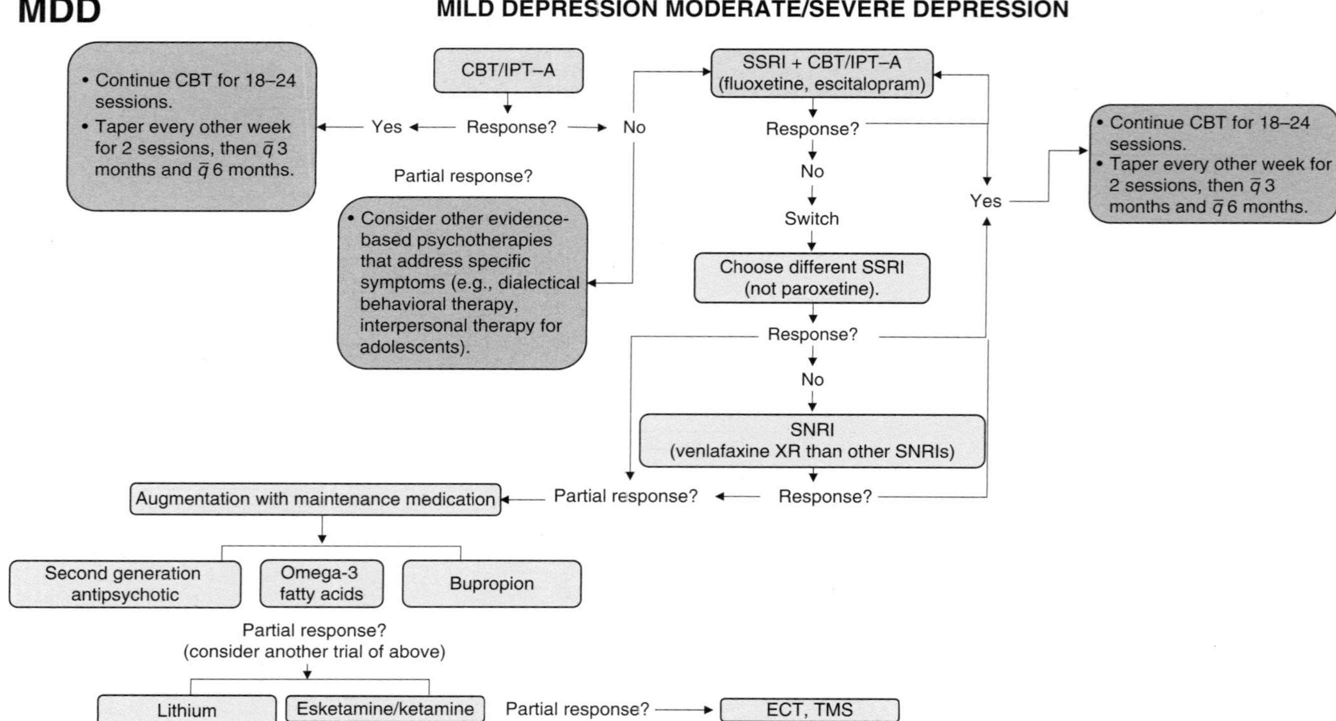

MILD DEPRESSION MODERATE/SEVERE DEPRESSION
CBT/IPT–A
Response?
Yes
No
• Continue CBT for 18–24 sessions.
• Taper every other week for 2 sessions, then $\bar{q}$ 3 months and $\bar{q}$ 6 months.
Partial response?
• Consider other evidence-based psychotherapies that address specific symptoms (e.g., dialectical behavioral therapy, interpersonal therapy for adolescents).
SSRI + CBT/IPT–A (fluoxetine, escitalopram)
Response?
No
Switch
Choose different SSRI (not paroxetine).
Response?
No
SNRI (venlafaxine XR than other SNRIs)
Response?
Yes
• Continue CBT for 18–24 sessions.
• Taper every other week for 2 sessions, then $\bar{q}$ 3 months and $\bar{q}$ 6 months.
Partial response?
Augmentation with maintenance medication
Second generation antipsychotic
Omega-3 fatty acids
Bupropion
Partial response? (consider another trial of above)
Lithium
Esketamine/ketamine
Partial response?
ECT, TMS

OCD

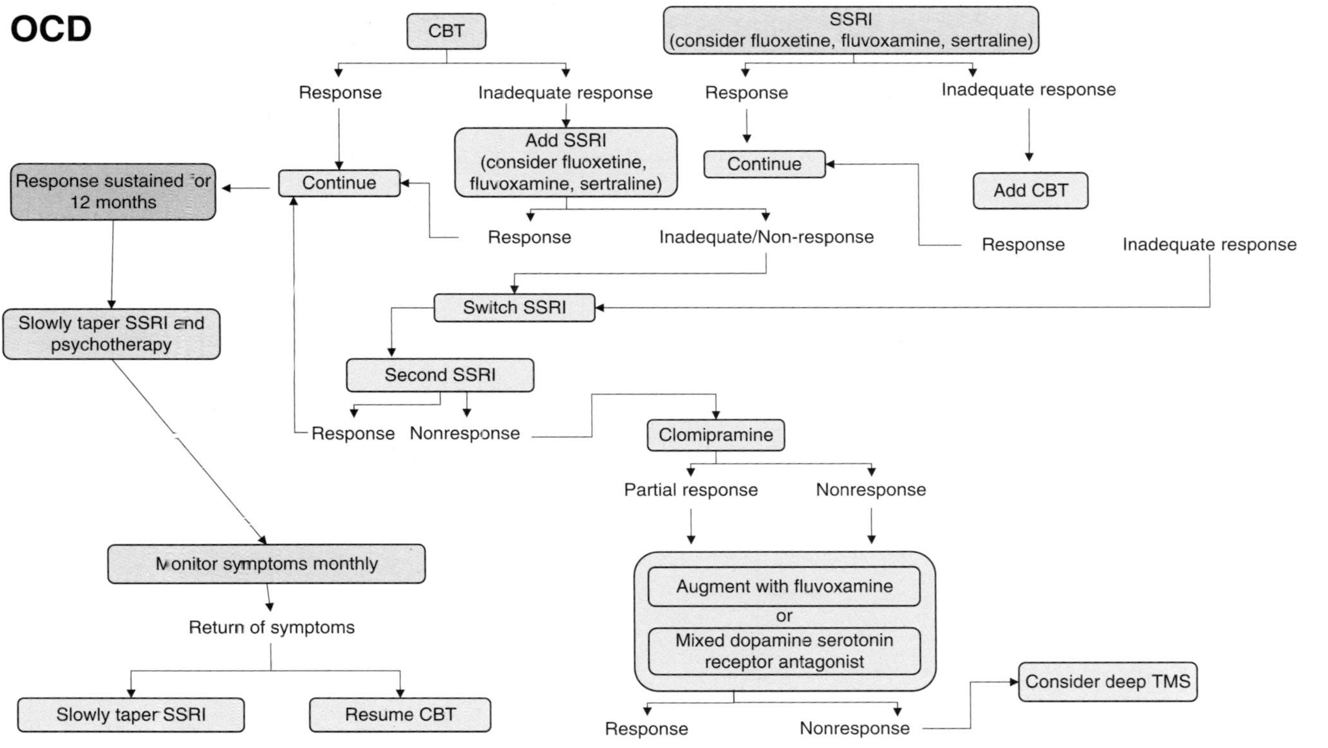

CBT
Response
Inadequate response
Continue
Add SSRI (consider fluoxetine, fluvoxamine, sertraline)
Response
Inadequate/Non-response
SSRI (consider fluoxetine, fluvoxamine, sertraline)
Response
Inadequate response
Continue
Add CBT
Response
Inadequate response
Response sustained for 12 months
Slowly taper SSRI and psychotherapy
Switch SSRI
Second SSRI
Response
Nonresponse
Clomipramine
Partial response
Nonresponse
Augment with fluvoxamine
or
Mixed dopamine serotonin receptor antagonist
Response
Nonresponse
Consider deep TMS
Monitor symptoms monthly
Return of symptoms
Slowly taper SSRI
Resume CBT

Stimulant Dosing Equivalents (Approximate)

Formulation		Regular methylphenidate
Concerta	18 mg once daily	10–15 mg total daily dose
	27 mg once daily	15–20 mg total daily dose
	36 mg once daily	20–30 mg total daily dose
	54 mg once daily	30–45 mg total daily dose
	72 mg once daily	40–60 mg total daily dose
QuilliChew ER	20 mg once daily	20 mg total daily dose
	30 mg once daily	30 mg total daily dose
	40 mg once daily	40 mg total daily dose
	50 mg once daily	50 mg total daily dose
	60 mg once daily	60 mg total daily dose
Aptensio XR	10 mg once daily	10 mg total daily dose
	20 mg once daily	20 mg total daily dose
	30 mg once daily	30 mg total daily dose
	40 mg once daily	40 mg total daily dose
	50 mg once daily	50 mg total daily dose
	60 mg once daily	60 mg total daily dose
Quillivant XR	20 mg once daily	20 mg total daily dose
	30 mg once daily	30 mg total daily dose
	40 mg once daily	40 mg total daily dose
	50 mg once daily	50 mg total daily dose
	60 mg once daily	60 mg total daily dose
Daytrana	10 mg once daily	10–20 mg total daily dose
	15 mg once daily	22.5 mg total daily dose
	20 mg once daily	20–30 mg total daily dose
	30 mg once daily	45 mg total daily dose
Cotempla XR-ODT	17.3 mg once daily	20 mg total daily dose
	25.9 mg once daily	30 mg total daily dose
	34.5 mg once daily	40 mg total daily dose
	43.1 mg once daily	50 mg total daily dose
	51.8 mg once daily	60 mg total daily dose
Jornay PM	20 mg once daily	12 mg total daily dose
	40 mg once daily	24 mg total daily dose
	60 mg once daily	36 mg total daily dose
	80 mg once daily	48 mg total daily dose
	100 mg once daily	60 mg total daily dose
Focalin, Focalin XR	10 mg total daily dose	20 mg total daily dose
	20 mg total daily dose	40 mg total daily dose
Azstarys (serdexmethylphenidate)	Begin with 39.2 mg/7.8 mg once daily	Any total daily dose

Formulation		Mixed salts amphetamine
Adzenys XR-ODT	3.1 mg once daily	5 mg total daily dose
	6.3 mg once daily	10 mg total daily dose
	9.4 mg once daily	15 mg total daily dose
	12.5 mg once daily	20 mg total daily dose
	15.7 mg once daily	25 mg total daily dose
	18.8 mg once daily	30 mg total daily dose
Dyanavel XR oral suspension and tablet	6.25 mg (2.5 mL) once daily	10 mg total daily dose
	12.5 mg (5 mL) once daily	20 mg total daily dose
	18.75 mg (7.5 mL) once daily	30 mg total daily dose
Mydayis	12.5 mg once daily	10 mg total daily dose
	25 mg once daily	20 mg total daily dose
Vyvanse (lisdexamfetamine)	30 mg once daily	10 mg total daily dose
	50 mg once daily	20 mg total daily dose
	70 mg once daily	30 mg total daily dose
Formulation		**Amphetamine base equivalence**
Mydayis	12.5 mg once daily	7.8 mg total daily dose
	25 mg once daily	15.6 mg total daily dose
	37.5 mg once daily	23.5 mg total daily dose
	50 mg once daily	31.3 mg total daily dose
Formulation		**D-Amphetamine equivalent**
Adderall XR	10 mg	7.5 mg
	20 mg	15 mg
	30 mg	22.5 mg
Xelstrym transdermal system	4.5 mg	5 mg
	9 mg	10 mg
	18 mg	20 mg
Vyvanse (lisdexamfetamine)	30 mg	8.9 mg
	70 mg	20.8 mg

2 to 20 years: Boys
Stature-for-age and Weight-for-age percentiles

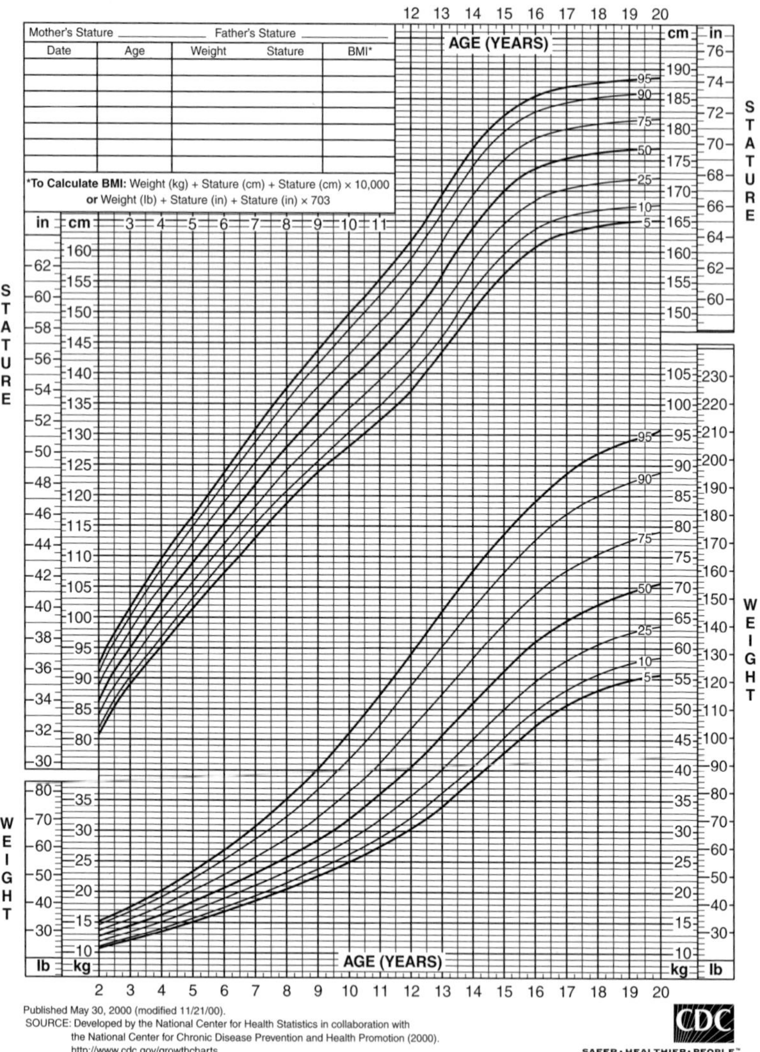

Published May 30, 2000 (modified 11/21/00).
SOURCE: Developed by the National Center for Health Statistics in collaboration with the National Center for Chronic Disease Prevention and Health Promotion (2000).
http://www.cdc.gov/growthcharts

CDC
SAFER • HEALTHIER • PEOPLE™

2 to 20 years: Girls
Stature-for-age and Weight-for-age percentiles

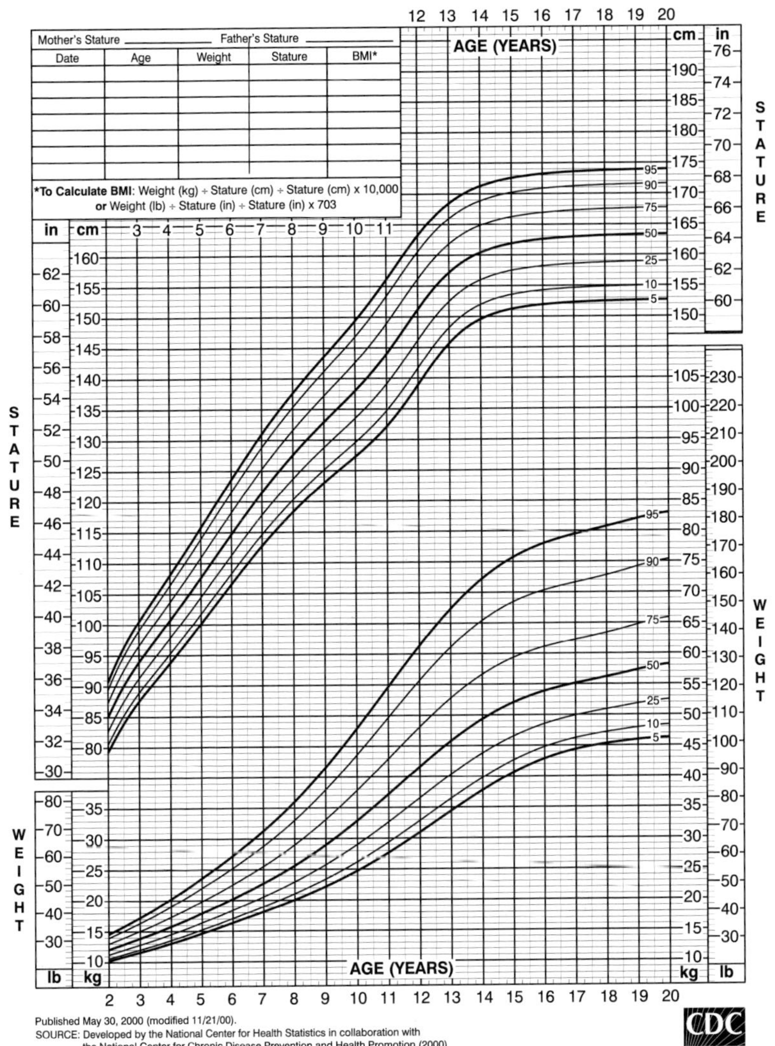

Published May 30, 2000 (modified 11/21/00).
SOURCE: Developed by the National Center for Health Statistics in collaboration with the National Center for Chronic Disease Prevention and Health Promotion (2000).
http://www.cdc.gov/growthcharts

CDC
SAFER · HEALTHIER · PEOPLE™

Index by Drug Name

Index by Drug Use

Commonly Prescribed For (bold for FDA approved)

Index by Drug Class

Abbreviations

5HT	serotonin
ADHD	attention deficit hyperactivity disorder
ANC	absolute neutrophil count
AUC	area under the curve
BEN	benign ethnic neutropenia
bid	twice a day
BMI	body mass index
BP	blood pressure
CBC	complete blood count
CBD	cannabidiol
CBT	cognitive behavioral therapy
CBT-I	cognitive behavioral therapy for insomnia
CMI	clomipramine
CNS	central nervous system
CPIC	Clinical Pharmacogenetics Implementation Consortium
CR	controlled release
CRP	C-reactive protein
CYP	cytochrome P450
dL	deciliter
DMDD	disruptive mood dysregulation disorder
DPNP	diabetic peripheral neuropathic pain
DRESS	Drug Reaction with Eosinophilia and Systemic Symptoms
DSM-5	*Diagnostic and Statistical Manual of Mental Disorders*, 5th edition
ECG	electrocardiogram
ECT	electroconvulsive therapy
EPS	extrapyramidal symptoms
ER	extended-release
FDA	Food and Drug Administration
GABA	gamma-aminobutyric acid
GAD	generalized anxiety disorder
GFR	glomerular filtration rate
GI	gastrointestinal
HDL	high-density lipoprotein
HMG	CoA beta-hydroxy-beta-methylglutaryl coenzyme A
IM	intramuscular
INR	international normalized ratio
IPT-A	interpersonal psychotherapy for adolescents
IR	immediate release

ITP	interpersonal psychotherapy
IV	intravenous
LDL	low-density lipoprotein
MAO	monoamine oxidase
MAOI	monoamine oxidase inhibitor
MDD	major depressive disorder
mg	milligram
mL	milliliter
mmHg	millimeters of mercury
MRI	magnetic resonance imaging
MRSA	methicillin-resistant *Staphylococcus aureus*
NDRI	norepinephrine dopamine reuptake inhibitor
NET	norepinephrine transporter
NMDA	*N*-methyl-D-aspartate
NNT	number needed to treat
NRI	norepinephrine reuptake inhibitor
NSAID	nonsteroidal anti-inflammatory drug
OCD	obsessive-compulsive disorder
ODT	oral disintegrating tablet
ODV	O-desmethylvenlafaxine
PD	panic disorder
PMDD	premenstrual dysphoric disorder
PMT	Parent Management Training
prn	as needed
PTSD	posttraumatic stress disorder
qHS	every bedtime
REMS	risk evaluation and mitigation strategy
SGA	second generation antipsychotics
SIADH	syndrome of inappropriate antidiuretic hormone secretion
SNRI	serotonin and norepinephrine reuptake inhibitor
SR	sustained release
SSRI	selective serotonin reuptake inhibitor
TCA	tricyclic antidepressant
TEAS	treatment-emergent activation syndrome
tid	three times a day
TMS	transcranial magnetic stimulation
TSH	thyroid-stimulating hormone
ULN	upper limit normal
WBC	white blood cell count